Remembering Margo

Remembering Margo

A Triumphant Life,
a Tragic Death, and
Life's Greatest Deception

Donzella Michele Malone

VANTAGE PRESS
New York

Parental discretion strongly advised.

The author's proceeds from this publication will benefit the Dr. Margo Shamberger Prade Trust Fund, established by the author for Dr. Prade's two daughters.

FIRST EDITION

Published by Vantage Press, Inc.
419 Park Ave. South, New York, NY 10016

Manufactured in the United States of America
ISBN: 0-533-15231-3

Library of Congress Catalog Card No.: 2005903680

0 9 8 7 6 5 4 3 2 1

For Kenya and Sahara, daughters of Dr. Margo Shamberger Prade; her mother, Ms. (Ma) Lillie; sisters, Frances, Veronica, Phyllis, Denise, and Edith; brother, James; nieces, nephews, extended family members, friends, colleagues, and the community she served.

Never to be forgotten!

Contents

Preface

It was a cool and rainy November morning in the modest city of Akron, Ohio. For most people living in this city the days, evenings, months and years are uneventful routines. Outside of work and family activities, daily life is business as usual. On this November day, however, a very special life would end, forever changing the lives of many living in the City of Akron and surrounding communities. The murder of forty-one-year-old Dr. Margo Shamberger Prade, a private citizen and popular family practice physician, would put the city of Akron, Ohio on the media map as one of the most heinous, newsworthy crimes throughout the nation. Over a six-year period following the murder, HBO, Hard Copy, Dateline NBC, Court TV, Jet Magazine, MSNBC, the Discovery Health Channel, True Crime, and local news stations across the state of Ohio broadcasted special reports and hour-long segments of the brutal slaying.

It was a cool and rainy November morning.

Then all of a sudden . . .

On Wednesday November 26, 1997, the day before Thanksgiving at 8:30 A.M., after completing medical rounds at Akron General Medical Center, Dr. Margo Shamberger Prade was on the way to work at her medical office. While driving, Margo made the last three phone calls of her life from her cellular phone. The first call was to Joyce Foster, Margo's office manager and friend. Joyce briefed Margo on the upcoming events of the day, including Margo asking Joyce to pull a patient's chart that needed her documentation for family medical leave. The phone call ended with Margo and Joyce sharing a joke . . . ***and their last laugh together.***

The second call was to Ms. Lillie Hendricks, Margo's mother. Ms. Hendricks was at home. Margo phones her: "Mama, are you up? Can you go by the house and pick up a check for Thanksgiving dinner? The check is in the kitchen cabinet. Pick up a turkey and whatever else you need." Margo instructed.

"Okay, baby. I'll see you when you get home," Ms. Lillie lovingly replied. Margo responded, "Alright, Mom." The check was for $160.00 and ***Margo never made it home.***

How ironic that the very person who brought Margo into this world would be one of the last persons she would speak with moments before her abrupt and savage departure from this world.

The third and final call of Dr. Margo Prade's life was to her car salesman, Robin, at the Rolling Acres Dodge car dealership. Margo wanted to discuss details of the new Dodge Durango sport vehicle she had on order. She jubilantly ended the phone call with, "Have a nice holiday!"

When Dr. Margo Prade pulled into the parking lot of the Professional Center West located at 1557 Wooster Avenue, she parked her winter-green minivan in her favorite parking spot alongside the metal fence, where she had uneventfully parked so many mornings before. However, today would be different. For the ***third and final time*** *within the past seven months of Margo's life . . .* ***the devil was on his way.***

As soon *as Margo parked her vehicle, she never had a chance to gather up her things and exit. With deftness and stealth,* ***her killer entered the van and was out in ninety seconds.*** *Within those ninety seconds a relentless scuffle ensued resulting in a scratch on the intruder's chin and a vicious bite mark on Margo's upper left arm. Because Margo was left-handed, it made sense that the bite impression would be on her dominant arm. The bite mark, however, would later only reveal an impression of the intruder's lower teeth. The intruder exited the van, leaving behind six bullet wounds in Margo's lifeless body; with—according to coroner testimony—four of the bullets administered* ***after*** *death occurred, portraying a* ***signature crime.*** *Although evidence showed Margo fought hard trying to save her precious life, her petite, fragile body could not survive such a brutal attack. The coroner's examination revealed that Margo had approximately twelve entrance and exit bullet wounds. The killer, on the other hand, being unsure of a successful hit and being on a timeline, took careful measures to lay Margo's body down on the passenger* *seat before exiting the vehicle. Therefore, should anyone happen by Margo's van in the busy parking lot before the killer left and before she succumbed, it would appear that Margo was not in the van at all . . . guaranteeing,* ***a death undisturbed.***

Margo did lie dead inside her van for at least an hour before her medical assistant, Lori Collins, discovered her body. Margo's eyes were open, and her pupils were dry. Her skin was slightly chilled, and her white lab jacket was drenched in blood. Joyce thought Margo had somehow hit her head and had passed out. While trying to revive her, Joyce happened to notice Margo's mouth was slightly gaped open, and there was yellow body fluid secreting from the right side corner of her mouth. Margo had already exhaled her last breath, her face had begun to turn ash blue; and in the final phase, the trauma to Dr. Margo Prade's small, five-foot body had caused her to urinate. When Joyce saw Margo was wet, she also knew ***Margo was dead.***

The old folks say when you die with your eyes open . . . you were not yet ready to go.

* * *

Dr. Margo Shamberger Prade was a very special human being. Like many who loved her, the grief that still lingers in my heart knows no boundaries, and spares no pain. The night before Margo's funeral, I sat at my computer to write her a good-bye letter. While writing, my heart ached with a pain so profound I thought ***I was dying.***

The brutality of the crime . . . shot six times . . . offered a distinct set of grief that reached far beyond my own comprehension. Nevertheless, it was time to say good-bye to my dear friend. Through the years, I had said good-bye to Margo so many times, and in so many different ways, and under many different circumstances. I had ***no idea*** *how to say good-bye to her* ***this way,*** *but I knew I had to. Margo would expect me to say good-bye to her. A decent and wonderful person, who exuded high morals, standards, and values, was the epitome of Dr. Margo Shamberger Prade's character. Tormented by continuous psychic pain and grief,* ***Remembering Margo*** *is inspired from many unintended pages of good-byes, hellos and pleas written to my dear friend af-*

ter her horrendous departure. Also included is a private stock of bibliotherapy, searching for some understanding AND truth to all the madness both preceding and succeeding Margo's death; and a ***desperate*** *attempt to purge the stress, pain, fear and grief this crime encompassed.*

I once heard it stated, "It is not how long you live, but how you live your life." ***Remembering Margo*** *is about the life, love, legacy and yes, that "infectious" laughter Margo bestowed upon all who knew her, but especially those who loved her. Dr. Margo Prade was a phenom. She was an asthmatic ball player who taught herself how to play softball right-handed, because at the time, left-handed softball mitts were an anomaly.*

As a family practice physician, Dr. Margo Prade was a woman who valued human life so much, that in her private practice, she would often provide free medical care to patients who were either indigent or those whose HMO insurance would refuse to pay for necessary tests, x-rays, or procedures. Margo would very matter-of-factly state to her medical assistant, "Well, she / he needs this test done so I'll pay for it! Order the test." Margo would personally absorb the patient's medical cost.

Remembering Margo *is dedicated to the contributions of a brilliant, BEAUTIFUL and young African American female who pursued her dream of becoming a physician. A woman who overcame the obstacles of an inner-city education, discrimination, racism and elementary school teachers saying, "Oh, honey,* ***you don't really think you*** *can become a doctor, do you?"*

Dr. Margo Prade's dedication to her profession, family, friends, and community was more than admirable. As a physician, Margo once escorted a close friend to New York City for a much-needed cancer surgery. Although her schedule was extremely tight and demanding, I remember her stating, "Don, ***I'm really busy.*** *I don't have the time to go to New York . . . but, she asked me to go with her and she has no one else to go. She needs the support." "Margo, you're a wonderful person, and I know it is appreciated what you are doing," I replied, admiring Margo's dedication to her profession, and to her friend.*

Finally, ***Remembering Margo*** *is a testimonial. Immediately after her death, Dr. Prade's convicted killer was given the* *opportunity to publicly profess innocence quite frequently via television specials, in news programs, and nontraditional magazine articles. Unfortunately, both the print and television media continue to award her killer this opportunity. Years after her death, the killer has continuously been allowed to shed doubt on the murder conviction, as well as devalue the phenomenal life led by this remarkable woman.*

After the conviction, the killer's family hired a man who—in his own words—professed to being, "a spy." This individual, named Boris de Korczak, began to develop fictitious evidence and assert erroneous "clues" about facts presented in the Prade murder investigation almost immediately after his hire, and long after the murder trial was over. In essence, Mr. de Korczak turned out to be nothing more than a bottom feeder seeking to victimize the killer's family even more, by charging "fees for hire." However, they were not the only persons who fell prey to de Korczak's unsubstantiated influence.

Once a respected local newspaper, the Akron Beacon Journal took on the complexion of ***tabloid journalism.*** *De Korczak manipulated the newspaper by spouting off insignificant theories.*

The newspaper began to print de Korczak's theories without ever researching the facts or validity of his assertions through investigation records, court documents, and the like. It was obvious that the Akron Beacon Journal's primary concern was to sell newspapers in sensationalizing a horrendous crime that had long been resolved. This effort by the newspaper and de Korczak, attempted to plant a suspicious seed within the community that the convicted killer ***may not*** *actually be guilty.*

The Akron Beacon Journal's disclosure of de Korczak's hypothetical evidence only launched an attack on the credibility of the outstanding investigation led by the FBI, the Akron Police detective bureau, and the remarkable prosecutorial talents of Michael Carroll and Alison McCarty in convicting Dr. Prade's killer.

Most disheartening of all, however, were the undergirded attacks by de Korczak on both the professional and private life of Dr. Margo Prade. Those attacks were emotionally disturbing to Dr. Prade's two young daughters, her family, colleagues and friends.

Due to the lingering hurt, grief, and disappointment over Dr. Prade's slaying, the media's involvement with de Korczak only angered the community Margo served even more. Whenever de Korczak would surface from the bottom of the pit spewing fictitious, unsubstantiated details about the Prade murder, the Akron Beacon Journal would print an article about de Korczak's theories. Thus began a noxious relationship between the Akron Beacon Journal and the "spy" who loved them. Together, they engaged in a writing campaign of articles, which very much resembled the popular 1960s television series titled, The Fugitive. The articles hinted that, "the real killer was still out there" and that de Korczak, by his own admission, "knew who the real killer was." The local newspaper massaged a relationship with de Korczak even though this man did not live in the Akron community, or the state of Ohio, and had never been heard of in the Akron community until hired by the killer's family.

All along, however, the articles—sordid and fictitious—would attack the pristine reputation and valued memory we all have of Dr. Margo Prade. Despite written and verbal pleas to the Akron Beacon Journal from Dr. Prade's family, friends, and community, some reporters of this newspaper continued writing the articles and turning the tables, ***making the killer out to be the saint, and the victim the sinner.***

Except for her killer, everyone who knew Dr. Margo Prade loved her. And, by the many articles that were written about Dr. Prade's murder and murder trial, those reporters knew she was well-loved in this community.

Sadly, if any one of the Akron Beacon Journal's reporters who engaged in the character assassination of Dr. Prade had had the opportunity to know her personally, I truly believe the negative articles never would have been written. Unfortunately, those articles were written, were discrediting to Margo's legacy, and emotionally disturbing to the senses of those living in this community. Essentially, the erroneous evidence from de Korczak's assertion should not have ***ever*** *been printed. Perverse and unsubstantiated, the information was not worth the paper ON which it was printed.*

Therefore, it is my hope that those who read ***this*** *publication* *will consider its contents as* ***Dr. Margo Prade's chance to speak*** *about her triumphant life as a living person,* ***and not just her tragic death.***

Names have been omitted to protect those who are innocent, ***and to protect the innocent from those who are not.***

Dr. Margo Shamberger Prade's killer was not interviewed for this publication. Her killer continues to have a chance to speak . . . she does not.

Acknowledgments

First, I would like to express my thanks to God for allowing Dr. Margo S. Prade to grace my life for twenty years with a unique and special friendship. Margo's friendship toward others was saturated with grace, poise, and an extraordinary kindness. Without that friendship, the reality of this publication would not exist. According to our friend, Joyce Foster, only hours after learning of Dr. Prade's murder, I stated, "I'm going to write a book about Margo." I *still* do not recall making such a statement to Joyce, however, there are many memory gaps from that horrific day. The statement was apparently made in Margo's office, when my senses were still paralyzed, trying to absorb the shock and to cognitively comprehend that ***Margo was just murdered.***

This book, first mentioned as a profound gesture of grief, has now materialized. The compilation of this project would not have been possible without the help, compassion, cooperation, patience, and consideration of a variety of individuals. Their contribution to this project speaks volumes. Without these individuals, Dr. Margo Prade's story would not exist, and her *voice and contributions to this earthly domain would have remained forever silent.* To the following persons, I express my sincere thanks, gratitude, and appreciation:

Ms. Lillie Hendricks, mother of Dr. Margo Prade, for your continued support and anticipation in asking, "Baby . . . when are you going to finish the book?" Sisters, Ms. Edith Shamberger, Denise Marks and Mrs. Frances Fowler; nieces, Ms. Dayne Arnold, Ms. Layne (Arnold) Farr; Ms. Sahara Prade, daughter of Dr. Margo Prade; Walter L. Hixson, Ph.D.; Judge Alison McCarty, Ms. Joyce Foster, Ms. Pam Foster, Ms. Jaquetta Poole, and Ms. Vickie Taylor. Dr. Thomas M. Anuszkiewicz, for his continued love, support, and inspiration; my son, Ian, for his love and patience with Mommy; my mother, Ms. Veralene Malone, for her encouragement; Mr. Aaron Malone; the Clerks Office at the 9th District Court of Appeals, Akron, Ohio; the City of Akron Law Department; the City of Akron Police Department; Van's Photo; Dr. Dinah Fedyna of NEOUCOM; Mr. Edward Duvall; Major Craig Gilbride of the Akron Police Department; Dr. Adolph Harper, Jr.; Cranston Edwards; and CeeJay Jackson.

I'd also like to thank the many friends, colleagues, and acquaintances who ***never failed*** to ask "How's the book coming?" whenever I would happen to see you. I thank all past and present students whom I've taught over the years for asking, "Is it done yet. . . . Is it done yet?" Finally, I thank all subsequent parties and individuals who may not be mentioned directly but who, without a doubt, in one way or another, assisted in the assemblage, process, and ***conclusion*** of this long awaited publication. ***Remember Margo*** for what she has done, and not *just* for how she died. May her spirit be blessed, and may the "spirit" bless ALL OF YOU!

(Letter written to Dr. Margo Shamberger Prade the night before her funeral. The letter, placed in her casket under her pillow, was near the right side of her head just above her ear, where the first bullet penetrated her skull.)

12/2/97

My Dearest, Sweet, Precious Margo:

I never thought the last laugh we shared ***would be*** *our last. I do not know who took your life away so swiftly and viciously,* ***but you do.*** *I am hurting so right now for your family, myself and all who love you. I hurt that someone felt they needed to take you away from us like this. I want you to know that your death will not go unavenged. If I have* ***anything to do with solving this horrendous crime, I will try my damndest to do so!*** *I know you will speak to us. I also know your spirit will continue to guide your two beautiful daughters in the direction you wanted them to go. I also know you were* ***very, very happy*** *my dear friend when you died so suddenly, and I try to take comfort in that. I also know heaven has a brand new angel! I pray your killer will be caught soon and punished as swiftly and viciously as he took your precious life! I'll always remember the good times we've had. Twenty years is a long time. It will not be easy for me, and I know I will never forget you. But I have years of wonderful, wonderful memories to cling to. We shared so much! I regret I never told you "I love you." I guess I just took for granted you would always be around. Now you are gone. Rest assured, you will never be forgotten, nor will your children. We will take care of them for you. Well, I could go on forever. There is so much I want to say to you, but I'm getting ready* ***to really start crying bad again*** *and I know you wouldn't want that. You're sweet that way. So, I guess I have to go. I don't want to, but I have to. I don't know* ***why*** *you had to leave us so soon, and it* ***hurts like hell*** *that you are gone so quickly! I love you. I'll miss you, and* ***I'll never, ever forget you!! Rest in peace my dear sweet angel, until I see you again!***

Love Always, Donzella

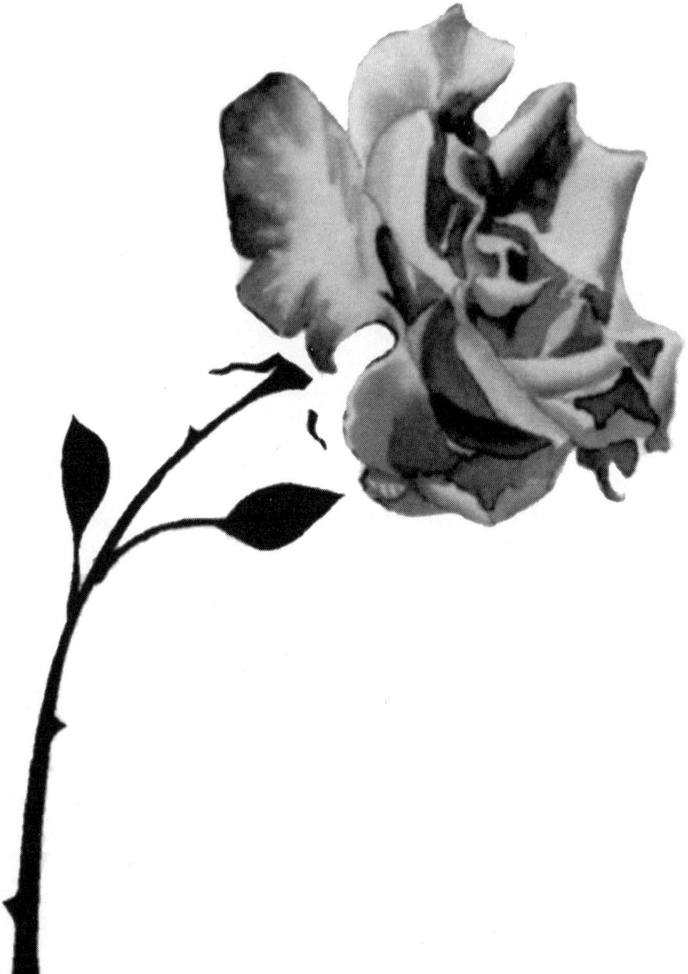

Introduction

I first met Douglas Prade when I was only twelve years old. I was an impetuous pre-teen, full of life and neighborhood friendships. At the time we met, I did not know his name, and had never seen him before. I only *met* him as a police officer.

I never forgot the encounter.

It was a warm summer afternoon. I was outside playing jacks with my best friend Dorothy. I had gotten my $5.00 allowance for the week and the money was burning a hole in my pocket. Dorothy and I wanted to go to Henny Penny's, a small fast food fried chicken store, but we were not in the mood to walk what seemed to be a long way to Copley Road.

While we were contemplating the walk to the store, I noticed my older neighbor, Jerome—who is now deceased, the victim of an unsolved murder—and his cousin, Roy coming out of the house. "Hey Jerome, where are you guys going?" I yelled. Before he could answer, I said, "How about giving us a ride to Henny Penny's? We'll walk back." Jerome looked at Roy for approval. Roy then looked in our direction, giving us the once over, and stated, "Sure, why not. But, I want *that one* (referring to Dorothy) to ride with *me*."

Being young and very unaware of his seductive intentions, Dorothy quickly jumped into Roy's car and I got into the car with Jerome. Off to Henny Penny's we went . . . so we thought.

While driving down South Hawkins Avenue, to my surprise Jerome and Roy began to engage in a drag race. They began a very dangerous, high-speed race northbound on South Hawkins Avenue. I was scared to *death*. My body became rigid, but I sat quietly and said *nothing*. The last thing I wanted to do was *distract* this young nineteen-year-old who was now holding my very life in his hands.

Suddenly, I heard the blare of a police siren. "Damn!" I

heard Jerome exclaim. "*Thank God,*" I whispered to myself. I was *so* happy the police was stopping us. I was *happy,* that is, until I met a very frightening police officer who, I learned later, went by the name of Douglas Prade.

Jerome and Roy stopped their cars about one and a half blocks from each other. Suddenly, *my door flung open.* A booming, fearsome voice yelled, **"Get the fuck outta the car!"** I looked up and saw a tall, slender, African American police officer, sporting a very angry look on his face. I attempted to plead my case, "But officer, I didn't do . . ." "Shut the ***fuck*** up!" he yelled, cutting my sentence off. I got out of the car shaking like a leaf, and wondering if he was going to address Jerome. After all, *Jerome was the one driving the car, not me!*

I stood quietly, trying to hold back tears, while the officer towered motionless in front of me. Standing nearly nose-to-nose in front of *me,* trembling, I attempted to plead my case again. "Officer, I just asked him to . . ." "I ***said*** shut ***the fuck up!"*** He yelled again. This time even louder.

The officer *finally* walked over to Jerome. He *calmly* asked, "May I see your license, please, sir?" I began mumbling under my breath, while delicately frowning at the officer. Why isn't he yelling and cursing at him! He was the one racing the car, not me! I'm just an innocent passenger. He can't possibly think I had anything to do with this! Nevertheless, I was happy he had gotten off my case and went over to the real culprit, who was Jerome.

While the officer was writing down information from Jerome's license, I saw another police cruiser arrive with another African American police officer, who I learned years later was one of Douglas' best friends. As I stood stunned wondering what I should do, the mean ole' officer began walking in my direction ***again***. I was ***petrified.*** "What is your name, where do you live, and who is your mother?" he bellowed. "My name is . . ." "Shut up! Don't you know he could have killed you!" He chanted more of a statement than a question. By this time, ***I*** was getting angry. Angry that this police officer was cursing and yelling at me for something I did not do, or had any control over. Now he is asking me questions, only to tell me to "shut up" before I can answer them. I said nothing else.

Shortly after that tirade, I noticed a police paddy wagon arriving about a block south of us where the other officer had stopped Roy and Dorothy. I began to tremble and was afraid for Dorothy and me. I'm thinking, *I* ***know*** *I'm not being arrested, here! I am* ***only twelve years old*** *and I did not do anything!* What will my mother think! Given the way the officer was treating me, I was sure we were ***all*** being arrested.

Looking down the road, I saw the other officer handcuff Roy and call for a tow truck for Roy's car. I learned later, through neighborhood gossip, that Roy had an outstanding warrant on him, and that is why he was arrested. The officer who stopped Jerome and me gave Jerome a ticket, and Dorothy and I were ***ordered*** into his police cruiser so he could take us home. I would have rather walked.

Although my home was just a couple of streets east of South Hawkins Avenue, the trip home seemed like the longest ride of my life.

"You fass-ass little Black bitches is all the same, looking for some thrill! Those guys could have killed you!" the officer shouted at us, continuing his tirade. The ride home consisted of both verbal assaults and insults.

During the entirety of the trip, this *police officer* cursed and yelled at Dorothy and me, calling us derogatory names supposedly ***all in the name of safety.*** Dorothy and I just looked at each other in dismay. The officer never asked us if we were okay. It never occurred to him that Jerome and Roy's drag racing frightened ***us.*** Now, **he was the only frightening reality** of this entire episode! I remember thinking to myself; he must ***really think he is something!*** The big bad Black police officer, cursing out two little girls and ain't a thing we can do about it . . . not one thing! I felt violated, hurt, and angry while I fought back tears.

When we arrived at my house, Dorothy and I jumped out of the cruiser, barely allowing it to stop. I ran into my house without looking back and Dorothy ran down the street to her home too. I was ***so*** happy my mother was at work, but at the same time,

I wished she was home so I could tell her what this police officer had just done to me and Dorothy.

My mother was ***always*** my savior, and my protector. I knew if she got wind of what this officer had done to her little girl, she would be downtown at the police station in a New York minute filing a complaint! However, she was not home and I was there alone, left to deal with my feelings of shock, hurt, and embarrassment. I was very upset and felt victimized that this police officer had assaulted, attacked, and assassinated my character. I had ***never been*** cursed at and chastised like that before, and had never had any encounter with a police officer. My God *I was only twelve years old.*

Little did I know that thirty years and many friendships later, *this very same police officer* would *again* touch my life in a very volatile way. Little did I know that this very same police officer would ***again,*** assault, attack and assassinate. This time, *again,* the crime would incorporate another one of my dear friends . . . the very young, *BEAUTIFUL* and *talented,* Dr. Margo Shamberger Prade.

Remembering Margo

One
Sunrise

On Monday September 17, 1956 at 9:00 A.M., a very special person was brought into the world at Akron City Hospital. She was a baby girl weighing 7 pounds, 2 ounces and relatively short for a newborn; only 18 inches long. The proud parents were Mr. and Mrs. David and Lillie Shamberger, and she would be the seventh child born to Ms. Lillie.

When leaving the hospital only one day after the child's birth, Ms. Lillie Shamberger and her bouncing baby girl who she had named Margo, were transported home by Evan's Ambulance Service because at the time, the family had no car. Upon arriving home, baby Margo was carried into the house in a gorgeous white picnic basket. The older siblings gathered around and gazed upon the family's youngest and latest new addition exclaiming, "She's so little!"

As a toddler, Margo had round chubby cheeks and dark brown curly (what African Americans call), *good hair.* Margo was so short and little that nearly every family member had a nickname for her depicting *short.* Her father called her "munchkin," and sister Edith teased her with "runt." Other nicknames, as "squirt," "snookum macknukum," and "baby" were soon to follow. Ms. Lillie, however, only called her, "Dumplin." It was not long before the Shamberger family learned that big things come in small packages, and that little Margo was small, but "sho nuff mighty!"

"The baby came here smiling and cheering," states Ms. Lillie. Margo smiled constantly and would make up cheers screaming, "yeeeeeahhh," while jumping up and down clapping her hands. When she would become angry, however, Margo would get on her knees and bang her head up against the wall or against the mirror until her anger was satisfied. "Stop! You're going to knock ***all*** the sense out of your head," Ms. Lillie would scold.

* * *

The head banging episodes obviously had the opposite effect. At age two Margo could read a book. Ms. Lillie thought for the longest time Margo was reading pictures in the books, until one day she discovered the small two-year-old was actually reading the words under the pictures. Margo's intellectual development soon became a central focus for the family. By the time she reached grade school there was no doubt, Margo was quite bright.

Throughout her formative years, Margo *loved school* and continued to excel academically. Margo was so dedicated to her education that she refused to be absent. One weekday, Margo was scheduled to have a tonsillectomy, and insisted her mother take her to school that morning until the time of surgery which was 10:00 A.M. Not only was Margo in school the day after her surgery, but also for every day thereafter, *Margo never missed one day of school.*

Margo's academic agility excelled to the point that after third grade, she skipped the fourth grade at Grace Elementary School, and headed straight to the fifth grade. According to Ms. Lillie, throughout her junior high and high school education, Margo earned straight A's. Margo only earned one B in elementary school and she cried when she received it.

At age fourteen, Margo entered the tenth grade at Central Hower High School. At that time, students who attended Central Hower High would major in specialized fields of study. Margo majored in drafting and was very active in extra-curricular activities, particularly cheerleading. Margo became a very gifted cheerleader and eventually became a cheerleading coach. Her cheerleading squad would often enter local and state cheerleading competitions. When the routine was over, Margo would end it with a magnificent split, a bright smile, and a clever wink at the judges to polish off the grand finale.

In her adolescent years, Margo was a typical teenager with many friends, but a very protective family. She was extremely popular with, and particular about her friends and associations. Although Margo would not—and, through the protection of older siblings—*could not* associate with "street-wise" teenagers, "She never looked down upon them either," Ms. Lillie poignantly asserts. As far as Margo was concerned, they were all living and playing in the same neighborhood together. Although she frolicked the neighborhood like any other kid growing up, according to sister Frances, "Margo was the studious type. She liked to stay indoors and read a lot. She loved books, she loved to read."

* * *

While attending high school and not quite seventeen years old, Margo met twenty-seven-year-old Douglas Prade at a local dance and invited him to her high school graduation. Although this was truly an exciting time in Margo's life, it was also a sad time. Margo's father had been very ill for a number of years, and she was afraid he would not last long enough to see her graduate. Even though Ms. Lillie and Mr. Shamberger were divorced when Margo was age four, he was not an absent father. Mr. Shamberger remained very much involved in his children's lives. As his illness progressed and took control, Margo's father told her, "I just want to live long enough to see you graduate from high school." Behind the walls of academia, however, David Shamberger's youngest and brightest daughter was massaging a brand new love interest. A love interest that never would have materialized had Margo's father not been consumed with his illness.

* * *

Douglas Prade accepted Margo's invitation, and attended her graduation. Margo spoke as valedictorian of her 1975 graduating class. *Nearly thirty years old,* and *donned in his police uniform* rather than casual clothes, Douglas attended the graduation of his teenaged sweetheart hopeful. No doubt, by wearing his uniform, he was expecting to ward off any age appropriate male classmate admirers Margo may have had. As if his age was not intimidating enough, Douglas deliberately and carefully positioned himself as an authority figure at Margo's graduation by wearing his uniform.

During the summer of 1975 after Margo graduated from high school, she took a summer job at the City of Akron Engineering Department. She was hired as a drafter.

Margo employed her drafting skills in designing a drainage pipe system that was to be part of a newly renovated area along Cedar Street near Akron General Hospital in downtown Akron. Before her employment was over, Margo completed the drafting plans and the pipe system was installed. Whenever she and her mother would pass by the area in the car, Margo would exclaim with proud excitement, "See those pipes, Mom, I did that!" When her tenure ended, Margo's employers asked that she stay on as a full-time employee. Margo was so intellectually dazzling and valuable to the team that they did not want to lose her talents. Although flattered, emphatic and excited; Margo asserted to her boss, "Nope, I'm going to attend medical school!"

* * *

While Margo set her sights on medical school, her relationship with Douglas also began to develop, but her mother disapproved and became concerned and warned, "Margo, I think he is too old for you."

"Oh, Mom, it's okay. . . ." Margo insisted. "Besides, by him being older, he is more mature. This way, I don't have to worry about him messing around and running around in the streets on me while I'm studying in college and medical school. I need someone I can *trust*."

Two
Aspirations Abound

At the tender age of nineteen and having never taken a chemistry course before, Margo entered medical school in an accelerated cooperative program between Kent State University and North Eastern Ohio Universities College of Medicine (NEOUCOM). Margo and her student colleague, Yvonne Patterson, were the only two African Americans pictured in the 1982 NEOUCOM yearbook as freshmen on their first day of medical school. Compared to the other students, Margo was *very* young and looked it.

In college Margo's wit, popularity and charming personality earned her the title of Homecoming Queen at Kent State University in Kent, Ohio. At NEOUCOM, Margo started the first multicultural center for racial diversity. That center is still in existence today. This was the beginning of Margo Shamberger Prade making an impact in the community she lived in. From the days of working as a drafter, well into her college career, it seemed that whatever ecological system she maneuvered in for any length of time, Margo Prade would leave something ***positive*** behind.

While in medical school full time, Margo continued to work part-time jobs at various places including the former O'Neil's Department Store in downtown Akron, and in doctors' offices throughout the community. Margo's parents were not wealthy, and by the time she entered college and medical school, her father had passed away. Ms. Lillie was working as a factory worker at the Chrysler Corporation in Twinsburg, Ohio while still parenting two of her seven children at home.

With her father being deceased, and having a working mother, Margo had to secure loans, work to pay her tuition through college and medical school, and attend medical school full-time. For anyone else, this would have been an unachievable, if not impossible task. For Margo however . . . no problem.

Margo continued to impress her college instructors and medical school professors. Her tenacity and determination was something to be admired. Although she had challenges, Margo persisted to be a bright and popular student throughout, gaining long-term friendships with other medical students along the way.

One such friend is Dr. Dinah Fedyna. Margo and Dinah Fedyna began medical school together in 1978. The two were part of the first class of medical students enrolled in the BSMD program. The program was a cooperative effort of undergraduate students from the University of Akron, Kent State University and Youngstown State University. According to Dinah Fedyna, "The students in the program were under tremendous pressure to cut the mustard."

Dinah came from Youngstown State University and she first met Margo at a medical school colloquium held at Kent State University.

Because the BSMD program was new, the school wanted to make a concerted effort to bond students from Kent State, the University of Akron and Youngstown State University together. The school accomplished this endeavor by creating colloquiums, which met a couple times per year. The purpose was for students from all three campuses to join in a unified effort to get to know one another, share ideas, frustrations and goals as they suffered through medical school together.

When Dinah met Margo on the Kent State campus, her first impression of her was that she was friendly, open and fun. Dinah asserts, "Even when she was overwhelmed, Margo never looked it, she didn't show it." The two later shared an anatomy class together during their first year of medical school.

Margo's medical school experience was not without difficult challenges. According to Dr. Dinah Fedyna, "We did not finish together. Margo did an extra year of medical school. I don't know whether she chose to take a leave, or they asked her to take a leave. She had some academic problems. We lost thirty percent of our class that first year. The first year was really hard." Dinah also believed, that part of Margo's difficulty derived out of "having to be there for Douglas" as well as devote time to her studies. During the second year, Margo was the only student who was married. After changing her name from Shamberger to Prade, Margo did not really socialize very much with her student colleagues after hours.

Margo's challenge in medical school was the first and only time she ever had trouble academically in school. She was, however, only nineteen years old entering an accelerated, full-time medical school program, while simultaneously earning a Bachelor of Science degree from Kent State University. This, along with working part-time jobs to help pay for school, was not a modest endeavor for a teenager to pursue.

Margo's academic challenges rendered her completing five instead of four years of medical school, along with the required three years of residency. Margo's chosen field of expertise was family medicine. Although Margo just *loved* infants and children, she did not specialize in pediatrics for one *very good reason* . . . Margo once stated in sincerity, "Don, I couldn't stand it if one of my babies or kids died, I couldn't practice medicine anymore if that happened." The eight-year journey was well worth the time, effort, and challenge Margo endured.

As Margo matured, she became intellectually resilient in completing her studies. By the time she entered residency, Margo was academically sound in her medical education, expertise, and skills.

In a candid interview, Dr. Dinah Fedyna shares what impressed her most about Margo as a medical student and resident.

"She wasn't afraid to question things in class, she could fit in very well with everybody, but she wasn't going to give up who she was either. She didn't *pretend* to be someone she wasn't. Margo mingled with everyone, but after marrying Douglas, [Dinah continues, smiling, and asserts she knows I'm going to quote her on this and, 'it is terrible'] I was never sure if she just didn't want to bring Douglas along when we did things, or if he just did not want to associate with us."

Three
Meeting of the Minds

I first met Margo while she was attending medical school. We actually met on the softball field. I had seen her around because she lived on Bell Street across from my maternal grandfather, Willie Lee Harris, who I would visit often. Margo and I never formally met however, until we started playing softball together.

It was the summer of 1979; a bunch of us women in our early twenties had gotten together to learn how to play softball. The Akron Chapter of the Black Law Enforcement Officer's Association sponsored our team. A friend, who was the wife of a police officer, had organized the team for "police wives" and other women who worked for the Akron Police Department. The friendship between Margo and I did not flourish right away because we were both vying for the same playing position, and we *both* knew that. Because we had nothing else in common, our relationship began as one of competitiveness. Although we never verbally discussed the competitive spirit between us, it was obvious to everyone else that this was an issue on the team.

One day during practice, I noticed Margo wearing a sweatshirt with the initials NEOUCOM written on it.

"Hey Margo, what do those initials stand for on your sweatshirt?" I yelled, while warming up with someone else.

"Northeastern Ohio Universities College of Medicine," she yelled back. "*You're in medical school?*" I asked with astonishment.

"Yup," Margo replied unpretentiously, while throwing the softball.

Curious, I asked, "What made you decide to become a doctor?"

"Well, when I was growing up my father was so sick and it

seemed like no one would ever help him. So, I told myself that when I grew up I was going to be a doctor so I could help people."

Not knowing her father was deceased, I then stated, "Well, I bet he's proud of you now, being in medical school and all!"

Margo smiled, hung her head slightly and humbly asserted, "Well, he's dead now. He was *really sick* in my senior year of high school and he had said he just wanted to live long enough to see me graduate."

"Did he?" I replied, feeling sad and identifying with my own feelings of having lost my father at age ten.

"Yes, but he died a week later," Margo replied.

"Well at least you had your father in your life longer than I had my dad in mine, be thankful for that," I responded, feeling sorry for both of us. At that moment, I realized that I was feeling both shocked and impressed in what seemed to be Margo's best-kept secret in becoming a physician, but I certainly understood what inspired her to take on such a monumental endeavor.

Nevertheless, I *still* could not believe this woman was in medical school because Margo laughed and giggled constantly! If Margo missed a ball in practice that she should have caught, she would burst out with a loud and bold belly laugh, *laughing at herself,* which would result in everyone else in fun, laughing at her. I repeatedly thought to myself, I do not *believe* this woman is going to be a doctor. *She is so silly!* And, because I was still contending with Margo for that softball position, I politely convinced myself that no one would take her seriously anyway, because she just giggles too much!

I could not have been more wrong.

* * *

One evening after a very hot, sweaty practice, we all went out for cold drinks. While there, we engaged in various conversations. I began talking about my first love, our fights, my catching him with other girls, and other "illnesses" of our relationship. Margo giggled and laughed at the events I spoke about the *entire time.* As we prepared to leave, Margo giggled and shouted, "Good gossiping Donzella!" From that moment on, Margo and I became the best of friends and it never mattered that she eventually earned that left-field position I wanted so badly.

On another evening during practice, I overheard Margo talking to another player saying, "He'll be here any minute now." I thought to myself, *finally,* I'll get to see who her husband is. At that time, I only knew Margo had a partner who was a police officer. We had been playing ball together for quite some time now, but I still had never seen her husband. I assumed she was married as some of the other women were; and even though I was working for Akron police too, I had no idea who her husband was.

Shortly after Margo's conversation, I noticed a car pull up on Storer Avenue alongside the softball field of Crouse Elementary School. "There he is!" I heard Margo exclaim with girlish glee. Margo lit up like a candle and I was sure she was going to drop her softball mitt and run up to him, then I would never get the opportunity to see who he was. To my surprise, she continued practicing and allowed the man to come to her. I glanced over and saw a tall, well-built man in a police uniform walking towards the softball field. My eyes followed him. As the figure became closer and closer, I recognized his face. ***"Oh . . . my . . . God, it's him!"*** I whispered to myself as my memory quickly reverted back to eleven years prior. I felt a familiar and haunting sting of butterflies in my stomach. "It's that mean black cop who stopped me and Dorothy on South Hawkins!" I whispered to myself.

Even though I was now twenty-three years old and much more mature, I still never forgot the horrendous encounter I had with that police officer. I *always* wondered why he treated Jerome with more respect than he did me, especially since I was just a young, female child. Now, I could not believe, and wondered *why* this exceptionally nice person was married to him. It was perplexing to me.

The man walked over to Margo and handed her something. Stunned at his identity, and trying to conceal my own, I had stopped practicing with my partner, stood motionless and watched the encounter the entire time; as if I was *spying on* a *suspect.*

"Take your medicine, go home, and lay down," I heard Margo yell at him as he exited the field.

"Listen at you!" the coach stated, teasing Margo.

"*I'm his* doctor," Margo lovingly replied. At that moment, it was obvious to me that Margo embraced a profound love for this man.

After Douglas left the field, I approached Margo in an effort to seek either an apology, or at least a rationale I could live with for what *he had done* to me eleven years ago. Besides, we had really become good friends now and Margo seemed nice enough that she *would* apologize for him if she had the opportunity to hear my story.

"Is that your husband, Margo?" I asked suspiciously.

"No, not yet. We're not getting married until I finish medical school." Puzzled, Margo asked, "I'm surprised you don't know Douglas, don't you work at the Akron Police Department?"

"Yeah, I do . . . for about a year now . . . but, I've never seen him there," I replied, with eyes peeled on Douglas making sure he was leaving the area.

"I thought I knew all the Black officers because there aren't many of them anyway," I continued.

"Oh, really? I thought ***everybody knew Douglas!***" Margo expressed with pride.

I thought to myself now is my chance.

"Well . . . actually, Margo, I did meet him once when I was twelve years old. You see me and my girlfriend . . ."

"Twelve!" Margo shouted, cutting off my sentence and giggling.

"Yeah, you see me and my girlfriend were in the car with my neighbor and his cousin. Then, they decided to start drag racing and your fiancé stopped us and then . . ."

"Girl! What in the ***world*** were you guys doing in a speeding car at twelve years old?" Margo asked with concern. "Those guys could have killed you! Your mother would have had a fit! I'm glad he *did* stop you guys. I'm sure it probably upset Douglas too! You guys could have really been hurt!"

I began to think my appeal to Margo for Douglas' actions would be futile, especially since her words were uncanny in their familiarity to Douglas', eleven years prior. Nevertheless, I felt driven to let her know that this man she plans to marry, had cursed at and called me everything but a child of God when I was only twelve years old! I attempted to plead my case again, just as I had eleven years prior with *him.* While throwing the softball with her, I continued.

"Well . . . Margo, it's not like we asked those guys to start drag racing, we just wanted a ride to the store and . . ."

"Girl!" she interrupted me again, this time with medical expertise. "You had better thank your lucky stars that Douglas stopped you guys and nothing happened to you. I've seen victims of car accidents come into the emergency room and it is not a pretty sight!"

It was obvious Margo was going to defend and protect Douglas no matter what I told her. By now, I believed the conversation was a moot point. I had already noticed her sincere admiration for him, and I felt she was smart enough to know where I was going with my conversation and she did not want to hear *anything negative about him.* Looking back, perhaps the attempted conversation was a surrealistic intent to warn Margo about the dark side of Douglas Prade.

Reluctantly, I tried to convince myself the point I was trying to make was no longer important now anyway, and because Margo responded with *genuine concern,* I also convinced myself that Douglas probably did react out of fear for me and Dorothy.

Victims of abuse often find ways to rationalize and justify their offender's actions.

* * *

As the years and our softball seasons progressed, so did the friendship between Margo and me. Although Margo became an extremely busy physician and mother, she never missed a softball practice or game the entire eighteen years we played together. Margo would even arrange her medical conferences around softball seasons and games. I began to gain a tremendous respect for Margo as a ball player. She was a true humanitarian; so unselfish and caring.

We played high-powered softball in highly competitive leagues. In the games whenever our coach would not play the weaker players, or would give them minimal playing time, Margo would always take issue with the coach. "I'll come out so they can play," she would plead to the coach. Margo was a very skilled softball player and would always play the entire game, but she believed everyone should get equal playing time, no matter what their skill level. One year, she threatened to quit the team in the middle of the season if the coach did not start playing every player in every game.

The care and consideration for others that Margo demonstrated on the softball field was an extension of her kindness as a physician, friend, mother, sister, daughter and *wife.* Margo's legend will forever live on in the hearts of a variety of softball players, black and white, throughout the City of Akron and Summit County. Many players grew to know and love her as that, "giggly doctor in left field." Margo would often say in slang terminology, "Don, I *luv* softball! It allows me to relax and release *all* my frustrations."

"Me too, Margo . . . me too," I replied.

Four
To Be Young, Gifted and Black

On December 29, 1979, at the young and impressionable age of twenty-three, Margo Shamberger married thirty-three-year-old Douglas Evans Prade. The marriage was Margo's first and Douglas' ***third.*** Douglas and Margo had a non traditional wedding. Douglas favored Afrocentrism; therefore, he and Margo's wedding ceremony was fashioned in African culture.

The couple dressed in African wedding attire, and had the traditional broom jumping ceremony. During the ceremony, Douglas' sister, Yvonne, was overheard by Margo's elder sister, Frances, stating, "Humph, I wonder how long *this one* [marriage] will last." Referring to Douglas' uniting in holy matrimony for the third time.

Even though Margo had planned to wait until she finished medical school to marry, for some unknown reason, Douglas and Margo married several years before Margo graduated from medical school. I was surprised Margo married before she finished school, since she had previously stated she would marry afterwards. Given they were living together, Douglas or Margo may have insisted they marry early. However, *Margo should have waited.*

* * *

Margo's accomplishments and success in her journey through medical school was not without varied displays of racial bias and discrimination. In her early years at NEOUCOM, both the medical school and the community Margo resided in shared in the demarcation of racial bias.

According to Ms. Lillie, when Margo first attended medical

school, and before she married Douglas, she and another white female student rented an apartment together. At the time Margo had no car and would walk to and from her classes. NEOUCOM located in Rootstown, Ohio was a rural, predominately white populated community. There were times when Margo would walk through her neighborhood, and cars would pass by shouting derogatory racial epithets towards her such as, "Nigger, get away from down here, you're not wanted down here!"

Margo, in the long run, also had problems with her roommate, when she discovered the roommate was growing marijuana in the living room of the apartment. When this occurred, Douglas moved Margo out of the apartment, back into Akron, and *in with him,* not back to her mother's home. Douglas and Margo's mother, Ms. Lillie, paid $500.00 a piece to purchase a car for her so she could commute back and forth to school.

The medical school too, was not without displaying racial bias. I remember a candid conversation Margo and I had one day in the office.

"Don, there were some days I *really did not think* I would make it through medical school."

"Why Margo?" I asked curiously.

"Well, there was just so much discrimination against the black students that it was just very difficult to take sometimes. White students would not be penalized whenever they came to class late, would not complete assignments on time, or would just miss class altogether. A black student *had better not even try that!* Girl, they would threaten to kick us out of school if we tried something like that!"

"Really, was it that evident?" I asked.

"Yes, girl! I used to cry a lot in medical school. I even went to Dr. Rita Robinson one day because I was so upset. She told me to hang in and to not give up," Margo explained. [Dr. Rita Robinson is an established African-American physician in Akron and surrounding communities.]

Margo's pep talks with Dr. Robinson obviously paid off for her. The support and encouragement of Dr. Robinson and others who had Margo's best interest at the helm, would help encourage and foster the unfolding of an indelible lifestyle and career.

While in her junior year of Medical school, Margo met Dr. Adolph Harper Jr. Dr. Harper was a very popular African-American obstetrician from Mississippi who arrived in the Akron, Ohio area in 1976, and began practicing in 1980. Dr. Harper's first impression of Margo as a young, and energetic medical student was that, "She was very charming, very likable, intelligent and a caring person. When I first met her, the very first conversation I had with her was about medical school, because this is what veteran physicians usually talked about with medical students. Margo said, 'school was tough.' "

Dr. Harper states he and Margo's friendship developed "at first sight" primarily because she was a black medical student, and him being a black attending physician, "I knew she was being faced with the same challenges I had already been through, and was going to be faced with some of the things I had already been faced with. This alone gave us some kind of an instant bond. I think I mentored her just by having already made it to where she still had yet to get. Students look at you and say to themselves, if they can do it, I can do it. So, I am sure I mentored her at least in that way," Harper admits.

* * *

When Margo graduated from medical school in 1983, Douglas along with Margo's family threw her a graduation party. I had been divorced for two years and had purchased my first home.

I remember retrieving the party invitation from the mailbox and feeling so much excitement for Margo. "She did it!" I screamed, while standing alone in my living room. I expressed so much exhilaration that if witnessed, one would have thought it were *my* accomplishment.

Smiling, I briefly thwarted my memory back to a recent softball practice where we were finishing up for the day. The coach was reminding us about the upcoming Saturday practice stating, ". . . and I want EVERYONE HERE!" Margo regretfully stated, "I won't be able to come on Saturday." Butting in, I stated, "And WHY NOT? Margo, we need everybody here to have a decent practice so we can win some of these games! We're playing our rival team next week and you know they always beat us! We can beat them if we get this team together for a decent practice!" Margo sheepishly stated, "I'm sorry, Don, I just can't make it, I wish I could, but I'll be graduating on Saturday."

To say I felt embarrassed, *and having stuck my foot* ***way deep*** *in my mouth,* would be an understatement, especially since Margo had NEVER missed a practice or game. Nevertheless, Margo took my unsolicited criticism in stride smiling as we all pummeled her to the ground screaming, jumping up and down, and hugging Margo congratulating her. It was quite a moment.

* * *

Margo's pending graduation party was the talk of our softball team, and the social circle we all operated in. In the shopping malls, at the hairdressers and on our jobs, friends and acquaintances alike, would engage in conversation about what we were wearing to the celebration and what gifts we had purchased for Margo. Everyone was excited about having her as a new, African American female doctor in town. Even people who already had doctors were planning to switch. When approaching Margo with the idea, she would just giggle and say, "You'd better stay where you are! I still have to do my residency!" What was even more exciting, however, was that *we all knew* Margo as a friend, a common resident in our community and a softball teammate. This accomplishment was a defining moment *for her,* and we were awarded the opportunity to celebrate the moment *with* her.

With all of her unpretentious grace, poise *and* softball playing, in our eyes Margo had definitely reached celebrity status, although she would never think of herself in that way. I was bursting with excitement and could not *wait* to attend Margo's graduation party!

The graduation celebration was at the Goodyear Local Hall #2. It was a warm Saturday evening and people were arriving in droves. The very first guest to arrive was Judge Joseph Roulhac, one of the very first African American Municipal Court Judges the City of Akron ever had.

The hall was beautifully decorated, iridescent with trimmings of a successful endeavor that was now complete. Everyone was well dressed, on time and eagerly anticipated celebrating this awesome feat with Margo, her husband and family.

Donned in a sleeveless, white, tight fitting sequin pantsuit outlining her small, petite frame and wearing silver high-heeled shoes to match, Margo was *dressed to impress.* Looking happy and radiant, Margo shined as bright as her smile while she greeted every guest to her celebration. Her long brown hair glistened in subdued lighting as it swayed from side to side across her shoulder blades when she walked. I whispered to myself, "This woman is simply perfect. She has EVERYTHING! A large, loving family, a wonderful husband, a gifted personality, physical beauty from head to toe; and now and medical degree!" I felt proud to be her friend and looked forward to celebrating with her.

As the party progressed throughout the night, many guests stood in line to grant Margo kudos for her achievement. One of the most memorable speeches was from Margo's sister, Phyllis Foster: "I'd like for everyone in the hall to please stand and give my little sister, Margo, a big hand," Phyllis humbly requested. "As a family, we are ***soooo proud of her!*** She worked ***soooo*** hard! And we are so very proud of her!" The crowd stood, and applauded. Then the whistles and cheers roared and began to drown out Phyllis' salutation to her baby sister, and the music playing in the background.

Margo ran to the middle of the dance floor like a little girl running through the playground, snatched a bottle of champagne off her table, threw her head back and turned the bottle up to her mouth with her left hand. The cheers and clapping became louder as she began snapping her fingers of her right hand, dancing to the music, rolling her hips like Elvis Presley, and *still* drinking from the champagne bottle. She was ecstatic as the crowd roared, "Go Margo . . . go Margo . . ." while she danced alone on the floor, relishing in the abyss of her accomplishment. At one point, the cheering and applauding became extremely loud; Margo had stolen the moment, mesmerizing the crowd with her champagne bottle and victory dance. Even with that, however, I could still faintly hear big sister Phyllis yelling, "We are soooo very proud of her!"

All of a sudden, Margo abruptly removed the champagne

bottle from her mouth, stopped dancing, and her eyes eagerly scanned the crowd searching. The clapping began to cease. Suddenly, we all thought something was wrong. With a surprised look on her face, Margo then shouted, "Wait a minute!" While gracefully gesturing her right arm to a table, Margo proudly gazed at the group sitting there and stated with a smile, "These are doctors too!" She then motioned for her medical school colleagues to join her on the dance floor. The crowd resumed applauding, whistling and roaring even louder as Margo's new colleagues joined her on the dance floor!

For me, this *unselfish* gesture of Margo asking her colleagues to join her on the dance floor was the most memorable moment of the entire graduation party.

Even though the accolades were meant for Margo and her alone, she simply *was not going to allow* the crowd to congratulate her, without congratulating the other new doctors. In her mind, they all deserved kudos for enduring the same accomplishment in realizing the most respectable outcome of higher education—the choice to practice medicine, cure illness and save lives.

Altruistic in nature, Margo's gesture to her colleagues exemplified the uniqueness of her personal characteristics; unprecedented characteristics *only Margo* could possess. I felt privileged to be her friend.

* * *

After Margo finished medical school, she and Dr. Harper would see each other at the hospital during medical rounds, or in the parking lot of the hospital. Harper smiles, explaining, "When we would see each other in the parking lot or the hallway, we would both look at each other and break out with this big smile because we both knew *we always had something* to tell each other. Then, we would just stand wherever we were and talk for the longest. She loved talking about her daughters and what they were doing. I was very interested in what they were doing too because with her being successful, and having such bright girls which I delivered, it gave me a sense of pride too. I always liked to follow her girls and hear what they were doing."

Although Dr. Harper delivered many other physicians'

wives children, from his recollection, he states, "Margo was the only female physician who I delivered babies for." For Dr. Harper, his pride in delivering Margo's children magnified the special bond they had between them. When seeing Margo walking around the hospital pregnant, he states, "Taking care of pregnant women period, gives you a special feeling. However, taking care of one that is your friend, colleague, and who is so loved by the community, who is such an integral part of the community; that gave me an even more special feeling. The feeling that I am going to help bring the life of *her* children into the world was really a special feeling," Harper confessed.

Margo and Dr. Harper had many patients in common after she completed medical school. Those patients would liken Dr. Harper to Margo stating, "You and Doctor Prade are a lot alike because you talk to everybody about everything. It seems like you don't mind talking to anybody!" Dr. Harper explains, "That is just the way I am, *I think* . . . but *I know* that is the way she [Margo] was. Margo never had a problem relating to *anyone.* Margo's patients *loved her, she was a charm to them* and they often stated they would not go to anyone else. Margo cared so much about her patients. She always wanted to do her very best for them and let them know how much she cared. Her patients were loyal to her, they gave her many referrals, and they thought she was the best!"

Dr. Harper, too, acknowledges the struggles that both he and Margo endured to make their marks in history as African American physicians in Akron, Ohio. Dr. Harper candidly admits, "I know Margo had challenges, because I had quite a few. I went to the University of Mississippi; we called it, 'Ole Miss.' At the time, they [medical school officials] still felt that medicine was a white, male's profession; being a black male, I didn't fit in, and I know with Margo being a black female, that was kind of like two strikes against her. Not only was she not a white male, but also, she wasn't a male, ***period.*** I am sure there were quite a few [negative] encounters she had to face being a black female. She evidently took those challenges in stride, did not let it hold her back, and did not let it stop her, and went on to become very successful!"

Five
A Kindred Spirit

During her residency, and now well grounded in her medical training, Margo had the opportunity to rekindle her closeness with Dr. Dinah Fedyna, when they both worked at Akron General Medical Center. In the third year of residency, Dinah was Margo's chief resident for the team, and this is where Dinah states she really came to know Margo. Dinah remembers Margo, "Hustling [in her work], while dealing with asthma attacks when she was pregnant with Kenya. We saw each other's patients, and I was able to see how she kept her charting, and got to see what they [patients] felt about her . . . and *they loved her even then.* Margo's patients loved her! She was a fearless advocate for her patients, which I think a lot of that came from her own self [determination]. She would take care of her patients and be there for them. Margo would protect her patients from the insurance companies, the sub-specialists and sometimes even from *themselves.* She would stand up for them! She would do this!" Dinah emphatically asserts, gesturing with her hands.

Dinah continues, "Margo would stand up to the medical consultants. Not only was she a [racial and gender] minority, but she *was tiny!* For Margo, she left an impression and people learned you had to listen to her. She *was not* just squeaking to squeak, she was squeaking for a reason and she was going to make sure her patients were taken care of! If one of her patients needed a procedure done, and the specialist would say 'no, I don't think so,' or, 'I think it can wait,' Margo would be right there, saying, 'No! I really think the patient needs to have this done.' "

Dr. Fedyna visibly exhibited a sense of pride while she spoke of Margo's challenges as well as her triumphs. *I* felt proud to witness Dinah's hand gesticulations, emphasizing pride in speaking of Margo's accomplishments. Dinah's expressions validated what I had always known about Margo Prade for twenty years; and what I wish to share with others . . . and that is, that Margo was a phenomenal individual, *a no holds barred, tenacious go-getter.* Moreover, even with Margo's pregnancy leave, Dinah proudly asserts, "She still managed to graduate from residency on time! She graduated with her class." And, Dr. Fedyna adds, "When Margo's internship was near completion, she took her State Board Medical Examination and passed it the first time around!"

* * *

Through tireless effort, Margo worked twenty-four hour shifts in residency and made outpatient hospital visits both while pregnant, and as a new mother. Throughout her medical school experience, Margo also periodically helped raise two special nieces, Layne and Dayne Arnold, and nephew, David Shamberger, who was with her the longest. Margo had a distinct and passionate adoration for her nieces and nephews. In the words of one of her twin nephews, Tony, "She was everybody's mother. One time I was having trouble with my wrestling and she made me get down on the floor with her and wrestle. At the end of that year, I took 5th in the state, and continued to place in state championships after that."

Margo constantly embraced her family with love and devotion. And, Margo never set any boundaries on her allegiance towards her family, patients or friends.

Niece Layne, ardently reflects on her first recollection of her aunt Margo . . . "She was a ray of sunshine. With me being so young, I just always wanted to be around her. . . . I wanted to *be like* her. She was lovable, and just had that energy! She always knew how to talk to us in the right way. Even if we just had a little scratch, she knew how to make us feel we would be okay. I can remember being at her [high school] games in 1975 when she was cheerleading, just watching her, wanting to be like her when I grew up." Layne admits that although Margo could not officially be their physician, family members could always call her and she would give them peripheral medical advice. . . . "What's wrong with you, do you have a cold? Well, go to the drugstore and get this, or get that," Margo would order. Even I knew Margo was *everybody's doctor* away from the office. If you knew her phone number, you could call her, any time, day or night.

Grasping her chest, Layne admits how proud she was of Margo. "I was so proud of her. I mean . . . for me to be able to go to school and tell my friends my aunt was a doctor just made me so proud. When I was in Erie Island Elementary school in the 5th and 6th grade, she came up to the school and talked to my health class about our bodies, how they worked, puberty and how we should take care of our bodies. As a class, the teachers would have to set the entire afternoon aside whenever aunt Margo would come to the school and speak. It was so exciting for me to be young like that, and have her come in and talk to my class. Sometimes I still see my elementary school teacher and she still remembers aunt Margo coming in talking to our class stating, 'Your aunt was so nice to do that, and I *still* remember.' " Layne goes on to confess, "I always knew aunt Margo was smart, but I did not know she was ***that smart*** until I was older and was able to see how she would chart all those charts, and see all those patients and how she was [so smart] academically!"

Layne had her own special talents, for which she also credits Margo as her inspiration. Layne had been a very gifted singer from the time she was a very young girl. Margo would always support her niece in her talent endeavors. Layne admits, "I wanted to be just like my aunt Margo. Since she sang, danced in dance groups and was a cheerleader, I emulated her and wanted to do everything she did. We would sing and act out scenes together, dress up and entertain ourselves, so I had talent all along. Being around aunt Margo just brought more of it out."

Margo's influence on her niece's talent made a profound impact on her life. In 1995 at the age of twenty-one, Layne's talent took her to New York City. There, Layne competed and won five contestant appearances on the hit show, Showtime at the Apollo, including three Amateur Night performances.

When Layne won her first appearance on Showtime at the Apollo, Margo packed up her kids and flew to New York City to support her niece. Layne laughs stating, "No one believes me, but, I am ***positive*** while I was up there on stage singing, I heard aunt Margo yell, 'That's my niece . . . that's my niece!' " Layne's success in New York caught the eye of the local media in Akron. Layne appeared in the entertainment section of the Akron Beacon Journal under headlines titled, "Akron's Arnold on the Brink to Stardom."

Margo and her entire family were ecstatic over Layne's success. Also at this time, my youngest first cousin Rodney Harris, had a comedy act that was taking off like a rocket. Both he and Layne were featured at different times in the local newspaper, and both were scheduled to appear in separate shows at Akron's Tangier nightclub. Layne was scheduled to appear with Akron native and pop recording artist, Howard Hewitt. Rodney headlined his show exclusively.

Margo and I often talked about how exciting it was to have close relatives on the fast track to stardom.

"Girl, by the time Sahara is of age, Layne's stardom would have paved a much easier way for Sahara!" I would often assert to Margo about her youngest daughter and the obvious talent she also had.

"That's what I'm hoping for!" Margo would respond with excitement.

When Layne decided to leave Akron and move to Atlanta to pursue her singing career, Margo's support followed. Layne candidly asserts, "I moved to Atlanta because after the Apollo theatre shows, the recording contacts and contract opportunities were much greater for me there. Aunt Margo co-signed for my apartment when I moved to Atlanta."

Layne still credits Margo with keeping her focused on her God-given talent of singing. "She would always tell me, you are the best singer, and no one is better than you are. I want you to be the biggest star. ***My niece*** is going to be the biggest star!" As much as Margo comforted and supported her family, Layne admits laughing, "If I needed some money though, she would make me work for it! Aunt Margo would say, 'If you need some money, then you'd better get in this office and do some filing or something for me.' Then, I'd go in and start doing stuff *all wrong*. Aunt Margo would kick me out of her office, give me the money anyway and say, 'girl, get out of here before you mess something up!' and we would both end up laughing about the whole thing!"

* * *

Daughter Sahara, the younger of Margo's two daughters, speaks of her mother's love in no uncertain terms that are more than convincing, and difficult to measure. Sahara cannot recall her very first memory of Margo, but having known her mother for at least six years, she committed to memory that:

"It was like *she was not real.*" Sahara's eyes sparkled as she spoke of memories from the heart. "She would always hug, kiss, and play with us. And I was just soooo spoiled! I was spoiled by her love and generosity. I mean, she was a generous person anyway, but she gave me anything; not just material things . . . but in her *love and generosity.* Everybody got the generosity from her, she was a very generous person. But I got it one hundred times over because I was her daughter and SHE LOVED ME!"

For her fourteenth birthday, Sahara had her mother's name wrapped in a sacrificial heart with the initials R.I.P. tattooed on the back of her left shoulder. Sadly, Sahara states, "It's been too long since I have seen my mother."

* * *

Margo not only embraced her family members with love, support and kindness, she treated each one of her patients as if they were family as well.

Patient Aaron Malone states he first met Dr. Margo Prade at age "Eight or nine." His first impression of her was that she was "A compatible person. She was nice and anybody could get along with her."

Because Aaron first met Margo away from the office, and on the softball field or other social settings, his immediate impression of her was that, "She was a fun person who giggled a lot! I did not become a patient of hers until I was about thirteen. When I would go to her, it was not like I was going to the doctor. It was more like I was sitting down with a person who knew what they were doing and knew what they were talking about, but it was just a friendly visit, rather than a doctor's appointment. I liked that because I never had to wonder what my doctor was going to be like, because I already knew Margo, and what she was going to be like when she came in the room. And . . . she would not leave that room until she knew I felt that I would feel better and had all my questions answered!"

* * *

Long time patient Vickie Taylor, had been a patient of Margo's during her entire medical career. Ms. Taylor first met Margo when she worked at Health Guard. Ms. Taylor met Margo by happenstance. Margo was listed on her insurance network group. However, Ms. Taylor did stipulate, "I was *looking for an African American doctor* who could treat my entire family."

Her first impression of Margo was that of a warm, friendly, and kind person. "She even purchased the first case of baby formula for my second son I gave birth to. He couldn't hold down any other type of formula. The special formula was extremely costly at the time. Dr. Prade was very sympathetic to my husband and me. My son was ill, dehydrated and was hospitalized for fourteen days. He could not hold anything down, and his bowels would not move. Dr. Prade called in a stomach specialist, Dr. Robert Stone, because no one else at children's hospital could figure out why my son would not hold anything down. He [Dr. Stone] told us our son's stomach was intolerable to the regular formula and needed to have this special formula. We were complaining, my husband and I, about the cost of the formula. Through Dr. Prade's kindness and generosity, she purchased the case of formula for us. We were contacted at home one day to come and pick up the case of formula from her office, that ***she*** had bought."

In hindsight, one could determine that Margo apparently not only wanted, but more importantly, *needed* to finish her residency on time. It was as if Margo herself, envisioned a harsh reality that her very existence of a healing spirit, enjoying a long and happy life practicing medicine and raising children would meet with a foreshortened future.

Six
Subliminal Messages

After Margo completed her residency in 1986, she began working at the Westside Family Practice medical center, located inside Akron General Medical Center. This is where Margo began her career as a full-fledged, qualified, and skilled physician. Margo's duties involved seeing her own patients and precepting the medical residents. Margo's precepting involved her being available to medical students for advice on their patients, as well as monitoring the resident's work and progress with those patients.

In 1986, Douglas, too, began climbing the professional ranks of his career in the Akron Police Department. I was still employed by Akron Police, and was one year into my new and much more satisfying marriage.

Margo and I were still playing softball together every chance we could. My husband sponsored our women's team with the business, and we were winning tournaments and racking up trophies left and right. As professionals, friends and softball players, we were really having a good time in our work and our play.

As time marched on, Douglas and I became closer friends. My friendship with, and *perception* of Douglas, was primarily fostered through my friendship with Margo. Even though Douglas and I both worked for the Akron police, I rarely saw or interacted with him. Douglas always worked the night shift, and except for my final two years at Akron Police, I always worked the day shift. Also, Douglas almost never attended any of our softball games, and the few times he did, he would make Margo so nervous if she made a mistake, that he became a handicap for her. Nevertheless, our friendship was apparent. We would attend many of the same parties, and after I remarried, the four of us would sometimes double date. Whether I was married or single, Margo and Douglas always seemed to be there for me.

Margo always spoke of Douglas in positive terms. She would offer him up as a support system if I (or someone else) were having problems, and if she thought he could help. Margo never hesitated to say, "I'll talk to Douglas, he'll help you," or "Ask Doug, and he will know what to do." Margo ***loved*** that man and she ***kept*** him on a pedestal for many years.

As professionals, Margo and Douglas began to acquire status and success within the community. They seemed to take in all the good things life had to offer. Together, the two embarked on what seemed to be the *perfect life.* People liked, respected and wanted to be in the company of the esteemed couple. Between the two of them, they ingratiated the community. Indeed, Douglas and Margo had all the trappings of a happy, fulfilled life.

Professionally, Douglas engaged in behavior which—for all intents and purposes—earned him celebrity status amongst his colleagues, friends and family. Margo's family, too, respected him to the utmost, and they were very proud of him. His personnel file reveals that after every single promotional exam Douglas sat for, he fought City Hall through legal battles and lawsuits over the lack of promotions of Black officers. After each legal battle, Douglas himself would be promoted.

In February of 1986, Douglas earned his Sergeant stripes. This was the first of three promotions Douglas would receive over the next ten years.

In June of 1992, Douglas was promoted to Lieutenant, and in February 1996 to Captain. Essentially, it became evident that Douglas Prade was indeed on the proverbial fast track to become Chief of Police.

Douglas also gained community and departmental respect for his role in a gun buy back program, he held the title of President of the Akron Chapter of the Black Law Enforcement Officers Association for several years, and gained notoriety in significant areas of law enforcement training and interdepartmental advancements. As Douglas' professional notoriety and accomplishments bloomed, *so did his ego.* When Douglas was truly at his professional best, *it seemed to only bring out the worst in him.*

For any other African American police officer, to master these professional accomplishments in such a short time would have been stellar achievements admired by many, and obtained by few. For Douglas, however, the promotions became *demonic influences* that cultivated a pervasive and diabolical ego, erased his superego and nurtured a persona that would reach catastrophic proportions.

One night while working the midnight shift, I witnessed a chilling incident over the police monitor that involved Douglas and two subordinate officers, just after his promotion to Sergeant in 1986.

The monitor was located in the Akron Police Department radio room. The structure of the radio room had every type of technology available. All incoming and outgoing phone calls were recorded and the audio and visual monitor recorded all arrestees who were brought into the sheriff's booking area by police. The monitor protected police from false accusations of brutality by arrested individuals, as well as deterred them from becoming overly aggressive towards prisoners. The monitor was on 24 hours a day, 365 days a year.

On this particular night, there were six of us working as communications technicians, and our police sergeant. There had been a very serious call involving an offender and a victim of some type. Douglas was the district 8 supervising Sergeant on duty. District 8 was West Akron and where the incident occurred.

The two officers were rookies and had somehow botched the call, even though they had made an arrest. Douglas, along with the rookie officers, escorted the prisoner into booking. What had previously been a quiet night . . . suddenly turned loud, intimidating and *ugly.*

"What the ***fuck*** were you guys thinking of!" Douglas bellowed in a horrific rage at the two officers. Startled, we directed our attention toward the monitor. "How in the ***fuck*** am I supposed to straighten this shit out now? You guys really, really ***fucked up***! Do you know that! " It seemed as though Douglas was screaming at the top of his lungs as he leaned over in the young officers' faces, nose to nose, *deliberately taunting them.* The officers stood motionless and said *nothing* while Douglas ranted and raved at them. Undressing them. *Humiliating them.*

Stunned, we continued to watch Douglas carry on this brutal attack on the subordinate officers. Our sergeant in radio was ignoring the entire incident. Dismayed, my colleagues looked at me as if *I was supposed to somehow explain* his behavior, but I was just as startled as they were. My colleagues were well aware that I had a close friendship with Douglas. I felt embarrassed and worried. Puzzled, I began thinking to myself while watching, what will happen when the officers complain on him. He won't *be able to deny it, the incident is right here on tape in front of God and everybody! Doesn't he realize or care that we are all watching this?* Then I thought, maybe he was so angry he did not realize how he was behaving, or just could not control himself. After all, if his officers screw up, he has to bear some of the responsibility too.

I was nervous and worried Douglas would get into trouble with his supervisors on this one, and in turn, cause public embarrassment for him and *Margo.* I had never seen him like that before.

Oh, how soon we forget. . . .

Like Margo, Douglas Prade was one of seven children, having five sisters and one brother. Socially, Douglas Prade was a quiet, reserved individual at parties and social gatherings, active only in taking pictures. Publicly, however, he appeared very cocky, controlled, and stoic. Professionally, Douglas displayed the mentality of Black Militancy and had the propensity to become violent, enraged and demeaning to whoever was in his path at the wrong time.

Records reveal that before joining the Akron Police Department, Douglas attempted a career in the United States Navy after graduating from John R. Buchtel High School in 1964. Douglas first attempted college at the University of Akron. He listed on his police application form that he attended the University of Akron for two years from September 1964 to June 1966.

However, Douglas also listed on his application form that on December 7, 1965 he enlisted in the United States Navy. The police department apparently never caught the date discrepancy between 1964 and 1966. Douglas' discharge from the Navy on November 3, 1967, although honorable, cited "emotional issues." After his discharge from the Navy, Douglas would attempt college two more times between September 1970 through June 1971, and 1980 through 1983, without—according to personnel records—ever obtaining a degree from either attempt.

On June 6, 1968 Douglas E. Prade was awarded an appointment to the Akron Police Department. The oval shaped tin pinned on the right-breast pocket of his uniform bared badge # 241. Douglas Prade was only twenty-two years old when he joined the Akron Police Department. At the time, he was married to his first wife, to whom, according to investigative reports, he was physically abusive.

Douglas Prade carried his abusive tendencies into his work as a law enforcement officer. Documents from his personnel file included evidence of him accosting women on traffic stops, overexerting his power with other professionals, and perpetuating an overall *dysfunctional level* of authoritative overkill. A confidential report written by Douglas, located in his personnel file earmarks the ***beginnings*** of this pathology:

Form 190P **For Inter-Departmental Use**

CITY OF AKRON, OHIO

POLICE DEPARTMENT

From: OFFICER DOUGLAS PRADE #241 DATE 5/21/69 4:45 P.M.

Report as written by Douglas Prade

TO: MAJOR ____, CAPT. ____

REF: DRAWING OF REVOLVER

AT 2:15 P.M. DATE, I WAS HAVING DINNER AT HOME WHEN MY MOTHER CALLED TO ME THAT SOMEONE WAS OUTSIDE ASSAULTING MY SISTER ____ 18 yrs. AS I RAN FROM THE HOUSE TO THE STREET, I OBSERVED MY BROTHER-IN-LAW AS HE WAS CHOKING MY SISTER WITH HIS HANDS. HE THEN THREW HER TO THE GROUND AND CONTINUED TO CHOKE HER. AS I WAS RUNNING TOWARD

HIM I SHOUTED TO HIM TO STOP AND HE THEN STOOD UP OVER AS IF HE WAS GOING TO STOMP HER WITH HIS FOOT, AT WHICH TIME I DREW MY GUN AND TOLD HIM IF HE TRIED TO KICK HER THAT I WOULD SHOOT. HE THEN LET HER UP AND STARTED TOWARD ME AND I REASSURED HIM THAT HE WAS AT A DISADVANTAGE AND HE THEN BACKED OFF.

HE APPEARED TO BE UNDER THE INFLUENCE OF SOME TYPE OF DRUG OR INTOXICANT AS HIS EYES WERE RED AND SENSE OF BALANCE LIMITED. HE ALSO APPEARED AND ACTED AS IF TO BE IN A STATE OF HYSTERIA. WHEN OFFICER___CAR#13, AND SERGEANT___ CAR#45 ARRIVED WE ACCOMPANIED MY SISTER TO HER HOUSE ON___AVE. WHERE WE FOUND WHAT WE BELIEVED TO BE MARIJUANA SEEDS AND LEAVES IN AN UPSTAIRS BEDROOM CHEST OF DRAWERS. ONE CASUALTY REPORT, AND ONE EVIDENCE REPORT WERE MADE AND AN AFFIDAVIT FOR ASSAULT AND BATTERY WERE SIGNED.

RESPECTFULLY SUBMITTED
OFFICER DOUGLAS PRADE #241

Only eleven months into his career as a police officer, Douglas awarded himself the first opportunity to draw his weapon on a private citizen. The nature in which Douglas drew his weapon is not necessarily odd or inappropriate. In fact, any skilled police officer might have reacted the same way given the same circumstances involving an active assault on a family member. However, Douglas had an advantage that the average citizen in the same situation would not have had; that being the use of his weapon, *and* the opportunity to search the assailant's home for something that had absolutely nothing to do with an assault that occurred at another location.

The weapon offered Douglas an extended measure of control over his brother-in-law to where *he had to "back off."* The extra trip to the home, however, in search of drugs that he obviously already knew or suspected was there, shows that Douglas was not willing to limit his power, authority or control in this incident, to the scene of the crime.

This event may have been Douglas' first exhilarating experience with having the ability to wield ultimate power and control over another. By using his weapon *and his position* as a police officer, Douglas was able to qualify the extension of that control. Thus, the pathology begins . . . does he love it?

Douglas' pathology would continue for years. The pathology, however, would be masked by career promotions, exceptionally bright and talented children; and a wife who had a thriving and successful medical practice.

The extramarital affairs—some of which, according to investigative materials, rendered children—and the celebrity status he obtained amongst his family, peers and colleagues only proved to exacerbate the beast stirring about in the belly of Douglas Prade. Unfortunately, Douglas never learned how to tame that beast.

Seven
The Vestiges of Time

Through the late seventies and beyond, I gained the utmost respect for Margo and Douglas as a couple, friends, parents and professionals; holding both in very high esteem. I was proud to place them both on pedestals. I would not engage in, or listen to any gossip about Douglas that would surface in the police department. Ironically, the gossip would seem to become more prevalent whenever Douglas was embroiled in a legal battle with the City of Akron, over promotions, or shortly after he attained a promotion.

I recall snapping at a white female colleague one afternoon who was dating a high law police detective.

"You know DZ . . . Douglas Prade is seeing some woman . . ."

"Shut up! I don't want to hear it because I don't believe it."

"But, I heard . . .."

"I said I don't want to hear it. That's all the people in this department do is gossip, I'm sick of it! Douglas is a loving husband and father. He would never cheat on Margo. You all are just jealous!"

Douglas and Margo were an admired couple, and it is not unusual for folks to cheer for your success and root for your failure. By them being a well established African American couple, some people were indeed, rooting at the very least, for Douglas' failure; especially within the police department *and* because he had the bravado to fight city hall . . . and *win*.

While she suffered through medical school, residency and beyond, Margo and I continued playing softball together. I was enjoying my career at the Akron police department while attending the University of Akron part-time, obtaining a degree in

Criminal Justice Technology in hopes of attending law school one day.

Douglas prided himself in having a wealth of community support both within and outside of the police department, as he fought to alleviate racial discrimination within the Akron police department. Over the years, Douglas' efforts eventually helped to develop a well rounded law enforcement institution; balancing out both racial and gender gaps that had hung around way too long. It was a job well done, and Douglas' resilience in this endeavor was outstanding and commendable. The results of Douglas' efforts to bring diversity into the Akron Police Department continues even today.

* * *

It was the summer of 1982. I had been married to my first husband in 1980 and divorced by 1982 living back with my mother. Margo called me on the phone: "Don, what are you doing this weekend?"

Annoyed at being "dateless" I answered in a dry tone, "I don't know. Why what's up?"

"Well, my brother James is in town and we're having a party for him over my sister Frances' house. Why don't you come?" Margo ordered.

Reluctantly, I replied, "Well . . . I don't know, I've never met your sister and I don't know where she lives. I feel uncomfortable going to someone's home I don't know. "OH, PUH-LEEEEZE!" Margo wailed, punctuating her statement with a giggle. "She's my sister, and you're my guest. That's all you need to know. I'll introduce you to her when you get there if it will make you feel better. You ain't doin' nothin' anyway so you may as well come on over. It'll be fun, Don!" Before I could give Margo an answer, she ordered me to write down the address and said what time the party started. Margo then playfully stated giggling, "You better come or I'll beat you up!"

I bolted out a laugh, shook my head stating, "Girl, you are craaa-zy!" Margo laughed and we both hung up the phone.

I felt privileged Margo thought of inviting me. Many times, married friends will not socialize with divorced friends. However, whether I was single, married, or divorced, Margo never changed her demeanor towards me. She was kind, considerate and seemed to always think of her friends through both the good and bad times of our lives. Margo was a refreshing detour to driving my emotions away from the periods of loneliness and frustration I experienced in being a divorcee.

Nervous about arriving alone, I did attend the party primarily because I did not want to disappoint Margo.

After taking a deep breath, I rang the doorbell of the quaint brick home located on South Hawkins Avenue, just south of Douglas and Margo's home. I could hear laughter and music coming from the basement. A middle-aged woman answered the door. "Hi, my name is Donzella, Margo Prade invited me to the party. Is Margo, or the lady or gentleman of the house available? I'd like to introduce myself to them." The woman smiled while directing me to the basement. "Sure. Come on in, Margo is downstairs, let's go find her."

Desperately trying not to fall from my super-high, high-heeled shoes, I carefully walked down the narrow stairs to the basement.

The party theme was unpretentious and veiled silhouette lighting. Simple but elegant party favors decorated the basement and tables. Everyone was well dressed and friendly. "Margo," the woman yelled. "A friend of yours is here." Margo quickly turned around from talking with a guest and saw me.

"Hey, Don! You look nice!"

"So do you, Margo! Well, I made it. I had no choice since you threatened me!" I playfully stated.

"Oh, girl!" Margo laughed. "C'mon, I'll introduce you to everyone. You probably already know most of the people here anyway!"

I could tell Margo was very excited. She grabbed my hand and led me through the crowd. I met her eldest sister, Frances and her husband Kenny for the first time. I also met all of Margo's sisters except for Denise who lived in California. I then met the guest of honor, her brother James. I had no idea Margo had so many siblings. After introducing me to her family, Margo led me over to an older woman sitting in a chair next to a younger male. She graciously stated, "This is Douglas' mother, Mrs. Prade, and his brother. This is my girlfriend, Donzella."

We all smiled and said hello to one another. Margo began to direct me to various corners of the basement pointing and stating, "The food is over there . . . if you like to play cards, there's a card game going on over there . . . the bar is over there and most of the people are just mingling around."

I knew Margo well enough to know that, as gracious as she was, she was not going to babysit me throughout the party, and she knew I did not expect her to. As I waded my way through the party, I realized, just as Margo had predicted, I did know many of the people in attendance. Margo and I parted ways for the moment, drifting in separate directions. I headed toward the bar while Margo worked the crowd, being the perfect hostess.

Margo had a smile that shined like summertime, and as I began to mingle, I could see her smiling and hear Margo giggling throughout the night as she engaged in conversation with various people. Margo was very extroverted; she had character fortified with charm and an unquenchable thirst for life. As if being kissed by the sun, Margo's personality, smile and giggle could ignite simple pleasures that lay in the most dormant of souls.

At one point during the party, I was walking through the crowd and heard a flat, obtrusive voice echo, "Don, hold it right there and look this way." The voice was Douglas wanting to take a picture of me. I stopped, posed and smiled as Douglas snapped the picture. Douglas *always* took pictures at parties, softball games, and social events. Oftentimes, Douglas would not engage in any conversation of length, if at all, with *anyone.* At parties and social events, he would lurk around like a dark shadow taking pictures of people who were mostly, if not all, women, all night long as if to purposely create a shield from interacting with others. Enigmatical and mysterious, Douglas was like a privately sealed envelope, that when opened . . . *would explode.*

After Douglas snapped the picture, I decided to go over to him and have *that discussion.* In a party setting with a friendly atmosphere, I figured now was as good a time as any. I intended to ask *him* about the encounter we had when I was twelve. Despite all the years that had passed, I just could not seem to let this thing go, and I did not understand why I was being so obstinate about receiving an explanation for Douglas' actions. I just wanted to feel a sense of comfort about it all, and not *still* feel so victimized by the encounter, especially since we were all friends now and so many years had gone by. I wanted closure. This time, I decided to take the plunge and approach *Douglas* for an explanation.

With deliberate steps, I walked toward Douglas.

"How's it going Douglas . . . are you enjoying yourself?"

"Yeah . . . yeah, it's a nice party," he responded tentatively.

I then purposely began giggling to myself in order to seek a response from Douglas as to why I was laughing. The giggle was a masked introduction into asking Douglas about that encounter we had had when I was twelve, and I wanted the issue to surface in a friendly manner.

I knew Douglas well enough now to know that, at the very least, he always portrayed a serious demeanor, even in party settings; and he seemed to master a *whole lot of self-control.* Douglas rarely talked to others, laughed or smiled. And, as he rose in ranks at the police department, his socialization with others seemed to decrease as well. On this particular night, I felt I needed to approach *this* subject both with kid gloves, and as an incident that was *funny now;* as opposed to how frightening the encounter *really was* when it actually happened.

The giggling approach did not work. Douglas did not ask or *care* why I was snickering in his ear. Nevertheless, I preceded on with my quest for comfort in this thirteen- to fourteen-year-old saga that continued to haunt me as my friendship grew with this interesting couple.

"Douglas, do you remember stopping a speeding car one time on South Hawkins Avenue about thirteen or fourteen years ago?" I asked.

"I've stopped a lot of speeding cars." Douglas replied in a very dry but articulate tone. As he continued snapping pictures, I continued to interrogate.

"Well, you'd remember this incident. I was twelve years old and you stopped these two speeding cars on South Hawkins Avenue. In fact, the one driver was even arrested. I know you remember! Anyway (I went on giving him the benefit of the doubt), you were soooo upset that me and my girlfriend were in the cars with those guys speeding, that you *really cursed* and yelled at us and it scared me to death! *Do you remember that,* Douglas?" I asked, still laughing in a desperate attempt to make this thing seem as if it was no big deal now, even though *it was.*

Douglas suddenly stopped snapping pictures, turned and looked at me and stated in a very cold, matter-of-fact tone, "***I don't remember*** that" as if I were making the whole thing up.

"Come on, Douglas, you *have* to remember *that incident!* How many cars with two young girls in them have you stopped speeding down South Hawkins in your career?" I insisted, using my police-like investigative persona.

"Don, I said ***I don't remember*** the incident," Douglas replied. This time, the tone was all too familiar. It rang with the same chilling demeanor he had used years earlier when he bolstered his authority in shouting, "I *said,* shut the fuck up!"

Although disappointed in his response and willing to take the conversation further, I was smart enough to let the issue go. It was obvious Douglas did not want to be reminded of the incident; although I did believe he remembered it. I had also decided that pressuring him to remember the encounter when he did not want to, was not worth jeopardizing the friendship. Again, I chose to rationalize Douglas' response. I figured because we *were* friends now, it *was possible* Douglas felt too embarrassed to admit he'd acted so horribly. Therefore, for the time being, I dismissed the subject.

"Oh, well, if you don't remember, then I guess you don't remember."

"No, I sure don't." This time, Douglas responded with a little more kindness in his tone. I assumed that since I backed off interrogating him as if I were a cop, he decided to back off the cruel demeanor in his responses.

I gave up on the issue for the moment. However, I knew I would ask again on another day, at another time. I just really wanted and needed closure to this thing that had grown geriatric with time, but was still very young and fresh in my mind.

* * *

Saturday March 21, 1998

Hey girlfriend. Margo, not to worry you but your family is in such turmoil. The evil Douglas has perpetuated is lurking all around and penetrating your family nucleus. Everyone is just fighting and arguing amongst themselves. It makes me cry. I'm trying to help as best I can in talking to different family members. I pray for some sense to all of this. Can you let your spirit shine down soon? I know that will help tremendously. If they could just hear, feel or smell you I know it will make a difference. Hurry up okay? I love you so much. Gotta go now.

I'm back. I thought I was finished but I forgot to tell you, both Pam and Paula had baby girls two weeks apart. They are both beautiful. And, guess what, Pam named her daughter, Sydney MARGO! She named her after you sweetheart, in memory of you! That just goes to show how much Pam loved you too. I know you would be spoiling them both if you were here! Margo, it is **SO** *difficult to be happy about anything these days. Your death was just so horrible, and for me, it is simply* ***unacceptable****! I try to think of how you would want all of us to be, feel and act; and try to go from there. But, it is just not working yet! Why?*

I have started watching old videotapes, enjoying seeing you alive and giggling in them. I guess it helps some, but yet, I'm not quite sure of the emotions I feel seeing you alive. Sometimes I want to cry, and other times I feel such pleasure from them. I don't know, ***maybe I'm losing it!*** *I guess I think I should feel either one way or the other. Maybe I'm just trying too hard to feel the same hurt, or some joy for having had you in my life for twenty-one years, or both. I just know I miss you and right now, I just cannot get over it. There is not a day that goes by I don't think of you, your death, or the horrible way you died.*

You were so ***undeserving of such a horrific death.*** *Did you suffer? Was the pain so great that you begged to die after first thinking of your children? I know they were the last thought you had. You loved them so much!*

Margo, do you remember when we talked in the office that day about how the good people always have bad things happen to them? Who would have thought you would be next on the list in that reality. I wish I had told you about my dream last summer of your funeral. I was so afraid for you girlfriend! Now I know why. Maybe if I had told you it would have made a difference. I'll never know now. Margo, I get angry sometimes that you didn't do anything about that bastard when I begged you to. Now you're dead! Couldn't you see what was happening? I could, and I didn't really know that part of him like you did. Maybe you felt a police report wouldn't have done any good anyway. ***And you are still dead anyway—by his cruel, evil hands.*** *Margo, do you know this man is just pure evil in human form!! He had the* ***nerve*** *to wave at* ***your mother in court last Wednesday****! That fucking bastard is truly a psychopathic killer!*

Well, I'm going to close for today. I'm starting to feel depressed, and I know you don't want that. You were always so happy and positive all of the time, even in your most unhappy periods of life that you kept hidden. How could someone like you, die like this?

Love, Donzella

Eight
Building Blocks to Success

After Margo graduated from NEOUCOM, she began her internship at Akron General Medical Center working the night shift in the emergency room. It was during this time that Margo became pregnant with her eldest daughter, Kenya Monique. I remember having a conversation with Margo one evening after a softball game.

"Well, Don, I don't think I'm going to be playing softball this fall," Margo stated.

"Why not?" I responded trying not to show my disappointment. I'm thinking to myself, I hope she has a REALLY good excuse with THIS ONE! Margo was an excellent softball player and extremely valuable to the team. Losing her as a player would cause a major deficit in the strength of our team.

"Well, I'm pregnant. I can finish out this season because the pregnancy is in its early stages, and the exercise will be good, I mean it is not harmful to the baby, but I will not be able to play fall ball. I'll be three months when this season ends."

Happy for Margo, I hugged her and then stated with concern, "But what about your internship? I mean you are working the night shift. Will that be a problem when you have the baby?"

Margo replied with confidence in a business like manner, "I'll be almost finished with my internship by the time the baby is born."

"Girl, you have just really planned your life perfectly!" Margo smiled, and seemed embarrassed by the comment.

Margo was probably the most unpretentious, unobtrusive and humble person I have ever known. One summer, our softball team had thrown a big end-of-the-season party at Goodyear Local #2. Our team had become quite popular, mostly because the

B.L.E.O.A. (Black Law Enforcement Officers Association) was our sponsor. Our team name was, the B.L.E.O.A. Bunnies.

At the time, we were one of the most talked about female softball teams in the Akron area, so we had no problem *packing the house* when it came time for the party. Identical to Margo's graduation party, it seemed as though all of Akron attended.

During the party, I had the opportunity to finally introduce Margo to my longtime good friend Rosemary, whom she had heard me talk about, but had never met; just in the same way Rose had heard me speak of Margo often, but had never met her.

"Rosemary, this is my friend and teammate Margo, Margo this is my best buddy, Rosemary!" I proclaimed, excited to *finally* introduce them to one another.

"Hi, Rosemary, nice to meet you," Margo greeted her smiling. Rose, in return, smiled back and stated, "Nice to meet you too, Margo!"

"Ahem! She's a doctor!" I stated with pride to Rosemary.

Rosemary reared her head back, bucked her eyes, smiled stating, "OOOOOH! How nice!"

"Don, *do not* do that! " Margo chastised me, slightly embarrassed. "What?" I reacted puzzled.

"I don't like it when people do that to me," Margo explained.

"Well, you *are* a doctor, Margo! And if you are not proud of it, that doesn't mean I'm not proud of you!"

"Well, it just makes me feel funny, that's all." Margo resigned apologetically.

I learned a lot about Margo that night. I learned that although she placed value on the very credo of her profession, she did not place herself in a light of high esteem in being a medical professional the way other people did. I also learned that as much as Margo would brag on another person's success, she did not welcome someone bragging on hers. Since Margo was my friend, I abided by her wishes, sort of. *I did not stop bragging* on her, I just stopped doing it in front of her! With future encounters, as soon as Margo would walk away from an introduction, I would lean over and whisper to the person, "She's a doctor!" Like Rosemary, the person was always impressed.

Margo *was impressive*. She was a down-to-earth,

no-nonsense person. She was a person who played a relentless softball game, laughed and smiled *all the time*, and was a dedicated professional who practiced medicine. Parallel to an oxymoron, Margo's personality and profession did not seem to go together. After learning of her profession, people would make statements such as, "She is so normal acting to be a doctor" or, "She is so little, cute and friendly, not stuck up like most doctors are!" Most people had experienced physicians as being pompous, pretentious and serious all of the time. Margo was the *complete opposite.*

According to Jane Freeman, an instructor and director of the behavioral science curriculum at Westside Family Practice, and who teaches interviewing skills to resident physicians, "Margo came to this residency already gifted with interpersonal skills. In her interview with patients, she was warm, supportive and sharp about what was going on with the patient. She did not easily get the wool pulled over her eyes. She was a great team player." Ms. Freeman also states, "my recollections of Margo are all fond, warm ones."

In her softball demeanor and her everyday life in dealing with family and friends, Margo *always* had the same conduct towards others as if she were working with a patient . . . warm, supportive and sharp about what was going on. Margo was creative, intelligent and capable of mastering whatever challenge she would encounter.

* * *

On January 7 1985, Margo gave birth to her first child, Kenya Monique, one year before she would graduate from her residency at Akron General Medical Center.

Margo and Douglas' life took on a distinct new meaning. They were now parents, although Douglas had traveled this route before with a son, Prescott, from his second wife. In addition and according to investigation records, Douglas also had an illegitimate daughter who was born two years *after* he and Margo married. A daughter Margo had yet to discover.

For now, however, everything that was to make life complete was falling into place for Margo when Kenya was born.

Margo was equally ecstatic about being a parent, as well as meeting all of the challenges parenthood was sure to offer.

I remember visiting with Margo one afternoon while she was convalescing after Kenya's birth. "Margo, she is beautiful," I asserted. Both Margo and Douglas were smiling, but Margo could not take her eyes off her new daughter.

"Well, how was it?" I asked, inquiring about the labor pains I thought I'd never experience.

"Girl, *it hurts* . . . and I had *back* labor!"

"Like I know what that is, Margo!" I stated, slightly annoyed. [Margo would sometimes speak in medical terminology during a conversation; just enough for one to not *quite* understand the full degree of her point, and to become just a little annoyed by it.]

"Well, back labor is extremely painful. Don, when you get pregnant, you'd better pray you don't have back labor!"

"Well, she is beautiful, Margo and, you look good already! Your weight has really come off fast!"

Because he was standing around listening, Douglas joined in the conversation, "I'm shocked you're saying that, Don, 'cause she wasn't giving up NO FOOD while she was pregnant."

Margo gave Douglas a sharp, nasty look, and scowled a deliberate, "Shut up!" at him, and she *meant* it. Don't mess with a woman's raging hormones after a recent pregnancy!

I did not want to stay long, so I prepared to leave.

"Well, Margo, I'm going to go now, I've got some things to do."

"Okay, Don. Thanks for stopping over."

Margo bid me ado, while cradling Kenya's tiny body in her hands and forearms, resting the tiny infant on her knees. Mesmerized by her existence, and without ever looking up from her daughter, Margo gave me a faint, "Bye, Don." I looked back at Margo while walking through her dining room to leave and witnessed a sight of true adoration glowing from Margo's face as she gazed upon her newborn child. The way Margo looked at Kenya, with Kenya's tiny eyes looking back at her, marked a permanent place in my memory.

I was thinking while driving home how wonderful it must be

to have given birth, to where the mother *visually displays* her love for that child through a simple gaze or facial expression. I never forgot witnessing that awesome encounter between Margo and her newborn baby, and I wondered if I would ever have the opportunity to experience what I had just witnessed.

Margo strived to be the perfect parent. She refused to defer to the fact that she was a busy physician as an excuse to not be all she could in her duties as a mother. Margo succeeded in that feat—just like every other challenge she encountered. Margo exemplified her desire to be a perfect parent when Kenya was born one year before she was to complete her internship at Akron General Medical Center.

After returning to her residency, Margo's assignment sometimes involved the night shift. She would insist that Douglas bring Kenya to the hospital at night in order to nurse her. She arranged her nighttime break to correspond with Kenya's feeding times.

Margo shared Kenya's nursing schedule one day in conversation. I was quite impressed at her tenacity and dedication as a new parent. I began to believe Margo was blessed with a rectitude that many people wish they possessed, and that few will encounter in one lifetime. I began to believe that Margo could do *anything*.

Nine
A Genteel Journey Awaits

After Margo finished her residency, she began working at Westside Family Practice Center located inside of Akron General Medical Center. This was Margo's first introduction into her medical career as a full-fledged practicing physician. As excited as Margo was about now being a practicing physician, and working for Westside, she still had dreams yet to be fulfilled.

According to Dr. Dinah Fedyna, Margo's vision in opening up an office had a distinct twist to it. Margo really liked the idea of fixing up an older house, and having the office in or near the neighborhood, she grew up in. Margo preferred an older house, as opposed to being in a newer building. Margo's desire to have a private practice in or near her own neighborhood, was, knowing her, a way of giving something back to the community she grew up in.

At this time, which would have been some point in 1987, Dinah was in a private group practice that she knew she did not want to stay in, and Margo was examining her options beyond Westside Family Practice. One day Margo and Dinah went to look at a big old house on Perkins Street, in hopes of things panning out well enough to where the two of them could go into practice together. According to Dinah, there was a lot involved, with the availability of loans to fix up the house and at the time, Dinah asserts, "there was not a lot of support from the hospital."

The house on Perkins Street did not materialize as a partnership for Dinah and Margo, and they both went their separate ways afterwards, but stayed in contact with one another. Dinah secured another private practice, and eventually began teaching at NEOUCOM, and Margo began working at Health Guard of Ohio shortly thereafter.

Health Guard was a Health Maintenance Organization (HMO) conglomerate, located on South Broadway Street in Akron, Ohio. Margo never surrendered her vision of a neighborhood medical office. The vision was temporarily deferred, as she pursued her career in practicing family medicine at Health Guard; and pursued the final additions on her personal life by becoming pregnant with her second daughter, Sahara Denise. Sahara was born on May 3, 1988 and Margo, being very close to her family of origin, proudly gave her sister Denise's name as Sahara's middle name.

After Margo joined the medical team at Health Guard in 1986 she met what would ultimately be her longtime friend and office manager, Joyce Foster, and medical assistant, Pam Brannon. From this point on, Margo's career as a private medical practitioner continued to soar, as did her friendship with both Joyce and Pam.

Health Guard had employed Joyce since 1982. She first met Margo when she joined the staff of physicians at Health Guard. However, Joyce's first meeting with Margo wasn't until Joyce ran a training session on a new phone system that had been recently installed, and she needed to train the doctors on how to use their phone cards.

When asked what was her first impression of Margo when she first met her, Joyce replied, "I liked her, and I was *so* glad we had a black doctor. For *years* I had been harping on them to get a black doctor because most of our patients were black."

Under Joyce's tenure, Margo was the very first black physician that Health Guard employed, and she was well received by all the other doctors. Joyce remembers a candid conversation with the medical director before Margo's arrival. "I was constantly on the medical director to get a Black doctor in here." The Health Guard medical director would sarcastically respond, "Well, do you want to go to school?" Then Joyce would respond with deliberation, "If I wanted to go to school to be a doctor, I would have been a doctor. You need to get a black doctor in here! All the patients are saying, 'where are the black doctors?' and they are coming to me saying it!"

When Margo did arrive at Health Guard, Joyce met a very

personal side of Dr. Margo Prade under the most demure circumstances.

Joyce explains: "I was working in member services, and I was upstairs one day because I had to take something to her [Margo's] office. I heard this noise, a loud noise coming from her office, and [in a whisper] I asked someone, '*What is going on in there?*' The person responded, 'Oh, she's just pumping milk for her baby.' Everybody always laughed because Margo would pump her breast milk at work for her new baby, and the machine was really loud!" Joyce explained with a smile.

Joyce then knocked on Margo's door and after a few seconds, a soft, kind voice invited her in. Joyce went into Margo's office and noticed Margo had been crying. Puzzled, Joyce asked, "What's wrong?" "My baby is sick," Margo responded. "What's wrong with her?" Joyce asked, concerned. Margo stated to Joyce that Sahara had a temperature, and although her mother was with Sahara, Margo was crying because her infant daughter was ill, and as her mother, *Margo wanted to be with her.*

Joyce sat and talked with Margo for a while, and explained to her that if she needed to take off work, "Then take off!" Interesting statement coming from line staff personnel, and given that this was Joyce's very first personal encounter with Dr. Margo. Undoubtedly, the most outstanding quality Joyce learned on *that day was, in her own words, "Margo was very dedicated to her patients, and she loved her children!"*

Joyce and Margo did not become close during the two-year period they worked at Health Guard. Not even after that candid moment in Margo's office. Joyce explains, "We didn't get real close, we weren't real close at all. We were social and Margo would invite me to a couple of her parties that I never really got to attend because I was rippin' and runnin' up and down the road playing bingo."

In early 1988, however, one of the employees had told Joyce they heard Margo was leaving Health Guard. Curious, Joyce went up to Margo's office once again, but this time she was on a *personal* mission. Joyce knocked on the door and waited for Margo's invitation to enter:

"I got a question for you."

"What?" Margo responded.

"I hear that you're leaving."

"Who'd you hear that from?"

"One of the employees, they said you were leaving and were going to open up an office. What I was wondering is . . . if I could give you a resume?"

"Yeah. Sure."

"Well, what positions do you have open?" Joyce asked, obviously enthused.

"Well . . . all my positions are open."

"I'd like to give you a resume. I'd like to apply for a position of office manager, which is what I have experience in."

"Well . . . okay. Bring me a resume and I'll have my partner, Ken Eugene, look over it. Then we will give it to Dick Moore." [Mr. Moore was the person at Akron General who oversaw the opening of Margo's private practice.]

After Joyce forwarded her resume to Margo, an appointment was set up with Margo, Dr. Eugene, and Mr. Moore. Before the interview was over, they said, "Put your notice in as soon as possible . . . you got the job!" Joyce was ecstatic.

Medical assistant, Pam Brannon, now Pam Foster, met Margo at Health Guard in 1986. Margo was one of the doctors for whom Pam did medical assisting and charting. Margo was pregnant with Sahara when she and Pam met, and Pam remembers Margo bringing her infant daughter in from time to time.

Pam's first impression of Margo was that, "She was real nice and quiet. The other doctors were, of course, loud and obnoxious, and Margo was the only female doctor in my group."

Pam noticed a uniqueness in Margo that was unparalleled by the other doctors. "Margo was very caring and cared a lot more about her patients than the other doctors there. She cared about her female patients, because she was a female. I thought she was a good doctor; she always took care of her patients," Pam asserts with admiration.

When Pam and Margo formed their friendship, Margo had asked Pam to join our softball team. Pam credits that union with two other factors as well; "We were the only females in my group of doctors I worked for, we had a good working relationship and (laughing) we both hated Health Guard and wanted to get out of there!" After Pam joined our softball team, it was quite apparent to the rest of us that Margo had a special relationship with Pam.

I thought it quite interesting and rather special that Margo could have such a close relationship with an employee after work, with whom she was their boss *during* work. It was unheard of, especially in the capacity of a Black doctor, and a White medical assistant! Margo, however, was not your everyday ordinary person. Her character alone, illuminated diversity in everything she either did or attempted to do. By merely being herself, Margo had the ability to teach others, without *ever being aware* of the lessons many of us learned from her.

* * *

Time was marching on, and our lives were advancing in various directions. The softball team seemed to become a permanent fixture year after year on ball fields throughout the city. Tom and I began building a home, and over an eleven-month period it took for the home to be completed, Douglas offered to do regular safety checks at night while he was working. Margo was increasing her visibility within the community, and working hard on plans for her own office.

Shortly after Tom and I moved into our new home, Margo and Douglas bought a beautiful home located in west Akron, on Mull Avenue. The home was complete with towering pine trees for privacy, and a walkout patio that led to a beautiful in-ground swimming pool. I knew the pool was primarily for Kenya and Sahara. Margo insisted on her girls knowing how to swim and swim well. Margo frequently involved Kenya, who was the eldest and most capable child at the time, in disciplined swim lessons several times a week, and engaging in swim competitions throughout the county. At their youngest ages, Margo was grooming her children for success. She once told me, "Don, I want my girls to be able to compete with *anybody, on any level, with anything.*"

I believed her. I also believed Margo's drive for her children to be successful would most certainly pay off for her and them, one day; because the Margo I knew, had *never failed* at anything.

Ten

The Business of Taking Care of Business

"Margo, how's the office hunting going?" I inquired during one of our softball games.

"Girl, this thing is something! I had to go down to a city council meeting and *present a case or argument* for why there should be a medical office building in West Akron," Margo replied.

"Where is the office going to be located?" I asked.

Margo responded with poise, "Doug and I own this old house on Wooster Avenue, and that area is becoming more commercialized. I want to have the house torn down and have a medical office building built. That way, I can bring in other doctors, that I know are needed in that area."

"Wow! That is a huge endeavor, Margo."

"I know, but it can be done. I've already contacted a builder who is interested, it's just about getting the city's approval now and going to all these *damn* meetings trying to convince the people in the neighborhood. Girl, there was this one lady there, a black lady, too, you know [a lady who was a political activist in the community]?"

"Yeah, I know her," I replied, frowning as if to say how dare she question Margo's motives.

"Well, she said, 'why should we let ***YOU*** build an office building right next door to ***MY*** house?' I just told her that I am a physician, I live in West Akron and a medical building is lacking on this side of town. I think there is a need for it. I also told her that other medical professionals like a dentist, gynecologist, a surgeon, and psychologist, which is Tom, are hoped to be in the building as well."

"Really?" I responded more than impressed with Margo's business sense. "Who is the psychologist?"

"Tom, *your husband, of course!*" Margo responded, yelling and laughing at the same time. "I was going to tell you guys one day!" Margo said, giggling with her belly laugh.

"I guess we never really thought of having an office, Margo, since we have offices in all the places we work."

"Yeah, but, every doctor needs a home office, Don. Besides, I have a *lot of patients* who I think need to see Tom, he'll get plenty of business!" Margo asserted jokingly.

"Well, what did [the lady] say after you answered her question?"

"She kind of rolled her eyes and said, 'Well . . . I guess it is a good idea, you convinced me.' "

Because this woman was older, African American and a known community activist, the woman was haughty in her demeanor toward Margo. The woman made it clear that it was young Margo's task to pay *her* deference in insisting that the medical office would benefit the residents of West Akron.

After the meeting, the woman approached Margo privately to give her blessing on the endeavor. Again, Margo's impressiveness as a businesswoman and a gifted physician prevailed.

"How exciting! Are you going to take Pam with you?" "Yeah, *if* she acts right!" Margo and I laughed as we headed toward the softball field to play defense. I took my place on the pitcher's mound, and Margo trotted to left field. I remember thinking to myself at that very moment . . . at every turn; Margo seems to reinvigorate her career . . . at every turn. How exciting!

That same year we were having difficulties with the softball team. We had employed a new coach and he seemed to be causing a division on the team between the white and black players. His behavior was suspicious, but we could not quite put our fingers on the problem. One day after practice, my mother called. "Don, this is Ma, did you guys have practice today?"

"Yes," I replied.

"Well, your coach (who lived directly across the street from my mother) just came home and a whole bunch of white girls from your team got out of his car and another car."

"What!" I shouted. I was livid.

"Yep, I don't know who he thinks he is, this is *your team,* and he can't invite you and Margo and the rest of you guys over after practice?" Mom stated, very deliberate and direct. Mom was sending me a message, and I knew what it was.

"I'll take care of it, Mom. Thanks for calling me and letting me know."

"Okay, baby. Talk to you later." Mom made her exit out of the conversation, just as quick as she entered it.

I phoned Margo right away. "Margo."

"Oh, hi, Don, what's up?"

"Mom just called and said Jim just pulled up in his driveway and all the white girls from the team jumped out of cars going into his house for a little *party* I guess."

"What!" Margo yelled, just as I had.

"Yep, Mom was looking at them while she was talking to me."

"That's it! We need to get rid of him, Don. I mean, why didn't he ask the rest of us to come over? We're part of the team, too! He is tearing this team apart!"

"I agree, Margo. We need to nip this in the bud right *now.* What should we do?"

"We need to fire *his ass, then* call the team and let them know that he is gone!" Margo suggested with a "street tone" in her assertion.

"Okay, well, I don't want to call Jim."

"I'll call him!" Margo replied in a very matter-of-fact tone. "Then, I'll call you back after I talk to him."

"Okay, I'll call the team, and we won't tell the others, they will find out when they see a new coach show up next week. If they don't like it, they can go, too!" I shouted. I was mad.

"Good, I'll call you back after I talk to him," Margo stated, and hung up the phone.

When Margo called back, she went over what she had said to the coach, and for all intents and purposes, he seemed to take it well. Margo had been very diplomatic with him, as I knew she would be. I wanted Margo to talk with Jim because I knew he would not get nasty with her. No one got nasty with Margo; she was too nice. After we discussed the firing of the coach, somehow, Margo and I engaged in a candid conversation about her and Douglas' relationship. This was the first time Margo had *ever even hinted* to me that she and Doug had problems. Margo mentioned divorcing Douglas, stating, "I'm the primary breadwinner in the family, so he would be the one that would have to move." I did not say much. I wanted to lend a listening ear. However, I did mention to Margo how young Sahara was, and suggested she and Doug seek marriage counseling to work out their problems.

In 1989, Margo moved into her new office building. Before the building project's completion, Margo had been in contact with my husband, Thomas, and he had expressed an interest in occupying office space.

Margo came to our home one Saturday afternoon, with architectural plans in hand, asking if we wanted to see the space available and make any changes. Tom was excited, so was I.

When we met with the builder a couple of months later, however, my demeanor toward the office had changed. I had had a miscarriage the day before and was not in the mood to be excited about any damn office! *I wanted the baby* I had just lost, not an office. Beforehand, I recall calling Margo one evening at home, as I often did, if I had a medical question or problem.

The phone rang and Margo answered in a melodic tone, "Hellooo."

"Margo, I'm spotting!" I answered frantic with my voice shaking.

"Don, just relax, it could be nothing. Now tell me, is the blood light or dark?"

"It's light."

"Are you feeling any pain?"

"No, just spotting."

"Okay, stop whatever you are doing, lay down and put your feet up. Tom will just have to fix his own dinner tonight, ya hear me?"

"Okay, I'll do that. Thanks, Margo."

"You're welcome, I'll call you tomorrow, but call me back if you need to."

"Okay." I hung up the phone and did exactly what Margo had ordered me to do. Nevertheless, my efforts were futile.

When Margo learned of the miscarriage she was sympathetic, but she also responded like a professional. . . . "Don, miscarriages are more common than you think. It's God's way of getting rid of a baby that was not going to be healthy in the first place. I had a miscarriage."

"You did?" I responded for the first time during the conversation.

"Yeah, after I had Sahara."

"Yeah, but you still *already* had *two children under your belt.* I have yet to have one and I'm getting frustrated! This is my second miscarriage in six months!" I replied, crying, and nearly screaming while trying to restrain the emotions that were surfacing.

"Don, I know you really want to have a baby, and you will. Look at it this way: ***at least*** you know you can get pregnant! Remember when you thought you could not even *get* pregnant? So, don't get so upset. . . . I mean try not to, okay?"

At that moment, even though I was sobbing, I felt so much respect for Margo. I appreciated her candor and support during my crisis. At that very moment, Margo comforted me in a way that no one else had been able to master, through either of my miscarriages.

The office plans and design continued to materialize for Margo, with Tom and me in mind. However, many of the other professionals, including us, were not prepared for, and/or were not amenable to the overall contractual factors involved in leasing space in the new office building. Except for the dentist, the remaining health care professionals Margo had hoped would move into the office building did not.

Margo, however, revered in her effort, was sure this endeavor would not be in vain. Having the assistance and blessing from Akron General Medical Center, Dr. Margo Prade opened up her brand new office located at 1557 Wooster Ave. Margo proudly named the building: The Professional Center West, and she and Dr. Kenneth Eugene occupied suite 101, located on the first floor. Margo had the office beautifully decorated in off-white and mauve. All the furnishing matched perfectly. The office gave off a dainty aura of pastels and professionalism.

Both Margo and Dr. Eugene had their own private offices located in the rear of the office. The office had a quaint kitchen area and Margo even had a full bath installed complete with a shower stall, specifically for the evenings we had to play softball. Margo had her office laid out in state of the art fashion.

Margo and Partner Dr. Kenneth Eugene moved into the new office, and began to establish their family practice.

One balmy autumn afternoon, Margo and Kenneth had their office open house party. Margo had also coordinated the open house celebration with Dr. Byrd, the dentist who occupied the office space across the hall.

Attending guests were introduced to and welcomed by the doctors and their staff. This was a smart business move. In this way, the potential to create and share new and existing patients was optimal for Margo, Kenneth and the dentist as well as their patients. When guests would leave Margo's office, she would say, "Be sure to stop across the hall and visit Dr. Byrd's office. Thanks for coming!"

Tom and I attended the open house. I was three months pregnant at the time, but looked to be nine, and was having difficulty surviving the celebration. I was perspiring profusely while trying to dance, celebrate and enjoy this momentous occasion with my dear friend. This night was special for both of us. After two miscarriages, I was finally going to have the child I so desperately wanted, and Margo finally achieved the ultimate goal of her career . . . having her own office in *her neighborhood.*

Margo served expensive champagne, hors d'oeuvres and desserts. People were in and out all night eating, dancing and celebrating . . . except for one person.

It was getting late, and the party had gone on for several hours. "Margo, where is Douglas?" I asked curiously. I could not understand why Douglas was not there, given that this event epitomized all the hard work *his wife* had endured to get to this point in her career. Douglas should have been present celebrating with us, *with her.* "I don't know where he is, Don, he should have been here by now," Margo responded, trying to mask her disappointment.

Although quite happy with her success, I could see the hurt and embarrassment in Margo's face that Douglas had yet to arrive. I felt hurt and embarrassed for her and did not pursue the matter any further. Instead, feeling awkward that I had even asked the question of Doug's whereabouts, I said, "C'mon, let's do the Monte Rail," which was a popular line dance that was somewhat outdated, but people were still doing it.

We began to dance and others joined in. Purposely standing next to Margo, I *pretended* that I could not keep my balance due to my large, pregnant girth. "Whoa!" I yelled, teetering from side to side.

Margo burst out with a boisterous belly laugh. Mission accomplished! I felt obliged to make Margo feel better. She was my "sista."

Late into the evening after visiting Dr. Byrd's new office, Tom and I went back over to Margo's party to say goodnight. My unborn child was pulling rank tonight saying, "It's time to go home and sleep, Mom." Margo's festivities were winding down. Just a very few of Margo's family members were present, and her new staff was beginning to clean up.

Douglas arrived, *in uniform.* Margo did not ask him where he had been. Tom and I spoke to Douglas, he and Tom shook hands.

"What can I do?" Douglas asked, while Margo was cleaning up. Barely making eye contact, Margo directed Douglas to start taking things out to the car. He did so, diligently. Douglas' timing and arrival was brazen and disrespectful, given that he never bothered to show up for his wife's celebration in the opening of her new medical office.

I walked over to Margo, gave her a hug, and said, "Goodnight, Margo. We had a ball! I'm soooo proud of you!"

Margo responded forcing a faint smile, "Thanks, Don. Now you go home a get off your feet. We don't want any problems this time with your pregnancy, I'm not havin' Dr. Lavin [who was my GYN during the pregnancy] yelling at me! Oh, don't forget to go over to Dr. Byrd's office."

"We already went over, Margo, his office is very nice. Good night!"

Tom and I left.

Eleven
And the Walls Come Tumbling Down

Margo was an astute and talented professional who placed no boundaries on the successes she sought to achieve. Even in her marriage, Margo strived for optimum happiness through immersing herself in Douglas, her children, her work and family. She would take fabulous vacations, two to three times per year; and would treat family members to vacations as well whenever plausible.

An unfortunate truth for Margo, however, was that the sanctity of the intimate family connections only existed within the confines of her relationship with her children, her family of origin and friends. One day, it would become apparent that Douglas wanted no part of Margo, their two daughters, Margo's family or friends; and that Margo would spend *years* trying to calm the quiet storm brewing in her marriage. The only area of their marriage for which Douglas had a stake in, was the *money* Margo earned and how he could use it to his advantage. For Douglas, the existence of any intimate, personal relationship in HIS WORLD only proved to feed the insatiable appetite he possessed for adulation, greed, infidelity and control that eventually, even for him, *became uncontrollable.* Douglas became his worst enemy, and his domineering behavior became the vanguard of his own destruction.

Absolute power corrupts . . . absolutely.

* * *

In the daytime hours, Margo's medical practice thrived incessantly. Margo was so busy, that she rarely—if ever—went out to lunch. I would often find Margo sitting at her desk during lunchtime, charting and trying to shove down a quick bite to eat.

In the evening hours after work, Margo would rush off to retrieve her two children, taking them to their activities; often needing the assistance of her sister Frances, especially when the children were very young and, if we had a late softball game. On Tuesday nights during softball season, Margo often showered and dressed for our softball games at work.

In the midnight hour, however, Douglas may have been visiting Margo's office while *he* worked. With deliberate deception, it was *rumored* that Douglas would often take women into *Margo's office* for quick sexual rendezvous, frequently setting off the office alarm system in the process. Whenever the alarm would trip on Saturday or Sunday, either Joyce, my husband or I would have to go to the office and meet the police there and call the alarm company. There was *never* anyone there whenever we would arrive.

Whenever the alarm would trip at night, perhaps Douglas would be the one to thwart additional police response. After all *he was the police, he worked the night shift and, he would be, "already on the scene."* No other ranking officer would have questioned Douglas' response to Margo's office alarm. He was a ranking officer himself working the west side of Akron and, *the building was the home* of his wife's medical office. A perfect combination, a perfect setup, especially since no one spied on ranking officers while on patrol. They were basically self-supervised.

In contrast, Margo would *never respond to her office alarm.* "Margo would not go to that office no matter what," explains Joyce. "I think she knew Douglas was taking women in her office after hours. One morning, I was the first one in the office. Someone had slipped a note under the door after we had closed the night before. The note was addressed to Margo, informing her that Douglas was taking women into the office after hours. This is why she would never respond to the alarm when it would go off, especially at night. I think she was *afraid* to let him see she had caught him."

Although certainly disturbing for Margo, those letters of ruse did not asphyxiate her capacity to practice good quality medicine. As physicians, Margo and Dr. Kenneth Eugene were the talk of the town. West Akron had never had a medical office building such as this; a brand new building staffed with African American medical professionals throughout. Like Camelot, Margo's effort of spearheading the establishment of the Professional Arts Building was history in the making. Unbeknownst to many, including myself, Margo was a hell of a business woman, and it showed.

When Dr. Eugene left the partnership after only two years, Margo's active patient list quickly grew to an astounding 7000.

Even with an enormous patient list, Margo still became actively involved in the community offering free medical exams to little league football teams, high school basketball teams and training workshops. In the late eighties during basketball season, Margo and I relentlessly followed the Central Hower girls' basketball team. My teenaged cousin, Dasha and Margo's niece, Dayne were both playing for the team, which was having a tremendous winning season. Given that Central Hower High School was also Margo's Alma Mater, following the team that year that her niece played for, and with them having a winning season all the way to the state championship was an exciting time for Margo. She would often have young Kenya and Sahara accompany her to late night games.

Once during a spirited game that was a real nail biter, Margo volunteered to keep the stats during the game. At one point during the game, I looked at her asking, "Margo . . . what are you doing?"

"Keeping stats."

"How can you enjoy the game if you are doing stats, Margo, especially at a time like this?" She just giggled. I then remarked annoyed, "Do you *just always have to be busy* doing something, Margo?"

I was annoyed with Margo for keeping stats because I wanted to engage in conversation with her about the intensity of the game. I felt I needed to be nurtured through the potential outcome of this game, and Margo was the person to do it. After all, she was usually the voice of reason in tight situations such as this, and Margo knew basketball, all the rules, penalties and what every foul meant. I needed to know from her, if the referees were cheating us or not when fouls were called. Nevertheless, Margo was a community person and would do *whatever* anyone needed her to do, in whatever setting she could contribute, if she could make the time. This, amongst other things is what made her a community icon specialty.

* * *

It was the third trimester of my pregnancy and I became ill. I was in school at the time. I missed the last three weeks of the semester and my final exam.

While in the hospital, Margo sent two vases of beautiful flowers, one from her and Douglas and one from the softball team. She had paid for both. After being discharged from the hospital, I went to the University of Akron to meet with my professor on what I needed to know for the final exam. While walking down the hallway, I heard a very familiar voice. It was Margo's voice echoing from a classroom in Olin Hall. I stood quietly by the door until her peripheral vision took notice. Margo glanced over while talking, gave me a quick smile, wink and low level wave camouflaged by her hip and the desk she stood behind, then continued teaching the class. At that time, I felt so proud to have a friend like her. Such unselfish professionalism, she was all over the place in the community, and never bragged about any of her services outside of her office.

Aside from her community contributions, Margo's professional demeanor with patients left nothing to be desired. Margo embraced each of her patients with medical knowledge, skill, dignity and respect. Dr. Margo Prade's patients simply *loved her*.

Patient Jaquetta Poole recalls first meeting Dr. Margo Prade in 1991: "I did not know of Dr. Prade before I met her. I came of knowing her through Dr. Harper." Dr. Adolph Harper is a very successful African American gynecologist in the community. He and Margo met on the elevator of Akron General Medical Center and had been very good friends since that time. Dr. Harper also delivered both of Margo's children.

Ms. Poole continues, "I was looking for a doctor for my newborn daughter and Dr. Harper recommended Dr. Prade for my daughter's shots or if she had a cold and things like that. Eventually, I became her patient, so did my husband and other family members."

Smiling, Ms. Poole recalls the first contact she had with Dr. Prade: "I remember it was the fourth of July and I was home by myself with my daughter. I had never met Dr. Prade in person. My daughter's belly button had fallen off, but her naval just did not look right to me. I called Dr. Prade and I was just frantic. I didn't know what to do, I was *just frantic.* I called her office number and they paged her."

When Margo returned Ms. Poole's phone call, without a doubt, she was a calming professional for a patient she had yet to meet in person.

"Dr. Prade, my daughter's belly button is not right! She doesn't look good!"

"Well, have you taken her temperature?" Margo asks.

"The only thermometer I have is the mercury one, I don't have a digital one, and it is hard for me to take her temperature because she is fussing and crying and she seems like she has a temperature!" At that time, Margo tried to tell Ms. Poole how to take her daughter's temperature. Being frantic and upset, the new mother could not read the thermometer, and Margo's instructions appeared futile. Wanting to be on the safe side, and knowing Margo, also wanting to calm the nerves of the brand new mother, she instructed Ms. Poole, "Well, okay, just go ahead and go to the hospital." Ms. Poole remembers the conversation; "She was *just so kind and sweet* over the phone. It was the holiday and I knew she was having something. I could hear the kids in the background, and it sounded like she was outside with the kids." Ms. Poole emphatically asserts, "For me, first impressions are the best, and in just talking with Dr. Prade over the phone, she was just so kind and caring, even though she had never met me before as a patient . . . or my daughter. When I did take Chanel in to see Dr. Prade for her check up and shots, she was just genuinely kind." When they finally met in person, Ms. Poole explains her very first impression of Margo. "I was *PROUD,* you know!" She states smiling, clutching her fists and placing them on her chest. "To know a Black woman who was a ***doctor***, and a person who was a real *people person.* There are so few of us who are doctors anyway, and to have a personality that attracts all of us when we want to be comfortable. I was able to talk with her and be personal with her."

Margo loved children. In her profession, Margo took great pride in caring for children as she did all of her patients. Ms. Poole remembers taking her daughter in for a routine check-up one morning, and Margo inquired, "Is she walking?" Jaquetta replies, "Yes, she's walking!" "Well put her down and let me see!" Margo instructed excited. Jaquetta placed her small toddler on the floor of the examining room, and Margo yelled giggling, "Look at her, she's walking! But, wait . . . her feet are too little to be walking!" Margo jauntily exclaims. Jaquetta laughing over Margo's excitement recalls, "She was *so excited*, you could tell she loved children and she had a special way with children. She would just talk to them."

With this being Ms. Poole's first child, Margo took care to educate mom about Chanel's diet as well. Indicating her love for soul food, Margo stated, "You know . . . you can feed her other foods. She can have [collard] greens and stuff. She can take that, she can eat little things like that now!"

As the years went on, Ms. Poole, her family and extended family members both became and remained patients of Margo's. Margo, too, had uncanny memory recall when it came to her patients, regardless of how long it had been since she had last seen them. In her own words, Ms. Poole asserts, "There *was never* a time when I was dissatisfied with the care Dr. Prade gave me and my family."

Jaquetta recalls trying to become pregnant a second time, and seeing Margo at Dr. Harper's office: "Jaquetta, you're not pregnant yet?" Margo asked concerned. "No." Jaquetta replied. "Humph." Margo spurted out in disappointment; very much in the same way she would often respond to me when asking, "Don, aren't you pregnant yet?" Margo loved children and wanted ***everyone*** to have kids, especially those whom she knew *really wanted children.* When learning of my pregnancy, Margo was just as excited *and cautious* as I was. And, because she was a physician, she would immediately spout off orders: "Don't wear high heeled shoes, lay off the caffeine, including chocolate and sodas; and do not read books that show you pictures and talk about birth defects. Those pictures will just make you scared and upset! Call me if you need anything or have any questions." Margo ended that conversation with a giggle stating, "Have fun eating all that good food, girl! Food tastes *sooooo* good when you are pregnant!"

Margo's private practice experience was indeed bittersweet. She took great pride in caring for her patients, having a staff that enjoyed coming to work for her and creating a work atmosphere that was fun. One Halloween Margo and her staff donned costumes portraying characters from The Wizard of Oz. At lunchtime, and still in costume, Margo and her staff surprised Kenya and Sahara by visiting their school, Our Lady of the Elms. The Catholic elementary school was gender specific for girls. Margo's children were startled, and playfully embarrassed. The teachers and students were ecstatic with laughter as Margo and her staff paraded through the classrooms. Margo was Dorothy, Joyce was the wicked witch of the West, and Pam was the good witch from the East.

Margo was a fun mom. She loved making her children happy, and making them laugh by making faces, dancing, singing and playing with them. She held *nothing* back from her children. Whatever they wanted, they got. Margo's children loved pets and had every type of domestic pet a child could imagine, including ferrets and rabbits. Margo loved her children more than anything and she spoiled them *rotten*. She offered volunteerism at their school and their extracurricular activities. Ubiquitous in nature, I often wondered how Margo ever found the time she gave her children, family, the community and her profession.

As Margo spoiled her children unmercifully, she also expected high performance from them both academically and with their activities. Margo had her children competing in swimming, gymnastics and theatre at very young ages. She also insisted her children earn A's in school. I recall a conversation with her in the office one day:

"I have to get on Kenya, she got all A's and one B on her report card."

"That's ***good*** Margo!" I exclaimed.

"Not ah! Kenya wants to be a doctor, and I told her if she wants to be a doctor, she has to earn all A's, all the time."

"Margo, she's ***only in the fourth*** grade!"

"It doesn't matter. If she gets used to earning all A's now, it will come easy to her later. It's the same with her swimming and gymnastics, that's why she goes every day to one or the other."

"That's a lot along with her school work."

"Yeah, but Don, I want my children to *always* be the best at everything! Besides, what else are they going to do . . . stay at home watching television?"

"Well, I guess you have a point there."

I admired Margo's parenting tremendously, to the point that after my son was born, I followed Margo's example early on with extracurricular activities for him as early as nineteen months, introducing him to gymnastics. I sent my son to Our Lady of the Elms preschool, as Margo did Kenya and Sahara, until he had to leave after kindergarten. Margo, in effect, taught me how to be a new parent, without even knowing. I felt very satisfied, secure and comfortable in emulating her style of parenting.

Margo loved people just as much as children, and had no problem expressing her affection to them. At Christmastime, she would splurge on gifts for her staff, friends and colleagues; as well as her children and family. Her office too, was overwhelmed with expensive gifts and cards from patients and colleagues during the holidays. I saw this as a community display of what Margo meant to others.

The first Christmas Tom and I shared the office with Margo, I was taken aback when I walked in one day and Margo handed me an oversized, beautiful Christmas basket filled with all the goodies one could hope for at Christmastime. "Here, Don. Merry Christmas to you, Ian and Tom!"

Margo loved Christmas and loved buying for others, making them happy. From that year on, we continued to exchange Christmas gifts, and Margo would exchange birthday gifts with friends, her staff and close acquaintances. During other times of the year Joyce states, "We just had a lot of fun. It was a joy going to work every day."

It was quite normal to walk into the office *every day* and catch Margo and her staff in the middle of hearty laughter about something, or *anything.* Margo *loved to laugh, and people loved sharing laughter with her.*

* * *

When Margo was at work, with her children, or on the softball field, one would never detect she lived in a constant state of incipience. For Margo, arriving to work anticipating another *note* found slipped underneath her office door; or an anonymous phone call during the day about Douglas and his sexual escapades with women became stressful and began to compromise the meaning of her marriage. Many of Margo's friends and family were oblivious to this part of Douglas Prade. Had I ever heard of him cheating on Margo, I never would have believed it. I believed Douglas to be a devoted, responsible husband and father and no one could have changed my mind about that, ever.

Nevertheless, Margo's marriage to Douglas was laden in marital skew, discord, control and unhealthy boundaries. Whenever, *if ever,* we went out, Douglas would always show up *in uniform.* Margo and I once attended a softball team members wedding reception. Margo drove and insisted on picking me up. After we spent about two hours at the reception, Douglas arrived in uniform, sat down at our table, ate and engaged in light conversation for a few minutes. Douglas then stood up and left. Not even ***fifteen*** minutes later, Margo looked at me, as if she knew I would be disappointed with what she was about to say.

"Well, I gotta go, Don."

"What! Margo, it is only ten o'clock! They haven't even cut the cake yet."

"I know, but I have to get up early," Margo defended herself sheepishly.

"Okay, can you at least wait until I find a ride home because I am not ready to go yet?"

"Yeah . . . sure, Don," she replied in an apologetic tone.

I was suspicious about Margo's urgency to leave, and I wondered if Douglas' brief appearance had *anything* to do with her wanting to leave in such haste. This interaction between the two of them was new to me, and although I was suspicious, I did not want to jump to any conclusions. On the other hand, if Margo had clinical rounds to do at the hospital in the morning, she would have probably said so. Margo had an occupational habit in that she would frequently recite her next day's schedule automatically, as if she was thinking aloud, or trying to stay ahead of her hectic schedule.

As fate would have it, my answer to the question was revealed over the next several years. Whenever Margo and I went out, Douglas would show up *in uniform,* wherever we were. I began to notice this pattern in his behavior. . . . Doug wore that uniform like a broad dimension of his control over Margo. *There was a message in the wearing of that uniform. The message* was overt to Margo, subliminal to others. . . . "To all persons who happen to be with her, *near* her, in admiration of her . . . KEEP AWAY." It seemed as though Douglas perceived *everyone* as a public threat to *his authority as a police officer* and to his control over Margo. All he *ever* had to do was just *show up.*

After the wedding reception incident, if Margo and I went out together, I would make sure I drove, or Margo and I would drive separate cars and meet at the designated place. The only way I would ride with Margo was if we were going somewhere out of town . . . away from Douglas *and his uniform.*

* * *

She arrived shortly after the Akron Police department's late 80's early 90's hiring campaign. For some time now, and thanks to the efforts of Douglas Prade, Akron police had been more diverse than ever in its hiring practices of both gender and racial minorities. Gorgeous, indeed. A fine and *young,* petite, woman, complete with light skin and long hair. This female specimen was just the way he liked them, young and *vulnerable.*

Her position as a *nice,* new female police officer was sure to tantalize. She fancied all interested parties, and all who would apply. Douglas was one of many to sample the fresh produce within a three-to four-year period. Once he had a taste of honey, and if the honey was sweet, it did not matter who else was in line for the tasting. *If* Douglas Prade wanted her, only he had her.

There was *an unspoken rule* amongst *all* officers; black, white, green with envy or melancholy blue . . . *you don't mess with Douglas Prade's black or white women . . . on or off the department's playing field . . . not now . . . not ever. Douglas did not allow it.*

Except for a *very* few cop friends, Douglas was not well received by many of his colleagues. He did not want to, *or care to* get close to any one of them. Douglas Prade isolated himself from as many people as he could, as much as possible. In many ways he was like a ghost, taking on phantom-like behaviors, covertly lurking around; never really being seen entering or exiting a place . . . but most certainly "showing up."

Many of the white officers loathed Douglas, they saw him as a black militant, always crying racism and discrimination. With many of the black officers he made them feel he was better than they were. Yet, in some ways the black officers needed and respected Douglas as their *hero.* He looked out for their causes and interests as well as his own, making sure they would receive the promotions they deserved. Consequently, black officers had to take the bitter with the sweet as far as Douglas Prade was concerned.

Nevertheless, his rising star in a system of rank and file, also gave Douglas the tools to intimidate other officers as well. Both personally and professionally if other officers crossed *his line* there was at least the *threat* of a consequence. Messing with Douglas' women would be crossing *his* line.

In an [anonymous] interview one officer states: "Once he [speaking of another officer and a woman living in an apartment complex in west Akron] found out Douglas was seeing her too, he stopped seeing her! He was afraid Doug would go after his job."

Unlike many of his police colleagues, Douglas did not engage in recreational sports of softball, golf, or tennis. He did not frequent the FOP lodge for after work socializing. He did not go to many of the parties held by police officers in their homes. No, Douglas' passion was working out in the gym, exerting his power and authority in the community, climbing the ranks of the police department and for sport, he *collected women.* Douglas was, in effect, a *serial womanizer.* Out of the aforementioned activities, it appears Douglas was most proud of his accomplishment in *lusting after women on a regular basis.* He apparently *enjoyed this extension of his manhood.* The *overkill* in his use of *authority* in the community ran a close second to his infidelity, especially if the interaction involved intimidating women:

[*Actual complaints from police file, reprinted and omitting identifiable information of complainants.*]

DATE: May 16, 1986
TIME: 8:30 *A.M.*

COMPLAINT OR INFORMATION REPORT

****** *****   ***ARDMORE AVE.***********

FIRST NAME MIDDLE LAST ADDRESS PHONE

NATURE OF COMPLAINT OR INFORMATION:

*****States that she was driving her young children to school this morning and she stopped at the Lawson's store on Storer Ave. to buy a few lunch items. She alleges that as she was exiting her vehicle, she was accosted by a black man who stated he was a police officer and showed her a police badge in an ID case, and accused her of running a stop sign. She alleges the man (Sgt. Prade) invaded her "personal space" by yelling at her almost nose to nose. She further alleges that he acted "like a wildman" and intimidated her physically to the point that she was "reduced to sobbing." She feels his actions were uncalled for under the circumstances.*

SIGNED: Lt. **********

COMPLAINT FORM Police Division Akron, Ohio **NO. 89 C 080 DATE:** 9/12/89

******** * **** *** Fried Av. Akron, Ohio 44320 ******

FIRST NAME MIDDLE LAST ADDRESS PHONE

NATURE OF COMPLAINT: *Ms. **** called the police to her home because she was being bothered by her ex-husband. The officers on the scene where Sgt. Prade, Officers ******, and *****. According to Ms. **** Sgt. Prade was rude and that he made several uncalled for remarks. Ms. ****felt he had a bad attitude for someone that was supposed to help her.*

******** * **** 9/12/89Lt. ******* 9/12/89*

SIGNATURE OF COMPLAINANT COMPLAINT RECEIVED BY: DATE

There was never any question within the department as to

why citizens' complaints against police officers were routinely "unfounded" or rationalized away by the investigating officer (i.e. "she [the complainant] should be thankful officer Prade did not give her a ticket," or "Officer Prade's actions reported by the complainant are completely contrary to my past experiences with him"). In other words, the improper behavior *did not happen,* and even if it did, it is *not worth getting a police officer in trouble* over, particularly one of rank. In the law enforcement community comrades rule, not citizens.

All the same, Douglas Prade's uncontrollable behavioral rages against citizens in the community did occur. Those rages occurred with young twelve-year-old girls, and with adult men and women. Douglas Prade's rage against women in the community became commonplace, as did the "unfounded outcomes" of those complaints that were laden with excuses by his superiors. Those outcomes, however, only proved to feed the *monster lying dormant* in Douglas Prade. One day, that monster would awaken; and once it began to move, the entire community of Akron Ohio, including the police department that routinely protected him, would meet with an *incomprehensible reality.*

* * *

In late 1990, my husband and I joined Margo in her office, leasing space that was vacated by her partner one year prior. Our company, which provided psychological counseling and assessment services, needed a "face." Margo made that possible for us when she did not have to. She could have easily inserted another physician in the office, made a lot more money and had more patients. Her gesture was **altruism at its best!**

Margo was pleased to have a psychologist located in her office, and she sometimes referred patients to him if she felt they had mental health concerns.

I had resigned from Akron Police in November 1988, wanting to finish my education, help my husband with the business and start a family. Ironically, Douglas was the officer who drove me home before the night shift ended on my final night of employment. At about 3:00 A.M. I was dispatching and radioed Douglas, then awaited a reply.

"Car forty-eight. . . ."

"Forty-eight go ahead. . . ."

"Signal eighteen to the front of the station, and go to channel four please. . . ."

"Forty-eight, copy that."

"Two forty-five." [Every radio contact between the dispatcher and the patrol car ended with giving the time of day.]

Channel 4 was the designated channel police personnel communicated on for private conversations between themselves, car to car, and with the dispatcher. When Douglas joined me on channel 4, I informed him I was going home early and asked if he could give me a ride home.

"Sure, ETA five minutes," he replied. When Douglas arrived, we had one of the most candid and pleasant conversations I can ever remember having with him during the drive home. . . .

"Well, Douglas, this is my last night working here, I'm never coming back again," I stated with an emotional lump in my throat.

"You're resigning?"

"Yes, but no one knows yet so keep it under your hat. I'm calling off sick tomorrow night to use up the rest of my sick time, and this place will never see me again!"

"Why?"

"It's just time for me to move on, Douglas. I mean, I like this job; it is very challenging and interesting, but it is a ***thankless*** job. I've been here eleven years and they are never going to make us supervisors as promised. I'm tired of being cussed out by people calling in, while I'm *trying* to help them. I can't seem to get pregnant and the doctor told me it could be both the stress from my job and school."

"Are you going to miss it?"

"I'm going to miss the friendships I've made, not the shift or the stress."

"What are you going to do now?"

"I'm going to finish school on a full-time basis. Tom really needs my help with the business, and hopefully, I can get pregnant. I know I'm taking a risk giving up part of my independence, and I really hate giving up the medical benefits, but I just really think it is time to leave here."

"Well, good luck."

"Thanks, Douglas."

The remaining ride home was uneventful in conversation. Even his portion of the discussion was *mechanical* at best. Nevertheless, I knew this is as good as any conversation will ever get with Douglas Prade. He would ask questions during normal conversation as if he was interrogating a witness. . . . *"Just the facts ma'am."* I knew Douglas was enmeshed in his position as a police officer and his *dedication* to the police force; therefore, his silence made me wonder if he had somehow thought I was *betraying* the department by "leaving my post." He was a Sergeant now, and very much into the authority and everything that position entailed. When we arrived at my home, I exited the cruiser with a gentle, "Thank you, Doug, I'll see you around!"

He then made a *very rare* comment in jest, "Well, you are going to need eight hours a day off work anyway just to clean that big ole house!"

I turned, smiled at him and replied with a sarcastic, "Yyyyeah . . . right!" He swung his head back laughing, in what again was a rare jovial moment for him, and drove off.

* * *

Shortly after we moved into the office, as a thank you, Tom planned a surprise. He told me to call two of my close friends, choose a date, and we would all go out for dinner and dancing. I phoned Margo, and my ex-brother in-law Cranston, with whom I was very close. As an occupational habit, Margo inquired: "Well, what are we going to do?"

"I don't know, Margo, dinner I know for sure, the rest is a surprise, I guess."

"Well . . . should we come over to your house, or what?"

"Tom says we'll pick you guys up."

"Well . . . okay!" Margo gave up interrogating me.

That evening, Tom played the surprise to the hilt. All the way to making me believe, we would certainly be laughed at by our friends. Tom succeeded in pretending that he believed three couples would actually squeeze into a Dodge Daytona, complete with several bottles of liquor. I felt like Piper Laurie, warning Sissy Spacek in the famed horror movie, *Carrie* stating, "They're going to laugh at you!"

At about 7:00 P.M. the doorbell rang. When I answered the door I saw a nice young man standing dressed in a black tuxedo, and a fancy white limousine parked in the driveway. I was ecstatic. It was my first time ever being in a limousine.

When we picked up Margo and Douglas, Margo walked out of the house smiling, gesturing her hands from side to side stating, "OOOOOOOOHHH, fancy!" Douglas was vacant, only examining the vehicle, giving it the once over as if he were looking for a hidden candid camera. When retrieving Cranston and his date, they were equally surprised, impressed and smiling while walking towards the limousine. We knew we were about to have the time of our lives.

The ride to Cleveland was eventful. We talked about the softball team. At the time, Cranston was our coach and he and Margo always differed in their philosophy of who to play in the games. Margo believed everyone should play every game, and Cranston believed in giving the best players the most playing time . . . and in playing to win at all costs. As their conversation grew, Margo became so irritated at her and Cranston's debate that she stated, "Well, then, I don't belong on this team." After her comment, it was time to change the subject, and we did. Margo began laughing at something that was said. The five of us were really having a good time laughing and talking, while Douglas seemed to be guarded more than anything else, bottlenecking looking out the windows, examining the outer surroundings as we traveled to Cleveland. I remembered thinking to myself, *Does he think we're being followed or something?*

Douglas had pretty much been silent during the entire ride. At one point, the five of us were laughing so hard, he leaned over and whispered something in Margo's ear. Cranston felt Margo's entire demeanor changed after that, and he always believed he overheard Douglas order Margo to "stop laughing."

Cranston never *really* cared for Douglas. He always felt Douglas hurt Margo's performance when he would attend the games. Cranston also contended throughout the years that Douglas was jealous of Margo.

*   *   *

They actually met in 1991. Margo became privy to the affair years later. Margo confessed her *entry* into their lives while explaining one of many reasons she was divorcing Douglas . . . for real this time. "If he was ten years older than me and I was too young for him, *she is definitely* too young for him at twenty years younger!" Margo explained with reality-based logic.

She had not only joined the police force as a pretty, *young thing,* according to investigators, she had also been around the block with several other cops before becoming pregnant. The pregnancy bore a son for Douglas; although during the murder investigation, she would later deny the child was his.

Douglas, on the other hand, proudly claimed the child enough for him to be no secret to some in the community, and to *many* in the police and sheriff's department. For Douglas this child was not a *maybe baby.* This particular child would eventually serve as a replacement for his eldest son, Prescott, who was caught up in, and died from an accidental shooting leaving the Inner Belt Lounge. This child, according to investigation records, was one of *at least* four children Douglas had fathered outside of his marriage. Coupled with the legitimate ones investigations revealed, Douglas Prade had *sired at least seven children, although he would only admit to five.*

This child was special. His mother was the woman Douglas was willing to keep along with, or *replace*, Margo . . . *forever.* With this child, he was the diligent father. The child lovingly called him "buddy" and Douglas made sure his new son attended the same private preschool as Kenya and Sahara. According to Ms. Lillie, "He wrote checks to the preschool to pay for his [the child's] tuition." On school days, he would pick up the child from school daily, *but would not pick up his and Margo's daughters,* Kenya and Sahara. An interview conducted in the investigation states: "Margo's kids were very upset that their dad would pick up [her] son from school and not them. This was never understood by the kids."

One can only wonder how Margo's children were expected to comprehend their father's behavior. The report goes on to state: "Margo's mother is very upset over the possibility of Doug having a child with [her.]"

According to Ms. Lillie, when asked by Margo, "How can you pick up that boy and not pick up your own kids?" Douglas' response was, "He don't ***have*** anyone else to pick him up."

Unknown to her at the time, Dayne, Margo's niece, was hired at the *encouragement* of Douglas to be the child's babysitter; and to exert his *marital independence* even further, Douglas would bring the child *home to Margo* Halloween night so *she* could take him trick or treating with Kenya and Sahara. ***An ego way out of control.***

* * *

Wednesday April 8, 1998

Hey girl! Well, I finally put your picture up today. I haven't been able to do that since you died. It has been a process for me. I put your pin with your picture on it up in my guest room some weeks ago, but I only go in there once in a while. This has been so hard for me Margo. I think of you every . . . single . . . day. Yesterday your mother was granted temporary custody of Kenya and Sahara. I saw them at Juvenile Court, I'm doing my internship there now. Do you know the media was there! I swear Margo your family cannot make any move without them on their tails! I really hope Frances takes the girls away from here one day. They will never have any peace in this town again.

I really miss you Margo. My life is so changed by your death. What are you doing? Are you alive somewhere else and can't tell us? Is there really a heaven? I know you are there if there is one! I'm looking at your picture right now, the one you showed me the last time we saw each other. ***You're so beautiful and look so happy!*** *I am so upset you had only four months of happiness; your life was certainly worth so much more! You meant so much to so many people, Margo. We all miss you, your laugh and your smile. I just really cannot understand this.*

Well, that bitch has finally shut her trap. Her ass is probably being sued by____ for starting that rumor that____killed you. No better for her ass. That bitch! Margo, she did a royal con job on you. But you didn't know street people and street mentality, so I won't blame you. But I can blame you for being hard-headed! You just wouldn't listen to people warning you about her! I know you're bright, but Jesus Margo, you didn't know everything! Now look where you're at!

Sorry, I don't mean to fuss at you Margo. I just really miss you and I am angry you are not here anymore. I want you back!

Love, Donzella

* * *

It was the night of the Black Law Enforcement Officers Association (B.L.E.O.A.) annual ball. All of the social and political "movers and shakers" in town attended the affair that was usually held downtown, at one of the finer hotels in Akron. I continued attending the yearly ball for several years after I resigned because the event was a classy affair and I still had friendship connections.

Political dignitaries were often on the program to speak, including the Mayor of the city. Douglas had positions in the organization where he would sit on the podium with the other guest speakers, making sure he was seated next to who was deemed *most important.* Many times, the Mayor would send someone to speak in his place, along with an apology as to why he could not attend. In the eleven years I worked for Akron Police, I never saw the Mayor make good on his invitation to the ball.

Those of us who were employed with Akron Police knew the inside scoop as to why the Mayor would never attend the ball. It was usually because the black officers were embroiled in some racial discrimination lawsuit against the city for not promoting black officers to high law positions; and Douglas was usually at the helm of the lawsuit.

The Mayor's chronic pattern of not attending the ball year after year exacerbated the black officer's contention that the City of Akron was racially biased against promoting black officers.

Nevertheless, the Ball always promised to be one of the best parties of the year, regardless of who did not show. Once the dance started no one cared who the dignitaries were, or if they even came. People dressed their best, and beauty and barbershops throughout Akron had great paydays on the weekend of the B.L.E.O.A. ball.

The adulterous culture of police work ran rampant within the department. Both black and white officers alike often gave way to the inevitable . . . the female groupies who loved the boys in blue. Retired police officer and friend, CeeJay firmly states, "Once we [police officers] put on that uniform, we get all the 'bootie' we want. A welfare chick, married or single mom, it didn't matter."

It was common knowledge that "unfaithful" officers attended the ball publicly with their wives; and some wives ***never attended*** at all. Some officers were ***bold enough*** to have several of their concubines attend the ball while their wives were there as well.

The mistresses mingled about the crowd in stealth, dressed to kill in *hoochy mamma* outfits, and *come fuck me* high-heeled shoes; making certain the statement, "I'm here for you," is heard loud and clear by their law enforcement lovers.

It was no secret that *some* officers would book hotel rooms for overnight stay with their wives, and book rooms for mistresses as well. When an officer would *disappear for any length of time,* it was suspected by those who knew, that he was in a room with his mistress while wives frantically searched for them. . . .

"Have you seen ____" "No!" The person—*usually another cop*—would answer and quickly move on before further interrogation would resume.

On the Monday following the ball, "cheating" officers would enjoy joking and laughing in the hallways about how they helped ***cloak*** for one another so they could *get with* their mistress in the designated room. Oftentimes, the officers would split the cost of rooms to be shared by all.

"Man, I had to go to the room when I did. She would have blown my cover if I didn't get on my job. You know how they are; they ain't gonna let you get through the ball with your wife there without fucking them before the night's over! And if you don't,

they'll fuck all your shit up at home! Next thing you know, you're gettin' put out the house and working ten extra [private security] jobs just to pay child support and alimony!"

Douglas had a high profile position with the B.L.E.O.A. He held the position of president for many years, and he was respected. *At least for this yearly affair,* he knew there was no way he would prevent *his wife* Margo, from attending nor did he want to.

This was an event where he *wanted* Black officers from across the state to know his wife was a popular physician. He wanted to be seen as the king of the ball, all the way around. *He wanted respect.* Margo's attendance at the B.L.E.O.A. ball as Douglas' wife was even more reason for other officers to *give him his respect.* Margo's professional position heightened Douglas' *importance . . . he knew it . . . he loved it.* The B.L.E.O.A. ball was a time Margo was not only expected, but also *invited to go with him.* This was one of many times Margo ***was not told,*** "You're not invited," when asking Douglas, "Can I go to the party with you?"

Douglas rarely attended parties.

* * *

The program portion of the ball was over and the dance had begun. Margo stepped onto the crowded hotel elevator in anticipation of visiting one of the many private parties being held in suites on the upper floors of the hotel. The elevator door opened and *she* entered. Giving Margo the once over with her eyes, sizing her up . . . measuring . . . comparing.

She spoke curtly. "You're Dr. Prade, aren't you?"

Margo glanced toward the attractive, petite young woman. She replied with a gentle and friendly, "Yes."

The woman looked away from Margo, never saying another word, and exited the elevator when she arrived at her floor, perhaps . . . *their floor.*

Margo's curiosity as to why the conversation did not go any further with an introduction such as, "Well, I'm so and so, nice to meet you," was overshadowed by a disturbing sixth sense that told her, *She already knows who I am, she just wanted me to know* ***who she is.***

Twelve
Journey Toward Perdition

During their eighteen years of marriage, Margo had endured and tolerated many marital infractions from Douglas. His sexcapades with women became out of control. *He* was out of control. His lack of financial commitment to the family he had once adored became commonplace.

Douglas had become a stranger to his family. He was rarely home, and when he was, ***he expected*** Ms. Lillie, Margo's mother, to stay and be the caretaker of the children, particularly if Margo was working late. Ms. Lillie states: "I had to stay there when he was home. I never knew when he was going to just get up and leave them babies there. Margo had a hard time with those kids. He only took them to their activities once in a while, and only if Margo asked him to, *and* only if *no one else* could take them." Ms. Lillie was Margo's rock. She was enormously proud of Margo and her successful family, and would do anything for them. Ms. Lillie cooked their meals, did their laundry and cared for the children in every way, including transporting them to and from their extracurricular activities if Margo was working late.

Douglas made it clear that transporting the children *was not* his role. Eventually, Ms. Lillie became somewhat of a permanent fixture in Margo's home, and Margo handsomely compensated her for that. However, when Douglas was around, things were a little different. One day while working, Margo discloses to Joyce: "I'm going to have to speak to Douglas about the way he treats my mother. He treats her like a *house slave* when he is there and I do not like that!" Margo did not confront Douglas with many issues for which she probably should have. However, when it came to Ms. Lillie, Margo's dedication to her as a daughter was limitless.

Douglas deliberately and *voluntarily* detached himself from his children as a father, his wife as a husband, and his home as a provider. When he came home at night, he slept on the couch. Douglas insisted Margo's income pay for *everything* including vacations, the children's tuition, their uniforms and extracurricular activities. According to Ms. Lillie, Douglas occasionally paid a few utility bills.

Margo's niece Dayne, angrily asserts, "I got so sick of every time we went somewhere on vacation, my aunt was digging down in her purse, paying for this, and paying for that. Douglas *never paid for anything!*" Dayne would often go on vacations with Margo and Douglas to babysit the children.

In Margo's own words of Douglas' absence from the family, she admitted, "Don, he doesn't even know what is going on with our kids half the time." He had abandoned them. She had had enough.

* * *

It was September 17th and Margo's 38th birthday when it became clear to me that all was not well in the Prade household. A bunch of us had gone to Cleveland to a popular nightlife area called the Flats. We were celebrating Margo's medical assistant Pam's bachelorette party and Margo's birthday. Pam had rented a limousine. She and three friends we had yet to meet for the first time, met Margo, Joyce and I after we arrived in Cleveland. Collectively, Pam and her friends were at least five to ten years younger than Margo, Joyce and I.

From the time we joined Pam we were having a good time. We began with an expensive dinner. Pam and her friends were very pretty, young white girls with perfect teeth, bodies and hair . . . the full bounty. And we didn't look so bad either. Three different shades of ebony beauty, dressed to kill and ready to take on Cleveland in good clean fun. Pam and her beauties lured young white and Latino males to our table not only at dinner, but in every place we went throughout the night. The few black males who were in the clubs were looking for and dancing with white women, but it did not matter. We all had more attention than we could handle.

During dinner, Margo kept making statements such as, "I hope we have this good of a time when I go out to celebrate my divorce!" The statement concerned me, however, I was not going to take the comment any further. I did not want to. Later in the evening while Margo was dancing, I quizzed Joyce.

"Why is Margo making those statements about divorce?"

"He treats her like shit!" Joyce replied.

"He is never, ever there for her, Don," Pam said with slurred speech from drinking.

"Oh? Well, at least she's having a good time tonight for her birthday!" I replied, bewildered.

"She's threatened to divorce him three other times but every time she tells him she's filing for divorce ***he starts crying*** and promises to do better. Then, he'll straighten up for about three months, and start his shit all over again!" Joyce continued, angry.

"That's too bad." This was the only statement I could conjure up. I was shocked at what I was hearing.

We continued our barhopping with the limousine driver in tow, and had guys following and approaching us all night long, some of which were flirting with Margo, Joyce and me, nonstop.

"Girl, these *young* white boys are OUT OF CONTROL!" Margo screamed in laughter, as we entered the limousine going to the next club. "There is *not one* of us who does not have at least two men hitting on us every, single place we go. It doesn't even matter to them that we are married!" She continued validating her observation. Perhaps the guys found the *marriage* detail to be even more of a challenge, or maybe a *safeguard,* should they happen to score.

Despite Margo's earlier statement about celebrating divorce, she did not allow the apparent breakdown in her personal life to interfere with her night. I had never seen her enjoy herself so much. The fact that twenty-five and thirty-year-old guys were constantly flirting and dancing with us did major stroking for her ego, and ours. It absolutely was a happy birthday for Margo.

We danced into the late night, early morning hours. At one point, Margo had walked up onto the stage in one club and was dancing so hard, I thought she was going to blow a gasket. She was exuberant in her whimsical movements, all while displaying feminine finesse. Joyce and I enjoyed watching her have such a good time. Margo worked so hard at her profession, and with her children, she ***rarely had time for fun, and she was rarely allowed*** to have fun. Douglas was extremely controlling over Margo's life. Since I was more accustomed to going out in Cleveland than Margo was, she called shortly before we left for the evening asking, "Don, how much money do you think I should take for the night? Do you think one hundred dollars will be enough?"

Throughout the evening, the attention was so profound, we made a rule that no one is to leave the club with anyone they do not know, no matter what. When the night ended, we had an entourage of men following us from the club, yelling, pleading for phone numbers, and *attempting* to grab us into staying and going with them. The limousine driver literally had to fight the men off and away from the car, yelling to us, "We have to leave this area and we have to leave now, ladies!"

"We can't find one of our friends," (who had apparently snuck away anyway) I attempted to explain to the driver.

"Well then ***look for her while I drive,*** but we have GOT TO GET OUT OF HERE RIGHT NOW OR THERE'S GOING TO BE TROUBLE. These guys want you ladies in the worst way; they are drunk, rowdy, *horny* and dangerous at this point. Please, ladies, I have to leave the area, now!" We could tell the driver was quite serious, and had no choice but to give in to his plea.

The fiasco was foreign to us, but apparently all too real for the driver. Nevertheless, we were on cloud nine from all the attention. Three black women, older than the four young white women we were with, in an all white area of Cleveland Ohio, partying and being vigilantly pursued by these young guys. The driver herded us into the limousine while he tried desperately to fight off the mob. Some bystanders were watching this ***amazing scene*** unfold. We felt like *celebrities running and ducking from the paparazzi.* The experience was intoxicating.

The young lady we could not find was located down the road a bit and we stopped to pick her up. Like a mother scolding her child, I chastised the young lady for leaving the bar and making us worry about *and* look for her; and I *was not* ***at all*** *kind about it.* When the limousine driver reached my car in the parking lot, we said our good-byes to Pam and her guests who were half conscious from the drinking and partying. The driver took them to a hotel in Lakewood, Ohio.

Joyce, Margo and I had had the time of our lives, and were oblivious to the fact that we ALL had to visit the restroom, and now it was too late. There was ***no way*** we could risk going back to the club, it was four o'clock in the morning, the club was closing and we would not have made it anyway.

The three of us shared desperate eye contact, "It's a long ride home," I pleaded, attempting to encourage the inevitable. The three of us looked at each other, busted out laughing, with Margo laughing the loudest. In unison, we descended into a dark corner of the parking lot; unbuttoned, unzipped and untied our clothes *and went.* With cars passing by occupied with unsuspecting occupants, *we went,* laughing the entire time. The longer we streamed, the louder we laughed. Although the parking lot visit was out of character for all of us, it was a unique evening all the way around; a night to remember, and one of the absolute best times I *had ever* had with Margo Prade and her staff.

On the ride home, we discussed our fun-filled evening nearly the entire time. We laughed and joked about what could have happened to three professional women arrested for *going* in a public parking lot.

All of the admiration and attention we received during the night eventually led to an unsettling conversation. Joyce and I listened while Margo echoed statements from the back seat of the car. Those statements made it all too clear that she was married but not in a marriage, in love but not feeling loved . . . had all the trappings of happiness, yet was unhappy. I felt sorrow for my dear friend. I became angry with Douglas, and disappointed in feeling that they no longer had a storybook lifestyle, and that their marital union may be in trouble.

Thirteen
Psychodrama

The early 1990s proved to be a fruitful and delightful era for Margo's practice. Douglas was rising the ranks of the police department with ease. Our softball team was on a winning streak and my son was born in June of 1990.

At least with our social circle, all seemed right with the world. Margo's children were as successful as they could be at their young and tender ages. Kenya, the oldest child, became a gymnast on the national level. Sahara was developing into a child prodigy in the performing arts, excelling in musical extravaganzas, dance, piano and theatre.

As Margo's children became more successful in their extra curricular activities, Margo had less time for friends and social events. Douglas was not *available* unless one of the children's events rendered them a trip out of town. Then, according to Dayne, "He would be packed and ready to go before anyone else."

Margo began to travel nearly every weekend with Kenya to compete in gymnastic competitions all over the United States, and Sahara was performing regularly at Weathervane Theatre in musicals and plays.

One day, Margo informed me the family was going to Hawaii to Kenya's gymnastics meet. I had already been to Hawaii, and was very excited for Margo before they left.

"Girl, you are going to love it!" I exclaimed. "The water is so blue it looks like God painted it with a giant blue crayon. When you see Hawaii, you'll know only God could have created a place so beautiful! And, the nightclubs, oh, girl! The nightclubs are just fabulous! You and Douglas will have a ball!"

"I can't wait to go!" Margo responded excited. After Margo

and her family returned from Hawaii, I could not wait to talk with her about her trip.

"Well, how was it? Did you go out, did you see Blow-Hole Mountain, did you go to a luau, the rock-n-roll dinner cruise . . ." I was asking questions so fast, Margo had to interrupt me just to answer.

"I didn't do anything at night, Don, but watch movies in the room," Margo replied with disappointment.

"What! You went ***all the way to Hawaii*** and did not even go OUT!" I gasped, shouting almost to the point of interrogation. "Why not, no babysitter?"

"No, we had a sitter. Some of the older girls with other families watched the younger kids in the hotel rooms while the adults went out at night."

"Why didn't you go out then, Margo?" I asked, more than curious now.

"Douglas didn't want to. He went to bed ***every night at eight o'clock, so he could get up in the morning and run!***" Margo responded with obvious resentment.

"Margo, I cannot ***believe*** you went all the way to Hawaii and did not *do anything!* If I were you, I would have gone out anyway with the other couples if Douglas did not want to go! I certainly would not have stayed in ***every night*** and watched movies for ten nights in a row. You can watch movies at HOME!" I responded in anger.

Margo did not respond, and I was angry that she obviously allowed Douglas to control her enjoyment—or lack thereof—on a once in a lifetime trip, which resulted in her staying in every night. I also wondered how embarrassing it must have been for her to listen to the other adults the next day relish in the "good times" they had had the night before. I also felt compassion and sadness for Margo. She did not deserve for Douglas to treat her that way. Much worse, Douglas sent a direct message to the other couples that he had absolutely no interest in being with them, Margo or in having a good time with them all in Hawaii.

Margo's confession of "a vacation gone bad" was very telling. I wondered why Douglas did not show enough interest in his wife to take her out on at least one date in a place as beautiful *and ro-*

mantic as Hawaii. Understanding that marriages can grow old and have their dull moments, if any place can renew the ***"spark"*** in a marriage, Hawaii can do it. I thought to myself . . . something is *very* wrong here.

For the first time, I wondered if Douglas had someone else, he would rather have been with in blue Hawaii. Douglas' behavior that Margo had described was so brazen and *naked* with disrespect; I really believed Douglas *must have* been having an affair. However, I certainly did not ask. I did not *want to know, and* only shared my thoughts with my husband. I did believe that marital skew had honed in on Margo's marriage and took a very comfortable seat in the lap of Douglas Prade.

Douglas' behavior became the benchmark of future concerns that surfaced about Douglas and Margo's relationship. I would discuss my concerns with my husband, as Margo shared various disappointments about her marriage with me. For the most part, Tom was noncommittal. One day, however, while in the office he detected a sense of sadness in Margo that in his own words, "Could not be ignored."

"How are you doing, Margo?"

"Alright." She looked up and responded with sad eyes.

"You sure?"

"Yeah."

Not believing her, Tom ended the conversation stating, "Well, if you ever want to talk in confidence about anything at all, *anything* . . . I'm here for you, okay?"

"Okay, Tom. Thanks," she responded, looking back down at her charts.

"Sure, no problem." Tom attempted to conjure a smile out of Margo by joking, "No charge."

Margo did not respond.

* * *

At some point Margo became aware that Douglas had a new relationship that was not going away, *whoever she was.* Douglas had been seeing her for going on five years now, and *their son* was four years old. Although Margo had filed for divorce several times before, she was serious this time. Margo's unhappiness had taken its toll. She broke down in the office one day sobbing while talking to Joyce, "I'm so unhappy!" Margo's unhappiness was apparent to others as well. Her appearance had suffered. She had gained thirty pounds and spent many of her lunch hours reading romance novels; whereby vicariously, she dreamed of wanting, needing to feel loved, and *respected* by the man she loved . . . her husband.

Margo's smile, which was a definite signature of who she was, descended into a forced effort when she greeted others. Moreover, when she thought no one was looking, her facial expressions winced in emotional pain. Unhappiness unfurled slowly but surely during the final six years of Margo's young life.

A disturbing metamorphosis was occurring, Margo's family, friends and staff became concerned.

I knew enough to know that no matter how close I was to Margo and Douglas, bringing up issues of her marriage was water *not to be treaded on* by anyone . . . not even a close friend like me. Besides, the history of our friendship had taught me one thing . . . that Margo *would never speak ill* of Douglas . . . for any reason, at least not with me.

I was surprised when Margo hinted at divorce one evening when she and I went to a Cleveland Indians game for her thirty-ninth birthday.

It was September 17, 1995 and Margo had season tickets to the Indians game. The tickets were a Christmas gift from another physician from the past year. I was driving to the game and Margo just came out with it, "Don, I'm going to be selling my practice to Akron General Hospital. I'm going to be forty next year . . . and *I'm not* happy. I'm going to need my own health insurance. I'm telling you this because I don't know what it is going to mean for you and Tom renting space in the office. They [hospital management] may want to move another physician in your space. I'll let you know way ahead of time though, okay."

"Okay Margo, sure. . . . I'll let Tom know," I replied, shocked that she was disclosing this to me, but not shocked at *what* she was disclosing. Unless Margo was *really angry,* or upset, she hardly even *hinted* at speaking ill of Douglas or their marriage to me, but would do so with others, primarily her staff and her mother.

"Margo, what's wrong?" I continued.

"I'm just not happy, Don. Doug just has no interest in us anymore. I mean, he doesn't even know what our kid's teacher's names are! He is so detached from us. Then when he is home, he'll walk in on a conversation me and the kids are having and make a comment putting in his *two cents,* and he won't even *make sense* with what we are talking about, and we'll just look at him like he is crazy! Just like tonight. Don, it is *my birthday* and I asked him to come to this game with me. He says, 'I gotta work.' Then I said, 'Well, *just humor me!*' Girl, he walked out the house and left without a word."

"Why don't you guys seek marriage counseling, Margo?"

"A black man! Puh-leeeze! Don, Douglas *is not going* to go to counseling! I tried to get him to go when Prescott died and he only went once that I know of!"

"Margo, I've felt you've been unhappy for some time now, even though you have said very little to me directly, but occasionally dropping hints from time to time. Let me ask you a question."

"Okay, what?"

"Is Douglas your first love? I mean, sometimes those first loves are the most difficult to leave no matter how bad they treat you . . . and, they are the *hardest* to get over. If he is your first love, this may be why you've taken so much shit from him for so long." I spoke with the intention of letting on to Margo that I knew more about her unhappiness than she may have thought I did, but was only willing to discuss it as long as she was willing.

"No, he's not my first love, but *he is* the father of my children."

"I understand totally. Well, Margo, you deserve to be happy no matter what. I'll let Tom know what we talked about," I replied, signaling to Margo, my part of this conversation was over. I loved Margo like a sister, and she was *always* a true blue friend to me. I really did care about what she was going through; however, I also felt very uncomfortable discussing *this particular* marital problem with her. I never wanted to put myself in the position for Douglas to approach me stating, "Margo said you said I should do this . . . or that . . ." and perhaps ruin the friendship I had with both of them. After all, fighting couples often make up with each other later on after they have "spilled the beans" to a friend and gotten their support in return through criticizing the opposite partner. In addition, given our early history, I still considered Douglas a friend. However, Douglas could also be very intimidating, at least to the point where one would not want to cross the line with him . . . even someone who he considered a friend.

In hindsight, I wondered if Margo thought I should have been more supportive in our conversation and probed further, out of concern. I *never took sides* when Margo would engage in a rare discussion of her problems with Douglas, and she knew this. I now believe Margo held back on what she chose to disclose about her and Douglas' relationship until she absolutely had to, and until the very end. That night, it hurt me to see someone as spirited, genuine and loving as Margo so unhappy on her birthday. It hurt to know Douglas was the culprit who planted that seed of unhappiness. I wanted to do something to cheer Margo up.

After the game ended, I talked Margo into us going over to the Flats to a popular dance club called the Mirage. I did not feel like dancing, just was not in the mood for some reason, but I felt Margo would have a good time if she danced. After what she had disclosed earlier, I wanted her to have good time, after all, it was her birthday. Margo had just begun to lose weight, and she looked ultra-feminine that evening wearing a black cat suit with a blazer.

We entered the club, and Margo was irritated at the $5.00 cover charge, given that it was after nine o'clock. Gesturing her hand in a throat-slashing move, she stated, "They need to ***cut*** that $5.00 cover charge this late!" I remember thinking to myself that as much money as Margo makes, ***why*** is she concerned about a five-dollar cover charge!

After we paid the cover charge, I noticed Margo taking down her ponytail and letting her long brown hair roam free. As soon as we sat down a young man came over to the table and asked

Margo to dance. Even though Margo danced the remainder of the night, through her facial expression she still seemed emotionally preoccupied. When we left the club, I could see unhappiness written all over her face. "Well, did you have a good time?" I asked, hoping she felt better.

"Yeah . . . it was okay. I didn't like that five-dollar cover charge, though." It was very unusual for Margo to complain about anything, especially something as insignificant as five dollars for someone who made the kind of money she made. I was convinced that her complaint about the five dollar cover charge was really a smokescreen for what was actually going on in her life.

* * *

Like the slow burn of a lit cigarette, Margo's marriage began to disintegrate into ash. She had put off divorce several times before, and for various reasons, including the 1993 shooting death of Douglas' son from his second marriage, *and* the death of his mother within months of each other. "I can't do this [divorce] to him now," Margo would explain the delay of her previous divorce proceedings to Joyce. ***"He needs me."***

After the accidental murder of Douglas' son Prescott, Margo and Douglas became closer. Like all children, Margo loved Prescott and helped finance his college education. On the morning he died, Margo closed her office, and we spoke on the phone. This was the first and *only time* I had *ever* heard Margo cry.

Months later in discussion, Margo would confess, "Don, I hate like hell what happened to Prescott. I cannot ***believe*** that bullet traveled all the way across the street and hit him while he was minding his own business. It was just his time to go. But . . . there is always something good that comes out of something bad," Margo explained while standing in our office, "Doug and I are a **lot closer** now since this happened. I was real close to leaving Douglas before Prescott died."

The divorce proceedings are on hold . . . again.

The central and most salient reason for Margo not divorcing Douglas sooner was her children. "I don't want my girls to grow up without a father in the home like I did," she would explain to

Joyce. Margo always wanted to do what was right for her children. She never once put herself before her children, and as a result, she suffered in emotional silence much longer than she should have.

* * *

September 17, 1998

Happy birthday Margo! I know you are not here anymore, but in my mind you are still alive. Today is your 42nd birthday. The only sad part is that instead of me bringing you a clever little gift, I'll be putting flowers on your grave. That bastard just does not know what he has done to us all, especially you. I hope to God he burns in hell for the rest of his life and in death! ***Margo, do you know through his lawyer he plans to put Kenya on the witness stand today!*** *He has no feelings for anyone but himself! You need to have your spirit come down now and make this right! Margo, he needs to pay for your death! I know you can help that happen. Have a great celebration today up there with God and the angels. Have an extra piece of cake for me. You know how I love sweets.*

Love, Donzella

* * *

By late 1996, Margo came to grips with the inevitable . . . her marriage had suffered irreparable damage. Margo came to realize Douglas had long since relinquished his "fatherhood" to their daughters, and why continue to endure a unity that had long been forgotten, for the children's sake, when he is not there for them anyway.

When Douglas became aware that Margo's intention to divorce him was authentic, he began to behave more like a father to Kenya and Sahara. He often offered to take the girls to their extracurricular activities . . . ***under one condition*** . . . he had to use Margo's van to transport. His excuse was, *his car did not have enough room to transport the kids to their activities.* Douglas would, on a regular basis, come to the office, take Margo's van and leave her his car. For the past several years, the cooperation Margo needed from Douglas but he would refuse to give was now ever-present. Now that divorce was imminent, he was available . . . *all the time.* Margo's office staff began to joke of Douglas' newfound commitment to his family calling him, ***"Disneyland dad."***

In January 1997, Margo filed for divorce from Douglas Prade. That *same week* Margo had an *uncontrollable* accident in her van on a snow-covered highway. The accident occurred *after* Douglas had used Margo's van. Margo and Kenya escaped serious injury, although Kenya did have a minor injury to her arm. At the time, Kenya was a national gymnast; therefore, any type of bone or muscle injury to her was very risky to her gymnastic career. I was unaware Margo was divorcing Douglas, and learned of the information when my aunt, who was also Margo's patient, called me one evening.

"Hello."

"Donna."

"Oh, hi, Aunt Hazel!"

She got right to the point of the call. "Hi. Margo is getting a *divorce*?"

"What! Not that I know of!"

"Well, I'm reading the paper right now and it is right here in the legal news!"

"Really?" I asked, flabbergasted.

"Yes!" Aunt Hazel proceeded in reading me the declaration.

"Humph! Well, I guess she'll tell me when she is ready. I know how that is . . . I've been there."

That evening I went to the office after closing, knowing Margo would still be there working late, charting. She was dressed in a powder-blue pantsuit and looked very thin. I walked up to her station, and sat on the floor next to her chair, exhausted from a long day of graduate school studies.

I spoke calmly and cautiously. "Margo, Aunt Hazel called me today and said she saw in the legal news where you filed for divorce."

Margo smiled sheepishly with a hint of embarrassment and replied, "Don, I just did not want a lot of people to know."

"Margo, I'm not a lot of people, I'm your friend, but I'm not upset that you didn't tell me. I know how hard it is to tell your close friends that you are divorcing. I remember when I divorced Larry. My closest friends, ***including you,*** were the last to know . . . remember? I think it is harder to tell close friends because you feel a sense of failure, especially to your friends. Then you start believing they are going to judge you somehow and actually see you as a failure."

"Yeah, I hear what you're saying, but your marriage didn't have an eighteen-year investment."

"Margo, it *doesn't matter how many years are invested,* the feelings are the same! It is the sense of failure, hurt, embarrassment, and the *loss* that makes you want to hide it or not talk about it. It is like a *death* . . . only it is the death of a marriage. You feel your friends are going to judge you. Margo, I am not going to judge you. I know you've been unhappy for a long time, and frankly, I was wondering what the ***hell*** was taking you so long to do this! Listen, you are young, successful, beautiful and ***very skinny*** now [she chuckles, embarrassed]. You have two beautiful children who, thanks to you, are as successful as they can possibly be for their young ages. Given all of this, why should you be unhappy in your personal life? I'll support whatever you do. I am your *friend,* Margo, and have been for over twenty years. I just want you to be happy. You ***deserve to be happy***!"

Margo looked at me apologetically, flashed a smile of relief and replied, "Thanks, Don," and we hugged.

From that moment on, Margo seemed to ***want*** to tell me everything that had gone on in her marriage over the years. She opened up like she had never done before, as if she was purging an infectious disease . . . a disease that had lay dormant inside of her . . . *consuming* her for so many years. She told me about Douglas' mistress of five years, and about how she caught him the day before their wedding with another woman. She literally opened up a storybook of lies, deceit and unfaithfulness. I shook my head in disbelief and listened in shock.

I had to ask, "After catching him right before your wedding, why did you still marry him, Margo?"

"Because, I just did not want to give her [the other woman] the satisfaction of having him."

"Well . . . you were young then, preoccupied with school and didn't know any better."

"I guess so. And this woman now is *way too young for him.* ***I*** was too young for him at ten years, she is *definitely* too young at twenty years!"

Margo went on for an hour disclosing Douglas' maltreatment of her and their marriage. I continued sitting on the floor next to her, listening in amazement as she disclosed a side of Douglas I never would have thought existed had the information not come from her. . . .

"He even had that woman swimming in my pool while I was away at a conference," Margo confessed.

I had so many questions. "What! Margo!" I exclaimed, taken aback at what she is telling me about Douglas, who I admired, trusted and *respected.* I was extremely stunned at the shameless disrespect he apparently had for Margo, the children and their marriage.

Fourteen
A Paradigm of Tribulation

After Margo engaged in what seemed to be full disclosure about she and Douglas' relationship, we both seemed to feel more at ease in sharing her personal life in conversation.

Nearly every single day thereafter when I went to the office, Margo had *something* to tell me about what Douglas had either done or said to her. This time, however, it was his more recent behavior that sparked concern. Furthermore, I noticed Douglas was starting to use Margo's van ***a lot.*** Now that all the cards were on the table, and in no attempt to mask my suspicion, one day I asked, "Margo, why is Douglas *always* using your van lately and leaving his car with you?"

"Well, he's offering to take the kids to their evening activities and said his car isn't big enough. It's okay, he leaves his car with me."

"So! What does he mean his car isn't big enough? He's only transporting at the most, two kids at one time. It's a full-sized car!"

"Don, I know. But I'm just trying to be amicable, we need to get along for the sake of the kids. Actually, he's doing more for the kids now, than what he did before I filed for divorce."

"Yeah, I bet he is. Douglas doesn't want you to divorce him, Margo."

Margo stated with gentle strength and resolve, "Well, it's too late now."

* * *

For the first time in their eighteen-year relationship, it was all too apparent for Douglas that this relationship was definitely ending. Now Douglas was on the emotional "hot seat" that he had placed Margo on so many times before. He really *was* about to loose that smooth ride on the *gravy train* he'd enjoyed for *so long,* for *too long.* Never having to pay for anything or to be a husband or father, all while doing exactly what he wanted, with whomever he wanted, *when he wanted.* ***It was over***!

I assumed both Margo and Douglas had agreed upon the divorce. Therefore, as a friend, I was always cordial and friendly when I would cross Douglas' path. After leaving the office one evening, we met in the parking lot. "Oh, hi, Douglas, how ya doin'!" I greeted him as friendly as I could. After all, I was happy for Margo, I had nothing against him, and their impending divorce was not my issue. He seemed at ease.

"Good, Don, how are you?"

"I'm fine. How's the job?"

"Oh, good. I just thought I'd run in here (Margo's office) and talk to Margo for a minute. Since she's losing weight now, I want to get her this exercise machine for her birthday!" Douglas sounded happy and content.

"Yeah, she looks good!" I replied.

"Well, I'll see you around, Don. Oh, how are Tom and Ian?"

"They're good!"

"Good. Okay, I'll see you."

I felt reassured that Douglas seemed to be at peace with the idea of the impending divorce, and apparently still wanting, at the very least, to be a credible confidant for Margo whenever she needed him. Why else would he buy her a gift? ***I could not have been more wrong.***

*   *   *

In late September 1996, Margo and I attended a UNCF fundraiser hosted by the Akron Black Firefighters. We were to meet her eldest sister, Frances at the affair. This may have been one of Douglas' very last attempts to salvage his and Margo's marriage. Sometime during the evening, he arrived, *in uniform* as he always did. I saw him enter the building while standing in the atrium talking with a high school classmate.

"Hi, Douglas!"

"Oh, how you doing, Don?"

"Good, how are you!"

"I'm fine . . . a little tired."

Adhering to routine I then stated, "Guess you want to know where Margo and I are sitting, right?"

Douglas responded with a cold, "Yes."

"Follow me."

I knew Douglas *expected* me to take him to Margo. I also thought Margo was *expecting him* given that he arrived there. I led Douglas into the ballroom, walking much faster than he because I wanted to get back to the people with whom I was chatting. Margo was sitting in her chair talking with the person sitting beside her.

"Margo, Douglas is here," I announced. "I'm showing him where we are sitting, he should be here in a minute."

"What did you do ***that*** for?" Margo snarled, angrily.

Stunned, I responded, "Because *I always have* shown him where we are sitting when I see him before you, remember? Margo . . . what's wrong?"

"He doesn't want to do anything with me at any other time, so he doesn't need to be with me tonight."

I did not respond, but it was clear that not only had I over stepped my boundaries by taking Douglas to Margo, but also given Margo's reaction, there was *still* something clearly wrong *with them.*

Margo's smile quickly turned to a scowl, and I felt responsible. Although this was usual, run-of-the-mill behavior for all of us, this time, I had done something wrong. This time, the reaction was not the same . . . ***for any of us.*** When Douglas sat down next to Margo, she purposely did not even *acknowledge* he was there, nor did he say a word to her. Perching like a statue in his chair, Douglas was attempting to declare his control one last time just by sitting next to Margo. Realizing the *aloofness* between them, I left the scene as quickly as I arrived, returning to the reception area.

A short time later, Margo came out into the atrium without Douglas. He followed not far behind. I observed Douglas go to one end of the lobby while Margo went to the other. I saw her talking and laughing with a young man. I assumed the young man was one of her patients, and I was very surprised Margo was engaging in conversation with him while Douglas stood nearby, absorbing every word he could read coming from her lips.

Compelled to glance in Douglas' direction, what I saw ran chills up my spine. Douglas was staring Margo down. I was sure Margo knew Douglas was watching her, a glare that intense could be felt from long distance. She did not look in his direction. She did not care. Obviously feeling defeated, Douglas left in a haste.

I felt ambiguous witnessing the interaction. On the one hand, I felt a sense of sadness for Douglas, on the other, I felt proud Margo stood up to him by not allowing him to control her enjoyment of a rare night out anymore. In her behavior, Margo made a public statement to Douglas, a statement I welcomed as well.

* * *

On April 1, 1997, Margo's final divorce hearing was held. She attended the hearing that morning *alone*. ***Douglas refused to go.*** When Margo arrived home after her divorce hearing, Douglas was sitting on the couch reading the paper.

"What happened?" Douglas asked Margo, without ever looking up from the newspaper.

"Well, we are divorced!" Margo replied definitively in a very matter-of-fact tone.

"Humph," Douglas muttered under his breath.

Margo puttered around, gathered up her things for work and began to walk out the door. While making her exit, Douglas stopped Margo, grabbed her arm and met her eyes with a piercing, livid glare. He stated with a ***cold chill*** in his voice, "You just ***do not know what*** you ***have just done!" Douglas' reaction*** *disturbed Margo,* especially since he had refused to attend the hearing. Feeling uneasy by the interaction, upon arriving to work Margo shared the experience with Joyce.

* * *

The Friday following the divorce, Margo, her staff, a dear friend, Giselle, and I went out to celebrate. We had planned the outing a week prior, and agreed we would all wear black jeans, although Margo wore brown. She was entitled; she was the guest of honor. The plan was to go to dinner first, then out dancing. I was running late from school and Margo called my home to ask Tom of my whereabouts. "Well, tell her we are at the Roadhouse restaurant in Montrose waiting for her," she instructed Tom.

I arrived at the Roadhouse. Margo had reserved a large table, and we had a very entertaining waitress. She was a young white girl with a very loud, and genuine southern accent. This waitress had a blast with us and apparently got a real kick out of being outrageous while perpetuating outrageousness in us throughout the night.

We handed Margo *Congratulations on Your Divorce* greeting cards, laughed, joked and celebrated the entire time. We were noisy and knew it, but did not care because the waitress both supported, and engaged in the rowdy behavior with us. We became concerned for the waitress' job and agreed to settle down for her sake until she informed us with a distinct and *very loud* southern drawl, "I don't give a shit, I'm havin' fun wit' y'all!"

We burst out laughing. When our food arrived, we were getting ready to eat, when Margo intervened, "Wait a minute," she ordered. Sitting right across from her, I looked up and saw Margo gesture her hands to her head and chest in the sign of a crucifix. With her eyes closed, and head uplifted, she raised her left hand to the Heavens and stated, "I have ***got*** to say my blessings first and thank God for sparing my life today."

After Margo finished her blessing in silence, I asked perplexed, "What do you mean, thank God for sparing your life today?"

"Girl, I almost got killed today. The brakes went out in my van on Noble Avenue and I swerved out of control and hit a pole! If it had not been for that air bag, I'd be gone. It hurt though," she said with a slight giggle.

"Really!" I said . . . shocked.

"Yeah. Don, that airbag hit me so hard it gave me a black eye. Can't you see all the makeup I have on my eye?"

"No, I can't tell, Margo. Besides, I have never seen you wear makeup, and actually knew you had it on, other than lipstick. You always look the same to me."

"Look real close . . . Don, do you see it?"

"No, Margo, I don't see anything *like* a black eye, you did a good job with the makeup. How did you get here?"

"I caught a ride, but can I ride with you when we leave?"

"Of course you can," I responded with angry suspicion, but did not want to spoil the fun we were having. I decided to hold my questions until I saw Margo the following Monday.

"Girl, I swear, ***that van is going to be the death of me***." Margo confessed.

"If you keep having accidents in it, *I guess it will,*" I responded, feeling anxious about what she had disclosed about this *second accident.*

At the end of our meal, we thanked the waitress for "jumpstarting" our evening. "Y'all come back now, I enjoyed waiting on you. You were the funniest customers I've ever had!" the waitress spouted in her southern drawl.

I saw Margo smile and wink at the waitress while shoving extra money in her hand. Margo's tip was over and above what we had already given the waitress collectively. After leaving the restaurant, Margo and I went to the car.

"I hope that girl doesn't *get fired* from her job because of us," Margo said laughing, but slightly concerned. I could hear the compassion in her voice.

"Well, I would think if the disruption was *that bad,* they would have asked her to stop what she was doing, and asked us to leave."

"Well, not necessarily. They knew they were making a lot of money off us between the food, and the drinks ***you guys*** ordered." While laughing, Margo emphasized, *you guys* as a friendly reminder she was not one to over indulge in alcoholic beverages. Margo did not need to drink heavy in order to have a good time. Margo got high off of life and laughter.

"Yeah, you're right about that. And the more she entertained us, the more drinks we ordered. Maybe it was all a plan from the beginning. The management has to know how friendly and outgoing she is . . . maybe she is the waitress they assign to large crowds, because she is definitely a crowd pleasing waitress." Margo and I both laughed at my analogy of the waitress and the restaurant's *perceived intentions.*

"Girl, you can sure tell you are in graduate school for counseling, you are just analyzing EVERYTHING these days!" Margo laughed, almost yelling.

"Well, at least if we're wrong, and she does get fired, she'll leave with enough money to tide her over for a couple of days until she finds another job. I mean . . . we left her a *really big* tip!"

"We sure did!" Margo agrees, while never letting on she had given the waitress extra money. Knowing Margo was very modest about her kindness toward others, I was not surprised at her generosity, and I never let on I knew she had given the waitress extra money.

Just like with her colleagues, Margo was known for her generosity towards others, and oftentimes was criticized by others for it. However, Margo was not some unintelligent, weak bimbo of which one could take advantage. She was instead, a *conductor of kindness;* and others benefited by watching, and learning *from her* how to generate random acts of kindness.

After we left the restaurant we headed to the bowling alley to retrieve another person who could not join us for dinner, but had planned to go out with us. While there, Margo befriended several children and began playing and laughing with them until we were ready to leave. Margo giggled and frolicked around the lobby with those children as if she was a kid herself. It was amazing to see the effect she had on them.

After we left the bowling alley, we headed to the newly renovated downtown Akron. Most of us had not gone downtown since its opening debut with new clubs, eateries and entertainment. It was Pam's suggestion we go, since she had already been downtown and was familiar with some of the clubs. Surprisingly, and unlike before, Margo was not concerned about going out in Akron. Margo had a self-directed, professional "rule" whereby she would not go out in Akron. The friends who knew her best understood that rule. Margo was a professional, and other than while playing softball, she had no desire to see any of her patients while on her own time, out on the town, enjoying herself. On this night, however, the rule did not apply, and did not seem to be an issue.

"Put some music on, Don," Margo requested.

"Okay, what do you want to hear?"

"Anything!"

"I just bought this CD today at Best Buy. It's Stevie Wonder's Greatest Hits."

"That's cool!" she replied, excited.

I put the CD on and turned up the volume. The first song was "***Signed, Sealed Delivered.***" Margo and I began singing the song in unison aloud. We intermittently faced each other, violently bobbing our heads like punk rockers whenever the point in time came to sing, "Signed . . . sealed . . . delivered. . . . ***I'm yours!***" Margo's hair was swinging back and forth, being combed by the wind of my Chrysler Siebring convertible. She clapped her hands, tapped her feet and snapped her fingers to the beat of the music.

It had been a long time since I had seen her so happy.

Fifteen
Reality Bites

The Monday following our night out, I made what would ultimately be one of many *purposeful* lunchtime visits to the office. Margo's staff typically went out for lunch, and Margo would stay in working on her charts. I was working on some documents for our business and thought this would be the opportune time for Margo and I to talk, since she and I would be alone for at least a half an hour.

Rather than *beat around the bush,* I just came out with it . . . "Margo, I need to ask you something. You know how I am. If I've got something on my mind, I need to discuss it no matter what."

"Okay. What is it?"

"Margo . . . do you think Douglas is doing something to your van . . . because I do. I mean this is the second life threatening accident you have had in four months. I've known you for twenty years and unlike me, you have ***never, ever*** had a car accident. Now, all of a sudden, you are divorced, Douglas uses your van regularly, and you have had ***two bad accidents***!" Margo offered an anxious giggle and said, "Well . . . I *hope* not."

"Well, I ***hope not too, Margo.*** Nevertheless, I gotta tell you, I'm becoming concerned about you, my friend! After all these years Douglas has acted as if you did not even exist. Now all of a sudden he is using your van, always running in and out of here, accusing you of dating around, reciting every move you make; I'm just concerned and worried about you, Margo."

"I know, Don. My whole family is concerned."

"Then why don't you do something? Girl, you make enough money to hire a personal bodyguard."

"I don't need a bodyguard! What would I look like going around with a bodyguard!" She started laughing. "Besides, I think once he gets used to the idea we are divorced, he'll accept it and go on about his business."

"Okay. Well, at least promise me you'll stop working here late at night after dark."

"Well, I'll try!" Margo accentuated the statement with a loud giggle that echoed, *If my work allows me to do that!*

* * *

Much to Margo's mortification, Douglas did not "go on about his business." Rather, he went on about *hers.* Shortly after the divorce, reality ***apparently*** set in. One evening, Douglas' awareness became quite succinct that Margo had actually divorced him and he no longer had control over her life. He was angry and his ego no doubt, emasculated. Margo was out of town at a medical conference in Atlanta, Georgia. Joyce had gone with Margo, taking advantage of an opportunity to visit her younger sister who lived there. While babysitting his children one evening, Douglas was fiercely annoyed that he could not exactly find Margo. *The private detective he had hired to follow Margo had apparently lost her.* With distinct vindictiveness, Douglas castigated his daughters stating, "I have a new family now anyway, and I *don't need you guys anymore.*" Kenya and Sahara wept at his remarks. Their father's words cut like a knife.

Upon her return from Atlanta, Douglas then rebuked Margo for having lost the private detective *she had no idea* was following her. He unflinchingly recited to her the type and color of the car she had rented, which hotel she stayed in, and how he knew Joyce did not stay at the hotel with her. Then, with faultless insolence he stated, "Yeah, you even talked to the [private detective] guy!"

In the months to follow, Douglas continued to stalk and harass Margo. For three months, he refused to move out of her home, stating he could not afford to move, even though at the rank of police captain, he earned a handsome paycheck. He made sure he always answered the phone when it rang, even when Margo was home. When Douglas finally did move, Margo had the locks changed, and a burglar alarm system installed. One weekend while away, Douglas coerced his eldest daughter into giving him her house key to make a copy, by leading her to believe that not only was Margo aware, but that she *approved* his request.

* * *

Seemingly, Douglas became jealous of Margo's *inner happiness,* and her willingness to go on with her life without him.

At the time of her divorce, Margo was maintaining the thirty pounds of weight loss she had gained over the years. She looked fabulous. Her emotionality returned appearing stable and secure. She had a skip in her step and a newfound freedom in her demeanor. Her signature smile, once overshadowed by emotional spoil and pain resurrected to new heights. Emotional turmoil and unhappiness was no longer a welcomed tourist in her life. Margo ceased reading romance novels such as, ***How Stella Got Her Groove Back***. No doubt, that book had something to do with a fresh and enhanced Margo Shamberger Prade. It was clear a transformation had occurred. Margo unearthed a personal new sense of self. A self buried too long underneath eighteen years of Douglas' control, infidelity, acrimony and indignation. Now, Margo had discovered *Margo.* She had arrived.

A revolutionized new energy unleashed in her, illustrating self-approval of the decision, *she* made to divorce Douglas. Anguished no more by the unenthusiastic emotions that lingered in her choice to leave her children's father, Margo was happy and exhilarated about her new look; and her peace of mind. She had it going on!

"Don, I just got so tired of being fat and unhappy. I was so depressed, I was using food for comfort." Margo bragged about how she walked every day, no matter what. With her very appearance alone, Margo was announcing a lucid statement that whatever had been tormenting her after the divorce, was either gone completely, or she found new resolve and peace to deal with the *disparaging emotions.*

Next to her children, maintaining her weight loss became the center of Margo's life. In addition, *for her children,* she attended and completed a program sponsored by the Akron Child Guidance Center titled, ***Guiding Families Through Divorce.***

Margo completed the program on February 15, 1997, only nine months before her premature, and wicked death. Everything seemed to be falling completely into place, everything . . . including *Margo's new friend.*

*　　*　　*

Myself, Margo's protective staff, her sister Edith, nieces Layne and Dayne and friends looked upon Margo's *new friend* with a jaundiced eye. Some of us warned, "Don't *trust her,* Margo. . . . For some reason, she is trying ***too hard*** to be your friend. . . . She is pushing herself into your life awfully fast. . . . How well do you even know her anyway? She is ***not*** your type of people. Margo, just what do you see in her anyway? Margo, ***do not tell this woman all of your business. . . .***"

Margo became visibly annoyed whenever *anyone* would say *anything* unconstructive about her "*new friend,*" or question the woman's motives for suddenly hurling herself into Margo's life. Given that Margo was now divorced from Douglas, everyone seemed to be even more protective of her, including her family. Margo had been shackled underneath the jealous and controlling claws of Douglas for scores of years. Therefore, as excited as she was about her new life, she was just as naïve on how to handle it.

One evening, Margo hosted a lingerie party. Encouraged by *New Friend,* Margo hired a male stripper who today is nationally known. At the time of the party, Margo's *new friend* claimed to be one of his agents. Big sister Edith expressed her concern afterwards.

"Margo, it's not like you to have a party like that." In speaking with Edith later, she stated, "Even though they [Margo and Douglas] were divorced, I was afraid Douglas would find out about the party, and that Margo had a stripper there. I was afraid at what Douglas might do if he knew."

"But she was divorced from him, the children were not home, and except for *New Friend,* everyone behaved in a tasteful manner, including the entertainer. Besides, she had a right to entertain in the home that she paid for!" I responded angrily.

"I know, Don, but that would not mean anything to Douglas,

and I did not want her to put herself in a position to make him mad."

Edith's statements were indicative of the control Douglas exerted over Margo, and how he extended that control well into their post-divorce lives. Even more telling, however, was Edith's feelings of *trepidation* over how Douglas might react when learning of Margo's party.

Although Margo was extremely classy and bright, her intellect fell short in one specific area . . . she was not well versed in her perception of *street people or street mentality.* Unfortunately, Margo's *new friend* was all that and more. She was an impious individual with glib intentions. *New Friend* quickly became a permanent fixture in Margo's life. The woman would flutter in and out of Margo's home as if she lived there, and would frequent Margo's office as if she was part owner; checking up on things . . . or perhaps, *checking up on Margo.* Closing in on Margo's private life, she knew everything Margo did, and with whom she did those things. The most notable peculiarity of *New Friend's* behavior was . . . she never accompanied Margo along with her other friends and acquaintances as part of the group, when we went out with Margo or met at social affairs. What was even more abnormal, however, was that *New Friend* would publicly proclaim to anyone who would listen, that she was Margo's *best friend.*

It is unfortunate that no matter how hard we tried; ***no one*** could convince Margo to distance herself from this woman. No one could persuade Margo that this woman was out to run some type of con on her; we just were not sure as to what. Good or bad, right or wrong, no one could tell Margo what to do or how to live *anymore.* Not even those who had her best interest at heart. Margo baulked at *anything* that bore the slightest resemblance of her being controlled. Sadly, Margo should have taken heed. This woman was *dangerous . . . very dangerous,* and it seemed everyone knew something *just was not right* . . . everyone except for Margo. It would later be discovered that Douglas was engaging in a nasty little fantasy of how to get rid of Margo . . . *forever,* and that *New Friend* may have been just what the captain ordered.

Sixteen
New Beginnings, Old Wounds

The summer solstice of 1997 breathed new life into the body and mind of Dr. Margo Prade. He clearly was a breath of fresh air that completed Margo's transition into single life. A professional friend and patient had introduced them.

"Don, I'm going on a blind date tonight!"

"What! A blind date? Well, that ***is*** original. I thought people only went on blind dates on television shows!" I remarked laughing.

"I know. Girl, I feel kind of silly going on one. You know, not knowing what he looks like or anything. But I do know he is an attorney."

"Oooh . . . nice, a ***real*** professional. That is what you deserve, Margo. Frankly, I'd like to see you be involved with someone who does not carry a gun for a living. Besides, it is not as if you go out to clubs or bars or anything. With the girls' activities, and your schedule, you really don't have time to join any singles clubs through church or within the community. Actually, now that I think about it, this is probably the only way you could possibly meet someone. Are you excited?"

Giggling, Margo responded, "I'm scared!"

Laughing, I agreed, "I would be too. No *black people* I know go out on blind dates! I mean . . . as a culture, do we even know how to do a blind date?"

"I guess I'll find out! I am really nervous though." "Well girl, have fun and let me know what happens!" I responded, while we shrieked in laughter as the conversation ended, and I left the office.

Margo's blind date went very well. Every day I saw her, she was glowing with happiness, sharing information, disclosing future plans. Along with those conversations, however, there were also telltale signs of stress and anxiety.

Daily, Margo would share her concerns over Douglas interfering with her life, complicating things at every turn, creating obstacles whenever and wherever he could. Nearly every day, Margo would share her latest drama-laden episode, and those episodes ***always*** involved Douglas.

"Margo, you've been divorced for three months now, why is Douglas still living in your home?"

"He refuses to leave and he won't tell me when he is leaving."

"Do you ask?"

"No. He is so mean and dogmatic, I'm afraid to say anything to him. I just look in the paper at night, find areas where apartments are for rent that I think he would like, and I circle them. Then, I set that section of the paper on the table so he will see it when he reads the paper."

"Margo, that is ***your house.*** He does not have the right to force his presence on you like this. I'll be damned if I would allow someone to live ***in my house,*** who is ***refusing to move, who I am afraid of!*** " I shouted, while Margo continued to rationalize. . . .

"I know. At first I thought he was mad about me being awarded the condominium in the Bahamas, *but he said* he didn't want it!"

* * *

"Margo, this has nothing to do with the condo, the kids, or even your house. Remember, he did not even attend the divorce hearing. This has to do with control and intimidation and him not letting you go on with your life! Why don't you call the police on him, and at least make out a report on harassment. As proud as Douglas is of his record at that police department, if you file a report on him, he is sure to back off. Or better yet, file papers to have him legally removed through the sheriff's department!"

"No! I don't want to start any trouble, Don!"

"Margo, the trouble has already started, and it is from Douglas! He has been harassing you for months! I mean, ***shit,*** you can't even receive personal phone calls in your own home, and somehow, he is spying on you. He seems to know every move you make! You know what else, he knows he can do whatever he wants to do to you and you are not going to do anything about it, he knows you *just that well.* He is using his position at the police department to hold you at bay!"

"Well, I'm thinking of moving anyway, Don."

"Moving! Where?"

"To Columbus, you know, start all over."

Without looking up at Margo, I made a statement that I later recognized was a very selfish remark.

"Girl, you'd better not leave me!"

I heard Margo offer a shrouded chuckle. When I looked up at her, however, I saw something much more significant . . . not her smile, but a look of desperation. Startled and somewhat distressed at the look on her face, I felt compelled to recant my statement.

"Margo, I'm sorry. If you move to Columbus, *you know* I will miss you. We all will. But . . . maybe you should move away . . . as soon as you can arrange things. It is not as if you will not be able to find a job, you *are* a doctor! Besides, the move will give me another place to visit!" I replied, pretending to be excited for her, but moreover, I was concerned. That look on her face scared me.

Margo did not comment. She did not need to. For months, I had been her confidant and sounding board in her post-divorce troubles with Douglas. For months, I had become increasingly concerned about his harassing behavior towards her. For months, *Douglas was not going away.*

* * *

"Hey Margo, how are you doing today?" Margo looked up in despair.

"Don . . . Douglas got in my face yesterday."

"What! Got in your face, what do you mean?"

"I mean *he got in my face!* He got in my face. He put his finger on my nose, pushed my head back, called me a fat-faced bitch, and said, 'I'll ***fuck*** you up!' "

"What! Margo, you have ***got*** to get Douglas out of that house! He is going to catch you at home one day alone, come in there and blow you away and then call his police friends over and say he found you that way!"

"I don't think____and____[Douglas' two closest friends] would go along with anything like that," Margo responded.

"Not the response I was looking for, Margo! Listen to me; apparently, Douglas is becoming ***emotionally unglued***. I know, Margo. I am studying adverse behavior material in school right now; and ***behaviorally***, this is ***not*** the Douglas I have known and respected all these years! Margo, I am worried. I really think Douglas is going to try to *do something to you because that will be his final sense of control over you!*"

Margo responded with an unequivocal and poignant, "Well . . . Don, then it will just be my time to go."

"Dammit Margo, don't be a martyr! Your children need you! Your family needs you! We all need you to stay in our lives, Margo! You have given up so much already in your unhappiness with Douglas all these years. Are you going to give up your ***very life*** to him too?" I replied with both physical and psychological fear.

Margo's reluctance to be proactive in her own safety made me that much more afraid for her life. It was obvious to me; she was not going to take any measures to stop Douglas' harassing behavior. It was obvious to me that Margo's fear of Douglas was so profound, she was afraid to protect ***her own life.*** I believed if these revelations were that obvious to me, then they were ***definitely*** obvious to Douglas. After all, by using aggression and control, Douglas was strident in how he dealt with people on a daily basis, including his wife. Douglas utilized antagonistic practices to manage people for a living. He was a police captain, and he was good at what he did.

One evening, I was power walking with a friend and softball teammate. Our children were on the same soccer team and she and I would walk around Hardesty park while the children practiced. We engaged in a discussion about Margo and Douglas' divorce, his refusal to move out of her home and the harassment Margo was enduring from him since the divorce.

"You know, I am so afraid for Margo that I had a terrible dream about her last night."

"Really, Don? What about."

"I dreamt I was at her funeral crying . . . I mean I was ***really crying, really hard.*** Obviously, the dream disturbed me to no end. I ***just wish*** Douglas would leave and leave her alone!"

"Humph . . . Yes . . . me too. I really hope things work out for her," she replied. We continued to power walk in silence pondering thoughts neither one wanted to share. We later resumed talking, changing the subject as we continued to walk.

* * *

In the late evening hours of ***November 24, 1997***, I saw, talked and ***laughed*** with Margo Prade for one final time.

"Margo, what are you doing here so late?"

"Oh, hi, Don, I had charting to do. How are you doing?"

Echoing the fear for Margo's safety that had taken up permanent residence in my own state of mind, I replied, "Fine, stressed out. It's finals time at school and I have a ton of work to do! Margo, do you see how dark it is outside; you should not be working here so late after dark, I worry about you. Someone could come in here and do anything to you and get away really quick in the dark!"

"I'm fine, I need to get these charts done."

"How was your trip to Vegas?"

"Oooh . . . girl! We had a fabulous time! Here is a picture of us."

Like a giddy teenaged girl experiencing her first love, Margo grabbed the picture from her desk smiling and handed it to me.

"Oh, Margo! This is the most ***beautiful picture*** I have ever seen! You are absolutely glowing! He is very handsome too! You are a very striking couple and you both look soooo happy! I am ***really*** happy for you, Margo, and it is about time!"

"I know, Don, ***I am*** happy too. I have not felt this way in so long, Don. Oh, that picture was taken at the MGM Grand at a show we went to!"

"I thought those seats looked familiar!" I replied, smiling.

"He is my baby . . . he is so sweet to me, Don. I cannot wait for you to meet him. He's going to have Thanksgiving dinner with us on Wednesday, and then I'm having a little dinner party on Friday so everybody can meet him, and I want you and Tom to come so you guys can meet him too!"

"Okay, cool! By the way, I have this awful pain going up and down my left arm. Should I be concerned, I mean . . . am I having a heart attack?"

"Can you move your arm?"

"Yes, see?" I gestured, moving my arm up and down, back and forth.

"Then you *ain't havin'* no damn heart attack, girl!" Margo shouted in black slang language, laughing all the while.

"Good, 'cause I have too much *damn* work to do before this semester ends!" We bellowed in hearty laughter as I continued down the hallway to visit the restroom, and check our mail.

When I returned, Margo was on the phone. I had no idea who she was talking to, yet; I knew the call was serious because she had a rare, stern look on her face. Because I had been concerned for Margo for some time now, I surreptitiously listened in on the conversation. . . .

"What did you say to her . . . [pause] and what did she say to you . . . [pause] and then ***What did you say back to her*** . . . ?" I was concerned about the angst in Margo's tone, and assumed she would be a while on the phone. I whispered to her, "Margo, I'm going to go now, I have work to do."

Margo held up one finger indicating for me to wait a minute; she covered the speaker on the phone and said with a smile, "Okay, Don . . ." she winked, "I'll see you tomorrow."

"Okay . . . bye, see you tomorrow!" I responded with a smile.

For us, *tomorrow never came.* The next time I saw that beautiful picture Margo had shown me, ***it was her obituary photograph***. The next time I saw Margo, she was ***embalmed and dead.***

* * *

On November 25, 1997, Margo arrived to work and shared a blunt and firm conversation with Joyce.

"I'm going to call Doug tonight and tell him I'm taking him back to court for more child support."

With concern, Joyce responded, "Oh, really? Aren't you scared to do that?"

"No, I'm not scared! He does not pay ***anything*** for Kenya and Sahara's school tuition, uniforms, extracurricular activities or anything. Yet, he is steadily paying for that boy's things, taking him everywhere, buying him things and telling everybody that is his son! So, I'm calling him tonight to tell him I want more child support for ***our children***!"

"Oooookay," Joyce responded with disquiet fear. Dreading what she felt would be an egregious, atrocious reaction from Douglas should Margo go through with her request.

The next day, Joyce never had the chance to ask Margo what Douglas' response was to her request. *Sadly,* when Joyce did speak to Margo, *she did not answer.* Margo would *never answer* ***anyone*** *again.*

Seventeen
Sunset

Time stood still the day forty-one-year-old Dr. Margo Shamberger Prade was murdered. If she did phone Douglas on the night of November 25, 1997, whatever transpired in that conversation is buried forever along with Margo at Mount Peace Cemetery.

On Wednesday ***November 26, 1997***, the morning ***after*** she was to have had the conversation with Douglas about receiving more child support and the day ***before*** Thanksgiving, Margo left home early headed to the hospital to conduct her patient rounds. Sadly, she would never return to her home, her children, family or patients.

Before leaving home, Margo grabbed her youngest daughter Sahara, *hugging her tighter than she had ever hugged her before.* Margo looks deep into the eyes of the nine-year-old child prodigy and stated, "***Sahara, whatever happens to me, I will always love you!***"

What, in ***God's name,*** could have caused Margo, a protective mother and positive thinker, to acquiesce **her very life** in a statement such as this to her nine-year-old daughter! Moreover, given her excitement about the new love in her life just two days prior, ***who or what could have possibly*** provoked her to resolve to such a *fatalistic affirmation*? These questions will forever haunt Margo's family and friends; but above all, her daughter Sahara.

Out of all the threats she received over the past eighteen years of marriage, perhaps this time, Margo received the *mother* of all threats. A repugnant threat so *powerful,* that it actually confirmed what would be her last day of life here on earth. A threat so *accurate,* that Margo at least *suspected* she would not live to see Thanksgiving Day. A threat so *vile,* that not only would it leave her lifeless; but make true a sobering prediction by Margo herself, that she would meet death in her van. A malevolent threat so *despicable* that it would end the life of a community icon who wanted nothing more than to live a common life raising two beautiful children, and dedicate her profession to saving the lives of others.

* * *

On Wednesday November 26, 1997 at about 8:30 A.M. a female housekeeping employee at Akron General Medical Center allegedly saw a man following, arguing with and harassing Margo while she attempted to do her patient clinical rounds. Although police investigators could never corroborate this story with any other hospital employee, the woman testified in Margo's murder trial of witnessing the altercation along with describing the man in question, in complete detail.

After Margo left the hospital, she headed to her office building, making three final phone calls from her cell phone. One to Joyce about her patient itinerary for the day, one to her salesman at Rolling Acres Dodge about the new Dodge Durango she had on order, and the final call to her mother, Ms. Lillie Hendricks about purchasing food for Thanksgiving dinner.

At about 9:00 A.M. Margo pulled into her favorite parking spot in the parking lot. Joyce was exiting the building to go to the bank, and the dentist across the hall was entering the building to see a patient, who ironically, happened to be Margo's attorney. Everything in the parking lot looked normal, as it did every other day of the week. What is *unbelievable* is that none of the people who worked in that building saw or heard *anything*.

Routinized behavior does not welcome disruption.

Margo's green mini van was sitting in the spot she always parked in. Joyce saw Margo's van and assumed she had missed Margo's rear hallway entrance into the office, while she exited out the back door of the building into the parking lot. What Joyce did not know, is that Margo never had a chance to exit the van. At the time Joyce was actually entering her vehicle, neither she nor the dentist who was entering the building noticed Margo's van which—for certain—had to be violently rocking and moving, as she incessantly fought for her *dear life* inside.

The horror of what happened within that vehicle can only be remembered and told by the person who, *without warning,* entered Margo's van . . . that is, the person who killed her.

What is clear, is that when the attacker left Margo's van ninety seconds after entering, a ferocious fight had ensued, leaving a scratch mark on the assailant's chin, and a sadistic bite mark on Margo's upper left arm.

The killer exited the van, but not before slamming six bullets at close range into the right wrist, skull and body of Dr. Margo Prade, invading the diminutive, delicate flesh of a community paragon; and *not before* laying her down on the seat, offering the appearance of an unoccupied vehicle. A nasty, bloody, and bruising scar sat centered on Margo's right cheek, disrupting an otherwise smooth and perfect ebony bronze complexion, compliments of Margo's favorite cosmetic, Mary Kay. The scar on her right cheek bore an uncanny resemblance to the *exact circumference* of the nose of a gun; indicating that the assailant forced the weapon against Margo's cheek with a vengeance; enraged, and *in all probability,* engaging in a few choice degrading and threatening verbalizations before execution. There is no doubt in my mind that in her very last moment of conscious thought, in her very last seconds of life, Margo most assuredly ***thought of nothing else except her children*** before death transpired.

* * *

At the same time Dr. Margo Prade was being slain, sister Edith suddenly became violently ill with stomach cramps while working across town in her station at the main branch of the United States Post office. Edith became ***so ill*** she was taken to the infirmary. Edith remained in the infirmary until Akron Police came to retrieve her, taking her to Margo's office. While riding in the police cruiser, Edith continued to plead with the police officers the entire time for an answer they would not furnish, but continued to drive toward Margo's office.

"What happened . . . is my sister all right . . . ***did Douglas kill my sister*** . . . tell me what has happened!"

This same day and before she heard the news of her youngest sister's murder, 3000 miles away and *three hours behind our eastern standard time zone* an incredible, disturbing and compelling sensation overcame Margo's sister, Denise, who resided in Reseda, California. Denise dropped to her knees and began praying uncontrollably. *She doesn't know why.*

At 7:00 A.M. in my home, I was quietly sobbing in the bathroom, while getting ready for school, thinking of how this day would have been my father's 72nd birthday had he not committed suicide on September 8, 1965 at the very young age of thirty eight. "Happy birthday daddy," I whispered with my face uplifted to the heavens, closing tear-stained eyes. A *melancholy morning that had only just begun. A morning whose day only proved to get worse as it went on.* A day when the eyes of ***many*** would continue to cry a river of tears well into the early morning hours of Thanksgiving Day 1997.

* * *

Between 9:00 and 10:00 A.M. patient Howard Brooks, was standing in the parking lot of the Professional Center West located at 1557 Wooster avenue. Margo had not started seeing any patients yet, so Mr. Brooks decided to go outside. While standing near the rear door entrance, Mr. Brooks noticed a car speeding like a bat out of hell from the parking lot, toward the driveway and disappear into the busy flow of traffic on Wooster Avenue. The only thing he can remember, is that the driver was a black male.

Margo's medical assistant Lori, decided to go outside and grab a quick smoke. After finishing her cigarette, Lori proceeded through the parking lot to retrieve a can of pop from her vehicle. Lori noticed Margo's van parked and that it appeared empty. She wondered why Margo had not yet come into the office . . . she had patients waiting! Lori approached Margo's van on the driver's side, peered through the window and was horror-struck. Blood is ***everywhere.***

Margo was slumped over, lying on the seat with her left arm hanging down over the side of the passenger seat and her head resting comfortably, *silently,* on the seat. Her white laboratory jacket was spotted with large, wide stains of fresh, wet blood located in different areas; one on the left side, underneath her arm, and one on her backside, in the left buttock area. Margo's lab jacket and cream-colored skirt were strewn about her body, as if a mini-tornado had hit, but only effecting the inside of the van.

The skirt was messed about, revealing knee-high stockings; an informative sign of a female professional too busy to fuss with panty hose in the morning. The contents of Margo's purse had emptied onto the floor. Loose change and other items were lying next to blood-stained carpet that marked the territory of a horrific murder, but nothing missing. Not even her cellular phone. The diamond tennis bracelet Margo wore on her right wrist laid on the ground in the parking lot, just outside the passenger side door of the van. The bracelet had been cut in half from the bullet entering her wrist, while Margo attempted to prevent the bullet's inward bound toward her head.

The killer, however, with relentless intent, shot *through* Margo's wrist, and the bullet rested in the base of the right side of her skull. That bullet, according to coroner testimony, did not kill Margo. It, however, "Severely stunned her or may have knocked her unconscious." *May have.* God, how she must have suffered. Labeled entrance wound #1, Margo's right wrist illuminated a large black hole outlined with a mass of thick black gun powder.

Unable to open the driver side door of the van, Lori cried out as she re-enters Margo's office, sprinting all the way. "***Joyce! Joyce!*** Margo's in her van and she's all bloody!"

While patients sat dismayed, Joyce yelled out, "Call 911!" Joyce left her office and ran to the parking lot. Joyce ran to Margo's van, opened the rear passenger door, threw herself over the front passenger seat. Joyce grabbed Margo's precious head, and cradled it with all her might in both hands. Shaking Margo's head, Joyce screamed, "Margo! Margo!"

Joyce looked up, and to the people standing around she shouted, "Get me a nurse down here!" Joyce was referring to the nursing professionals who worked in the Visiting Nurse Office on the second floor of the building. Still holding Margo's head, Joyce summarily canvased her body and noticed urine on Margo's skirt, and yellow fluid seeping from the corner of her mouth. Margo's face had begun to turn blue and her eyes were open, but vacant and dry. Joyce shuddered at the reality of what her medical training has certainly revealed, but what her consciousness wanted to conceal and deny. Joyce waited until the nurse arrived, and remained hopeful.

The nurse felt for a pulse. There was none. Rhetorically, Joyce trembled and whimpered to the nurse, "Has . . . she . . . expired . . . ?" Somberly, the nurse answered, ". . . Yes."

At that moment and without warning, shock overcame Joyce in a fury as she took off running, thrashing her arms and screaming through the parking lot like—in her own words—"*a crazy woman.*" Joyce ran around in circles waving her hands, quaking her head from side to side and . . . ***just . . . screaming***. She darted around the parking lot screaming, until one of Margo's patients intercepted her. A large woman, having heard Joyce screaming, had apparently come out of the office to see what was going on. She grabbed Joyce out of nowhere, held her close to her bosom, and began praying . . . and praying . . . and she prayed some more.

The dentist next door who Margo was so proud to have joined her in the new office building, came out into the parking lot, realized what was going on and seized Joyce from the patient who was comforting her. He clinched Joyce in both arms and used his strength to contain any involuntary physical gyrations that may manifest from her trauma. With calm persuasion he stated, "Come on . . . Joyce . . . let's go back inside . . . come on . . . Joyce . . . come on . . . go back inside."

After going back into the building, Joyce went into her office and took three nerve pills right away, and began to take care of business. She called Margo's answering service first and had operators put all calls to the office on hold . . . indefinitely. The only calls that eventually came in were the ones on Margo's private line . . . the calls Joyce *dreaded* to answer. Those calls came from Margo's mother, and from the new love in her life. The first ring was from Margo's mother. . . .

"Joyce . . . this is Ma Lillie. VeeDee [nickname for Veronica Drake, Margo's older sister] just called and said she heard on the news that there was a doctor shot on Wooster Avenue!"

"Yes . . . there was . . . Miss Lillie," Joyce answered with grave conviction.

"Well . . . ***is my baby alright?***" Ms. Lillie asked, hoping for an answer that will not threaten her very existence.

"No . . . Miss Lillie . . . no . . . *your baby is dead,*" Joyce yielded a crushing waft of shock to Ms. Lillie.

"What! *Well . . . what am I going to do . . . what am I going to do . . . what should I do . . . what* ***can*** *I do . . .*" Miss Lillie bade a pathetic plea.

Joyce tendered a forlorn response, *"I . . . don't . . . know."* Miss Lillie hung up the phone, and in her own words she stated, "I don't remember anything that happened after that phone call. My mind went blank."

Abrupt and absolute shock renders post traumatic stress.

The next phone call that rang in on Margo's private line was from Columbus, Ohio. It was the man who had quickly learned to respect, admire and love Margo Prade. The man who, in just *one more day* was to meet Margo's entire family. The man who could not wait to spend Thanksgiving Day with Margo and meet her family.

"Joyce, [*New Friend*] just called me and said something happened to Margo! ***What has happened to Margo?***"

"She was shot . . . she's dead." Joyce slowly surrendered the dreadful news. He began screaming and slammed down the phone.

Joyce felt awful in having had to tell two people who were so important in Margo's life *on the phone* that the one they love is dead . . . murdered . . . ***slaughtered***. People who hunt for a living do not shoot their prey as many times as Margo was shot.

An equally disturbing afterthought for Joyce was how swiftly *New Friend* knew of Margo's murder, in relation to how hastily she had notified Margo's companion. Moreover, *how* did she know how to contact him at work, out of town?

* * *

Pam, Margo's medical assistant, who was affectionately referred to as the "baby" of the office personnel, was in her kitchen preparing Thanksgiving dinner. Pam was five months pregnant with the child she would later name, Sidney ***Margo*** Foster. Pam loved Margo. Not only was she her employee, but also her friend.

"We just did things together, not all the time, but we did things together. Whenever Margo went on vacation she would always bring us something back, she loved doing that. On our birthdays and Christmas, she'd give us cash, and of course, I loved that." Pam poignantly admitted her boss' kindness toward them.

"Even on Christmas when we were supposed to just do the gift exchange and buy for the person whose name we had drawn, Margo would always buy everyone something anyway. We'd tell her, 'You're not supposed to be doing that, Margo!' "

And on days when Margo was not in a good mood, Pam would warn Joyce, "Stay away. . . ."

"Oooookay," Joyce would reply as they both snickered.

The snickering would occur because when Margo was in a bad mood, due to being angry with Douglas or the kids, it was only reflected in her sharp or direct tone. Her demeanor was ALWAYS demure; therefore, one could never determine from Margo's physical behavior if she was upset. And they would listen as Margo would complain about how she took Kenya and Sahara to a NBA basketball game and state, "I spent three hundred dollars on junk!"

"You know, Margo, you cannot buy what they are going to need later on in life," Pam would scorn. "I loved those kids to death, but they were brats," Pam admitted.

"I felt bad for Margo because she would always complain that she never spent enough time with her kids, even though I ***always thought*** she was with them, to be as busy as she was, she was always with her kids. She ***loved*** her kids," Pam acknowledged.

"We had it good in the office. We were self supervised, and we all knew what our job was and did it. Rarely would Margo have to call a staff meeting; and when she did, it was to reiterate minor things on how she wanted the office to run. But, there were not too many times that we did not laugh and just cut up in that office. It was the best!" Pam reflected.

* * *

On that fateful morning when Pam's phone rang, all future good times to be had in that office, came to a crushing end. A full and complete halt. Pam had taken the day off, she had an appointment with her OBGYN in the morning, and was back home preparing Thanksgiving dinner in the kitchen with her mother. Her husband, Wayne, was asleep. A City of Akron Firefighter, he had worked the night before. Joyce called and Pam answered the phone.

"Hello."

"Pam . . . it's Joyce. I have something ***terrible*** to tell you. Are you sitting down?"

"No, I'm not sitting down."

"Well . . . you should sit down, Pam," Joyce commanded.

"No . . . I'm NOT sitting down . . . what do you want to tell me?"

"Margo's . . . ***dead.***"

"That's ***NOT EVEN FUNNY,*** Joyce! Why would you call me and say something like that!" Pam fired back, yelling at Joyce. Pam does not remember what Joyce said after that. However, she does remember Joyce making a believer out of her, and *not wanting* to believe what Joyce had just told her. Pam hung up the phone crying, while her mother was trying to ask her ***what in God's name was wrong.*** Pam ran in her bedroom to change clothes screaming, crying, "***Margo's dead! Margo's dead!***" Her screams woke up her husband's peaceful slumber.

"What are you doing?" Wayne asked, startled by Pam's screams.

"I have to go to Margo's office . . . ***Margo's dead!***"

Shaken, Wayne leaped out of bed. "What are you talking about! Well . . . you can't drive!" The only event Pam recalls after that was Wayne actually driving her to Margo's office.

Like many of us, to some degree Pam has mental gaps as to the succession of events as they unfolded on that day. Deadened to what actually happened or to what was actually said, *after* that godforsaken phone call.

Psychic numbness.

Some time after the discovery of Margo's bloody and bullet-ridden body, her good friend and patient Brenda arrives at the office. Brenda had been called by her cousin who was also the dentist's secretary. Brenda idolized and respected Margo for all that she was as a person, for her commitment to her profession as a medical practitioner, and for their friendship.

A gifted and bright registered nurse, Brenda desperately wanted to follow in Margo's footsteps. However, due to circumstances beyond her control, she settled for becoming a nurse practitioner. Under Margo's supervision, Brenda was completing her externship working in Margo's office several times per week.

Brenda received a phone call from her cousin Sharon, that something horrible is going on at Margo's medical office. When she arrived and learned of Margo's murder, Brenda began to ***vomit uncontrollably.***

*   *   *

It was the first and only time I had ever missed a class. I was scheduled for a glamour photo shoot at eleven A.M. I attended my morning class and although anxious about it, decided to skip my afternoon class in order to get home and to my appointment on time.

I already had my black teddy and black panty hose on underneath the lime-green sweat suit, and had my hair wrapped underneath a little league baseball cap. God, I hated going out in public tacky like that, but this was the quickest way to get ready for my photo appointment after leaving class and after running the errands I needed to before going home.

"Tom is going to love this portrait," I whispered to myself. I had to be photographed that day in order to get the portrait back in time for Christmas. I only needed to stop home and apply my make-up accordingly.

After leaving class, I went to the main post office to check our P.O. Box to see if any of our contract people had decided to pay us. They had. I would also say "hi" to Edith before I left the post office because she was usually around in the lobby area whenever I would go there . . . that day she wasn't.

I left the post office, went to the mortgage company to pick up a check for the completion of our basement. After nine years in our new home, we decided to finish the final one-third of it, making a comfortable, livable lower level. Margo was so happy for us when I told her about the plans and when the project would be finished.

"Girl, we're having piped in surround sound music, and we're thinking of an indoor pool. We want to have a Christmas pool party!"

"Good! Let's have a Christmas party next year, Don!"

"Okay, it's a deal!"

"I'll split the cost with you and Tom!"

"Great, and you can invite whoever you want, I mean . . . I know you don't hang around any thugs or skank, so we won't have to worry about that."

We laughed. "It will be a great party, Don!" Margo shared her excitement.

"Yes, it will. I cannot wait! It's going to take the contractor about six to eight months to complete the project."

"Cool, we'll have plenty of time to plan the party!"

The party did materialize, but without the attendance of Dr. Margo Prade and her guests. The only remnant of Margo's presence was her picture, illuminated by a white Christmas candle atop a wooden table. Reminiscent of what should have been. I wanted to remember her in spirit. I wanted my guests, all of whom knew her either personally or through the media, to know she should have been there. I wanted my guests to know I wanted her presence, if only in spirit.

* * *

Time was running out. I had to get to this appointment on time. The traffic to and from the mortgage company was much busier than normal. I was rushing. While I walked in the back door the phone was ringing.

"Hello," I answered in an obvious rushed tone.

"Hello . . . Donzella . . . this is Deb."

"Deb? Deb who?"

"Debbie ____ from the reunion committee."

"Oh . . . hi, Deb, I just walked in the door. I have an appointment that I need to get to. . . ."

There is an *uncomfortable* silence. Much to my chagrin, and at the risk of sounding rude, I had to continue the conversation. After all, this was not a person who calls me, or who I talked with on a regular basis. At the same time, I did not want to hurt her feelings by being impolite.

"Well . . . what's up? I'm kinda rushed, Deb."

"Well . . . I know Margo Prade is your best friend. Right?"

"Yes."

"Well . . . honey . . . you know my daughter is a 911 operator. . . ."

"No. I didn't know that." I responded annoyed and thinking, *Do I need to know this now while I am in a hurry. What is the point . . . I have to go*!

"Well . . . honey . . . Margo has been shot."

"What!" I screamed, startled at what she had said. Although I do not remember the statement, Deb told me some months later during a reunion meeting that at that moment I stated:

"Did he kill her . . . did he *actually* kill her!"

What I do remember screaming is, "Was she shot at home . . . is she alive?"

"Honey, I don't know."

"Was she shot at the office?"

"I don't know."

"Is she dead!"

"Honey . . . I don't know *anything.*"

"Well, I have to hang up and call the office!"

"Honey . . . the office is not taking any calls."

"Well . . . then . . . I have to go over there!" My anxiety was rapidly building.

"Well, okay, but honey . . . why don't you pray with me first."

"Debbie!" I shouted, "I don't have time to pray. . . . I have to go and see about my friend!"

"I know honey . . . but please let me ***have prayer*** with you first before you leave." [Debbie knew Margo was dead, but did not want to tell me. Being a very spiritual woman, perhaps she did not want to be the bearer of the bad news.] In what felt like a scream to the high heavens, I stated, "***Goddammit***, Debbie . . . let me off the goddamn phone! I've got to go! Now!"

"Okay . . . okay . . . but at least take down my phone number and call me later after you get home. Promise you'll call me."

Exasperated from what I'd just heard, "Okay . . . give me the number!"

Debbie gave me the number and I wrote it down as fast as I could and hung up the phone, without saying goodbye. I ran out the door, jumped in my car and drove toward the office. While driving, my angst was building at a speed unmatched by the speed of my car. I purposely took the back roads, driving like a bat out of hell, not wanting to get stopped by the police or any red lights. I began to tremble, rock, cry and scream out, blathering words that I could not even understand. I had quit smoking, but wanted a cigarette. Bad.

I picked up my cell phone and dialed my girlfriend Rosemary's number at work. No answer. I then called her home and her daughter, Raquel, answered the phone. I began screaming. . . .

"Raquel, this is Donzella! Margo has been shot. I don't know if she is dead or alive. I called your mother at work but there is no answer. Find your mother . . . call your mother and tell her!"

"Oh . . . no! Okay . . . Donzella . . . I'll find her."

I make a second call to my husband. He was working in Canton, Ohio at the Stark County Jail. By now, I was engulfed in an uncontrollable screaming frenzy, and driving at least 70 mph through surface roads in modest neighborhoods.

"Hello, clinic."

"This is Mrs. A to Z . . . I need to talk to Doctor A to Z, it is an emergency . . . ***my friend*** . . . his colleague . . . Doctor Prade . . . has been shot!"

"Oh my God! Hold on. . . ." The voice dropped the phone.

By the time Tom got to the phone, I was less than two minutes away from the office.

"Hello."

Hysterical, moaning, and crying I shrieked, "Tom, Margo has been shot! I don't know if she is dead or alive, I don't know where she was shot . . . maybe at home!"

"Calm down . . . you're hysterical . . . you're going to have an accident! Where are you?"

"On Diagonal Road, headed to the office!"

"Well, calm down, be careful! I'll be right there!"

I continued driving, allowing those mechanisms in my brain to kick in. The ones that protect us from the injuries psychic pain can cause.

"Okay . . . okay. I know she is shot . . . but she is not dead," I told myself. "I'm going to walk in the office, and she is going to be being worked on by the paramedics. She is going to be shot in her right arm, that's all." I never once thought for a minute Margo would be dead. Death *never entered my mind.* In my mind, she was shot in her right arm, this is the only thought my mind allowed me to think. This was the only thought I *could* believe . . . visualizing Margo lying on her office floor, in the lobby area, talking with a paramedic while he worked on her arm, with people standing all around. I visualized the shooter having already been taken into custody. After all, it was broad daylight, people everywhere. There is no way a person could walk into a doctor's office, shoot them and just freely walk away.

Upon arriving at the corner of Frederick Boulevard and Diagonal Road, I saw Margo's van atop a flatbed tow truck, traveling east on Wooster Avenue. Unbeknownst to me at the time, her corpse was still inside the van.

"Well, there's her van," talking aloud to myself. *Okay . . . well . . . then she must have been shot at the office! They must be taking her to the hospital, and don't want to leave her van in the parking lot overnight.* I began to employ that graduate school analytic assessment that Margo had accused me of making use of lately with every thought process.

While turning the corner onto Wooster Avenue one block from the office, I see what seemed like hundreds of police cruisers. People were scurrying around the office building lawn and in the driveway like ants on an ant hill, and television cameras *everywhere.*

"What the *fuck* is going on here!" I talked even louder now to myself, straining to see further than my position on the road would allow. Then, that emotional mechanism in my brain kicks in again.

"Okay . . . well . . . it is not every day a doctor gets shot in Akron, that must be why the television vans are here. It's newsworthy."

My angst is now at its peak as I sped up onto the front lawn, park and jump out of the car and ran toward the building. Abruptly, I stopped running remembering that I had my purse, which contained checks in it, and my cellular phone visible on the front seat of the car and did not lock the door. In my hysteria, I ran back, retrieved my purse, and locked the car door.

I briefly noticed a plainclothes police officer tightly holding a large man who was in obvious panic. I later learned while watching the news, that the man was Margo's nephew, one of sister Frances' twins, and the officer was Adrian Johnson, a detective and high school classmate of mine.

Running into the building, and not remembering talking to anyone outside of the building, I learned one year later while watching Margo's murder on the television show, *Hard Copy*, that a detective was yelling to me, "She's dead . . . she's gone . . ." and I answered in a screaming voice, "Is she dead?"

The moment the officer told me Margo was dead must have been the moment that trauma wailed a swift left hook to my psyche. The information he gave me—that Margo was "gone"—did not register at all, or affect my present state of consciousness.

I ran down the hall and into the office. Uniformed and plain clothes police were everywhere. I see Margo's staff; Joyce, Pam, Tajauna, and Pam's husband Wayne sitting on the lobby sofa. Pam and Tajauna had tear-stained eyes. Joyce was just sitting next to them.

"***What happened?***" I snarled at Joyce in disgust.

"Margo pulled in the parking lot this morning and before she could get out of her van, someone got in and shot her," Joyce responded perfunctorily, with a blank stare, not looking at, but looking through me.

"Okay . . . where is she?" Joyce looked up at me as if to say, what do you mean where is she.

"Joyce, where is she . . . where is Margo . . . what hospital did they take her to?" Joyce continued to stare through me in fated silence, not saying a word, just staring, her head slightly trembling.

"Joyce! Where is Margo?" I began to scream.

"She ***is alive . . . isn't she? What hospital did they take her to, Akron General, City . . . what hospital . . . Joyce, she is alive . . . isn't she?!***"

With an engrossed, unoccupied but purposeful gaze, and never looking away from me, Joyce slowly and meticulously shook her head, "***no.***"

At that moment, I *totally* lost control of my faculties. The screams coming from the very pit of my larynx, echoing off the waiting room walls I could not recognize, or contain. This information—*Margo is dead*—surreal in nature, literally attacked every single sense I have; taste, smell, hearing, touch and sight; in a manner that seemed to threaten my physical state. I felt a corporeal numbness, manifested by emotional strain that I had never experienced before; a haunting and stabbing pain that caused my knees to buckle, and I fell to the floor, rolling around as if I was on fire without flames . . . perhaps I was.

At one point, I remember sitting up on my knees, salivating, crying out of control and screaming to Joyce, ***"Who did it! Who killed her?"***

Again, Joyce offered a featureless, self-effacing stare. She shook her head, "no" while barely speaking above a melancholy, trembling whisper, "They don't know."

"It's broad fucking daylight! And . . . a busy parking lot!" I shrieked . . . at the top of my lungs. "You mean to tell me nobody saw anything!" I screamed at Joyce, demanding a logical answer to this ***madness*** I was hearing. Again, Joyce shook her head to an unambiguous, "No." I lost it . . . again. I began earsplitting shouting . . . babbling, even louder this time, thinking, not only is my dear friend dead, but no one even knows who ***did it!*** This was illusory and deplorable! My only reaction, involuntarily was to resume rolling around on the floor kicking, crying and screaming like a dying bug on its back. What I *do not* remember is implicating suspects. However, two weeks after Margo's murder, during a conversation, Brenda said to me:

"Donzella, you were sitting on your knees, rocking back and forth like you were praying to Mecca. You shouted out names stating, 'I told her this was going to happen!' I was standing right behind you, Donzella, and I could not believe what you were saying. I said to myself, why would she say something like that! Donzella, I swear, I would not lie on you about something like this."

"Brenda, I don't remember saying *anything* like that!"

"You were in shock, Donzella. I'm so sorry, but you did say it. I would not make up something like that."

"I know you wouldn't, Brenda . . . but I just do not remember saying that. Why can't I remember?"

"I'm so sorry," Brenda replied in all earnestness.

Like many who were close to Margo, those gaps in memory of certain events of that day will forever remain hidden somewhere in our brains—for protection.

What I do remember is eventually getting up off the floor. *Something came over me. A feeling of defiance. Immediately, I stopped sobbing, stood up, brushed off and straightened out my clothing. I wiped the tears from my eyes and the mucus running from my nose with the sleeve of my sweatshirt. Slinging my purse over my left arm, I lifted my shoulders back, held my head up high and began marching . . . like a soldier* going into the battlefield. I marched into the foyer by the rear door facing the parking lot. The parking lot Margo had just been annihilated in. The parking lot where she parked her vehicle in the same spot for nearly ten years. The parking lot that she proudly entered so many days prior, helping to heal the sick and save the lives of others. The parking lot that where on *this day* after speaking to her loving mother for the last time, Dr. Margo Prade fought a valiant fight, but *could not save her own life.*

I noticed a high-ranking police official, who I knew well from working for years at the Akron Police Department. He was standing at the rear door, his eyes canvassing the parking lot. I approached, still sniffing a combination of tears and mucus back into my head.

"Do you remember me?" I ask.

"Yes, yes I do. . . ."

Cutting off his sentence, and trying to be quiet but firm in my questions, I began interrogating *him* about who he was questioning for this heinous crime. I wanted to speak quietly because there were too many cops around. The last thing I need is someone going back telling . . . discussing what I was saying to the Captain . . . police officers are notorious for gossip and innuendo.

The high-ranking officer proceeded in telling me all who had been to the scene; including Douglas, who had been there, fainted and left.

Quietly fuming, I stated, "I'm not asking how people reacted! I'm asking *are you questioning* Douglas Prade about this murder?"

The official then gestured his head for two line staff detectives to take me into the dentist's office across the hall for further questioning. The questioning was short-lived. I had screamed and bawled myself into a tremendous headache and was unable to be helpful, even after they had asked for, and the dentist had given me something for pain. I can only remember jabbering about how happy Margo was, and how she, "Just wanted to be happy."

The detectives understood the emotional and physical impact of the situation, they'd been there before.

"I can't talk . . . I'm sorry . . . my head *really* hurts . . ." I confessed I had literally screamed myself into a tremendous headache.

The detectives handed me cards stating, "It's okay. This is not the last time we are going to talk to you. Call us if you can think of anything. We'll be in touch."

When Tom arrived, I was standing in Margo's waiting room. I felt someone touch my shoulder and I turned around. Crying, I spurted out to my husband, "She's dead! Babe, Margo is dead," and began to cry hysterically all over again.

"Come on back into our office. You're in shock. You're just standing here in the middle of the floor shaking, come on in the back."

Tom led me to the back to our office and immediately began to attempt to control my grief—force of habit from his work.

"You need to settle down and stop crying . . . the focus is on her family now . . . control yourself."

Not understanding at the time, that this was the only way Tom knew how to console me, I was very angry at his dismissal of my grief, believing it was something to be controlled, rather than acknowledged. I remained angry for several years. What my husband did not understand was that I did not need him to be a psychologist trying to control a hysterical client, not with this. I needed him to be a supportive husband, let me cry. Let me scream. Let me beg almighty God for this horror not to be true. Let me process the pain I was feeling in the only way I could. Let me grieve.

Picking up the office phone, overwhelmingly distraught, I had enough presence of mind to call and cancel my appointment with the photographer. He stated he was just listening to the report of the murder on the radio as we spoke. He offered his condolence, "I am so, so, sorry. . . ." Then we hung up.

A new neighbor of ours, Karen, suddenly appeared out of nowhere. She rushed into our office, kneeled down on the floor in front of me, grabbed my hand closed her eyes and began to pray. Karen then looked up at me, and stated something to the effect of, "We do not always understand the Lord's plans for us. . . ."

"This is not the Lord's work," I snapped, crying and cutting off her words. "This is the ***devil's*** work! If God intended Margo to die now, she would have gotten ill or had a car accident . . . this is the devil's work! Don't blame this on God!" Just that quick, my pain had immediately turned to anger. Bona fide anger. Anger that, in many ways, still exists.

Before leaving the office, Joyce and I shared a moment together. It was the first time we had interacted since her telling me Margo was dead; and was the beginning of a closeness we had not previously shared, but continue to share to this day. Joyce was not crying. She was more traumatized than anything. In fact, a couple of months passed before Joyce *could* cry. When she did, however, she cried for a half an hour straight, while in the company of a Victims Assistance counselor. Joyce cried so hard, for so long, that the counselor began crying with her. The fact that they cried together, indicates that the counselor not only empathized with, but also *felt* Joyce's pain, and perhaps her own sense of loss.

Joyce and I sat inside one of Margo's examining rooms, holding hands tightly as if we were trying to conjure up and draw from each other's strength to get through this nightmarish day. Without looking at one another, we sat and stared into the abyss of sorrow. While we talked, Joyce revisited and reviewed step by step, her finding Margo in the van, bloody and inert.

"Were her eyes closed . . . at least," I asked Joyce beginning to sob again.

"No . . . they were open. . . ."

". . . Then she really wasn't ready to die. . . ." I responded with conviction.

"Well . . . whoever killed her, I hope they realize their life is over, too," I snarled.

"Um-hum . . . it sure is." Joyce agreed with composed resolve.

Sometime before our conversation ended, I apparently said to Joyce, "I'm going to write a book about Margo. I don't know how long it will take . . . but I'm going to write a book." Joyce and I hugged each other tightly, and Tom and I prepared to leave and go home. My eyes were so swollen from crying, and I was so distraught emotionally, Tom wanted me to leave my car and get it another day. I said, "No, I can drive, I'll just go slow."

* * *

After all the uniform police, detectives and victim assistance personnel finally left 1557 Wooster Avenue, Margo's death was officially confirmed a homicide and her van became the *official crime scene.* After it had begun to rain, the van had to be taken away in order to preserve the crime scene. Otherwise, my dear friend would have still been in the parking lot when I arrived. It would have *destroyed me* to actually see Margo dead like that.

The city of Akron, Ohio and surrounding communities began to gasp for breath as they systematically learn throughout the day and evening hours via radio, television and word of mouth reports regarding the shooting death of 41-year-old, Dr. Margo Shamberger Prade.

With everything Margo contributed to our community, and for all that she meant to so many people, especially her children, this was the ultimate insult. For so many people, Margo was more than a doctor, friend, colleague, daughter, mother, sister, aunt, and relative; she was an inspiration.

Dr. Margo Prade's prized life ended with her last day of work beginning at Akron General Medical Center, checking in on her patients; individuals who, next to her children, were the center of her world. Doctor Margo Prade's workday met with a despicable ending, with her riding on the butt of a flatbed tow truck; lifeless inside the vehicle that *she projected* would cause her to meet her demise.

A sobering, nauseating reality.

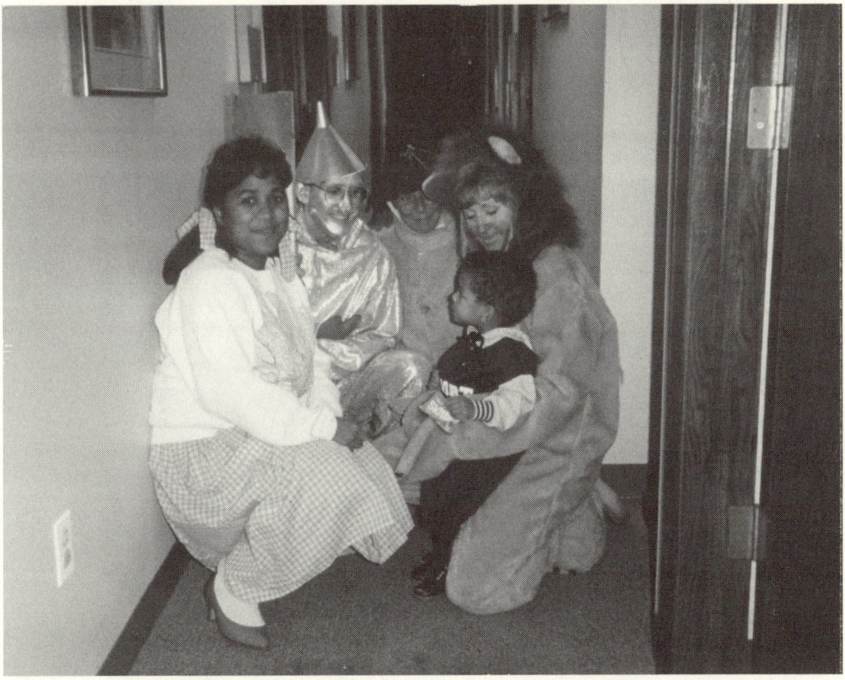

Dr. Prade and staff, at her office, dressed as characters from *The Wizard of Oz* in 1992. Child photographed with them is the author's son, then two years old.

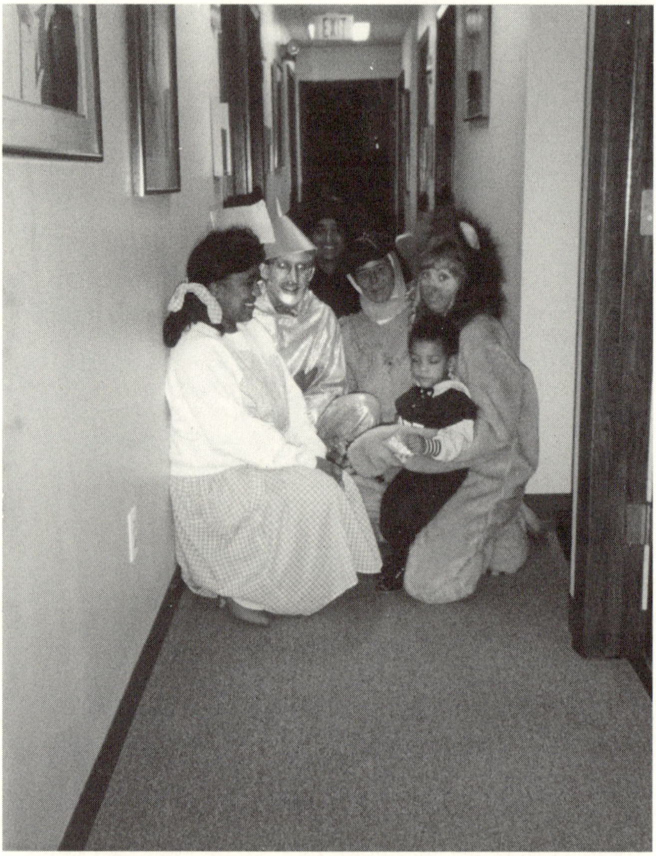

Dr. Prade and staff, at her office, dressed as characters from *The Wizard of Oz* in 1992. Child photographed with them is the author's son, then two years old.

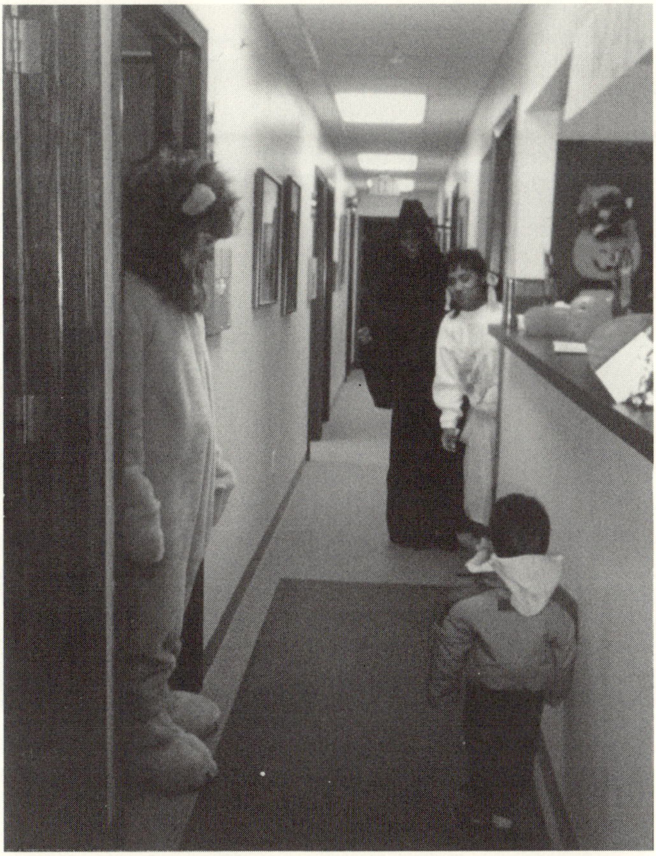

Dr. Prade and staff, at her office, dressed as characters from *The Wizard of Oz* in 1992. Child photographed with them is the author's son, then two years old.

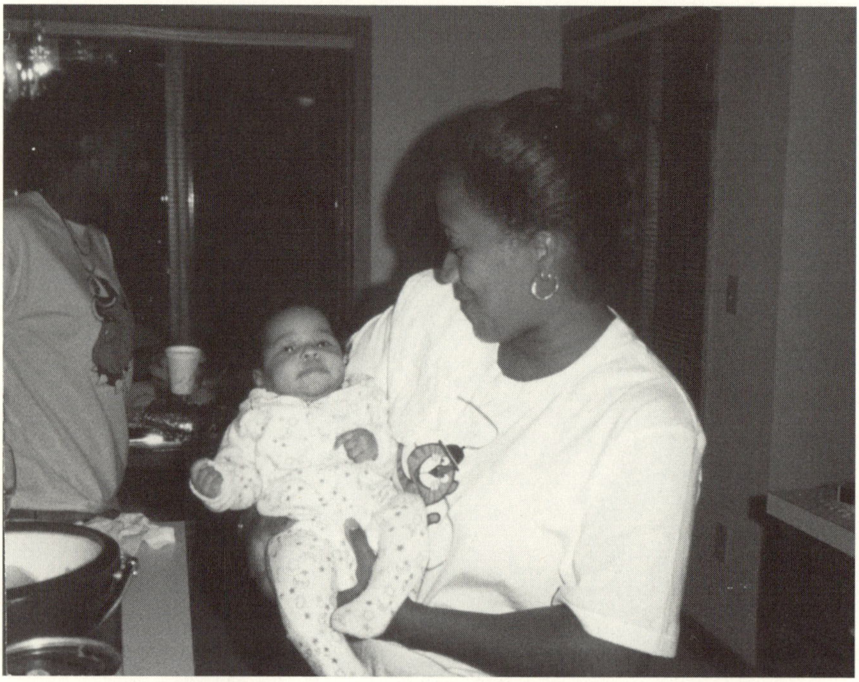

Dr. Prade with newborn daughter Sahara Prade, 1988

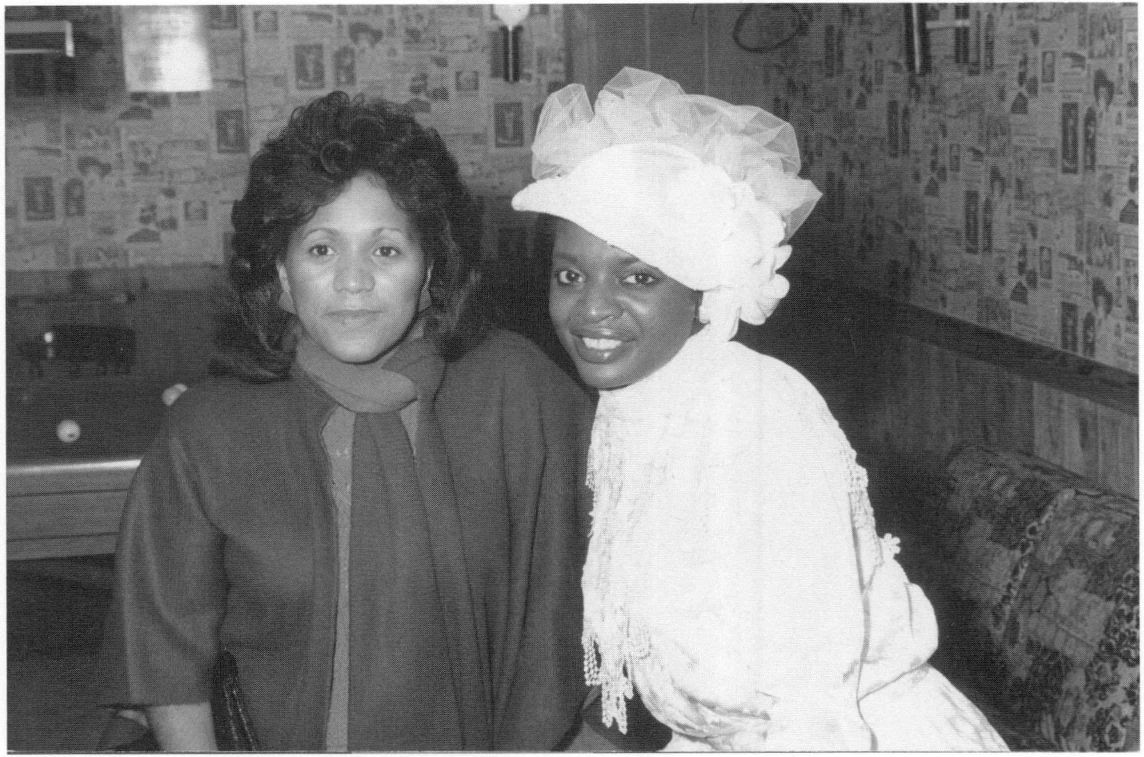

Dr. Prade and I at my wedding reception, September 14, 1985. Dr. Prade refusing to smile due to having braces on her teeth.

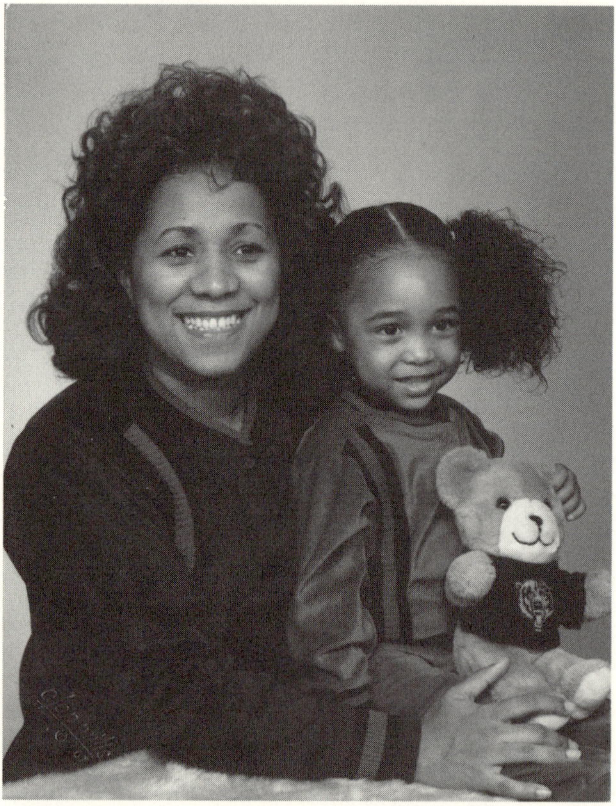

Dr. Prade and eldest daughter Kenya Prade

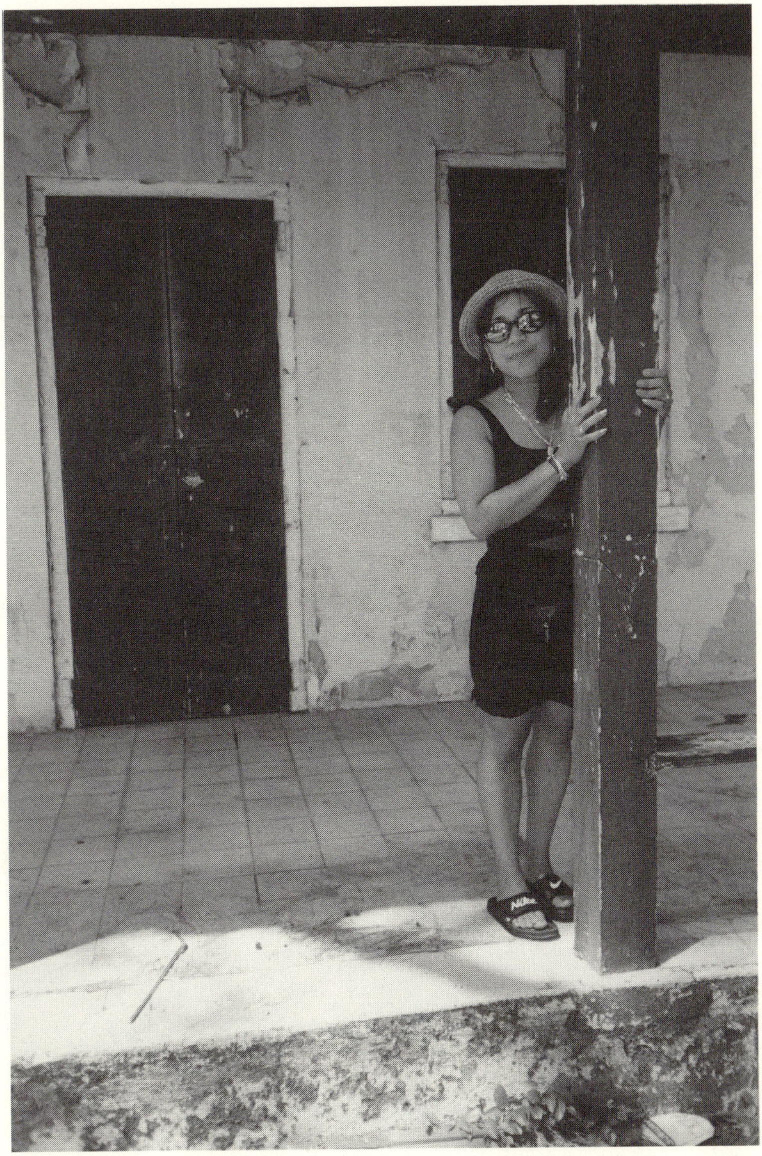

Dr. Prade on vacation

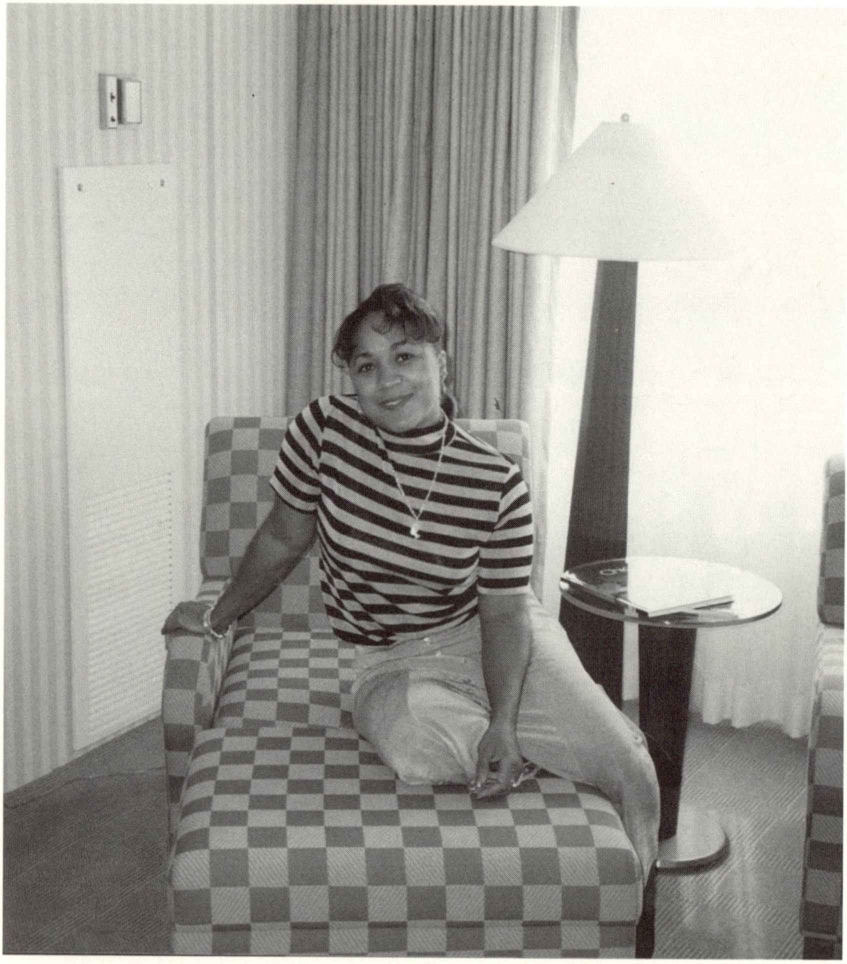

Dr. Prade relaxing at home

Eighteen
All Aboard the Insane Train

The crowd of police, victim assistance personnel, onlookers and other personnel from various offices within the building slowly began to scatter. Outside, teams of reporters in mobile news vans from Channels 43, 5, Fox 8 News and Channel 3 news interrupted drivers in automobiles, and pedestrians on foot throughout the city, forcing microphones in their car windows and faces, hoping for sensational responses and verbalizations worthy of the five and six o'clock evening news.

"I just couldn't believe it . . . I just . . . could . . . not . . . believe it!" an African American male stated standing on the sidewalk.

"It's horrible . . . just awful," a woman obviously shocked, said from her car while the reporter held the microphone through the driver's window.

One radio station's early report stated, "*A Doctor Margo Prade was found shot to death today in her minivan in the parking lot behind her medical office building. It is reported she was shot several times . . . an apparent suicide.*"

This was the beginning of many erroneous reports with accompanying, "whodunit" campaigns. This was the beginning of the inauguration of an untrustworthy *new friend,* budding with deceptive tentacles *and* a cloud of suspicion hanging over her head. This was the beginning of a stunned and polarized community. A community both creating and divided over theories of who murdered the divine and respected Dr. Margo Prade.

Over the next several weeks, and well into December, the marquee on the front lawn of the office building, the front and rear doors leading into the building, and even the section of the metal fence that Margo parked beside, were inundated with bouquets of flowers. Someone had tied a large purple ribbon on the fence; symbolic of a purple heart of heroism, marking the very spot where Margo was executed. A colleague of Margo's, Dr. Marta Roth, voluntarily went to Margo's office the following week to clear up her patients charts, examining lab results and x-ray reports.

* * *

At the time of her murder, Margo and Douglas Prade had only been divorced for seven months. The rule of thumb in criminal education is that in a murder, family members become the number one suspects. With this murder, you're not only looking at a newly divorced ex-husband, but also a high ranking decorated police official who worked in Internal Affairs. The victim, a well established physician, who earned an admirable salary. Robbery was ruled out immediately. It was obvious from the crime scene, that Margo was not robbed. It was not a viable rationale either for the crime to have been an early morning random act of violence; especially for this very busy part of town. Lastly, it was apparent Margo had been shot several times at close range, which for all intents and purposes, depicts a signature crime . . . *someone wanted* her dead. That someone, however, unbeknownst to them, was surreptitiously caught on tape entering and exiting Margo's van within ninety seconds, by the Rolling Acres Dodge dealership security camera that faced the office building parking lot, and the same area along the fence where Margo parked her van.

* * *

Upon exiting the parking lot onto Wooster Avenue, I saw my good friend, Cranston, driving at a snail's pace past the building, looking. He saw me, too, turned around and caught up in the right lane alongside me. I rolled down my window. Crying again, I yelled out to him.

"Margo's dead!"

"I know, Don . . . you going home?" he said with sadness.

"Yes, will you please come over?"

"I'll follow you there."

* * *

When Tom, Cranston, and I arrived at our home, Tom poured all three of us a strong drink. Cranston and I sat down at the kitchen table. Cranston sat quietly, keeping me under surveillance making sure I was not getting ready to have the big one. Tom couldn't sit so he stood. He took a gulp of his drink and said, "The community has really lost something today. . . ." He took another gulp. "This is the ***biggest damn loss for this community,*** and everybody is going to *want* it to be Douglas!" I began to cry profusely.

"Well, he was threatening her, and harassing her lately," I responded in angst and tears.

"That does not mean he killed her," Tom insisted.

"Everybody loved Margo, Tom . . . who would want to do something like this to her!"

"I'm just saying everybody wants it to be Douglas, right away, because people are going to want this solved, right away! I know he was mean to her lately . . . doesn't mean he did it!" Tom persisted in anger.

I briefly left Tom and Cranston; they were talking anyway. I went upstairs and called my mother in California.

"Hello," she answered with concern in her tone, voice shaking.

"Mommy," I begin crying, "Margo's dead. . . ."

"Oh . . . God! ***Then it is true,*** it's really true! Lil [a family friend who lives in Akron] called me a while ago and told me. I told her *I was not going to believe* such a thing until and ***unless you called me*** . . . Oh God, Don . . . ! Try to hold on baby . . . please, I know you are not okay. . . . I don't want you to have a heart attack . . . please try. . . ."

"No . . . I'm not okay . . . Mommy . . . I can't . . . ***my heart hurts so bad . . . I don't understand why someone would.*** . . ." Grief began to escalate again, and I began wailing and crying uncontrollably.

My mother began to cry along with me. Without actually saying goodbye, we hung up the phone. Mom has always been modest about her emotionality when she is pushed to the brink of crying, and being a mother, she did not want to upset me further by my hearing her cry. Mom was crazy about Margo and was very proud of her accomplishments, like many who knew her.

Cranston stayed for an hour or so. We hugged and he left saying, "I'll be in touch, Don."

The telephone began to ring, and ring and *ring* . . . before, during and after the news programs. Margo's murder was the top news story on every channel in Northeast Ohio. Our phone would not stop ringing, friends thwarted their rides home from work to stop over, and my home became grand central station for the next ten months. One of the last phone conversations I had the night of Margo's murder was from one who would later be labeled, "My Detective," in any future conversations with both Joyce, and Margo's family.

"This is detective King . . . how is your headache? Can you think of anything else?"

Due to the nature of the crime, potential suspects, shades of paranoia that encompassed all who were involved in the investigation or with Margo, we engaged in a desperate effort to preserve the integrity of the investigation. Joyce, Margo's family members and I adapted an unspoken doctrine to never speak the names of our detectives to each other, or to anyone. Whenever we spoke to one another about the progress of the investigation, and if we were still working with a detective, we would state, "My detective told me this," or, "My detective told me that." To this day, we are still unaware of who those detectives were.

For two people who were once a celebrated couple in the Akron, Ohio community, a couple who were revered and treasured, their lives swiftly became fodder for celebrity tittle-tattle surrounding the murder of Dr. Margo Shamberger Prade. Margo and Douglas Prade became the object of a major murder investigation involving Akron Police Department's most elite detectives and the local FBI.

Margo's distinguished life was beset by the scrutiny of both the radio and print media frenzy. The radio stations broadcasted whichever "whodunit and howdunnit" rumors that churned throughout the day, and whichever rumors were the most popular. The print media at times, made use of sensational tabloid journalism. Compliments of the Akron Beacon Journal. Douglas, on the other hand, was portrayed by the media as the grieving ex-husband. A father now flanked by two motherless daughters, twelve and nine years old. A father who will now have to endure raising two young children on his own.

* * *

Vee Dee, Margo's older sister calls. I had not spoken with her in years, not since she babysat my son when he was an infant and toddler.

"Donzella . . . it's Veronica." I began to cry.

"Here," I heard her say to someone in the background, "She's crying."

Ms. Lillie gets on the phone, asking me if I'm coming over.

"I can't come over there now, I don't want to . . . I'm too upset."

"Oh . . . baby . . . I know . . . when will you come over, I want you to come over?"

"I don't know, maybe tomorrow," I said, not remembering it was Thanksgiving Day, and I would be out of town at my in-laws'.

"Okay baby . . . don't cry . . . I'll see you then."

Recalling that I could not go over to Margo's house the next day, I called right back and Douglas answered the phone.

"Hellooo . . ." Revulsion hit me immediately. I'd never in the twenty one years I'd known him, heard Douglas sound so happy on the phone. He sounded like he was living it up at a damn party with a drink in his hand, even though he did not drink! I was pissed that he did not sound sad at all!

Knowing Douglas knew my voice, and without returning a kind hello, I ask for Margo's mother, not knowing Ms. Lillie's last name was Hendricks.

"Can I speak to Ms. Shamberger please."

"You mean Ms. Hendricks?"

"Ms. Shamberger . . . Margo's mother."

"You mean Ms. Hendricks . . . ***don't you?***" he responded, with sarcasm.

I'm thinking, "***Cut the fucking bullshit, Mr. Happy!***" and without realizing it, raise my voice.

"Can . . . I PLEASE . . . SPEAK . . . TO MARGO'S MOTHER . . . PLEASE! LET ME TALK TO MARGO'S MOTHER!"

Suddenly, Douglas' voice turns from a warm Mr. Happy, to an unnerving Mr. Ice Man. He states unyieldingly, ". . . Hold on. . . ."

At that moment, I knew the twenty plus years of friendship were over between Douglas and I. ***We both knew it.*** The line had been drawn in the sand and it represented betrayal . . . for both of us. I was gravely aware that my anger, pain and grief had unveiled the doubts I had of his innocence. Doubts revealed in a way I had not planned, and did not want to feel, at least not this soon. He knew I was no longer in his friendship camp the way I had been after his and Margo's divorce, he knew that perhaps if he was guilty, his secret was not safe with me. We both knew that now, "The fight is on . . . mother fucker . . . it's on!"

* * *

For months to come, I was exceedingly angry at everything and everyone; including any deity who wanted to take responsibility for this evil, or who could have prevented it. Even if I did not want to, I *had* to put my faith in God that my family and I would live through this insanity, and that no one else would get hurt before this crime is solved. I had to be careful, and stay aware of my surroundings at all times. "Watch what you say and who you say it to. *He* is very well connected." A good friend and attorney advises during a phone conversation the evening of Margo's murder, even though I had not even hinted at who I felt was responsible, I didn't *know* who was responsible. I also kept hearing the same clicking sounds on my phone, sounds that went on for two weeks; therefore, I felt my phone line was tapped. I found my friend's warning interesting, especially since I did not tell her or *anyone* who I thought killed Margo. My sister called later that evening.

"Do you think her husband killed her?" she asked, not beating around the bush at all.

"I'm not saying anything . . . I don't know . . . I hope not."

* * *

On Thanksgiving Day, we arrived at my in-laws in Pittsburgh in the early afternoon. Dinner was being held at Tom's aunt's home this year. The members of Tom's family who had the pleasure and opportunity of meeting Margo over the years were appalled at the news of her murder.

"I can't believe it," my mother-in-law said. "She was so nice, so pretty and so smart . . . how awful!"

"That's terrible! Was it a drive-by?" asks my naïve brother-in-law, as if drive-by shootings are the only way black people in America are killed regardless of their profession, status in the community, and geographical location; and as if Margo would even be in an area where drive-by shootings were prevalent. I was quite angry with him adhering to this stereotypical assumption first, without considering any other possibility. However, I was too distraught to address the statement, which was probably a good thing.

Being overwhelmed with concern for justice in this awful crime, I could think of nothing else. I could speak of nothing else. I knew I would not stay at the dinner long at all, in fact, I wanted to leave then. Too much emotional torment and grief to be festive.

During Thanksgiving dinner there were various conversations taking place that I was totally oblivious to. I had sunk deep into a dazed state of mind. Every once in a while, someone would wake me up with a perfunctory, "Do they know who did it," or "Where did it happen?"

I asked Tom to take me to his parents' home after dinner, but not before speaking with my cousin-in-law, Ronnie, who is a district attorney in the city of Pittsburgh. We go upstairs to a private room and talk.

"Ronnie, what are the chances of someone being arrested for a murder if no concrete evidence is ever found like the gun or bloody clothes, but the person constantly threatened the victim, and is a high ranking police officer?"

Ronnie paused in thought. "Well, most crimes today are solved without the smoking gun, so to speak." He went on. "I mean most criminals don't leave evidence lying around anymore, but they are convicted on circumstantial evidence."

"Well how much weight would be given to evidence that only involves verbal threats and nothing else? I mean . . . I doubt the investigation will ever find any physical evidence like a gun or bloody clothing."

"Well, believe it or not, we once convicted a guy of murdering his girlfriend, even though the body was never found."

"Really?" I responded with a glimmer of hope that dear Margo might get the justice she deserves.

"Yes, this woman's body was never found. Therefore, not only did we not have any evidence of a murder, we did not even have a corpse."

"Then how was he convicted?"

"Strictly on circumstantial evidence. On testimony from the victim's friends, co-workers and family that he had always threatened to kill her and get rid of the body."

"And he was arrested and convicted?"

"Yes. We convicted him on aggravated murder."

"Thanks, Ronnie."

"You're welcome. I'm so sorry about your friend."

We hugged before leaving the room. I returned to Tom, my son and the rest of the family and asked Tom to take me to his parent's home. He did, no questions asked. After he left, I got into bed and cried myself to sleep.

The next morning, Tom knew I was anxious to get back home, and his parents understood. While driving, I called Ms. Lillie to tell her I was on my way home from Pittsburgh and would be over as promised. Douglas answered the phone and I tried to be diplomatic.

"Douglas, this is Donzella. Is Ms. Lillie or Phyllis [Margo's sister] there?"

"NO."

"Do you know when they will be back?"

"NO."

"Well . . . how are you doing?"

"I'd be fine if people would stop going around talking about stuff that they don't know what they're talking about."

"Humph." This is the only remark I could conjure up.

"You wouldn't happen to know anybody who is doing anything like that would you . . ." he asked in a veiled threat.

"No . . . I don't, and I'm not sure what you're talking about, but I haven't heard anything. I've been out of town." I waited for a response, but did not get one.

"Okay, well, I promised Ms. Lillie I would come over today. So, would you please tell her when she gets back, that I'm on my way back home from Pittsburgh, and I'll be there in about three hours?"

"Well . . . they [the police] are over here right now with all kinds of search warrants and whatnot! So, it won't be necessary for you to come over here," he said with indignation. I offered a rhetorical, "Okay." Knowing I was going over anyway.

After sharing mine and Douglas' conversation with Tom, he suggested I refrain from going over to Margo's house.

"Babe, I don't think it is a good idea for you to go over there if he doesn't want you there."

"No, I'm going! I promised Ms. Lillie. Besides, if Douglas does not want me there, for whatever reason, then he'll have to ask me to leave in front of all those people. Then he'll look kinda guilty . . . don't you think? Anyway, there is an old saying . . . you keep your friends close, but your enemies closer. Right now, I consider Douglas the enemy with the way he is acting. I haven't said anything to anyone, so why is he talking to me and treating me like that?"

"Maybe he is just upset. Maybe people are whispering around accusing him because everyone *wants* it to be Douglas! Well, it's your call, but please be careful if you go over there."

"I will. But, if people are going around accusing Douglas, it hasn't been me. So, I still don't know why he is acting like that . . . unless the police are telling him who has implicated him, which would be quite inappropriate and dangerous. Don't you think?"

"Yes, very dangerous . . . because *if* he did do it, now other people's lives could be in danger as long as he is free."

*   *   *

I had baked a sweet potato casserole before I left for Pittsburgh, for the purpose of taking it to Margo's house. On the way there, I stopped to buy a bottle of wine. While in the store, people were discussing Margo's murder while standing in the checkout line. I could hardly bear to listen.

Upon arriving, Phyllis opened the door.

"Hi, Don."

"Hi, Phyllis," I replied hugging her.

Phyllis took the wine and the casserole stating, "I'm going to have Douglas open this."

I took a deep breath and walked through the door of my dear friend's house, knowing I would never be greeted by her smiling face again when ringing the doorbell to her home. With this thought, my heart sank into an unimaginable pain that was difficult to manage. However, I knew I needed to face Douglas. I could not allow him to scare me away for whatever reason he thought was needed. After greeting those who had gathered in the living room, I asked someone, "Where is Douglas?"

The person, who I later learned was Margo's sister Denise from California stated, "He's in there," pointing toward the family room. Denise's face was drawn and traumatized.

Dreading every step, I went to greet Douglas. He had stated his position loud and clear during the last conversation we had on the phone . . . "don't come over here . . . ," and I was defying him. According to his colleagues, people did not defy Douglas Prade; and if you choose to do so, you paid for it. I was willing to pay whatever price. After all, Margo had already paid the ultimate price for defying *somebody,* and maybe it was him.

I approached Douglas in what felt like slow motion. He was sitting down in a chair, opening the wine I had brought while talking with an attorney. This attorney was very popular in the Akron community at the time, and was often known for his political and social activism for the African American community. I spoke to him first, then to Douglas. Douglas seemed *surprised* to see me.

"Hello, Douglas." I bent down and hugged him during the greeting. He hugged me back, but the embrace was not recognizable. It did not *feel* like all the others we'd engaged in over the past twenty years. No, this embrace was *chilling*, hardcore and bitter. The tremendous strength and power of his touch disturbed me. I had never felt anything like it before in my life, not even with all the previous hugs from Douglas over the years. No. This embrace was quite different. It was unkind, unfriendly, and *frightening*. I could not help but notice the physical command of the embrace. I could not help but consider, that if Douglas had indeed killed Margo, there was no way she could have competed with the physical strength this man possessed. I could feel the credence of pure muscle. I couldn't even imagine feeling the force of untainted rage behind that kind of physical supremacy. The experience *unnerved* me to where at that very moment, I *believed* I was hugging a killer. I would need to test the waters just a bit more.

I pulled away from him, couldn't stand what I was feeling. I wanted to vomit, right in his lap! Instead, I began the test.

"Are you okay, Douglas . . . are you doing alright with the girls?" I asked with veiled care and concern.

"I'm doing ***fine!***" he replies, peering at me, *bolstering* while pounding his chest like King Kong; and visibly restraining an urge to yell and rear up from his seat! "I'm doing just fine with my girls. I'm going to take care of them. ***ME! Nobody else!***"

"Okay . . ." I responded, looking at Douglas wondering if he *realized* how revealing his remarks and body language was. He stopped looking at me, before I stop looking at him. This was a good thing, but would not be the last time we would exchange this particular type of eye contact.

The test was finished, and was a good time to make my exit. I returned to the living room to formally meet Margo's family members I had never met. I introduced myself to Margo's sister Denise. "I remember you, I met you one time at Margo's co-ed softball game," she said. Margo had named her team *Dr. Prade's Rx* The name ideologically true to *her* prescription of what a team meant—that being, everybody plays.

I sat next to a woman named Karen, who I'd known from high school. We spoke, and began conversations. Karen shared with me how she and Margo had grown up together as children, and would walk to grade school together.

"I always knew she would grow up and make a lot of money,

because she was counting pennies even then!" Karen reminisced. Then Douglas walked in the room, did not talk to anyone, and walked back out. Karen and I watched him the entire time. After Douglas left the room, *something* compelled us to look at one another.

"Are you thinking what I'm thinking?" she asked.

"I don't know what you are thinking, and I'm not going to say what I'm thinking." We left it there.

Shortly thereafter a lady walked through the door without ringing the doorbell. It was *New Friend*. She quickly scanned the room while holding a paper bag. Someone walked up to her and said, "Let me see."

She pulled an enlarged picture out of the bag. "Oh, how nice," the lady said. I walked up to look at the picture and *New Friend* quickly snatched it away from me saying in a huff, "I'm going to show Douglas!" and stormed into the family room.

For the remainder of the evening that I was present, neither *New Friend* nor Douglas *ever returned from the family room. New Friend* never came back into the room to converse with Margo's family members or friends. In the days to follow, *New Friend* seemed to have no interest in consoling anyone, except Douglas.

I also learned that *New Friend* was very much involved in *participating* in Margo's funeral plans. With all the family members Margo had, to say I was perplexed at *New Friend's* involvement in Margo's funeral plans, ***and*** the behavior she displayed toward me would be an understatement.

The resentfulness *New Friend* displayed was the second time I had been in her company since Margo's death and she treated me like the plague. Moreover, *New Friend* had also told a mutual friend of ours that, "Douglas was going to have a '*talk*' with me because I ran up and down the office building corridor the day of Margo's murder yelling, "Douglas killed Margo, Douglas killed Margo"; and that she witnessed my doing this, even though no such event ever happened; nor was she at the building when I arrived there. Why did she lie on me, and why is she now all about Douglas, when she was ***supposed*** to be Margo's good friend? ***I smelled a rat!***

*   *   *

"Hello, oh, hi Mom!"

"Baby it is way past midnight. I knew you were up, what are you still doing up!"

"I'm working."

"Baby, you are just working too much, staying up too late and just trying to do everything! You goin' too fast and just doin' too much. You need to slow down some before you cause yourself to have a heart attack and die! Then I would have to finish raising Kenya and Sahara . . . I'm too old to raise them children!"

Margo giggles and states, "Yeah . . . but YOU WILL. In fact, if ***anything*** *happens to me mama,* ***you will*** *raise Kenya and Sahara."* Margo instructs in all sincerity to her mother, ***just two weeks*** before she was murdered, and perhaps *after* receiving an abundance of threats and murderous innuendos.

On November 29th, the Saturday following Margo's murder, her eldest sister Frances who now resides in Las Vegas, accompanied sister Edith, Joyce, Douglas and Margo's attorney, to Margo's office to begin clearing out things. They wanted all of Margo's medical books to be packed up and given to Brenda, and all the softball trophies given to me. While walking in the building, Douglas shot a threat at Frances.

"I know y'all think I had something to do with this but I didn't. Y'all better respect me, too . . . , or you will ***never see*** Kenya and Sahara again!"

According to Joyce, once inside, Margo's attorney made a safe and legal statement to Douglas, offering advice deemed to be in everyone's best interest. She told him given that she represented Margo in their divorce settlement, it may be a conflict of interest for him to be in the office at that particular time, while they were going through Margo's personal and legal papers.

With recrimination, he remarked, "I know y'all think I killed her. ***I don't give a damn what y'all think***!"

At that moment, Edith went ballistic and began screaming to Douglas ***"I'm going kill you! I'll kill you!"*** Edith apparently had to be restrained.

Even if Douglas had not killed Margo, the audacity and insensitivity of his remarks were reprehensible, threatening and indignant. Given that he had already taken a lie detector test *and* had been cleared, his behavior was even more mystifying. Having been a cop for twenty-nine years, he had to know that in crimes like these, everyone who was remotely close to the victim is a potential suspect. Moreover, Douglas had his own list of suspects he gave to the police. Therefore, why the incensed behavior? He had to know that given the camaraderie rooted in the police department he so loved, and given the previous public infractions he had gotten away with, he *had* to believe that he would be the very ***last person*** the police would suspect with any seriousness. He had to ***believe*** that giving him the lie detector test was simply a formality to ***rule him out, not in,*** as a suspect. No police officer in the history of the Akron Police department had ever been investigated for a crime such as this, why would his colleagues start with him, a police captain?

If nothing else, Douglas' remarks to Frances and Margo's attorney clearly demonstrated an irony to his previous reaction of fainting after he arrived at the scene of the murder. The behavior also demonstrated he had no love for Margo at all. No empathy for the loss that his two young daughters would now have to bear; no sadness over Margo's brutal murder, and absolutely no remorse if he, in fact, was the killer.

Nineteen

Good-bye . . . Dear Friend

Monday night December 1, 1997. I was up very late, burning serious midnight oil, could not sleep at all. I decided writing Margo a goodbye letter would help. It was the night before her funeral and my grieving was in a horrible state. After writing the letter I called Joyce. Somehow I figured she was not asleep either.

"Joyce, are you asleep?"

"No . . . not at all." Choking on tears, and voice trembling, I told Joyce about the letter and asked if I could read it to her. "Yes . . . of course you can . . ." She responded in a soft, somber tone. I read the letter to Joyce, I felt I needed her approval. A goodbye letter to Margo had to be perfect. After I finished, Joyce offered a solemn, quiet approval with barely speaking above a whisper, "That is so nice, Donzella."

"Do you really think it is okay?"

"Yes, she would like that."

The following day, Tuesday December 2, Dr. Margo Shamberger Prade's funeral was held at the Arlington Church of God, with Reverend Ronald Fowler officiating. Reverend Fowler, a community statesman in his own right, is Margo's Sister Frances' brother-in-law.

The funeral lasted six hours. It was the longest funeral I had ever attended *in my life.* On this very cold and dismal day, patients, friends, relatives, colleagues and onlookers, lined the sidewalks for blocks encircling the church, there to say good-bye to a community icon. The information involving Margo's murder had become so newsworthy and sensational, that some attended the funeral out of sheer curiosity. Attendees of Margo's funeral had lined the sidewalks long before the funeral cars arrived at the church.

We left early, 9:00 A.M. "I am not going to stand up for my dear friend's funeral!" I cautioned Tom, since he has a tendency to run late. Before leaving, my neighbor Karen made an early morning phone call.

"Are you alright? This is going to be a long, hard day for you." She then suggested, "Let's have prayer. . . ."

At the request of Margo's niece Layne, I purposely did not wear black. Perhaps symbolic of Margo's bright and colorful spirit, Layne demanded, "I don't want nobody wearing black!" While crying on the phone the day before.

Ironically, we met up with the funeral cars while coming off of the expressway. "Follow the funeral cars!" I instructed Tom, almost in a panic. "This way, we won't have to wait in what is sure to be a long line!"

My young son was tense, sad and full of questions he did not want to ask, because mommy and daddy were sad too. He loved his "Auntie Margo," and could not understand *how or why* she could die this way. At seven years old, this was his very first funeral ever, and the first day of school he had ever missed since having the measles at age four.

Upon arriving at the church, we still had to wait in line for about one half hour, until the funeral directors seated the family. It was rainy, cold and sleeting. The weather conditions were impeccably similar to the weather on the day Margo was murdered. People had arrived early. I overheard one woman say to another, "I've been standing out here since 9:30 this morning."

Inside, television cameras, uniformed and plain clothes detectives were quietly stationed in all four corners of the sanctuary and outlined the vestibule and aisle ways. Cranston was the first person I saw upon entering the door. I later learned that at my mother's request, he was waiting for me. Looking at one another and without speaking, Cranston and I just grabbed hands and held on tight. Tom, Cranston, Ian, and I all held hands in a single file as we slowly made our way to Margo's casket. This was the saddest day I had experienced in my life since my father's tragic death and funeral in 1965 . . . *so much pain and sorrow.*

"That's my baby . . . that's my baby!" Patient Jaquetta Poole heard Ms. Lillie cry out as she was led down the aisle toward

Margo's remains. "I will never forget that sound, hearing her cry out like that!" Jaquetta admits.

The casket was powder-blue, and paradoxically, Margo was dressed in the same powder-blue outfit she wore to Douglas' son, Prescott's, funeral just a few years prior. The inside hood of her casket bore a beautiful brushed script message written in bright blue lettering:

Remember Me From The Things I Have Done.

While walking past the front pew, I saw Ms. Lillie, Kenya and Douglas. Ms. Lillie's chest was heaving up and down to the beat of heavy sobbing as she cradled Kenya in one arm. Kenya was crying heavily. At only twelve years old, unfortunately, I *knew* what she was feeling. Douglas was not showing any emotion at all. As much as I wanted to greet him *I couldn't.* My body would not allow me to embrace that cold chill I'd felt in him before; ***not today! Not*** here while Margo's embalmed corpse looked on. For now, my husband shaking Doug's hand had to be enough from my family. I could not believe how Douglas was just sitting there stoic, as if he were waiting for all this hoopla nonsense to be over with, so he could get on with his life. His demeanor made me feel sick.

Ms. Lillie looked up at me, and I remember reaching toward her with one hand, while Tom held the other tightly. As I reached for her, I remember hearing a yelping, bawling sound come from deep inside of me . . . an *aching* sound of pain I'd never made before, and never knew existed inside of me. Tom squeezed me tight as if he thought I was getting ready to let loose something he would not be able to control.

I filed past Margo's casket. She looked so pretty, even in death. Frances was standing guard, making sure no one touched her baby sister, and when I tried, she said, "not uh" waving my hand away. I understood. If everyone who wanted to touch Margo had been allowed to, the funeral would have never ended and her body would have been a mess. I sought to stand next to the casket longer and never leave Margo, but the line was too long and people were waiting. We walked toward the pews that were roped off for "Doctors only." As soon as I saw Joyce and Pam sitting in the pew behind where we were getting ready to sit, I asked Joyce for one of her nerve pills.

"Have you ever taken one of these before?"

"No."

"Don't you *ever tell* Tom I gave you this!" she warned.

"I won't, I just know I *really* need it." I reached out and grabbed Pam's hand and squeezed it really tight. She was composed but sobbing hard. Overwhelmed with grief, neither one of us could speak. All we could seem to do was just squeeze hands. With the help from the accompaniment of mucus and tears I swallowed the nerve pill . . . it seemed to help.

As the funeral calling hours progressed, Margo's casket became filled with memorabilia. There was everything from an expensive Chicago Bulls jacket from her good friend Eddie Ponder, who is now deceased, to family photos. Margo loved the Chicago Bulls, but specifically, Michael Jordan. Margo loved Michael Jordan so much, she would get angry if anyone said a negative thing about him, ever!

Margo's casket was so filled, she was nearly covered with various artifacts. Eddie Ponder must have passed by Margo's casket at least twenty times. He would walk by, then get back in line again. Since we sat very close to the front, I would just get up whenever the mood hit me, and walk up to Margo. Both black and white softball friends and foes from years gone by, attended the funeral in droves; hugging me, each other and offering condolences.

Surreptitiously, *New Friend* was prancing around Margo's funeral like it was the party of the year. No sadness appeared on her face, in her demeanor and apparently not in her heart, only gaiety. I could not understand why and how she could be so celebratory over such a tragedy involving someone who was *supposed* to be, according to her, her *best friend.* From where we sat, I was in a position to watch everything and everyone. Particularly Douglas. A mutual friend walked past Douglas without greeting him. *New Friend* chased her down, grabbed her hand stating, "Aren't you going to say something to Douglas?" while leading her back to greet him. I was very distraught at the time, and paid little consideration to this interaction. Then, I noticed *New Friend* in a rear hallway talking and laughing with a guy who I recognized to be the stripper who danced at Margo's lingerie party. I became angry and voiced my concern to Tom, "How *dare* her invite a *stripper* to Margo's funeral! He didn't know Margo, he was only hired as entertainment at her party! How dare her! *What* is wrong with this woman!"

"Relax babe, you're just upset." I was not *just* upset. I was ***completely disturbed*** by the inappropriateness of what I saw! I instantly acquired a stress headache and was ready to open up a can of whoop-ass on somebody!

* * *

Upon exiting the church, a final viewing was offered for Margo's family members only. The casket was placed near the exit door. Tom, Cranston, Ian, and I stood up to join in the final viewing line. Someone approached me from behind and grabbed my arm. When I turned around, it was my cousin Rodney Harris who, like Layne, was on the brink of stardom with his comedy. Rodney had also grown up across the street from Margo at my grandfather's home. His eyes were blemished and sad. All we could do was hug each other. Before walking away he whispered, "I love you, cousin, hang in there."

While filing past Margo's casket for one final time, I secured my letter under her pillow. All other memorabilia had been removed earlier just before the eulogy. I did not want my letter to be confiscated so I retrieved it before it could be removed. I was insistent that the letter be buried with Margo. While sobbing intensely, I leaned over and kissed Margo's unpleasantly cool face as many times as I could before leaving her. I looked up and saw Layne standing at the head of Margo's casket . . . the niece Margo had literally, in many ways raised and mothered over the past twenty years. I was crying so hard I could not speak, I could only look at Layne in sorrowful disbelief.

Standing next to Layne, I saw an attractive black female. It was detective King, who I had spoken to at the scene of Margo's murder. As our eyes met, I could actually feel my facial expression *pleading* with her to *find the bastard who did this!* Her eyes never left mine. She gestured her left hand to her ear with the telephone sign. I read her lips to say, "I'm going to call you."

At that very moment, I felt an astounding sense of relief overcome me. A feeling I had not felt since this madness began. I actually felt justice was on its way.

Upon exiting, I hugged many people, including Giselle Ponder, Eddie's wife. Giselle was not crying, but appeared to still be in shock perseverating over and over again, "We're going to miss her . . . we're going to miss her . . . we're . . ." I noticed a man crying profusely in the doorway. He looked to be Margo's new companion. I recognized him from the picture Margo had shown me the Monday before her murder. I approached him to clarify his identity, give him a hug, and to tell him, "Margo was happy when she died, and she was happy because of you!" He shook his head to greet me and stated he remembered Margo mentioning my name to him. Then, as if he truly believed what I was saying he stated, "Thank you." Before leaving the ceremony, *Mr. Happy invites him over to the house.*

Joyce did not attend Margo's burial. "I just did not want to see them put her in the ground," she confessed. I did not attend the burial either, but for an additional reason. The funeral went on for so long, I had only one half hour to get to the University of Akron. President Bill Clinton was speaking on campus the following day, and my department had selected me to attend the open forum as a student representative. Due to high security concerns, had I not gotten my ticket before five o'clock, I would not have been able to attend the open forum.

After retrieving the ticket, I did not go to the funeral dinner, to Margo's home or anywhere else. I went home. I took off my dark sunglasses and looked in the mirror. After six hours of crying, my eyes were nearly swollen shut. I looked awful! There is no way I *would* have gone anywhere looking like that! I went upstairs, undressed, crawled into bed, curled up in a fetal position, called my mother and cried some more.

At her home and during the evening of Margo's funeral, Ms. Lillie and other family members were met with yet ***another***

tragic blow to the family. The family had left the church from having dinner, and had stopped by sister Edith's home. Margo's brother James stated he did not feel well, which was understandable after the day's events. Only a couple of hours after her burial, and possibly due to his shock and grief, after arriving at Margo's home her brother James, the eldest child in the family, suffered a massive stroke of the brain and was rushed to Akron General Medical Center; the very hospital his baby sister worked at for nearly twenty years.

James' wife, a registered nurse, eventually had him moved to a hospital back home in California where a craniotomy was performed. To this day, James is still alive and living in California, ***but does not remember his baby sister Margo is dead.*** When he comes to visit Ms. Lillie in the summertime he asks, "Where's Margo?"

"She's not here right now," Ms. Lillie responds.

"Okay." James acquiesces, but still not understanding Margo ***is never coming back.***

An hour or two later, he'll ask again. . . . "Where's Margo?" Ms. Lillie will offer the same answer as the one before . . . "She's not here right now."

This question and answer narrative will go on throughout the day. Ms. Lillie doesn't mind. She enjoys *remembering* her youngest child not being home because she is working, rather than because she is dead. I've asked Ms. Lillie if she will ever tell James the truth.

"NO! I'm afraid it will kill him. You know, out of all my children, he was the one who encouraged Margo to go on and date Douglas. I think if he remembers Margo was killed, it would *kill him.* I don't want to lose another child. When he visits, I won't even take him to the cemetery with me. I don't *want* him to remember Margo's dead."

Twenty
And the Dead Shall Speak

Gossip ran amuck in the days, weeks and months following the murder of Dr. Margo Prade. Some rumors became so rampant, they actually took on their own life form; having arms, legs, standing up . . . walking and talking all over town. One rumor, however, never seemed to ever really have closure, not even after Dr. Prade's killer was convicted. It was the rumor that there were *two people* who entered Margo's van on that fateful day . . . a man and a *woman*. Moreover, once the bite mark on Margo's left arm became publicized, the "woman rumor" had even more credence.

"It had to be a woman! No man would bite a woman like that unless they're gay! Men are too macho! Men don't bite in the middle of a fight."

These comments were whisperings that lingered about town as people engaged in their daily activities. Margo's murder captivated the uninformed, and fascinated the ill-informed. Unfortunately, those ill-informed individuals continued to feed into an erroneous rumor that the female culprit involved in the murder was one Delphenia Gilbert, the wife of a prominent attorney, career woman and mother. "Someone had sent a letter to the police and the FBI, saying that I pretended to be Margo's friend, but that I hated her," Ms. Gilbert reflected in a Dateline NBC interview.

It has never really been quite understood as to why this particular rumor took on an alien life form that lived on for weeks on end. Even other professionals within the community, whom would be thought to know better, engaged in this rumor's journey through the thoughts and minds of the community. I, however, never believed in the rumor and would not allow those who called my home to mention it. Often the phone would ring with someone on the other end, sizzling with sensational innuendos:

"Donzella . . . I heard that Del . . ."

"Stop! I don't want to hear it!"

"But everybody's saying she . . ."

"Everybody's ***WRONG!*** Why would that woman, who is a wife, mother, and has a successful career want to kill Margo so savagely? Use your head! It doesn't make sense . . . it just doesn't fit and I don't want to hear it. Besides, all these false rumors are just going to throw the police off and prolong their investigation of the real culprit and people need to stop spreading them! I want Margo's killer caught as soon as possible and this stupid shit will interfere with that!"

"Donzella . . . I know Margo was your best friend but you have to believe that if ***everybody's*** saying . . ."

"Listen to yourself! Don't you think that woman would have been arrested by now if the rumor was true? I don't want to hear it anymore! Please do not call me with this again . . . please! I've got enough to deal with right now! I'm cutting ***everybody off*** if they keep calling me with this shit! I . . . DON'T . . . BELIEVE . . . IT . . . OKAY!"

In addition to being overly annoyed with the callers of, and contributors to the rumor, I also felt empathy for the Gilberts. I would not have wished the "who murdered Dr. Margo Prade" rumor on my worst enemy, even though I had none accept Douglas; and in my mind, he ***was*** the killer.

Margo *was so well loved that* some members of the community actually developed murderous intentions themselves over the dreadful crime. It was not uncommon to take notice of people submitting to true confessions and subtle mumblings stating, "If I knew who did this . . . I mean actually *knew* for sure . . . they would not make it to trial! I'd kill the son-of-a-bitch myself! I loved Dr. Prade!"

I could not *imagine* how the Gilbert family dealt with folks looking at them with a jaundiced eye everywhere they went. According to an article in the Akron Beacon Journal titled, "Gilbert's Fight Back," Ed Gilbert stated that, even in church one Sunday another member glared at them and gestured their fingers with cocking a gun and shooting them. In ***church!*** Sometimes *hypocrisy* knows no boundaries.

I felt so bad for the Gilberts. Attorney Gilbert once represented me in a case against my sergeant when I worked for Akron Police. I wanted to do something helpful. One day I pulled into a gasoline station pay phone, looked up their phone number and called. By this time I was extremely paranoid and not sure of my suspicions that my phone line was tapped were real or Memorex. I left a message on their answering machine. I did not leave my name, but wanted them to know that at least *one person* in Akron *disbelieved* this cruel and invalid rumor. I had hoped the phone call would make the Gilbert's feel better.

What was most perplexing about the Delphenia Gilbert rumor was that it became so authentic that at least one Northeastern Ohio radio station actually broadcasted her arrest. The station was eventually sued by Attorney Gilbert.

How did the Delphenia Gilbert rumor begin? According to investigator Craig Gilbride, an anonymous female sent the letter to the Akron Police Detective bureau and the FBI implicating Ms. Gilbert. At the time, there was only one female who fit the category of someone who would want Margo gone, and it ***was not*** Delphenia Gilbert. In addition, many other people were implicated in Margo's murder including me, my husband and Joyce.

Just about anyone who was remotely close to Margo became a suspect to either rule in, or rule out. So why did this particular rumor explode like thunder and travel like lightning? Those of us who were close to Margo and her case will never really know the answer to this question. However, I believe the general public was so infuriated by the scandalous murder of Dr. Margo Prade, that they ***wanted swift and certain justice, and they wanted it*** to the point that they were willing to employ any plausible revealing factor, and willing to *sacrifice anyone.* Given this, I chose to travel about town incognito. Due to continued media coverage, I purposefully went out and purchased a black trench coat, wore black clothes, sunglasses and hat. Everywhere I went, except for school, people who knew me, also knew I was close to Margo and Douglas. People wanted to hear the story and ask questions. When I wore all black, I was at ease and unnoticed; just the way I wanted it. My graduate school colleagues and professors were merciful, and only asked, "How are you doing?"

There was not a grocery store, beauty shop, department

store, bus stop or any other public arena a person could enter and the murder of Dr. Margo Prade was not being discussed in the background.

The phone calls too, were continuous. People like my long-time friend and retired police officer Cee Jay, would call on the phone almost daily; primarily due to my mother's request that he "check up on me."

"Douglas is a lot of things . . . but kill Margo! I don't think Douglas would do no shit like that!"

[silence]

"Don . . . you there?"

"Yeah . . . I'm here."

"I *said* . . . I don't think Doug would do no shit like that! Doug is too smart to do something like that. He would not be that stupid. There is no way a cop would do something like that, 'cause he would be the number one suspect . . . he automatically *knows* he would be the number one suspect especially since he was married to her!"

However prompted, I had to remain silent in my true convictions.

"Well, whoever did it, their life is over too . . . and I hope they get arrested soon and burn in hell for what they've done to Margo! She did not deserve to die like this. God did not intend for her to go out like this!" I began to get emotional, as I often did when people would call.

"I know that's right! Margo didn't deserve to die like that. Hell, Everybody *loved* Margo . . . plus she was a doctor too . . . she was our shining star! You can't find one person in Akron to say anything bad about Margo! This shit is fucked up, Don!"

He continued, almost yelling. "Shot six times! Hell, *nobody* I know, not even my enemies deserve to die like that! This is some ***fucked up shit!"*** He paused.

"Shit!" he concluded in anger. "I'll see ya. . . ."

"Okay."

Realizing our emotions beginning to surface and not willing to share them with each other today, CeeJay and I hung up the phone until the next time we dispensed our *grief and anger management therapy on one another.*

*   *   *

Margo's lifeless body had been hosed down, washed and ready for examination. Even though rigor mortis had begun to set in and her body was clean, a massive pool of blood lay beneath her head. The blood flowed past her neck towards her shoulder blades. Margo's right arm lay to her side, and her left stretched completely out extending beyond the gurney. Her corpse was riddled with bullet wounds. Margo's right wrist, labeled entrance defense wound #1, bore an incredible large black burn with a hole in the middle. The force of the bullet was so intense, that it shot the tennis bracelet off her arm. That same bullet entered the lower rear of the right side of Margo's skull, just to the left of her ear. The wound looked to be the size of a quarter, and according to coroner testimony, [that bullet] "did not kill her," but may have severely stunned her or rendered her unconscious. In essence, Margo *suffered dearly,* experiencing twice the amount of pain she should have from that first projectile. Her suffering however, had just begun. The bullet that actually killed my dear friend was the one that entered her torso.

The slug swiftly pierced Margo's beating heart, flitting around like a pinball. In a fraction of a second, the bullet crafted four holes in Margo's heart. In those seconds however, according to coroner testimony, Margo did, in fact, experience "excruciating pain for four to six seconds before death occurred." And finally, according to coroner testimony, Margo's killer shot her four more times "***after***" death occurred. Those bullets ravaged her upper back, breasts, buttocks and pelvic area. In no uncertain terms, this was a signature crime with emotional wrath and detestation written all over it. An unrelenting crime that had gone on for ninety seconds. A fight to the finish with results deliberately gone unnoticed for at least an hour, because that is the way the killer wanted it.

The original "whodunit" scuttlebutt in the community favored a murder for hire theme . . . a worst case scenario, and a random act of violence as best case scenario. No one, however, wanted *to believe or even entertain* the thought that someone would *intentionally* kill Dr. Margo Prade or *want* her dead. Moreover, criminal justice theory would suggest that a hired killer would have rendered one to two bullets in the temple for a quick and painless death, and a robbery suspect would have stolen something. A random act of violence most likely would not have occurred in such a busy parking lot and probably would have accompanied a robbery. If a down and out citizen of the neighborhood was having a bad day and wanted to be violent towards someone, that someone probably *would not* have been Margo, she was too *well known and loved* in the community; and their victim most likely would have been cussed out or assaulted.

No, this murder was no accident and was most certainly premeditated. At the very least it was a crime of passion, and at the most it was *planned.* A calculated and flagrant action that spiraled many in the community into a point of no return. This crime sent many of us in the community into an abyss of darkness that overshadowed the serene glow of daylight for many days, months and years to follow. Nevertheless, ***there is no perfect crime,*** and this particular murder had *someone's* name ***and*** an *unusual set of prints* written all over it.

"Look at my arm . . . !" The corpse of Dr. Margo Prade seemed to broadcast without speaking. In every single position she was turned on the gurney to examine and retrieve bullet fragments from her body; Margo's left arm was outstretched . . . chronicling the events of her murder that was just a few hours old. Margo's arm offered up a peculiar kind of evidence. A dying declaration identifying a sadistic killer . . . *her killer.*

Margo was left-handed and this time, her left arm gave her strength in achieving justice. Metaphorically speaking, I believe even in death, Margo's left arm remained true to being a dominant force of strength for her by guiding investigators to the one and only significant piece of physical evidence. Her nail beds had been removed in order to examine underneath her fingernails, looking for any foreign blood particles or skin tissue not belonging to her DNA. The blood covering her lab jacket was also tested. However, because Margo had bled profusely, it was determined that her blood may have washed away any other identifiable foreign blood or tissue.

The bite mark on Margo's upper left arm, however, was so

horrendous, and so vicious that it penetrated both her lab jacket and blouse, and left a deep impression in her skin. The mark left such a cavernous impression, that forensic dental expert Dr. Lowell Levine was able to make a waxed dental impression from the mark. That particular evidence at the very least, put Margo's killer at the scene of the crime and therefore, ultimately led to his arrest. Dr. Levine's forensic skill rendered him notoriety in the famous sexual assault case of sports announcer Marv Albert a few years prior to Margo's murder. Once again, his skill in forensic dentistry helps bring justice to all that is ugly in the world. The conviction rendered in Margo's murder case, however, was not won on the bite mark alone; although without that evidence, some folks still believe because Douglas was a police captain, the case would have gone unsolved.

Twenty-one
The Investigation

To say the investigation into the murder of Dr. Margo Prade was a daunting task would be an understatement. And, after the investigation's completion and the killer's conviction, nearly every single detective who was on the case, and who was eligible to retire, did. Given the volume of horrendous murder cases they had processed over the years, detectives Duvall, Myers, Gaines, and White, to name a few, had the wind taken out of their sails with this case. Why? Because this one was different.

Regardless of what many officers may have thought of Captain Douglas Prade, whether they liked him or loathed him, investigating a fellow officer for murder is a task no officer would want to perform. It was the first time in the history of the Akron Police Department that an officer was investigated for murder; and because of this, the detectives investigating the case were under tremendous stress, pressure and scrutiny from every angle imagined.

One evening shortly after Margo's funeral, I phoned her home to speak with Ms. Lillie. I knew Douglas would probably answer the phone and I was prepared for that. What I was not prepared for was the conversation that took place.

"Hi, Douglas . . . how are you doing? This is Donzella. I was just calling to speak to Ms. Lillie if she is there, and to just see how you all are holding up."

Coldly, he responded, "Yeah, I've been meaning to talk to you. *I heard what you said.*"

*   *   *

"Excuse me, what are you talking about? I haven't said anything to anybody!"

"I heard what you said . . . *to the police.* I would appreciate it if you don't come around here anymore or call over here."

"Well . . . I don't know what you have heard or who you've been talking to, but I will *certainly abide by your wishes.*"

We hung up. It was too late in the evening to call Detective King, but I phoned her the next day. By this time, even phone calls to the detectives were short, discrete and spoken in "code."

"Detective King speaking."

Without giving my name, I state, "Something's come up!"

"We'll be over."

"Okay." We hung up.

Several hours later Detective Miles, arrived at my home. Detective King was on another assignment. I tell him about my conversation with Douglas, told him how I considered his directive a *threat* and asked what I should do.

"Do I need to carry my gun with me now everywhere I go? Because I will! I'm going to tell you right now, I loved Margo but I am not like her in many ways. If I think someone is out to get ***me***, I'll get *them first* before they *will ever* get close enough to get me! I have done nothing wrong here and I certainly do not deserve to be another murder victim . . . and I won't be! I have a family!"

"As a police officer, I cannot legally tell you to carry a concealed weapon. But I can say do what you feel you can to protect yourself. I mean . . . we are watching our backs too. Someone broke into our offices and went through the trash cans looking for notes on the case. Now, we have to memorize as much information as we can, or type the information on a home computer, save it on a disc and place the disc in a locked drawer away from the department. And, every time we come to your house, we take a different route to make sure we are not being followed." I decided because my son was so young, and except for my going to school, he along with his friends was always in my car. I decided I would never want small children to witness something as horrific as a gun fight while they're in my car . . . you're talking major childhood trauma now. I decided to put my faith in God, and just be extra careful and aware of my surroundings wherever I went.

On another evening after returning home from Margo's, Ms. Lillie was accosted by a black male in the dark of night while entering her home. After fighting the man off, he dashed away as readily as he had appeared. Ms. Lillie lived in her home for over forty years without incident. Now, all of a sudden she is accosted. Was this attack a coincidence or contrived? If any person knew ***everything*** about Margo's personal and professional life, it was her beloved mother, Ms. Lillie. To this day I believe Ms. Lillie's attack was a warning . . . perhaps to keep her mouth shut, or at the very least for her to be afraid enough to mask whatever she'd planned to disclose to the police. Hence, another investigation had to take place simultaneously that now involved Ms. Lillie.

The question was never answered, but the question remained . . . was the attack on Ms. Lillie orchestrated to throw the police off from investigating Margo's murder even if for a few days? This killer needed to be caught . . . and soon! This was *serious.* Like a bad dream that one could not wake up from. Not only had Margo been savagely murdered just one week earlier, but now it appears everyone's safety may be in jeopardy; including the police and perhaps particular members of Margo's family as well as her friends.

In the weeks that passed, the local newspaper too, added undue pressure for the detectives' investigation by printing confidential information gathered in private interviews. The information was being leaked to certain members of the press, and the reporter printed information that could have botched the entire case had the wrong information been printed. Eventually, the Chief of Police publicly issued a gag order, which included punitive reprimands for any police personnel suspected of talking to the press.

* * *

The initial investigation into the murder of Dr. Margo Prade began immediately after her murder. According to Craig Gilbride, "Along with the interviews at the office, we canvassed the surrounding neighborhood immediately after leaving the scene, asking questions and passing out our cards." Douglas was also given a lie detection test almost immediately, and was told by authorities that he passed the test.

As a courtesy to the family, Akron Police did not thrust their investigation into high gear until after Margo was buried. When the investigation began, however, the detectives went into it full throttle, including utilizing the efforts and skill of the FBI from the beginning, to the end. Because the department was potentially looking at a high ranking internal affairs police captain as a possible suspect, and because the *public was looking at them,* it was necessary to employ the FBI to help preserve the integrity of the investigation. This was one case where detectives could not leave any stone unturned, or leave any assumption to question. With this case involving the murder of a popular Akron Physician, who was freshly divorced from her police captain husband, to the public, you are not only looking at a possible cover-up by the captain's colleagues, the entire Akron Police Department may also be publicly sporting a shiny new black eye should Douglas actually be the murderer. This was a very difficult time for the image of the Akron Police Department, and for those garnered to bring justice to this heinous crime.

Duvey

His father was a detective sergeant for the Akron Police department, and he grew up knowing many of the older detectives. After joining the Akron Police Department at the youthful age of 21, Ed Duvall, affectionately called, "Duvey" by many, was the youngest police recruit in his class.

Ed Duvall retired from Akron police in May, 1999 after thirty years of service, moved to Columbus, Ohio and went to work for Maureen O'Conner at the Ohio Attorney General's office. Ms. O'Conner was the Summit County Prosecutor in Margo's murder case. Ed Duvall was no stranger to the pressures and perils of police work. By the time he retired, he had been involved in a county public corruption case, four shootouts in the line of duty—two of which were fatal, and multiple car accidents which rendered him fourteen hospitalizations.

In 1973, officer Ed Duvall was assigned to the homicide division of the Akron Police Detective bureau. In May of 1977, he made sergeant. However, he remained in the detective bureau. In 1992 Duvey was promoted to Lieutenant and was asked by the

Chief of police to start an Internal Affairs Unit, for which Douglas Prade became a member. Hence, for the majority of his career, Ed Duvall had been investigating crimes against persons and crimes committed by police.

To say he was a seasoned, senior homicide detective at the time of Margo's murder would be an understatement. Lieutenant Ed Duvall was undeniably, the ***detective's detective.*** Duvey was no stranger to investigating high profile cases, or to bringing high profile dignitaries to their knees if crimes were committed. In 1979, while working in the detective bureau, then Sgt. Ed Duvall and his partner were directly involved in an investigation involving public corruption in Summit County, Ohio. That investigation led to the arrest and conviction of several high profile individuals, including Common Pleas Court Judge James Barbuto, the then county sheriff and auditor; an Akron Police Captain; the secret service officer for the Summit County prosecutor's office and the county coroner. At the time, this investigation was one of the top ten in the country, and was a three year endeavor from 1979 to 1981. The case involved white slavery of black women who had gone before judge Barbuto for misdemeanor crimes such as shoplifting, prostitution, drug abuse and theft. In effect, the judge was running a plantation of prostitution out of his courtroom, in exchange for suspended sentences.

Ed Duvall and his partner received several awards, including the International Association of Chiefs of Police Parade Magazine Police Officer of the Year Award, the B.L.E.O.A. Award for Criminal Justice and one national award for their bravery and investigative efforts in the case. The investigation, however, was not without personal peril. Duvey and his partner received information from FBI intelligence in Cleveland, Ohio that there was a $10,000 per man, hit out on him, his partner, and the chief of police. The case was so high profile, it not only reached national news, the case brought famed newsman Geraldo Rivera to Akron, Ohio and I remember asking for and getting his autograph when I saw him one afternoon in the lunch room. The Barbuto case put Akron, Ohio on the media map throughout the country.

Unfortunately, eighteen years later Lieutenant Detective Ed Duvall would be involved in yet another fall from grace, high-profile, media-worthy case, again involving another Akron Police captain. But this case was different. According to Duvey, "This case was more emotionally gut wrenching than any other case I've ever worked . . . *any other case.*"

Douglas Prade was the second officer assigned to the Internal Affairs department. He was assigned to IA by the chief of police, after the murder of his son. At the time, Ed Duvall was the only other IA officer. Duvey stated, "Honestly, I have to say I was not happy with the chief's choice. Even though I, like everybody was devastated by the fact that an officer rolled up in his cruiser only to find his only son had been shot. But, Doug did not like white people too much, I didn't feel as comfortable with him as I did my other partners," [some of who were black, as Duvey named them]. "We were work associates, we were not friends, we did not go out after work, but we were very cordial to each other. I did most of the investigation work, and he was very comfortable doing the review of paperwork. I will say when we were working on a case together, we were always pretty much in agreement with the assessment of the case results." Duvey clearly and candidly emphasized, however, "but we *were not at all friends.* After work, he went his way and I went mine. That was a very difficult time in my life because I have *always enjoyed* a great relationship with my partners. I mean, you spend more waking hours with your partner than you do with your family when you include extra jobs, working overtime etcetera, etcetera. Doug never shared conversation with me about his personal life. . . . I mean his most dominant conversation with me about his personal life was about his two girls, Kenya and Sahara . . . about their accomplishments and achievements. But, very limited conversation about Margo, or her practice. Unfortunately for me, I didn't get to know Margo in-depth and in detail until ***after*** she died."

* * *

On November 26th 1997, Lt. Ed. Duvall had just put the finishing touches on another public scandal case involving the successful conviction of an Akron Police Deputy Chief. According to Duvey, "The scandal ended with a meeting with the top brass of the NEC World Series of Golf, on how we were going to address extra job assignments in the future, to help alleviate their fears that no one would be bilking them out of their money again."

Duvey recalled where he was at the time he learned of Margo's murder. "I was in my office up in the Juvenile division. I was called and ushered into the chief's office. When I opened the door, no one had to say anything . . . and you could just see it on everyone's faces that they were in shock. The chief told me Dr. Margo Prade had been found shot at the office and asked if I could go out and find Doug and notify him. I went and got Bill [Douglas' longtime friend] who was also visibly shaken up, took my car and we go out to an address that Bill had off Jacoby road in Copley, Ohio to his apartment. Bill was in shock. He really cared about Margo . . . he thought a lot of her. I'd seen Bill in combat conditions, where he was shot for the second time. But I'd never seen him like this . . . I thought a lot of Bill, he's a great guy." Having known Douglas lived through and survived the tragic death of his son, at the time Duvey could only feel sympathy for Douglas. "I'm thinking, how are we going to break *this news* to him. . . ."

As it turned out, the two were not able to find Douglas' apartment, and even though they were the police, they had no jurisdiction in Copley, and due to privacy issues the management would not cooperate. After calling back to the station to find a possible address, they learned Douglas was already *on the scene* of Margo's murder. Upon arriving on the scene, Duvey recalls, "You could tell by the body language of the people standing around, that this was *not good.*" After entering the dentist's office across the hall and seeing Douglas, Bill went directly to him. Duvey, although emotional, felt he would be more useful outside with Lieutenant Mary Myers, who was commander of the person's unit, and in charge of this homicide.

Because of his experience in investigating homicides, but also not wanting to interfere with Mary's investigation, Duvey asked Mary, "Has anyone asked Doug for his weapon? You know we have to do that even though he is a police captain. We have to take custody of his weapon and we have to make sure that weapon is checked." Lt. Myers concurred and they both approached Douglas. His weapon was in a fanny pack in his unmarked cruiser which was on the scene. Lt. Mary Myers gave custody of the weapon to Duvey, and he recalls, "I know it was distasteful to ask a fellow police officer for his weapon under these circumstances." Duvey then left the scene so that the weapon could be taken to BCI (Bureau of Criminal Investigations) to be test fired, even though at the time, Duvey states, "I did not know if she [Margo] was shot, stabbed or what, but I wanted to make sure. But, it was a two-fold thing: Number one was to protect the Akron Police Department so no one could say, hey we are showing favoritism to a fellow officer, and number two, if in fact . . . heaven forbid, that he [Douglas] lost it [the gun] or was involved in this [murder] that we had the evidence if he drove up to the scene with it [the gun]." After Duvey returned to the police station, he had Douglas' weapon tagged into evidence and turned it over to the two pawn detectives and ordered them to take the weapon immediately over to BCI to be checked. This was the extent of Lt. Ed Duvall's involvement in the murder case of Dr. Margo Prade on the day of her murder. He would, however, later be asked to return to the investigation and he did . . . with a vengeance, examining all the mysteries intertwined in this crime.

The big mystery, according to Duvey, was the car. "We know exactly what time he turned on that cruiser when [Douglas' mistress] paged him [about the murder]. As soon as he turned on the key, the radio comes on, it registers with the police station and it marked that as the first time that day that [cruiser] had been turned on. It took him exactly six minutes to get from his apartment to the scene of the crime, but he did not use *that* car [as the getaway car]. According to Duvey, "The clothes Douglas wore (which had to be covered in blood), the car used and the weapon were all probably confined in the car [used in the murder] and later taken out. *Which is . . . there is no question about it, still a mystery.*" Those mysteries coupled with informational leaks to the press and the doubt perceived by some officers that the chief of police, who was one of Douglas' best friends, would somehow compromise the case made for an overwhelmingly complex investigation assignment. However, according to Duvey, "To me, he [the chief] was appropriate. He never articulated anything. What I got from him was 'do your job,' when I was called back in on the case."

Gilbride

Major Craig Gilbride joined the Akron Police Department on September 12, 1977. He spent four years as a patrolman and was transferred to the detective bureau working the rape, robbery and homicide unit from 7 P.M. to 3 A.M. He was promoted to Sergeant in 1986, spending two years as a supervisor in the narcotics bureau, and some time in the radio room. At one time, I had the pleasure of having him as my sergeant on the night shift before I resigned. It was during that time, that my colleagues and I began to affectionately call him "Gilbride."

In 1992 Gilbride was promoted to Lieutenant and in 1995 to Captain. In 2000 Captain Craig Gilbride was promoted to Deputy Chief of the uniform sub-division and still holds that position today. Major Gilbride is one of very few officers who worked on the Prade case, who has not fully retired.

Craig Gilbride was nine years Douglas' junior on the police department. The first and only time he and Douglas were paired up to work together was during an internal investigation of a ranking officer which involved prostitution and money laundering. At the time, Craig Gilbride was a captain and commander of the narcotics bureau, and Douglas was commander of platoon four the 7:00 P.M.-to 3:00 A.M. shift. IA was tied up on another investigation, and the chief of police paired the two together to investigate the scandal.

Gilbride's initial opinion of Douglas was that he was very intelligent and well spoken, and they actually tested against one another for the captain's exam. "Personally, I never had a problem with Doug. I didn't know him that well, and he was very closed-lipped . . . very closed-mouthed. I knew who he was and would obviously say hello, how are you when I would see him."

However, while working together for that short period of time, Gilbride admits, "I was working with him at the time [of Margo's murder] and I didn't know he was divorced." Not only did his colleagues on the department not know he was divorced, but neither did Douglas' closest friends . . . including his friend and Chief of police, Ed Irvine.

The fact that ***no one*** who Douglas communicated with on a regular basis and/or was friends with knew he and Margo were divorced, gives wonderment as to why he held on to the secrecy of his divorce, particularly when divorce is somewhat commonplace amongst police environments. This gives rise to the question . . . was Douglas' reluctance to disclose his divorce to his friends, in fact, part of a calculated scheme to make Margo's execution look a lot like a random act of violence, an angry patient or some kind of personal vendetta?

* * *

When the call came in of the shooting at 1557 Wooster Avenue, Captain Craig Gilbride was at an off-site location of the narcotics division, he had his radio on in the office when the call went out over the air. After hearing the call, Gilbride called into Chief Irvine's office and spoke to his administrative aide, Harold Craig.

"Hey, what the *hell* is going on?" he asked.

"Hey, we think Margo Prade has just been shot!"

"Well . . . I'm at the narcotics office . . . do you need any assistance out there . . . ?"

"Start rollin!" the chief instructed Gilbride, through Harold Craig.

Unlike Duvey, from that moment on, Gilbride was involved in the murder case of Dr. Margo Prade. Even though Gilbride and Douglas were actively working together at the time, the irony of not knowing that Douglas and Margo were now divorced, eventually raised enough suspicion amongst investigators that at the very least, *Douglas needed to be examined with a "jaundiced eye."*

"Everybody was out on this one." Gilbride defined the magnitude of police response to the murder scene of Dr. Margo Prade. "Not just for the fact that she was [believed to be] a police officer's wife, but also the fact that she was a doctor too." At the time of Margo's death, never in the criminal history of Akron, Ohio, had a physician been murdered in broad daylight, and in cold blood.

There were no immediate impressions in Gilbride's mind as to what may have caused a distinguished physician to be murdered so savagely in broad daylight as she arrived to work to practice one of her many talents . . . to heal the sick. "God only knows what the possibilities could have been at that point, it could have been an attempted car jacking, an angry patient . . . who knew?" Eventually, it just became a gradual progression, try to keep an open mind . . . I mean you hate like hell to think a policeman killed his wife, particularly a high ranking police officer . . . but as things started to progress . . . who wanted to kill Margo Prade? Who had a *motive* to kill Margo Prade? I just couldn't see it! In that investigation, and I mean we interviewed tons and tons of people, we could not find one person to say a bad thing about that woman, and THAT is unheard of!"

For a person to have had as much exposure to the public as Margo Prade had, exposure to people from just about every realm of society and every walk of life; from patients to softball players, a large family, colleagues, friends and no foes to speak of, after interviewing over approximately 400 people, no one had an ill word to speak of regarding Margo Prade. *It was as if she was a saint.* Nevertheless, according to Gilbride, "Anything that moved that day [of the murder] was stopped and questioned. We canvassed the neighborhood but did not come up with anything." After that, Gilbride stated, "It was not raining, but it was drizzling. She was slumped down on the seat, and no one could see her. I told the guys, hey, we cannot pull her out of this van. I gave an order to leave her in the van, put the van on a flatbed [tow truck] and it is all one contained crime scene."

Gilbride asserted, however, "The one thing that I really keyed in on during the investigation though were those audio tapes where she was being . . . I mean her phone was tapped. It really brought out how controlling he [Douglas] was and you know . . . without knowing the guy's background or home life, you would never know he was that controlling . . . but boy, he was!"

The audio tapes were not the only tapes discovered during the investigation. There was one more tape that was not immediately recognized . . . a video tape that belonged to Rolling Acres Dodge. The video camera was positioned in the rear parking lot of the dealership as a security camera, to capture anyone who may tamper with or actually attempt to steal any of the vehicles on the lot after hours. That camera, however, was situated in a way where it partially taped activities in the parking lot of the medical arts building. Because Margo routinely parked alongside the fence that separated her building from the dealership parking lot, that camera, unbeknownst to many, surreptitiously caught her murder on tape and *in action.* ***Hence, there is no perfect crime.***

After leaving the scene, Gilbride joined others at the coroner's office for Margo's autopsy. Margo's corpse stayed at the coroner's office for four days. The initial examination however, may have been the detectives very first clue, that this murder was beyond a doubt, a crime of rage and passion. "Every time we took off a layer of clothing, another [bullet] fragment fell out. I did not realize she had been shot so many times." Lt. Mary Myers ardently admitted during an interview. Over the next three months, and three days from November 26th 1997 to February 23rd 1998, the investigation into the murder of Dr. Margo Prade grew more intense.

As suspicions, paranoia and rumors grew, over who murdered Dr. Margo Prade, authentic fear came along for the ride. To make matters worse, the local newspaper continued their charade in reporting any and all information, real or Memorex, substantiated or unsubstantiated, and whether or not they had permission from the police department to print it.

As the investigation grew more intense, so did leaks from the police department, leaks from one police officer exclusively, to one journalist in particular. That journalist became reckless in his reporting and could have actually put many lives, including mine, in danger. When leaks to the press became overwhelming, the investigation was downsized by chief Edward Irvine to just five ranking detectives: Lt. Mary Myers, Lt. Ed Duvall, Capt. Craig Gilbride, Lt. Beth Daugherty and Detective Paul Calvaruso. Gilbride explained, "when you get a case of this magnitude, let's face it, people are going to talk . . . people are going to want to talk and people want to know what the hell is going on. I know the line staff detectives' feelings were hurt [for being taken off the case], they felt people were looking at them as the source of the leaks to the press. But they were out here too, putting their ear to the ground trying to find out whatever they could." Gilbride continues, "It [the investigation] just got too big, with too many people and as time went on, we just really had to downsize the amount of people working on the case." The irony of the downsizing effort however, was that according to a *very* reliable source, whose name will not be mentioned in this publication, the leak to the press was a high-ranking captain, not a line staff detective. Fortunately, that captain *was not* one of the final five detectives who finished the investigation.

Gaines

Detective Donald Gaines, was a twenty-three year veteran of the Akron Police Department. He was officially assigned to the investigation December 3rd 1997 by Lieutenant Mary Myers and Captain Mullins to investigate several anonymous letters. One letter was addressed to the police department and the FBI. The second letter was addressed to Captain Douglas Prade, but was sent to Margo's home. According to investigation file material, those letters were directing the police to investigate Delphenia Gilbert, the wife of a prominent attorney. The fact that someone went as far to implicate a person who was not even *remotely* involved in this murder, gave even more validity to the fact that either Douglas himself acted alone, or he may have had an accomplice, or at the very least, someone was desperately trying to thwart the investigation in another direction. But why? More importantly, *who* would create such an erroneous hypothesis? One rationale for the Delphenia Gilbert theory was that because Dr. Margo Prade was so well loved in the community, there was a general consensus that people *wanted* her killer caught . . . and caught now! And the person who started the rumor probably believed it would take off like a rocket, masking or at the very least, slowing down the process of looking at the real killer. It did. That theory, however, never explained why the finger was pointed at Mrs. Gilbert.

What did explain the "woman theory" however, was that whoever did kill Margo, also *knew she was bitten.* Men typically do not bite someone in the midst of a struggle. Biting during a fight is more indicative of female behavior and therefore, the rumor gave more *credence* to a plausible theory that a woman was the killer. Within the community, there was also looming and jaded suspicion hovering over the head of the newly divorced ex-husband, who just happened to be a police captain, who had one mistress for sure, and perhaps more. What was interesting, however, was that with Douglas being a high ranking black professional in this city, typically the black community would have been in an uproar just by the mere fact that he was a viable target to investigate. Typically, and because Douglas' position on the department earned community respect, the black community would have been proactive and infuriated, screaming about a conspiracy scheme of a "modern day lynching of a black male professional by the white power structure." The black community in Akron Ohio is not a passive community when something goes wrong that smacks of racial bias . . . they speak out. This time, ***they did not.*** In fact, the black community in Akron was *grippingly silent.*

Nevertheless, unfortunately the "whodunit" letters caused Mrs. Gilbert to be investigated in a more intense fashion; including taking bite mark impressions, hair samples, and saliva *and* blood samples from her. Mrs. Gilbert however, was not alone. Many others, including Margo's friend and office manager Joyce Foster, was also ordered to give dental impressions. I was questioned by Detectives King and Miles if I was, "Jealous of Margo" and if Margo and my husband were, "having an affair." I was also asked if I "owned a gun," and "can we please see it?" My husband, too, was questioned separately, but in my presence. He was asked if he and Margo were "having an affair." Therefore, all kinds of *friends* and colleagues had either been implicated at some point and time in

Margo's murder, and/or were seeking to be ruled in or ruled out. Nonetheless, the interrogation and investigation procedures imposed on those of us who really were her true friends were in some ways perplexing, and indicated that perhaps *someone* wanted to derail this investigation in the worst way. Ironically, I felt a personal sense of relief and comfort being questioned in the suspicious manner that I was. I knew I loved Margo, and that I did not murder her. Therefore, if I were to be questioned in this way, then *for sure,* they were going to look closely at Douglas.

Assuming she had been questioned as well, I always believed *New Friend* had a hand in at least *some* of those suspicions and rumors . . . pointing her own finger, which led police to question Margo's true friends.

Douglas Prade's locker located at the Akron Police Department, had been searched twice during the course of the investigation. On the first search, Detective Gaines was accompanied by Lt. Ed Duvall and Douglas Prade. At that time, Detective Donald Gaines was not looking for any specific item, the locker just needed to be searched. The first search on February 6, 1998 did not render anything specific. Detective Gaines went back to the locker alone about two weeks after the arrest of Douglas Prade on March 5th 1998. He returned to the locker particularly due to the fact and according to his testimony, "there was just so much stuff in that locker, that I needed more time to just take my time and go through each piece and each garment that was in that locker."

It was at that time, Detective Gaines discovered what would eventually be marked states exhibits 1, 2 and 3, retrieved from the top shelf of locker 112, of the Akron Police Department. Those items caught Detective Gaines' attention because of the outside abbreviations of "360 and T E L E," earmarking the partial home address of Margo Prade and the first four letters of the word . . . *telephone.* That discovery, evidence of an electronic stalking which began in 1996, became one of three critical pieces of evidence in Margo's murder trial.

Obstinate Trepidation

It was early February 1998. One afternoon, the phone rang . . . like it had constantly for close to three months now.

"Hello."

"It's me."

"Oh, hi, what's up?" I asked with butterflies in my stomach hoping to hear good news, not anything bad. I was just about burned out on bad news, and believed I had already acquired a stress related illness such as heart disease or cancer, that had yet to surface "I just want to let you know, they're getting ready to let Doug come back to work."

WHAT! "How can they do that!"

"This is what we're hearing. Some of us have gone to the Chief and told him we did not think this was a good idea, and how it could severely hamper our case. It's policy. We're being told that if he has not been charged, we cannot legally keep him from returning to work." In an instant, and in an effort to cope with what I was hearing, my emotions took a tailspin out of control. I began dropping "F" bombs like they were going out of style.

"Fuck policy! Policy has to be bent sometimes, and this policy may very well get some more people killed! So now what are we all supposed to do! All of us who have probably implicated him? Sit up all night long and wait for him to arrive while he's working the night shift? Sit and wait for him to come and blow all of us the hell away, too? Shit!" The caller gave no answer, but offered a very professional, "I'll keep you posted."

"Okay," I responded, scared and dismayed. "Now, what? I gotta be Annie Oakley! Sit up all night toting my gun!" I screamed aloud alone as I dialed Joyce's number. I told Joyce about the phone call.

"Just be really careful wherever you go. Don't even go out at night. I know I'm not," I warned.

"I won't, girl. I can't believe this!" Joyce said, seeming to be in as much shock as I was. "I just cannot believe this . . . how can they *allow this*!"

Not only was Douglas permitted to return to work when he was ready, and after his *bereavement leave,* he was also permitted to leave the state, including traveling to Louisiana to Kenya's gymnastic competition.

Douglas actually did return to work. According to Ed Duvall, "he had been back for about a week, going through in-service training. He had been assigned to services to help with policy and procedures while this [the investigation] was going on, but he was actually working for about two days, in the services department during the day time."

Douglas was physically working for Akron police during a time when he was now the ***strongest*** suspect in the murder of Dr. Margo Prade. Allowing Douglas the freedom to move about as he wished, and allowing him to return to work, may have been another strategy by the police to get Douglas to relax. However, in the world of psychotherapy, the best predictor of future behavior is past behavior. Basically, once you have murdered someone, it probably is a lot easier to commit murder again. With the city allowing Douglas such leverage, it only made those who implicated him in Margo's murder and those who were *investigating* him, feel more vulnerable, less safe, and even more psychologically distraught. Now, I was certain the Akron police department was either not going to, or *could not* protect *any of* us. Next to learning of Margo's murder, ***It was the worst feeling in the world.***

The next morning, feeling as if the police department was not going to shield us from harm, I felt the need to be proactive in my own safety and the safety of my family. I made a call to the Mayor's office. I did not give my name, and asked if their phone lines were taped. The lady answered, "No, they are not."

I went on to lodge my complaint stating, "There are certain people in this community that . . . until the police find out who committed this murder . . . they may be in danger if this man is permitted to return to work. I don't see how you can let him come back to work in this capacity especially since I believe *he is still a suspect* and no one has been arrested!" The woman was very kind and understanding of my concern.

"Have you voiced your complaint to the chief of police?" she asked.

"You sound African American, are you?"

"Yes."

"Well, do you read the Reporter newspaper?" (a newspaper for the African American community).

"Yes."

"Have you seen the front page of the Reporter newspaper today?" I asked, angrily.

"No, I haven't seen it yet."

"Well, he's on the front page of the Reporter newspaper standing behind the chief posing at the B.L.E.O.A. ball last weekend . . . smiling!" Near tears, I shouted a statement rather than a question. "Now, would *you* call the chief! Why the ***hell*** would I call him! The chief is one of his best friends!!"

"I understand. I'll forward your complaint, ma'am."

"Thank you!" I looked at the photograph in the Reporter again after hanging up the phone. This time, I actually *examined* it. Talking to myself aloud, I said, "*Uh huh . . . I know what you did here. You never smile and pose for pictures . . . you were always the one taking pictures . . . and in twenty years . . . you have never worn a beard . . . ever! You are once again* ***revealing*** *yourself Douglas Prade, and with the beard . . . you are trying to conceal yourself . . . a frantic attempt to camouflage the monster inside you that killed poor Margo . . . through this photograph you are telling us a story and you* ***don't even know it.***"

The photograph actually looked as if Douglas, unbeknownst to Chief Irvine, walked and stood behind him while he sat for the photograph, without the Chief ever being aware of his presence. Douglas' pose in the photograph looked to be purposeful and for *public consumption, not because the Chief of police asked him to pose with him.* There were other pictures floating around from that night. Photographs of Douglas in a tuxedo, with an interestingly patterned cummerbund; and his mistress standing at his side with a custom made dress, that *matched* his cummerbund. Rumor had it, that Douglas had his mistress' dress and his cummerbund professionally tailored . . . paid for through money from Margo's insurance policy.

According to Gilbride, after the complaint to the Mayor's office, "That's when he was put on administrative leave, and shortly thereafter, we actually made the arrest."

* * *

The search for evidence intensified in the first three weeks of February 1998, and all arrows began to point to Douglas Prade as the person who killed Dr. Margo Prade. Through their searches, a bank deposit slip had been found with several numerical deductions on it from an amount of $75,000. That was the exact amount of Margo's life insurance policy, and by early February, Douglas had *yet* to pay for Margo's funeral expenses. The phone rang. . . .

"Hello."

"It's me."

"Hi Ms. Lillie . . . what's wrong. . . . ?"

Upset, she responded, "I just got another notice from Stewart and Calhoun [Funeral Home], and Douglas ***still*** has not paid for my baby's funeral. Why won't he pay for it? He cashed the insurance policy! I can't pay for it, I don't have that kind of money!"

"He doesn't care, Ms. Lillie . . . he just doesn't care. I'll call the detectives . . . try not to worry about it."

"Well, there is something else . . ."

"What is it?"

"I don't know what is going on, but he is walking around here wearing his guns!"

"Really?"

"Yes!"

"Well, I know it is scary, but don't worry. It is not unusual for off duty police officers to wear their guns, okay? And, I will call my detective and let her know about the funeral bill."

"Okay, will you call me back?"

"Yes, I will."

Actually, it was not atypical for officers to wear their guns while not at work. In fact, during the time I worked for Akron police it was a requirement. However, through all the years Ms. Lillie had been around Douglas working, cooking, cleaning and babysitting in their home, she *had never* actually seen Douglas' guns on his person in such a visible fashion. Although I did not convey my beliefs to Ms. Lillie, I believed Douglas was sending her a very silent and *threatening* message. A message very similar to when she was accosted at her back door by a stranger shortly after Margo's murder. A message that she and I still believed may have been orchestrated by Douglas.

After Ms. Lillie's phone call, I phoned the detective bureau and informed Detective King of Margo's funeral expenses having not been paid. At this time, Detective King was not only someone I was working with professionally, but she had become my emotional confidant. Detective King found the information to be quite interesting and promised to pursue the matter further with her supervisors, and she did. Detective King called back within several minutes with more questions I could not answer about Margo's insurances; such as what company the policy was with, were there any other policies I knew of, etc. The information about the insurance policy, coupled with Margo's funeral expenses not being paid may have eventually been added to the voluminous vat of circumstantial evidence against Douglas Prade. However, before it was all said and done, there was one more disturbing phone call from Ms. Lillie. It was early afternoon.

"Hello."

"It's me . . . somethin's goin' on!"

"What is it, Miss Lillie?" I asked in earnest anticipation.

"Douglas and *New Friend* just left here, dropping a bunch of kids off for *me* to watch, so they can go to Youngstown to the dentist."

"What? The dentist! With all the dentists in Akron, why do they need to go to *Youngstown* to see the dentist? And why is *New Friend* with him? I thought she was *supposed* to be Margo's good friend! Anybody who was Margo's good friend would not be hanging out, and going out of town with Douglas right now the way she has been doing!" I was furious.

"Like I said, somethin's goin' on . . ." Ms. Lillie replied.

Something was *definitely* going on. By now, those of us who were close to the case were aware that Margo had been bitten. We knew Margo had been bitten because Joyce had to submit teeth impressions as part of her being investigated. One could only wonder now why in the middle of the afternoon Douglas was traveling all the way to Youngstown, Ohio to a dentist's office, and ***why*** was *New Friend* accompanying him?

Other key pieces of evidence were the audio tapes found by Detective Gaines. Those tapes revealed a clear effort to clandestinely stalk Margo electronically by taping all of her phone calls, including her most personal calls to patients and friends. From as early as 1996, Margo's home phone conversations had been secretly taped. The bite mark on Margo's left arm was that of someone's bottom teeth only. Douglas' bottom teeth were stationary, his top teeth were not. Margo only had an imprint of someone's bottom teeth on her lab jacket and blouse which penetrated all the way through to her left arm. And finally, it was revealed by Detective Ed Duvall, "Douglas never passed the lie detector test. We just told him he passed it to get him to relax . . . he never passed it." In hindsight, what is even more telling, however, was Douglas' response when he received the call that he had *passed* the lie detector test. According to Ms. Lillie, Douglas began crying spontaneously stating, "I *knew* I *could* pass it . . . I knew I *would*!"

Closing the Door

Detectives investigating the murder of Dr. Margo Prade worked in excess of 16 hour days. By early February, the investigative team had been downsized from the original fourteen detectives who worked the case from the beginning.

The five detectives were Capt. Craig Gilbride, Commander Mary Myers, Lt. Beth Daugherty, Detective Paul Calvaruso and after February 6th 1998, Lieutenant Ed. Duvall. The team was called, Eagle Command, under the leadership of Craig Gilbride and Mary Myers.

Mary Myers, a twenty-one year veteran, had the task of compiling, cataloging and indexing information, clues and leads. This was not a small task. In a thirty-day period, 1,100 calls had been made to the detective bureau in reference to the Margo Prade murder. Commander Myers was a tenacious detective who was working on her Ph.D in psychology at the time. In the beginning, Commander Myers was not easily convinced Douglas was the killer of Dr. Margo Prade.

"About two weeks into this [investigation] my detectives are telling me that he's [Douglas] a real potential suspect and I'm saying, I don't think so. I really don't think so. I really don't think he would do this to his wife." After irrefutable evidence began to surface however, Mary Myers could not be stopped in her relentless pursuit for solid evidence and, ultimately, justice. She had her investigators working day and night; sometimes well into the wee hours of the morning, behind locked doors. One afternoon two detectives approached her.

"Mary, Mary . . . Mary can we please have two hours off?"

"What's the matter?"

"Mary, we haven't done any shopping for our wives and it's Christmas Eve."

Commander Myers stated in a newspaper interview, "I about cried."

Detectives Daugherty and Calvaruso of Internal Affairs had worked the Prade murder case full time and had contributed all along. In addition to other tasks, Ed Duvall also was in charge of looking for evidence of wiretapping Margo's phone calls. Calvaruso was assigned to search Douglas' personal and professional records.

By the time investigators began closing in on Douglas Prade, detectives from Eagle Command continued to meet with challenges from their own colleagues. "After we got him [Douglas] out of that building [from returning to work] I decided to take his city-owned vehicle. Psychologically, we wanted to further reduce the sense of power he thought he still had," stated Ed Duvall.

"You can't just take a captain's car from him!" Duvall met with opposition from a fellow captain, who was unwilling to admit to himself that policemen can and *do* commit crimes.

"We can take the car and we're doin' it!" Duvall insisted, staying the course.

"Well, I have to clear this with somebody."

"We're taking the car!" Duvall responded.

As rumors spread throughout the department that Douglas (having been returned, then removed again from working) may be the prime suspect in the murder of Dr. Margo Prade, so did the dark humor that police officers often engage in. There were running jokes amongst line staff officers who began referring to Douglas Prade as “Captain O.J.,” referencing the O.J. Simpson trial that reached national headlines involving the murder of his ex-wife, Nichole Brown Simpson.

Twenty-two
The Arrest

On February 5, 1998 Chief Irvine, Captain Craig Gilbride and Lieutenant Mary Myers went to Summit County Prosecutor Maureen O'Conner to brief her on the status of the case. At this point, all investigative arrows were pointing toward Douglas Prade as the prime suspect in the murder of Dr. Margo Prade. The detectives were now on a very slim timeline. This meeting with Prosecutor O'Conner was the most crucial meeting because within a few hours, Douglas Prade would be returning to work as commander of the patrol division's 7 P.M. to 3 A.M. shift, and his very presence at the department could, and most certainly *would* have impeded the investigation. Due to Douglas' high-ranking status, he would have gained access to the investigative materials, witnesses, etc, and there ***was no way*** any subordinate officer would tell him, "I can't tell you that" or "I won't let you see that." Also, Douglas had began traveling out of state on the weekends with his daughters to gymnastic competitions, and no one wanted this fish to get away.

On February 6, 1998 Chief Edward Irvine assigned Lt. Ed Duvall full time to the Margo Prade murder case.

"I got the call to go down and see Chief Irvine. When I arrived, there sits Doug. He'd been back for about a week, I think. He had been in in-service training. He had been assigned to services to help with policy procedures. So when I come down, walk into the third floor chief's office, there sits Doug Prade! I go into the door, shut the door and the Chief says I'm assigned . . . my job is to do a controversial, confrontational interview with him and put the facts on the table and see how he [Douglas] handles it. Me and Don Gaines."

To say Duvall felt awkward would be an understatement.

"He [the Chief] tells me this and here Doug is sitting only thirty feet away! But the Chief is between a rock and a hard place, too. You have to understand, all the investigators are very uneasy about Doug being back to work . . . and very uneasy about seeing Doug on the third floor when they're doing investigations. You have to understand, this is a whole lot different from investigating a homicide on Wildwood Avenue or Work Drive! There is a big difference when your homicide suspect resides at 217 S. High Street!" (Address of the Akron Police Department.)

Regardless of his reservations, Duvall did as he is instructed with one request, "I told the Chief I wanted Beth Daugherty and Calvaruso from I.A. (Internal Affairs) on my team. I was the old dog and was used to investigating homicides. Beth is very analytical . . . she and Calvaruso. Calvaruso was not only analytical but could also put things together with common sense. They both had the internal affairs experience and I loved the way we worked as a team . . . and . . . I . . . well . . . I just had to have them. So he [the Chief] agreed they could be on the team." On this particular day, the Chief wastes no time updating Ed as to what he wanted from him on his first day of full-time assignment to the Prade case.

After hearing the Chief's instructions to interview Douglas, Ed Duvall and Donnie Gaines took him up to the sixth floor detective bureau into an interview room. Donnie Gaines was assigned to Ed at that time by the Chief because he was a good street cop, and in his own words, Ed stated, "I love Donnie, we worked together for many years at Rolling Acres mall."

When Douglas was summoned to the sixth floor detective bureau for questioning, many of the line staff detectives who worked on the case from the beginning, including Detective King, were in the rear hallway outside of the room within earshot distance. Ed and Donnie were sitting at the table. Ed began the interrogation.

"Doug, I've been assigned to this case, we have to read you your rights."

"Good," Douglas responds, obviously accentuating his approval of *good and proper police work.*

Feeling uneasy and emotional, Ed was looking down under

the table, with Douglas' leg iron staring him in the face. Ed was thinking to himself, *This is the same gun we have.* Looking the devil right in the eye, rather than away, Ed continued.

"Doug, we have good reason to believe that the bite marks found on Margo are yours . . . and Doug . . . there is a very high probability we are going to arrest you for the murder of Margo."

Douglas slammed his fist on the table, Ed remembers. "He got pissed!"

"That's bullshit, who said that!" Douglas responded.

"Well, we have forensic odentologists who say that your teeth are the ones that made those marks. . . ."

"That's bullshit . . . experts lie, they get paid to lie all the time!" Becoming hostile, Douglas began to rise up out of his seat. Donnie Gaines took notice of Doug's movement and began to question him.

"Well, what are we *supposed* to think, here?"

"Doug, do you have any other weapons, other than the ones Mary and I took?"

Ed continued, speaking calmly to get Douglas to calm down and *sit down.*

"Oh yeah, I have a couple in my locker, they've been there for years and I don't know what [type] they are."

"Can we go down and look in your locker, Doug?"

"Yeah."

"Well . . . we'll go down and look. But we just want to let you know these bite marks are lookin' like you're the donor. We'll get back to you. . . ."

Douglas Prade has now been put on notice regarding the murder of Dr. Margo Prade. Douglas Prade no longer gets to look out the window and see his city owned vehicle, the vehicle that was *his* police status symbol of a stellar career. That vehicle had been confiscated and was now being processed for evidence in a homicide. According to Ed Duvall, "That car should have been taken three months before, but it wasn't. So we corrected that."

Again, however, the day Ed decides to confiscate Douglas' city vehicle, he meets with resistance from the same captain. This captain was on the case from the beginning and was the person I approached at the scene the day Margo was murdered. He is the same captain who, according to Ed, had made the statement earlier, “A police officer cannot commit murder!” Perhaps *his* type of police officer cannot commit murder, but this captain failed to realize Douglas Prade was a different breed of cop and a lethal, atypical kind of creature.

“Well, you can’t take it now . . . it’s three months later!” the captain insisted.

“Just because you ***fucked it up [earlier], don’t mean I can’t un-fuck it*** . . . and we’re takin’ that vehicle!” Duvall responded rebelliously.

“It was a very difficult and emotional thing,” Ed asserts. This case had pitted captain against captain, officer against officer, family and friends of Margo against one another and the community against the local newspaper, media and the like. This case left a dark cloud of distrust hovering over everyone who had even the slightest relationship with Dr. Margo Prade and/or Douglas Prade.

* * *

Later that evening, Ed Duvall received a call from Donnie Gaines about the audio tapes found in Douglas’ locker. After retrieving the tapes, Ed had them slowed down for clarity. Sitting at his desk one evening, Ed Duvall listened attentively and heard several sounds of a telephone dialing, a phone line ringing and eventually the angelic voice of Dr. Margo Prade.

“*Oh . . . my . . . God!* We hit the hoogly moogly! He’s been *tapping* her [home] phone line and taping her calls!” Duvall said aloud to himself.

Now, Ed Duvall has an *alarming* new perspective on the pencil pusher, astronomical figure of a community cop. He has the perspective of a control freak electronically stalking his wife. “It was a case like no other,” Ed asserts. “I’ve never had a case, where the victim speaks out in her own words . . . and you not only have a dedicated doctor talking to her patients, but you have a school girl . . . a giddy school girl . . . an aunt, a highly respected aunt . . . you’re [present company] on there as a friend talking to her . . . but we don’t know ***how*** he taped her.”

Based on a tip, investigators conduct another search of the

storage shed on the premises of Margo's property. They retrieve a total of six more tape recordings from a brown grocery store bag, which had been missed the first time around. All were Margo's phone conversations. Detectives also retrieved a tape recording machine. In total there were 435 taped conversations of Margo.

What detectives ultimately had through those tape recordings, the information amidst all other conversations between Margo, her patients, friends and relatives . . . was a ***dying declaration from the grave*** of Dr. Margo Prade . . . "I know he [Douglas] got in my face Wednesday. . . ." Margo stated to her mother in conversation.

"He did . . . !" Ms. Lillie responded surprised and concerned.

"Yeah . . . and I told him, you need to step back out of my face . . . you need to ***step back*** . . . *you're too close!*"

Monday February 23, 1998

Hey girl! How are you? Well, three days less and 3 months after your death, they got Douglas! I knew he killed you from the very moment I learned you were dead, well, after I came down from my shock and hysteria. I can't believe that evil prevailed in someone in this way! I guess I never really knew him, but you did. I miss you so much Margo. Margo, to put this thing simply, ***you fell in love with the wrong man.*** *I see your smile and hear your giggle almost every day. I sometimes even forget you are dead. I have braces on my teeth now. So, I know how you felt those times when you didn't want to smile at the camera. I do the same thing now. I always thought though that when you didn't smile that your braces did not matter because you were so beautiful anyway—braces or not! I am so glad the police arrested Douglas! I hate that bastard for killing you. Your children need you so right now. Your Mom is doing the best she can, and that is not bad at all. I'm going to try and integrate myself back into the children's lives. You know, Douglas had cut me and your sisters out of their lives; and anyone else who he felt "peeped his hole card!" That bitch was never your friend Margo! She is so vicious and has been up under Douglas since the moment you died.* ***Do you know she***

never cried publicly when you were murdered, but cried when Douglas was arrested! *What a fucking bitch she is! I wish I could kick her ass and get away with it. Well, I'm going now. I have an early day tomorrow. I just wanted you to know that* ***justice has been served,*** *so far anyway. I pray he pleads guilty or is convicted. Margo,* ***there was no one else who would have done this!*** *I think that is why it really did not take the police long at all! Talk to you soon. Love, Donzella.*

On Monday Feburary 23, 1998 the person believed to be responsible for the murder of Dr. Margo S. Prade was arrested. Ironically, while driving to school this particular morning I had a premonition, one of many I'd had over the years. I actually *felt and stated to myself while driving,* "Douglas will be arrested *today.*" I remember staring at the building of the police department as I drove past it, talking aloud to myself stating, "You guys are going to do your job today . . . you are going to arrest that bastard for killing my friend today!" My belief was intensified by Ms. Lillie having called me that Saturday prior.

"Detectives say they going to make an arrest soon."

"Really! I sure hope so!" I responded emotionally drained, but elated.

"Well, me too but I hope they call me first so I can go up there and get my babies (Kenya and Sahara) outta that house!"

Ms. Lillie's concern was all too real and telling. Her statement told me that as much as she may not have wanted to believe, and until now, she had *never* expressed it; it was abundantly clear to me that Ms. Lillie believed Douglas had murdered her daughter . . . her ***youngest daughter*** . . . **her precious daughter**.

The karma of the day continued. It was lunch time and I was standing in line in the cafeteria waiting to make my lunch order. The line was long and I was getting frustrated because as graduate students, we only had an hour for lunch, then back in the class room we go; and these days it did not take much at all for me to become frustrated or to just flat out lose my temper altogether.

While in line, an elderly African American woman walked

up to me, a woman I'd never seen before in my life. The lunch counter was very crowded, but the woman walked up and spoke to me. . . .

"Oh honey, isn't it wonderful! They have made an arrest in the Margo Prade Murder case!"

"What! Are you sure?" I asked the woman, astonished and grabbing her arms.

"Yes, dear, I'm sure, they arrested her husband . . . the chief of police is going to announce it at one o'clock this afternoon in a news conference!"

Emotional, I responded, "Thank you . . . ma'am . . . thank you so much for telling me this . . . she was my dear friend!"

"Really?"

"Yes!"

"Well, honey this should be good news for you then. . . ."

"Yes it is!"

The woman then disappeared just as mysteriously as she appeared, as did my place in line and the money I held in my hand. To this day, I have no idea what happened to the money I held in my hand to pay for my lunch. Feeling both liberated and in disbelief at the news, I checked the clock in the lunchroom, it was 12:45. I hurried up to the class room taking the stairs, bypassing the elevator. I ran down the hallway, intending to ask my professor permission before class started, to take the afternoon off given the news I'd just heard. As I approached the class room, I saw Katie, a classmate who attended the night classes, and who worked as a Victim's Assistance supervisor. When I saw Katie, I knew the news was true. Given her day job, and her nighttime class schedule, there was *no other reason* for her to be standing at the classroom door at one o'clock in the afternoon.

"Katie . . . is it true, some woman told me downstairs that Douglas has been arrested . . . is it true!" I asked nervous, emotional and voice shaking.

"Yes . . . that's what I came up here to tell you, Donzella."

"Oh . . . Jesus . . . I've got to leave . . . I've got to get to Ms. Lillie . . . wait . . . for me."

"I will," Katie responded with kind sincerity.

I went into the class room, my professor is physically in

Cleveland, Ohio teaching on this day. With voice shaking, I speak to her through the distance learning monitor. . . .

"Doctor Faria . . . I just found out the police arrested my girlfriend's ex-husband in her murder . . . may I please be excused for the afternoon class . . . ?"

"I figured you would want to be excused, Donzella . . . certainly."

"Thank you!"

"You are very welcome," she responded smiling with a sense of pleasure in her tone, and apparently was already aware of the news perhaps through Katie.

As I exited the room, classmates both returning from lunch and those who had eaten lunch in the room, hugged me, became tearful and offered congratulations. The interaction was very emotional. Many of my classmates voyaged through the long grieving process with me after Margo's death; and many of them shared my angst over her murder in wanting her killer captured. Many of my classmates had gotten to know Margo through the stories I shared with them at lunch time about me and Margo's friendship before her murder and in the later months, about her ex-husband not wanting to "go away," and my sharing with them the fear I had for Margo's safety.

* * *

That morning, Douglas E. Prade was arrested for the murder of Dr. Margo S. Prade. Police detectives were stationed nearby at Margo's home, and at Kenya and Sahara's schools. They wanted to take precautions in the event Douglas decided to go berserk and try to take out his children; the classic murder suicide retreat of many killers involved in crimes of passion once they have been unveiled. The detectives meticulously planned their route, and moment of execution in arresting Douglas Prade, even down to the most finite detail of having him followed throughout the day until the point of the arrest. The media, for some unknown reason, still being a friend to Douglas, would report the arrest as if Douglas "turned himself in." He did not, but he was arrested without incident.

I went directly to Margo's home and Katie met me there. I

sat with Ms. Lillie, and Edith, and waited for Kenya and Sahara to come home. I wanted to be a support system for them after they heard the news of their father's arrest. People were sure to fill up the house fast as the news spread, and they did. Apparently, some time after Douglas' arrest, Margo's phone rang and niece Dayne answered.

"Hello."

"Hello, this is *New Friend,* who is this?"

"This is Dayne."

"Oh, hi . . . I heard on the news that Douglas has been arrested . . . is this true?"

"Yes, it's true."

According to Dayne, *New Friend* then yelled something to the effect of "Oh, no," began crying and hung up the phone.

Dayne found it to be quite interesting that she never witnessed *New Friend* cry over Margo's murder, but broke down crying in learning about the arrest of her murderer. Justifiably, the interaction angered her.

Within fifteen minutes of arriving at Margo's home, television cameras and reporters were already setting up shop, some incognito, and some openly in the park directly across the street from Margo's home. A Fox 8 News reporter knocked on the door. Edith got angry.

"Don't answer the door, if we don't answer it, they will all go away!" "Edith, they are not going to go away," I responded. "They are not going anywhere until someone talks to them."

"Well, they can stay out there all night! I'm not talking to them!"

"Well, this is news and they are reporters. They ***will*** stay out there all night until someone talks to them . . . so, if it's okay with you all, I will go out and talk to them." I volunteered.

"I will too," stated Margo's twin nephew, Timmy. Holding hands we walked outside and spoke to the media about the arrest of Douglas Prade. It was going to be a long night.

That evening returning home from Margo's house, there were twelve messages on my answering machine. The first one was from Margo's elder sister Veronica.

"Donzella . . . it's Veronica . . . they're over there arresting Douglas right now!"

One evening phone call in particular made to Ms. Lillie was quite disturbing. It was Douglas. He was calling to tell Kenya and Sahara to mind Ms. Lillie and do everything she tells them to do. Douglas' phone call ended with a very brazen statement to the mother of his murder victim. "You know grandma . . . the *only mistake* I made was . . . I don't *really* have an alibi. . . ."

The audacity to make such a remark to the woman whose precious daughter you've slain just three months and three days prior; once again, laden with contempt, Douglas Prade's conceit still has no restrictions and shows no remorse. Although at least for now, his self-centeredness has lost the opportunity to be *free.*

The Arraignment of Douglas Prade was taped and televised on the evening news. Like many others in the community, I ***wanted*** to actually see Douglas Prade in "jailhouse orange overalls," his appearance akin to the many common criminals he'd arrested over time as a police officer. As a friend and as my friend's husband, I was extremely angry and felt tremendously betrayed by Douglas, and the murder he chose to commit. Now, I detested him, and wanted to witness him receive the beginnings of his *just desserts.* More importantly, I was livid at ***why*** he chose to assassinate Margo as opposed to just accepting the divorce and walking away; *allowing* her to live out the remainder of her life and finish raising their wonderful, thriving children. Home alone and glued to the television, I waited for the six o'clock news. I wanted and *needed* the sense of elation and closure I thought the news coverage would bring . . . it did not.

Douglas walked into the arraignment room, sat down in the chair, and looked down while scooting the chair forward, making sure it was situated correctly. I found this gesture to be quite peculiar. I'm thinking, you are being arraigned for murder, why do you care if the chair is positioned correctly! I realized Douglas' gesture with the chair was a conditioned response of the control he personified for so many years. Control that enabled him to be the kind of cop ***he*** wanted to be; control that seduced others into giving of what he wanted from them . . . control that twisted this cop's mentality *out of control.*

As Judge Carla Moore read Douglas the charges against him, she asked, "do you understand the charges?" Douglas answered with a quiet, solemn and emasculated, "Yes." At that moment, realizing I'd never seen him so weak and vulnerable, to my surprise, I burst out crying screaming to the television, "Oh . . . Douglas! Just ***look*** at what you have reduced yourself to! All for what . . . for what!!" I was taken aback by my reaction. I had ***wanted and expected*** to feel elation, justice and closure. Instead, I felt a sense of sadness, *injustice* and the opening of a fresh wound of hurt, pain and grief. This time the emotions were not only for Margo and the way she died, but for Douglas too and the friendship the three of us shared over the last twenty one years. I felt hurt, miserable and confused, rather than overjoyed with a sense of resolve.

* * *

Tuesday, August 11, 1998

Hey sweet face! How are you up there in Heaven? Is there really a Heaven, Margo? I've been dreaming about you a lot lately. I think it is because your trial is approaching. I have to meet with the prosecutors on the 19th and I am scheduled to testify on September the 8th. You know Margo, you died on what would have been my father's birthday, and he also died suddenly and tragically like you did. The two of you are buried in adjacent lots, and you both have November 26th on your tombstones. Also, I will be testifying against Douglas on September 8th which is not only Tom's birthday, but the same date my father died tragically. Is this all some uncanny strange coincidence or some type of mystic reality? Two people who I loved dearly have such strange life and death connections with one another. I can hear you saying, "I don't know, Don, but it is strange."

Margo, I miss you so much! I don't cry as often as I had been but I do still cry. I'll never stop crying! I so much wish you were here. It is not so much that you died so soon, but it is the way you died, so viciously and brutal. This is what is so unacceptable. We all miss you so much! Well, I have to go now. I'll let you know how my meeting with the prosecutors went.

Love, Donzella

Twenty-three

Every "I" Dotted and Every "T" Crossed

After the arrest of Douglas Prade, the responsibility of a successful outcome lay with the Summit County Prosecutor's office, even though the investigation was ongoing and evidence was still being collected. This *was not* going to be an easy case to prosecute.

Douglas was nearly a thirty-year police veteran, with a wealth of police expertise, training and knowledge behind him. Douglas' personnel file revealed scores of commendations, FBI and numerous other specialized law enforcement training certificates he'd earned in trainings held throughout the country. Therefore, just as he was highly educated enough to investigate and uncover hidden evidence in difficult cases; he also *knew how to hide* evidence in a manner where it could never be found.

Douglas hired well-known defense attorney, Kerry O'Brien, who interestingly, during the plea phase of Douglas' legal procedures, described Margo's murder as, "a domestic situation that could have or apparently got out of hand [control]," placing at the very least, a *familiar* person at the scene of the crime from the onset.

The Prosecutor's office too, housed a myriad of talented and skilled attorneys. Under the auspices, leadership and supervision of Summit County Prosecutor Maureen O'Conner, veteran assistant prosecutor Michael Carroll and prosecutor Alison McCarty joined her on a prosecutorial journey neither of them would *ever* forget.

Alison McCarty was an attractive, energetic and skilled prosecutor whose mother's presence in the courtroom reminded her to "speak up" while practicing her craft. Ironically, just like Margo, Alison was soft spoken and petite, and exuded a beautiful, kind and friendly smile that made one feel comfortable and relaxed. Even Ms. Lillie told her repeatedly, "You remind me so much of Margo." Spry in her ascribed legal talents, Alison's shoulder length blond hair glistened underneath the lights in the courtroom after the trial began.

In a candid one on one interview with Alison McCarty, she revealed her sense of how this case needed to be approached:

"Once I became involved in the case, it was clear to me, that we weren't going to have the kind of evidence you had necessarily in a normal murder trial. So I pretty much determined that I had to *understand this relationship* [between Margo and Douglas] and how his actions contributed . . . I mean how his actions would . . . [pause] . . . why he would have done the things he did, and why he didn't do the things he didn't do. . . ."

"Like what?"

"Well, for instance why . . . um . . . why he didn't actually physically beat her, he just threatened her. Well, why *didn't* he beat her? Because that's unusual."

"Yes, it is. But I think he did not beat her because he *knew* Margo was intelligent enough not to become that kind of an abuse victim. I mean, she was a professional in the healthcare arena who came into contact with people every day. Plus, *Douglas knew* if he had ever hit Margo, that would be his badge. He was not stupid! He *knew* Margo would not have put up with that! I remember hearing that after the divorce, while Margo was out of town, he apparently slapped Sahara in her face! Well, I believe he slapped Sahara, because he *really wanted* to slap Margo, but could not . . . at least and get away with it!"

"Another question I had was what drove him to actually kill her? There had to be some triggers. I felt these were questions the jury would want answered. And to me the only key to answering those questions was to understand the *relationship,* understanding who *they were.* I learned more and more about her [Margo] which I did through interviewing Lillie, and you, Joyce, Frances, Edith, and Frances Ellison. I mean all the family members and some people in the police department also, I pretty much determined that Margo was an extremely brilliant young woman who met him, *unfortunately* very young in life, when she was still at a point in her life where she fell under his . . . um . . ."

"Spell."

"Yes . . . spell . . . exactly. He was ten years older and I don't think he was looking for monogamy, I think he was looking to hitch himself on to her star. He saw what she was, and what she was gonna be . . . that she had goals, she was polite, she was so popular and just loved by everyone who knew her and he wanted to be attached to that and he wanted to be able to *take credit for that and he did.* I remember when he testified, he said he helped Margo write her valedictorian speech . . . I mean . . . give me a break! So basically, when it came to Douglas, she was somewhat powerless to deal with him. She was very passive and very submissive. She discovered throughout her marriage that she was not happy, but it was one of those things where she *wanted* to keep her family together and decided she would just make the best of it. It wasn't until she started approaching her 40th birthday that she realized she did not want to live this way anymore, and if she really wanted to give her daughters a picture of what love could really be like she needed to make some changes. I mean they were growing up and able to recognize what was going on between them . . . and I really think her losing weight had a lot to do with it [divorcing Douglas]. It did so much for her psyche. I know, I've gone through those weight loss cycles and it does something for your psyche. I think it totally changed her attitude, she started to believe she really could find someone, and she really could have a life. Of course, it was the worst possible thing she could have decided as far as *he* was concerned."

In this excerpt, Alison adequately describes what I believe to be a *true confession* to what Margo's life was like being married to Douglas, as well as the type of *thief* he actually was. Douglas was not your common, everyday thief who steals from the store; but rather a thief of hearts. A thief of mind, body, soul and spirit. A thief of one's *being.* Through interviews and ingenuity, Alison was able to gain unique insight into Douglas' intentions as a husband, as well as the schismatic relationship that he coveted in their marriage.

At the time of Margo's trial, Alison McCarty had been a prosecutor for about eight or nine years. She and prosecutor Mike Carroll had already tried a couple of big cases together. Therefore, both were well qualified, *and needed to be,* in order to try this case with all the mysteries and unanswered questions contiguous in it. The media too, was constantly hovering over their shoulder, as well as the shoulder of the Akron Police Department while they continued to gather more evidence. Because there was *no room* for error of any kind, Alison and Mike Carroll had weekly meetings with all the police detectives on the Prade case, and prosecutor O'Conner lead the investigation which, according to Alison, "is unusual after the case comes to our office."

* * *

Alison was known for her "flare" and she had a very good track record for winning cases. Mike, on the other hand, was more of the quiet, reserved type. On the other hand, he possessed a gentle strength in his prosecutorial talents. An extremely tall and handsome alpha male, when he spoke he could make even the shyest witness sit up and take notice of him. The two were such opposites, they were nicknamed, "Fire and Ice" by their colleagues in the prosecutors office.

Alison admits that the Prade case was extremely hush-hush within the confines of their office. No one knew *anything* except Prosecutor Maureen O'Conner and senior prosecutor Mike Carroll. One evening, Mike invited Alison to Rockne's restaurant for drinks after work, which was something, according to Alison, they rarely did. A few cocktails later, Mike disclosed to Alison out of the blue, something she had wanted to hear some weeks prior, but was under the assumption Maureen O'Conner would be trying the Prade case.

"I got my next case."

"What?"

"I have my next case that we're going to do together. I know what it is."

At that moment, Alison knew it was going to be a big case because Mike always involved her in the big homicide cases and they would often try them together. And, Alison confessed: "I wanted that case, *I wanted to be on that case!*"

"What case you talkin' about?"

Mike looked at Alison and stated, "What do you think?"

Alison whispered to him . . . "*Prade?*"

Mike nodded and Alison asked, "Who's the defendant?"

Mike looks at Alison in no uncertain terms, and she replied astonished, "*It's . . . Prade . . . ?" And Mike nodded.*

Alison asked, "Well . . . what's the evidence?"

Mike whispered . . . "*He bit her!*"

"*Oh . . . !*"

"Don't *say anything,*" Mike instructed Alison, and she did not utter a word to anyone.

For Alison, the bite mark evidence was not enough, and it makes sense that a skilled prosecutor with a winning track record would be concerned about what they did not have on Douglas Prade.

"Mike, we don't have a lot of evidence . . . we got no gun, we got no clothes . . . we got no car . . . we don't have any way to tie the murder weapon to the defendant and we got one weak eyewitness, and I do *mean weak* . . . that's it!" Alison asserted the complicated facts of the case to Mike Carroll. Consequently, the prosecution team traveled to FBI headquarters in Quantico. There an FBI behaviorist completed a personality profile on Douglas to assess certain characteristics. That profile revealed a distinctiveness of the *type* of killer he would be, including an assessment on how Douglas viewed women in general. That assessment guided the team to have Alison be the one to question Douglas when the time came. For a conniving man like Douglas Prade, and the perspicacity he *never ceased* to portray, based on his profile, the team felt if Douglas was questioned by a female, especially an assertive female like Alison, if he was going to break under questioning or show some semblance of emotion—hopefully anger—only a female would be the one to bring that behavior to the surface.

Wednesday May 6, 1998

Hey, girlie, how's it going? I wish you could answer. Well, I finished graduate school. I graduate this Saturday. I'm relieved but, I sure wish you were here to share this with me. Margo, it is so hard to be happy about anything. I know you would want us to all go on and enjoy our lives. But it is difficult, very difficult. Our basement is finally finished. The construction took six months. Remember how we talked about having a party when it was finished. Margo, you left so fast! Many of us, your friends, just cannot understand or accept this. Jodi called me the other day; she was so depressed saying she couldn't stop thinking about you. Neither can I. None of us can Margo. We loved you so much! I never wanted anything as much as wanting you to come back. ***I just cannot understand this!*** *I can't stop crying either. I still cry over you. I want to see your pictures of how douglas killed you. I'm not capitalizing his name because he doesn't deserve it!! That bastard! I hope he burns in Hell! Love, Donzella*

Monday 6/29/98 Ian's 8th birthday

Hey, Baby girl: Well, much to my chagrin, I meet with the prosecutors tomorrow to prepare for your murder trial against Douglas. Margo, how life has turned out for all of us with this heinous crime! You know I am not prepared to deal with this shit! I hate so much that this animal killed you. I told you though in my first letter that if I could do anything to help solve this crime that I would do my damnedest to do so. So, I guess here it is. I have to testify against that bastard, and for you, in your behalf! Margo I know you are tired of hearing this but I wish so much that you had taken precautions against this man hurting you. Why didn't you listen to me? ***I knew he was going to kill you!*** *You know your kids needed you, and they still do. Sahara cries for you daily! How can you bear this? Well, it is not like you can change anything now! I know you know Sahara is crying! We are all* ***crying,*** *Margo! I look at your picture daily and I just cannot believe you are dead and that I will never see you alive again except in videos. This shit is fucked up! How am I supposed to go on after all of this is over? This is wrong, Margo. My baby, Ian, even wants to see you again. He told me yesterday that if he could see you* *again he would give you the biggest and longest hug ever! Last week I dreamt of you for three nights in a row, were you coming to me then? The dreams were so pleasant. I was so disappointed when I awoke and realized they were just dreams. Margo, I miss you so much. I drink every chance I get. What the hell is happening to me because of this? Love Donzella*

The bite mark evidence along with the offender profile was not going to be enough to convict Douglas Prade of the murder of Dr. Margo Prade. Another avenue had to be explored. That endeavor involved probing into the very psyche of Douglas Prade.

According to Alison, "I'd heard of Margo Prade prior to her murder, but I did not know her. I didn't get on the case until February. I remember reading all about it [the murder] in the newspaper. And I remember Doug Prade testifying in the grand jury for me a couple of times; and I remember just feeling so sorry for him because of the Prescott thing [the accidental murder of Douglas' son] and boy . . . does that go a long way . . . when you have something like that happen to you! I mean the good will that he [Douglas] got from that . . . and I remember having a lot of good feelings about him. And I remember reading about Margo's murder in the papers thinking, *Oh God, I really hope it is not her husband!*"

Because all circumstantial evidence did point to Margo's ex-husband, Alison, Mike Carroll and the prosecutors office had to dig deeper into the everyday life of Douglas Prade. The only way to do that, was to question potential witnesses who would actually be involved in the murder trial.

"What's your take on *New Friend?*" Alison asked during the interview with her and Mike Carroll.

"I am so glad you asked me that!"

"Why?"

"Because, I was beginning to think I was the only person who felt something peculiar was going on with her since Margo's death. She is *always* hanging around Douglas and running in and out of Margo's home like it is hers, and trying to be *real close* to her kids even though she was *supposed* to be *Margo's best friend*, at least that's what *she is telling people*! No best friend of

Margo's would be carrying on with Douglas the way she has been. Anyone who was truly her best friend, knows this man probably killed her!"

"So . . . what's your take on her?" Alison asked again refocusing me back on the question at hand.

"I think she was . . . screwing Douglas . . . you know, having a relationship with him! I honestly do!" Alison looked at Mike. Charily their eyes met but they said nothing to each other. I become curious.

"What?" I ask, darting my eyes back and forth between the two of them.

"This is not the first time we've heard this," Alison replied.

"Good! Like I said, I thought I was the only person who was feeling those vibes," I reiterated in tears.

"You know, I've been hearing rumors."

"Well, there have been lots of rumors over these past months," Alison replied very business-like.

"Well, but this rumor never seemed to go away like the others." I replied with voice shaking trying desperately to subdue an emerging, uncontrollable crying episode.

"What rumor is that?" Mike asked.

"That there was a man ***and*** a woman in Margo's van. Is this why you asked about *New Friend* . . . is ***she*** *involved in Margo's murder?!*" Now, ***I am*** crying almost uncontrollably.

"Right now, we are just focusing on Douglas."

At this point I am livid at *New Friend and* her spurious betrayal of being Margo's best friend, and I truly wanted her to be punished in some way for *whatever* part she may have played in this tragedy.

Yet, I still felt a sense of relief when Alison stated, "We're just focusing on Douglas right now," because in my heart of hearts, I felt even if someone else was in the van with him helping to subdue Margo, I *believed* Douglas ***actually did the killing*** of Margo and I did not want that issue to be clouded at all, especially with the jury when the time came; and not even at the expense of stringing up *New Friend,* which for me would have been a welcomed pleasure.

There were other interesting details in the preparation of

this trial, including a large bulletin board in the interviewing room of the prosecutors office with Margo's picture on one side, and Douglas' on the other. Douglas' side had arrows drawn from him, to ***numerous*** women positing labels stating, *"possible relationship."*

September 7, 1998
Hey, Baby Girl.

*Well, Margo, tomorrow is the day I testify against Douglas in your murder trial. Margo, over the years you have touched my life in so many special and unique ways. Never did I think you would touch my life in such a way as this! The other day on the news, I listened to your voice on a tape recording that was played in court. You were telling your mother that Douglas had really scared you and that "he got in your face," like you told me he had done. But you told him to get out of your face and that he was too close. Margo, I don't believe that Douglas ever hit you, I know that is something you would never tolerate. I only feel bad that the one time he did opt to really put his hands on you—**he killed you!!***

Well, it is my turn now. I told you in the very first letter I wrote you that if there was anything I could do to bring justice to your murder I would do it. So, tomorrow is it. For me, _____, ________and______, we're all going to try to bring in our little piece of justice for you Margo. I know you'll be there too, won't you? Just like, you have been all along. It was so refreshing to hear your voice on those tapes; they brought back a sense of life to you. I miss you, but I know you'll be there tomorrow too. Love ya! Wish me luck and strength.

Love, Donzella

Twenty-four
The Trial: Witness for the Prosecution

The audience gasped, and an eerie silence filled the Summit County Court room, veteran Judge Mary Spicer presiding. One juror hung her head in an effort to avoid the dreadful remnants of Margo's murder, and Ms. Lillie abruptly covered her eyes with both hands as Alison pulled Margo's blood drenched laboratory coat from the brown paper evidence bag. Ironically, one visible area of the lab jacket that was not covered in blood was the thick black label bearing the name, ***Margo S. Prade, M.D.***, the experience was extremely sobering.

Douglas sat stoic and controlled . . . no emotion . . . no reaction . . . no interest in the exhibit of Margo's bloodstained lab jacket. I watched Kerry O'Brien, who sat behind Douglas, lean over and whisper something in his ear. A moment later Douglas took a tissue out of the Kleenex box sitting on the defense table and *pretended* to wipe a tear from his eye. *That delayed gesture just sunk your ass with the jury! He actually had to tell you to show some emotion, you cold and heartless bastard!* I whispered to myself.

* * *

I had testified that morning. It was September 8th 1998, and I attended the afternoon session of the trial. The hallway was filled with lawyers, witnesses and spectators alike. The court room was just as crowded, with added occupancy by television cameras and news personnel.

Lori Collins, Margo's medical assistant, had moved away after the murder; she could not take the trauma and felt she needed a change. Lori had been flown in to testify. Meeting up in the hallway just outside of the courtroom, we hugged and I noticed she was wearing one of many buttons with Margo's picture on it that had been created and circulated throughout the community by a faction of Margo's friends, who I was not overly involved with at the time. Employing my undergraduate criminal justice education and experience, I addressed the wearing of the button.

"Lori, you need to take that button off," I instructed in a very matter-of-fact demeanor.

"Why?"

"You can't wear that into the court room while you testify. It could taint the jury. We have come too far now and we don't want *anything* to cause a mistrial." Margo's attorney who was standing with us, and who was also scheduled to testify, concurred. After Margo's attorney and I shared a hug, Mike Carroll approached me. He was smiling enough to conjure up some degree of reassurance in me, but he also wanted to make sure I was ready to battle. After all, the last time we had an encounter, I was a sobbing, blubbering mess in his and Alison's office.

"Good morning, Donzella."

"Good morning, Mr. Carroll."

"Mike . . . please."

"Okay . . . good morning, Mike."

"Are you ready?"

"As ready as I'll ever be . . . I guess . . . I'm nervous."

"Ah . . . it will be a piece of cake. Don't worry . . . just answer all the questions directly and loud enough for the jury to hear you, okay?"

"Okay."

"I'll come out and get you when we're ready for you to take the stand."

"Okay," I responded tentatively, shaking. I should have known then that when I actually got on the witness stand, the journey was not going to be a pleasant one.

September 8th 1998 was the only day of the twelve days of testimony I was in the courtroom as a witness and a spectator. I was permitted to sit in the audience after my testimony ended, and I did not attend any other days of the trial thereafter. After nearly one year of this saga I'd been through a lot and psychologically, it was beginning to weigh heavily on me emotionally and physically. My personality had changed. I was angry, short-tempered and would curse and drop "F" bombs—a word I once forbade myself to use—at the drop of a hat. I would pick arguments with strangers out in the community over the slightest indiscretion—like cutting in front of me in line at the grocery store—and would be ready to physically fight them. I did not at all like the person I had become. More importantly, I did not like the fact that I *allowed* Douglas to have that kind of control over me due to what he had done. Douglas Prade and the heinous crime he perpetrated on my dear friend, was the sole origin of my *new persona,* and I felt the more time I spent in the courtroom gazing at him for God knows how many more days, the more exacerbated my personality would become. I wanted and *needed* to work on getting my old self back. I did not want Douglas to have that kind of control over my language and behavior anymore. Since the moment I learned of Margo's murder, I had turned into a veritable cursing machine . . . it was time for it to end. I wanted and *needed* this trait in me to end.

Purposely missing the remaining days of the trial was a good way to start recovering the kind and compassionate personality I once had, that had gone astray for ten months. The day I testified also happened to be my husband's birthday *and* the 33rd anniversary of my own father's tragic death. My husband could not attend the trial, so a good friend of ours, who is a law professor, attended in his absence and in support of me.

Ten months of stress, grief and psychic pain took a comfortable seat alongside me on the witness stand, and spontaneously purged itself from my system at will during testimony. At a time when I should have been most composed, I was not. Distraught and emotional, it was all I could do to get through my testimony as Mike Carroll questioned me about my long-term relationship with both Margo and Douglas, his accomplishments within the police department as a police officer, and about the many warnings I gave Margo when my fear for her life became more than a notion. It was all I could do to fight through overflowing tears to bring my little piece of justice to the sad ending of my dear friend's life. Douglas however, attempted to add his level of condescension as he glared at me with piercing, hateful eyes during an "objection" break fostered by Kerry O'Brien. When Judge Spicer ordered both attorneys into her chambers over O'Brien's hearsay objection, Douglas used this time as an opportunity to speak to me in silence through his eyes while I sat in the witness chair. His glare was vindictive and impudent, and forceful. Telling me how betrayed he felt at my testimony and how if he got away with this, I could be next on his hit list.

I have always believed, that no matter what, one must look the devil in the eye, so he knows exactly where you are coming from. So I did. That morning, I *anticipated* a stare down contest from Douglas if he got the chance, as did my husband who, as a forensic psychologist, is well versed in working with the criminal mind. He offered his advice.

"No matter what, when he glares at you, and he will, DO NOT *look away . . . whatever you do, do not look away from him . . . okay, babe?*

"Okay. I already expect him to try and intimidate me, he has done it before, and I'm ready."

"When did he intimidate you, when you were over Margo's after she was killed?" he asked, angrily.

"Well, that . . . and when I was twelve, remember I told you about that?"

"Oh, yeah . . . I do remember. Okay . . . well, good luck and be strong . . . love you."

"I love you too. Happy birthday."

To my surprise, it was not at all a difficult task to exchange stares of betrayal with Douglas. Our stare down duel seemed to go on forever and so did the conversation we seemed to share:

[Douglas] If I get away with this, you're next!

[Me] What the hell are you staring at? What! You feeling betrayed now? You do not know the first meaning of betrayal you cold hearted bastard. Why don't you ask your children what betrayal means to them!! I feel more betrayed than you could ever imagine! And, I am ***certainly much more*** *pissed off than you are right now! You did this, not me! We are sitting here because of*

what YOU DID! You committed the ultimate betrayal by squeezing the life out of Margo for eighteen years, then when she said, "I've had enough" you ***took*** *her life. Now, you're mad at me and want respect! Revenge? I don't think so and if you do get away with this, it might be in* ***your best interest*** *to leave town, because I'm not going anywhere! In fact,* ***none of us are going anywhere . . . but you are!***

The stare down competition ended with Douglas *looking away from me first,* which is what I wanted, what I *needed* and what I anticipated. I refused to be intimidated by him *again,* ***I was not twelve years old anymore!!*** I was willing to engage in this duel of sultry eye contact as long as he was, and frankly after what he had done, it was time for Douglas Prade to know that people just were not in fear of him anymore. I was too angry *with* him, to be afraid *of* him. If anything it was *time for Douglas to live in fear,* fear of spending the rest of his natural life behind bars; and if that didn't happen, then at the very least, it was time for him to fear for his own life!

Alison McCarty and Mike Carroll built a solid circumstantial case against Douglas Prade. Extremely composed, Joyce offered a distinct and appropriate character assassination of Douglas; testifying to, amongst other things, his demeanor towards Margo. Out of all of Margo's friends and family, Joyce probably knew the most intimate details of Margo and Douglas' marriage and the most sordid connections of his extramarital activities.

Many other witnesses for the prosecution included Lori Collins, Margo's medical assistant who first discovered her bullet riddled body; Margo's baby sitter testified as to how Douglas would call interrogating her on the phone as to Margo's whereabouts after the divorce whenever she was out of town. Margo's attorney testified as to how irate and verbally abusive Douglas became toward Margo during a visit in her office while discussing details of their divorce. Margo's new companion provided disturbing details of how he believed the brakes on his vehicle had been tampered with one evening when he left it in the driveway while he and Margo took her daughters out for the evening. Longtime friend Frances, testified as to how she advised Margo to "get a gun" to protect herself from Douglas. Other witnesses included Ms. Lillie, niece Dayne Arnold, sister Frances; and an Akron General Medical Center employee who testified witnessing Douglas harass Margo while doing her medical rounds at the hospital the morning she was murdered. Robin Husk, the car salesman at Rolling Acres Dodge testified he saw Douglas staking out Margo's medical building parking lot on November 26th, 1997 just before the murder. When asked why he did not come forward sooner during the early stages of the investigation, Mr. Husk replied, "I was afraid." Mr. Husk also testified to Douglas' physically stalking Margo going in and out of the building on various occasions, to the point the stalking became humorous entertainment amongst his colleagues at the dealership.

The only physical evidence the prosecution had was the bite mark left on Margo's arm. Dental expert Dr. Lowell Levine, nationally known for his work on high profile cases, stated the bite mark impression looked like Douglas Prade's but did not want to stake his reputation on it stating, "there are certain characteristics that are similar to his, although I'm hesitant to say these are his with certainty." This testimony, perhaps unexpected by the prosecution, left the door wide open for reasonable doubt, on the *only piece* of physical evidence the prosecution had. On the other hand, prosecutors gained amnesty with *slam dunk* testimony from local dentist, Tom Marshall: "Ultimately they [teeth] matched. My conclusion that the bite found on Margo Prade was made by Captain Prade."

Other key evidence presented to the jury by the prosecution was the bank statement belonging to Douglas that had been enlarged for purposes of testimony. On the backside of the statement, Douglas had subtracted his bills from the amount of Margo's life insurance policy totaling, $75,000. Douglas *never paid* the $7,000 for Margo's funeral either, however, that information administered by Margo's family, surfaced too late for the prosecution to enter it into evidence.

The prosecutions other ace-in-the-hole was one key eyewitness, patient Howard Brooks. Mr. Brooks, one of Margo's elderly patients, stayed with the same story from beginning to end. He testified seeing Douglas leaving the parking lot of the medical office building in a speeding car the morning Margo was murdered. Mr. Brooks, who is now deceased, emphatically and deliberately pointed to Douglas in the courtroom stating, ***"It was him . . . it was him!"***

The Defense

Believing he always needed to be in control, as expected, Douglas took the witness stand in his own defense which no defendant is ever required to do. And, as forecasted by the psychologist who completed Douglas' profile, Alison did get a *slight* rise out of him during questioning about Margo's intentions to divorce him several other times previously, and how he had fathered several other children outside of their marriage. Trying not to rise from his seat, Douglas launched a scoffing, "Did she . . . did she?" when Alison questioned him about Margo's intentions to end their marriage, and revelations of his sinister side. That behavior was exactly what the prosecution was hoping for, and exactly what the FBI behaviorist predicted.

Douglas had an answer for *everything,* for every piece of damaging circumstantial evidence, he had an answer. For every witness against him, he had the perfect textbook answer. When asked about the audio recordings, Douglas offered a pompous and articulate, "Margo was interested in a way of keeping track of those [patients] calls. She had asked me to tape her phone calls because she needed to ***tighten up*** her record keeping and documentation." Articulating an answer to insinuate Margo was somehow inept in her record-keeping, and she needed him to help keep her on track. What an insult! Even if that were true, why would a physician as bright and ***ethical*** as Margo ask him to do something as illegal as taping people without their knowledge? In response to the tape recordings, a juror from the Prade murder case who was interviewed on the popular Dateline NBC Program discretely and emphatically stated smiling, "After the first day, we got the point . . . she was a very nice person . . . she was a sweet person . . . she was a good doctor . . . and she had ***no clue*** she was being tape recorded . . . end of story."

When questioned about being jealous about Margo beginning to date, Douglas replied, "I was happy for her. *I bought* all of her new exercise equipment." Again, Douglas is relishing in *reassuring himself* and the jurors, that *Margo still needed him,* even to the extent of helping her become physically attractive through exercise, for a new partner. Douglas did purchase Margo's exercise equipment, but it was long before she divorced him or began dating. Although it was not revealed through conversation with the jurors, I always wondered if they detected that psychologically, Douglas *persisted* in taking credit for *every facet of who Margo was as* well as the accomplishments she made in many areas of her life; and, if his flawed assertions had any influence on their decision.

*   *   *

The only real credible witness Douglas had in his defense was a neighbor from his apartment complex. A young, attractive blonde named, Kathleen Lynch. Ms. Lynch was to be Douglas' key alibi witness. She testified that on the morning of November 26th 1997, between 9:10 and 9:12. Douglas was still in the gym working out when she left. However upon cross-examination from Mike Carroll, Ms. Lynch admitted she could not ***exactly*** pin down what time Douglas was in the gym after 8:40 A.M. So, why was Ms. Lynch a witness? According to records, Douglas approached Ms. Lynch shortly after Margo's murder asking for her help in identifying him as being in the gym of their apartment complex the day Margo was murdered. "Someone killed my ex-wife, I'd appreciate it if asked, you would verify that you saw me here on that day."

Ironically, Douglas must have forgotten that little encounter with Ms. Lynch when he phoned Ms. Lillie on the night of his arrest stating, "You know, Grandma, my only mistake is that I do not have an alibi." The other irony to Douglas having this particular witness is that Douglas spent his very *career* on postulating confrontational racial inequities; playing the race card before every single promotion he earned, insisting that the white establishment was intent on keeping at least *this* black man down. Now, he is depending on a white woman to save his ass!

Fortunately, the prosecution was able to poke enough holes in Ms. Lynch's testimony by getting her to admit she could not say for sure what time Douglas was in the gym. And as far as travel time goes, detectives drove every conceivable route from Douglas' apartment to Margo's office; encountering red lights, stop signs and all types of high and low traffic volumes. Through it all, detectives determined the trip *still only took six minutes.*

The only other witness Douglas had with any credibility at all, only proved to botch his defense even more. A dental expert who attempted to demonstrate that Douglas was "incapable of biting anything" had him bite down hard on a piece of hard thick material. Upon jerking the piece from Douglas' mouth in open court, his upper false teeth pulled away from his gums and out of his mouth. Again, I could not believe Mr. Egomaniac, had reduced himself to this level of humiliation on national television. Nevertheless, when trying to literally get away with *murder,* one must at the very least, be humbled at some point.

The defense's biting demonstration illustrated nothing more than a freak show, and only further proved why there was only ***one set of teeth*** on Margo's arm, and why those teeth matched the teeth imprint on Margo's arm. Douglas' bottom teeth were stationary, *his top teeth were false.* The bite mark on Margo's arm matched that of Douglas' bottom teeth.

Ex-Summit County Coroner William Cox tried his luck too by testifying the killer had to be right-handed. That testimony did not hold enough water to rule out Douglas as a left-handed killer.

The last ditch effort by the defense was to have the jury see Douglas standing next to a jade green minivan, the exact replica of Margo's van. They were attempting to discredit the Rolling Acres Dodge videotape that surreptitiously caught the killer on camera. Consequently, after all the enhancements that were performed by the Bureau of Criminal Investigation, that video tape was simply too fuzzy to really determine the *size or sex* of the person who entered Margo's van on that fateful day, and a juror stated, "It was the equivalent of a Sasquatch tape!"

"He snuffed her out! Don't let him get away with it!" Passionate and nearly shouting, Alison instructed the jury on the 12th and final day of trial. This case and Margo had made a permanent mark in her heart. She used Douglas' covert tape recording of Margo against him. With an idea from detective Beth Daugherty, Alison played excerpts of Margo's voice, echoing from the grave . . . Margo the friend . . . Margo the daughter saying, "I love you Mom. . . ." Margo the mother and Margo the doctor. Alison then meticulously ended her summation playing Margo's voice saying, "Mom, he got in my face . . . he scared me." The final stream Alison played in those recordings was the impious, chilling and heartless voice of Douglas echoing, ". . . testing . . . one . . . two . . . three. . . ."

The jurors took only four hours to reach a verdict. After the guilty verdict was read, the courtroom erupted with screams and applause. Judge Spicer asked Douglas if he had anything to say. With brazen disregard, he turned his back on the Judge, pointed his finger and admonished the audience, then addressed the prosecutors stating, "you made a very good circumstantial case, and I commend you for that, but I'm telling you, you have convicted the wrong man!" Douglas professed his innocence stating, "God, Margo and the person who killed Margo knows that I am innocent!" It is amazing how the most despicable murderers tend to find God, only ***after*** they have committed the most scandalous of crimes.

After Douglas turned his back on the Judge and scolded everyone in the courtroom, members of the audience were given the opportunity to address him and the crime he'd just been convicted of. Margo's maternal aunt, Ida Sanford blasted Douglas for killing her special niece in a way that only an older aunt born in the south could. She gave Douglas an old-fashioned tongue lashing he is sure to never forget. Margo's dear friend Brenda, looked Douglas straight in the eye, scolding him stating, "she [Margo] was irreplaceable!" Margo's sister Phyllis, spoke of Douglas to the media after leaving the courtroom, tapping into the very core of his betrayal to the family stating, "We've loved

Douglas for years! How could he do this!" In the final analysis, the courtroom drama that became the top story of the evening news for the past twelve days came to an end with Judge Mary Spicer sentencing Douglas Evans Prade to the maximum life sentence of twenty years, for the murder of Dr. Margo Shamberger Prade, and six years for the wiretapping.

Douglas Prade saw himself as Margo's knight in shining armour. I also believe that, for what ever reason, Douglas Prade lived with a dark empty hole inside of him, a hole that would never be filled up, regardless of how hard he tried. When Douglas entered Margo's van on that fateful day, he was ***committed to killing*** her. After all the threats and stalking over the years, Margo never once filed a police report on him because she did not want to stain his career. We know now that perhaps that was a mistake on her part, and she might still be alive had she filed a complaint. Nevertheless, once Douglas entered Margo's van, he *had* to exterminate her; if he didn't, an assault complaint would have meant his badge *and* his career and he knew this. For Douglas, murdering Margo was supposed to make him feel better emotionally, feel more like a man who is always in control, and, get away with the murder all at the same time. However, there is no ideal crime; and as human beings we do not take another person's life just to make us feel better. When one does cross the line of deception to the point of committing murder, payback is imminent.

The trial is over and the conviction rendered. Douglas Evans Prade learned he would spend the rest of his natural life . . . in prison. The prosecution rested the case of the State of Ohio versus Douglas Evans Prade; and with all appeals exhausted, he will be eligible for parole in the year 2024, at the ripe old age of 76. The gun, the getaway car and what ***had*** to be Douglas' bloody clothing were never found. And, the rumor about the man *and* woman being inside the van while Margo was being killed, was never substantiated *or* discounted.

After the verdict, Ed Duvall finds Ms. Lillie and they engage in a lengthy embrace. Later, standing alone near a flagpole, and probably smoking a cigarette, Ed Duvall broke down and cried.

"I broke down like a baby, this case was for the kids." Referring to Kenya and Sahara. Had Margo Prade not fought for her life, and had Douglas Prade not lost his temper and bit her, Detective Mary Myers stated, "He might have gotten away with this." A juror concurred, "He [Douglas] was a very good witness . . . well spoken. I don't know that I would have convicted him without the bite mark."

* * *

September 24, 1998

Hey, Baby girl!!

They got that ***bastard today!! Douglas was convicted today of your murder and sentenced to life!!*** *I'm so happy. But I'd trade it all to have you back!! You probably seen him saying he didn't do it in court today. But we all know he did it.* ***There was no one else. Everybody loved you, Margo.*** *I don't know how we will go on without you but, it will be a lot easier now.* ***Rest in peace AND JUSTICE NOW MY DEAR FRIEND. I LOVE YOU AND HOPE TO SEE YOU AGAIN ONE DAY!!***

LOVE, DONZELLA

The evening of September 24th 1998, after the conviction of Douglas Prade; under the headship of Dr. Robert Denton from the local Victims Assistance Program and Margo's Pastor, Reverend Ronald Fowler, The Arlington Church of God held a closing ceremony on behalf of Dr. Margo Prade and her family. The ceremony was held at 7:00 P.M. and I arrived late due to work and traffic. The church was at full capacity, similar to how Margo's funeral had been. There were police detectives in attendance who had worked tirelessly to bring this case to justice; relatives, friends, patients, family members and colleagues of Dr. Margo Prade were all in attendance.

While walking down the church aisle toward the front pew, attempting to hold back tears, my peripheral vision caught a glimpse of someone approaching. I looked up. With arms outstretched and watery eyes, it was Alison McCarty. With immense emotion we embraced and sobbed; and although it was difficult to speak, I remember whispering in her ear, ***"Thank you . . . Alison . . . thank you so much."***

A large photograph of Margo sat on an easel in front of the pulpit where her casket was positioned ten months prior. Margo's youngest daughter, Sahara, played the piano while her friend sang a gospel hymn. Layne too, resonated a beautiful song in memory of her special aunt, hoping to help bring her sense of closure to the gap of grief, pain and suspicion our community had lived with for so long. Still today, however, for many of us, those gaps of grief will *always* remain slightly propped open.

Twenty-five
The Aftermath

The wind is swirling in a vicious torrent of leaves, rain and debris, earmarking the beginnings of what promises to be a mean and nasty winter. The fury of the wind is so intense, people can barely walk down the street without being blown away. Dogs are running against the wind as if it is the end of the world, and car windshield wipers are on full throttle . . . the weather today is showing no mercy and newscasters are warning, "If you don't have to go out today . . . don't!" It is going to be a long and treacherous winter.

Despite the weatherman's warnings, Ms. Lillie pulls into the cemetery driveway, jumps out of the car barely shifting the gear into park, leaves the drivers door open and runs towards Margo's grave screaming, "I'm coming baby . . . I'm coming . . . Mama's coming!" The whirling wind has nearly covered her baby's gravesite with leaves and debris; and the wind is about to carry Ms. Lillie away to the adjacent plot. With bare hands, Ms. Lillie frantically cleans off Margo's grave.

From that winter on, ***every*** year, Ms. Lillie has on order an expensive blanket for Margo's grave; something to keep her plot clean and in Ms. Lillie's heart and mind, something that will keep Margo warm from the winter months ahead. "It is expensive, and I can't really afford it, but I don't want her to get dirty and cold," Ms. Lillie explained in sorrow.

There is not a day that goes by, no matter the weather, that Ms. Lillie does not visit her youngest child's grave . . . her baby's grave. And on Margo's birthday, one will always see a string of balloons tied to the vase that sits atop her tombstone. Some people who live in the neighborhood also know exactly where

Margo's grave is located, because they see Ms. Lillie there . . . every . . . single . . . day.

"I don't think that is healthy for her," one woman stated to me in conversation.

"Who are you to say?" I responded protectively. "Perhaps it is the daily visits to her daughter's grave that might be what is keeping ***her*** from dying from a broken heart, or from losing her very mind to grief. She knows she has to finish raising Kenya and Sahara, that is what Margo wanted. I think Ms. Lillie is doing whatever it takes to deal with this thing. None of us have a right to say how someone else should process their grief. What may be unhealthy to you, might be very healthy for Ms. Lillie!"

"Yea, I guess you're right. Sorry."

"Okay. Thanks."

For daughter Sahara, having to deal with her mother's death is a daily struggle, and is a constant reminder that she must stay focused on her goals and aspirations to be a singer, actress and marine biologist. "I want to be the first person to train a great white whale," Sahara asserts. However, it will be difficult without having either one of her parents in her life for support and guidance.

About her mother's death, Sahara also asserts, "It really doesn't make any sense to me, that she had to die like that, and it makes me look at him [Douglas] in a whole different way." Sahara's feelings are epitomized through episodic anxiety attacks at least once a year.

Like many of us who loved Dr. Margo Prade, we are feeling a melancholy day coming on. A stressful day that will be defined on how well we can cope until bedtime. It has been this way every single November 26th since 1997, the day Margo was murdered. I call Joyce, or she calls me. I call Ms. Lillie, or she calls me. I've called Margo's nieces, Layne or Dayne or they may call me. In essence, there has never been a November 26th that has gone by since the murder of Dr. Margo Prade, that close friends and/or relatives of Margo's have not been drawn into the grief *and memory* of that horrific morning, needing to still share our heartache with one another.

On November 26th 2001, as much as I tried to avoid it, I called Ms. Lillie in the early afternoon hour.

"Hello." I could tell who the person was on the phone, and they were crying.

"Hi, Edith . . . this is Donzella. I just called to talk to your mom. How are you?"

"Not good, Don (sniffing)."

"I know. . . ."

"Momma's not here, the school called and she had to go and see about Sahara. The ambulance had to take her to the hospital."

"Oh, no! I'm going down to the hospital. Are you okay?"

"Okay . . . (her voice quivering from crying), I think you should go down there, Don, I can't go, Don . . . you go. They are probably still in the emergency room. I'll be alright . . . eventually."

"Okay . . . I'm on my way. This is so hard isn't it?" I ask choked up.

"Yes, . . . it is."

Upon arriving at Akron Children's Medical Center, after parking I entered through emergency. I stopped at the doctor's desk and asked where Ms. Lillie Hendricks or Sahara Prade was. The young male physician pointed across the hall and politely stated, "They're in that room. You know, I knew her mother . . . Dr. Prade . . . she had patients here . . . what a tragedy."

"Yes . . . it is isn't it."

I walked into the room and Sahara was lying in bed staring at the ceiling with Ms. Lillie sitting by her side. I didn't ask what happened. I already *knew* what happened . . . it was the same thing that happened every year prior since November 26, 1997, or September 17th, Margo's birthday. It was the same thing that has happened on one or both of those days . . . for the past four years . . . an anxiety attack and/or conversion reaction. It is the same sorrowful reminder of the loss of the beloved Dr. Margo Prade, and the grief and sadness renders a fresh cut with a sharp knife.

I spoke with Ms. Lillie about what the doctor's diagnosis was, but being a mental health professional myself, I already had a pretty good idea. Walking over to Sahara, I put my arm around her shoulders, leaned over her bed and laid my cheek on her pillow next to her cheek. Without either of us speaking a word, our tears joined together as they trailed down Sahara's right cheek. There was no talking, there ***is*** nothing that can be said to make this feeling go away for this child. Ms. Lillie says, "She was stiff as a board when the paramedics put her in the ambulance. They had to pick her up . . . she was just crying and stiff as a board. . . ."

Later, an older African American woman entered the room. She seemed to have appeared out of nowhere. She began to explain to Ms. Lillie who she was, that she had lived in the neighborhood where Margo grew up, and how she remembered Margo from when she was a little girl. The woman began to tell a heartwarming story of how she would give Margo cookies if Margo would sing a song for her. The woman asked that we all have prayer together. We joined hands around Sahara's bedside and prayed. The woman then disappeared as mysteriously as she appeared in the room. It was the strangest phenomena.

Margo's children and family will have to live out the remainder of their lives not accepting, but ***coping*** with the reality of living without Margo. Those coping mechanisms have and *will* continue to take on various forms as time passes on. For now, several of Margo's sisters are on anti-depressant medications, and brother James is afflicted with an organic brain injury that will never allow him to remember his youngest sibling is dead, or ***how*** she died. Given that James was the one sibling who approved of Margo's dating Douglas when she was just a young teen, perhaps the memory loss pertaining to her death is God's ***blessing,*** rather than a curse.

Ms. Lillie longs to dream of her daughter but cannot, and every Thanksgiving, sister Frances lovingly sets a place at the dinner table in memory of her youngest sister Margo.

When the pressure of losing both parents becomes too much for Margo's children they often remind Ms. Lillie in sorrow, "I don't have any parents." Ms. Lillie responds, "You don't have parents but you do have family."

January 23, 1999

Hi, Margo:

It's been some time since I've talked to you. I miss you so, and your children need you so! Kenya's going through her peer thing, she wants to change schools and go to Buchtel. We are trying to talk her out of it, because that is not what you would want. I think she is mad at me because I don't agree with her leaving the Elms, but it is not the first time. I've also been teaching her how to drive, we go out on Saturdays. I'm going slow with the driving lessons though. She did very well last semester, obtaining a 3.5 GPA, in spite of all the trauma with you and Douglas. I really hate him for what he did. Did you think he was going to kill you, Margo? I think you did at some point and time. I think you really felt he would end your wonderful life.

I put your picture back up. It doesn't bother me as much as it did right after Doug was convicted. I think I wanted justice so bad, that I really didn't have time to just grieve your death. So, after his conviction, I felt so much sorrow and grief, that I had to take your big picture down. Joyce said she did the same thing. This whole mess was and still is a mess! I really miss you Margo, and I still cry sometimes. It seems just like yesterday that you were murdered. I remember that day so well. It is so vivid in my mind. But you know what, you still looked pretty lying on the gurney in the morgue, even though your face was scarred with what looked like the nose of his gun. He pushed that gun so hard into your cheek that he tore your skin open didn't he, Margo? Well, he is suffering now. He has Bell's Palsy and I heard he has been beaten. As far as I'm concerned, he cannot suffer enough for what he did. He took you away from all who loved and needed you. Well, I'm getting sad now so I better go. Tom and Ian are doing great. Ian misses you too. We all do. I wish you could come back to life. I've dreamt about you so much at times. Some weeks I have dreamt about you nearly every night. What's that about. Are you coming back to me in my dreams because that is the only way I can ever communicate with you now? Your mom says she hasn't dreamt of you yet, but wishes she could. Take care until we talk again. I love you girlfriend and I'll keep watching over your little ones.

Love, Donzella

Twenty-six
Remembering Margo

To remember Dr. Margo Prade is to remember her journey through life as an astral performance.

For Alison McCarty, this murder case *humanized Margo's life* for her, and left impressionable footprints in her heart:

"I listened to those tapes, it was my job to listen to those tapes and they just blew me away. I would just keep listening to these tapes and I would tell Mike, 'this woman is just unbelieveable!' People had said to me, 'no one ever said a bad word about her.' And I said, well, she is a murder victim now, no one is going to say a bad thing about her. Then they would say, 'You don't understand, ***there is nothing*** bad out there on Margo Prade! We have interviewed everybody and there is nothing bad out there!' So I listened to those tapes with an ear to see where her flaws were . . . there were none. She didn't talk about anyone else . . . she wasn't negative about anyone else, she would console Brenda who was going through her cancer treatment . . . she would giggle all the time, laugh and make jokes . . . I mean, she was hilarious! I would laugh out loud when I would listen to those tapes by the pool with my daughter over the summer. I couldn't believe it. I remember thinking, if I'd known about her, I would have taken my daughter to see her" [as her doctor].

"Did you ever cry?"

"Oh . . . I cried a lot at home at night about this case. The stress, the worry . . . I thought about Lillie and what this case had done to the family . . . and when I was writing my closing argument . . . I cried, and I almost cried when I was delivering it."

Alison emphatically relates how, and more importantly, ***why*** this case became so important to her. It was not just another win for Alison . . . it was ***justice*** for Margo, Ms. Lillie, her children, her seven thousand patients and family.

Seven years after her murder, Judge Alison McCarty still attends the Victims Assistance Christmas tree candle light services for victims of violent crimes in honor and remembrance of Dr. Margo Shamberger Prade.

As a compassionate physician, Dr. Margo Prade is remembered by a young woman, who wishes to remain anonymous, who did not know Margo personally and had never heard of her before their encounter.

It was in 1985, Margo was moonlighting at a Rapid Response medical treatment center. The woman had been severely beaten by a man who mistook her asking him for help, as a romantic advance. When the woman refused his sexual advances he beat and nearly killed her. Several days later the woman sought medical treatment. The woman states, "I was not honest with Margo as to what happened. I was afraid of exposing myself to a stranger and afraid of being judged by her." Margo did not push the issue of how the woman obtained her injuries, she just treated the injuries, but obviously did notice the fingerprints around the woman's neck, where the man had nearly choked the woman into unconsciousness. After treatment and before leaving the center the woman states, "Margo stepped out of her role as a doctor and talked to me as a *woman.* She handed me her card, and wrote her home phone number on it. She told me if I ever needed to talk, to call her day or night because, 'no woman ***ever*** deserves to be beaten!' "

Today, this woman believes the significance of her encounter with Margo on that day did not reveal itself until after Margo was gone. When she heard of Margo's murder, "It stopped me in my tracks because she didn't deserve it either! I realized that this remarkable woman saved my life in so many ways without me even knowing it, and without my ever having the chance to tell her. The greatest irony for me, is that her death took on a spiritual level and in silence, [after her death] I *thanked* Margo Prade rather than leaving the experience in an ironic state now that she was gone."

Colleague Dr. Adolph Harper listens to a patient as she cries over the loss of her dear Dr. Margo Prade, stating, "What am I going to do . . . what am I going to do . . . ?" "I could not help her because I did not know what I was going to do for myself. I still have so much depression, anger and confusion. I had never felt like this before. A wrong has been committed and it can't be righted! I've lost loved ones through death, but I have never, *ever* experienced feelings like this before."

Dr. Adolph Harper expresses his desire for Margo to be remembered as, "Loving to laugh!" And that her death "Was a community loss. She smiled and laughed with people constantly. This community lost a great doctor. I loved her and hate she is not here anymore. I want people to remember Margo Prade as a person who was ***for real.*** She cared about people, she liked them, she *loved* them, and she did not pull any punches. She cared about her people and her patients because she truly did! It was not a front. She would talk to anybody! Margo never thought she was too good to talk to people, touch them or associate with them. She loved people and wanted to do the very best for them. She did not use her position as a doctor to believe she was better than anyone, all people were equal and the same in her eyes. She was fun and never represented herself as being prejudiced, racist or discriminatory towards anybody! For these reasons, I will *always* remember her as one of the ***greatest people*** I ever came in contact with. And, I know she is probably looking down smiling right now, or probably laughing because Margo loved to laugh! If you did something around her, Margo would laugh at you. Don't think she is not going to laugh at you because she will, and I loved that about her too!"

* * *

At age thirteen, daughter Sahara Prade, Margo's prodigy child who is an aspiring entertainer, offers what she believes the biggest influence her mother has left her. "Her intelligence. She was such a smart person. Even I would wonder how is she doing this; taking care of all of her patients, two kids, and a husband. Even now, I look around this house and I just want to give her a big hug because I see some of my friends and how they live . . . and

I'm just so happy I had her in my life for the short time that I did, and that I had the type of mom that I had."

Sahara wants people to remember that her mother, "Cared about everything, and everyone. That she would not do anything to hurt anybody. She was the perfect example of a good person, and everybody wanted to be around her and everybody wanted to be seen with her, and that it is really an honor that I got to be her daughter." As a doctor, Sahara candidly states, "She cared so much about each one of her patients. She would go out of her way just to see them. It's not that she would not spend time with me, [being so busy] it is just that . . . she would get my grandma to take care of me, just so she could go out of town to see how one of her patients were doing. I wasn't mad at her for that, I was happy for her because she was such a good doctor. As a friend, Sahara states, "She ***was my best friend***, I go to the cemetery once a week. She was *unbelievable.* She was just so *incredible* that . . . it was like she wasn't real . . . like she wasn't a real person . . . it was like she was an ***angel***." And about her father, Sahara adamantly states, "I used to look at him as someone I could depend on. Now, I look at him in a totally different way. I only see him as someone who is in jail. I love him, but I hate him for what he did! I mean, I don't know how he could do that to her, she was such a good person. She never did anything to hurt any body, and she ***never did anything to hurt him.***"

Patient Vickie Taylor, who eerily disclosed, "She [Margo] although she was still smiling, looked like death was upon her when I was in her office the Monday before she was murdered. It was very strange, I told my husband about it," offers an unwavering remembrance of Dr. Margo Prade stating, "She was an inspiration! I mean, I look at her and what she had done with her life as a black woman, a career woman, a doctor . . . and I feel empowered to keep going until I finish school. She was truly an inspiration for me. I have her picture on my desk, and I look at it every day!"

Remembering Margo means remembering that she possessed so much goodness, that ***she is*** difficult to describe. Everything that is superior and virtuous in the world can be associated with Dr. Margo Prade. Even in death, it is as if Margo Prade still wants us to do what is right.

Until she died, as an adult, I had never visited my father's grave. Now, when I go see Margo it is as if she is saying, "Thanks for visiting, Don, now go and see your dad." And I comply. My father is buried not more than thirty feet from Margo, and paradoxically, they ***both*** have November 26th printed on their headstones; his birth date and her death date.

As for Douglas, he will no doubt remember Margo just the way he left her . . . lifeless and bloody in the van she herself prophesized would be the death of her. And, should he forget that image, he can always pull out the photograph he so willingly snapped of Margo lying dead in her casket. A photograph reflecting the spoils of a war, a war between good and evil, where evil reigned victorious. Douglas Prade will have plenty of time to relish in his remembrance of Margo, remembering the final sense of control he *just had to have* over her precious life. Most people understand that in marriage, the words, "Until death do you part" is not intended to be a license to kill your spouse. Those words do not give one ***permission*** to engender death upon the other.

Douglas Prade believed he possessed *everything* Margo encompassed, and that she owed her accomplishments to him; her career, her popularity, her money, their children, and ***even her life.*** I'd like to think that while waiting for his parole hearing, Douglas Prade will spend those days thinking not only about what he has done to Margo, but what he has done to their *children.* I'd like to believe that his nights will continue to have reel to reel flashbacks and reruns of the day he killed Dr. Margo Prade. I'd like to think Douglas Prade is not only still suffering from the attack of Bell's Palsy he had shortly after he was convicted, but from symptoms of Post Traumatic Stress Disorder like the rest of us; only that his is so much more ***profound.*** I'd like to think of Douglas Prade waking up in night sweats after seeing himself in a nightmarish, murderous frenzy killing the mother of his two beautiful children. Moreover, I'd like to think that Douglas Prade's ego has taken a tremendous blow and that there will ***never be a day*** pass where those nightmares won't continue to haunt him all through the days, and the remainder of his life here on earth. After all, given that he still has the privilege of **living,** why should his days and nights take in any pleasant experiences or memories? Whatever the case, Douglas Prade's torment will never compare to that of his and Margo's children, her mother, family, friends and patients.

* * *

May 7, 1999

Hey, girlfriend! It's been quite some time since I've written to you. You have been in my thoughts though, you've never left, and never will. I've also been submitting writings to your memorial website. YES, my dear friend, two of your patients, Drs. Martha ____ and Rosalie ____ created an electronic memorial in your name. Your picture is on there too. Your girls are doing well, They are so tall now! Ian said he saw your face in the clouds this morning. I'm sure he did! Margo, we all miss you so much. I wish you could come back in some way and I actually know it is you. Joyce and I are having a hard time with it. When we go out, we drink a little too much and are hung over the next day. Then we vow we will watch one another and not do it again. But, the same thing happened the next time. Where will it all end? I love you girl. I'll talk with you soon.

Love, Donzella

A Heartfelt E-Mail from Ed Duvall

12/4/2003. 6:53:24 PM Eastern Standard Time

Donzella:

I did get your phone msg., but I have been a little under the weather this week. Actually went to the Doctor today and got some medicine to make me all better . . . 4 1/2 years later and Maureen O'Conner is an Ohio Supreme Court Justice, Craig is a Deputy friggin Chief, PHD Mary is retired and at AU and Cal and Beth are Captains. WOW a lot has changed. What has not changed is our desire to see that Douglas remains where he is until he is a feeble old sick man.

I realize it was really traumatic to rehash this story but it is something that truly needed to be done. You just keep plugging cause I know that Margo is watching from above and the story needs to be told over and over again about a cold blooded individual who took away this very blessed soul. I think about Ms. Lillie and the girls just about every day. She [Margo] truly was placed on this earth to be a mother and a radiate love. Thanks for your tenacity, I hope the book helps many out there who may have doubt whether to report abuse or not. I enjoyed seeing you in my new home town and I just can't believe I have been down here for 4 ½ years. If you should need something my home phone is (omitted) and the cell is always working unless I'm playing sick boy in bed.

Luv ya man, break a leg, hope to see you on Oprah telling this compelling story . . . Duvey

Epilogue

This story is a testimonial of the triumphant life and tragic death of Dr. Margo Shamberger Prade. There are those who will choose to love me for it, and those who will choose to hate me. It is, however, my story; one that needed to be told at whatever cost.

It is only now that this publication is complete that I can, with acute awareness and presence of mind settle on why I actually did write this book:

First, since the death of Dr. Margo Prade and even seven years thereafter, she *still* has only been known as a murder victim through any and all media coverage. I desired for Margo and ***all of her life's accomplishments and commitments,*** including that of a magnificent parent, and physician to be recognized. Second, although many people will refuse to acknowledge, these past seven years since the conviction of Douglas Prade, there are still *whisperings of suspicion* in the community as to whether or not he *really did kill Margo.* It is my hope that this publication is at least one vehicle needed to help put such suspicions to rest. Third, I never felt a sense of personal closure in the death of my dear friend, she left too fast; or in the conviction of her killer. And, I always felt offended when MSNBC would air Margo's murder year after year, obviously making money each time this crime is aired on national television. To my knowledge, none of the news programs or documentaries that have highlighted this horrendous murder, have ever compensated Kenya and Sahara Prade in a monetary fashion while they continued to sensationalize their mother's murder, and father's arrest and conviction. It is my hope that this publication can assist them financially in their future scholastic and career endeavors.

Finally, because they were so young when their mother was murdered, Doctor Margo Prade's two daughters *deserve* to know all of the *wonderful accomplishments* she achieved in her short life. Dr. Prade's daughters *deserve* to know how much their mother was loved in the community, and how much she loved life. Dr. Margo Prade's children *deserve* to know she was truly a gift from God!

It has taken tremendous effort to process the grief, anger, psychic pain, and acceptance that have suffocated me for the past seven years over Margo's murder; and many times when I have wanted to write and ***finish*** this book, I could not. It wasn't until recently on December 25th 2004, that I realized why. My friend and dance instructor, Sid, revealed so profoundly to me that, "You couldn't write to finish the book, because then you'd have to let her go again, and you are not *ready* to let her go a second time." Not only was he correct in his assessment, that statement alone was the push I needed. I completed this project in the five weeks following.

Now, I'd like to believe that my work is accomplished, and I *have* let Margo go in a positive realm; a realm that we all wish to release our loved ones in when they die; although I will never, ***ever*** forget Margo and the positive way in which she touched my life. Yet, I feel I can continue on with my life's journey; on the optimistic course it was intended to take before that detour of Margo's murder intercepted. I believe, too, if there is such a place, that Margo *is in heaven* and is somehow appreciative for what I have done.

There are those who have stated, "As tragic as Margo's death is, it was just her time to go." However, I believe God is too good and NOT THAT GREEDY to have taken Margo so soon, and in the way she met her demise. She was a saintly healer, a loving mother, daughter, friend, and wife. I believe the good do not necessarily have to die young, and that ***murder is never "God's will."***

Once having the life of Riley, I do not believe God intended for Margo's children to suffer the pain they share in having lost both parents within three months and three days. I do not believe God intended for young Sahara to experience severe anxiety attacks every September 17th and/or November 26th crying, "I miss my mom!"

I do believe, however, that Margo has watched over and

guided many of us; especially her children as best she can from where she is. Margo *loved* her children, and as a side note, she loved basketball star Michael Jordan. She once stated, "If it is the last thing I do, I'm taking my babies to see Michael Jordan play ball." Not surprisingly, she accomplished that goal too.

God knows Margo's children were placed at risk for serious self-destructive and antisocial behavior once they lost both parents. Even so, her children have prevailed in triumph through all the tragedy.

Daughter Sahara Prade debuted in the film, "Antwone Fisher" directed by and starring Denzel Washington in Cleveland, Ohio on October 3 & 4th 2001. October 4th is Ms. Lillie's birthday and this was a magnificent birthday present for her. The film aired in December 2003, and Sahara is in the final scene of the movie where Antwone Fisher meets his family.

On July 17th 2004 Sahara placed in the top ten of the "Beacon Idol" contestants. Beacon Idol was a contest created by the *Akron Beacon Journal* patterned after the Fox Network hit reality show,*American Idol.* Sahara went on to compete in the *American Idol* tryouts held in Cleveland, Ohio on August 3rd & 4th, 2004. Entertainment is a gift that Margo saw in Sahara very early in her life; and what Margo set her up for by enrolling her in Miller South School of Performing Arts. As of December 2004, Sahara is now sixteen years old, has earned a 4.0 GPA on her last grade card, and has completed two demo CD recordings. With the grace of God, her mother's perseverance *and watchful eye from above,* Sahara is well on her way to stardom.

* * *

On October 11, 2002, eldest daughter, Kenya, symbolic of her mother's popularity in becoming homecoming queen while attending Kent State University, was elected to the Homecoming Court at Buchtel High School. In June 2003, Kenya Prade graduated with full honors and a full scholarship to college. She is now attending Kent State University in the school of nursing, possibly with future sights on NEOUCOM. Both schools are her mother's alma maters.

The murder of Dr. Margo Prade, had a significant negative

impact on the Akron area community, not just her patients, family and friends. Thanks to the love, strength and determination of Ms. Lillie, a whole lot of love from family, friends, Margo's colleagues and the Akron, Ohio community, Margo's daughter's have remained steadfast on their paths to success. Achievement is a foundation their mother laid for them years before her death.

* * *

In the years following the murder of Dr. Margo Prade, there have been numerous celebrations, benefits and recognition ceremonies honoring the life of Dr. Margo S. Prade:

In the spring of 2000, The Women's History Project presented to Margo's family, the Woman of the Year, "Women as Healers" Posthumous Award in the name of Margo Prade, M.D. The award reads. "*For a woman who made a lasting and significant contribution to society.*"

In 2002, The Lunzy Armstrong Award from the South Rangers was presented to Dr. Margo S. Prade posthumously. The South Rangers is a community little league football team.

On May 14, 2003, NEOUCOM honored Dr. Margo Shamberger Prade in a benefit titled, "The History of Family Medicine." A Dedication of the Department of Family Medicine Memorial Wall. In total there were seven physicians memorialized, with Margo being the second youngest.

On February 26th, 2004 NEOUCOM held a Black History Celebration titled, "A Memorial Tribute." The dinner honored the memory of Margo S. Prade, M.D., class of 1983 and Neal Frost, M.D. class of 1988. Margo's family was presented with a beautiful memorial keepsake glass statue. The inscription reads: "*Dr. Prade, A beacon of light that still shines on.*" A $2000 scholarship award in the name of Dr. Margo Prade was also established to be awarded to a deserving minority student.

On May 26th 2004 Margo became a "Hall of Fame" inductee by the Central-Hower Alumni Association, Margo's high school alma mater.

Margo is featured in the Shirla McClain Gallery for accomplished African American Women of Akron. The gallery is located in Buckingham Hall at the University of Akron and

Margo's stethoscope and doctor's bag accompany her portrait encased behind a glass wall.

Finally, on Friday, May 21, 2004 under the love and leadership of Margo's sister Phyllis Foster, the very first Margo Shamberger Prade Scholarship Foundation dinner celebration was held. Monetary scholarship awards were presented to two deserving graduating high school seniors. This effort had been a vision of Margo's sister Phyllis in the years following Margo's death. The keynote speakers included the Mayor of Akron, Donald Plusquellic, and his wife Mary, who was also an honorary chairperson. Former prosecutor and now Judge Alison McCarty spoke overwhelmingly as to how she got to know Margo as a delightful spirit; and Deputy Mayor Dorothy O. Jackson was the Mistress of Ceremony. Retired detectives from the Prade case, including Dr. Mary Myers, also attended.

Margo's niece, Layne Farr, sang two beautiful selections; one being "I Believe I Can Fly" by R. Kelly and Margo's daughter Sahara sang, "Hero" by Mariah Carey. Sahara's voice and lyrics harmoniously reflected everything Margo wanted for her talented young daughter. As the striking lyrics soared from her tongue, there wasn't a dry eye in the place. Finally, when Sahara synchronized, "*You are the wind beneath my wings . . .*" the Mayor wept.

Dr. Margo Prade was the spark that lit a bright light of hope, trust and good health in her patients. A maniacal killer named Douglas Evans Prade, snuffed out that spark. In killing Margo however, Douglas chose his own road to hell. His actions marked the ending to the life of an intelligent and dedicated police captain now living out the remainder of his years behind prison walls. Rumor has it that Douglas is teaching illiterate inmates how to read, obviously an avenue for him to still seek respect, adulation, and the need to be needed. Unfortunately for Douglas, he fostered his demise when he became ***fixated*** on "winning" rather than "accepting" the inevitable divorce between him and Margo. Whatever his accomplishments are behind bars, they can never, ***ever*** compare to that of the beloved Dr. Margo Prade.

I believe Margo has indeed watched over us all, and she has been the driving force behind my chronicling this project. I believe Margo's spirit has watched over her two daughters, ensuring that they complete the positive pathways she set for them. I believe that Dr. Margo Prade's accomplishments will be remembered by many young scholars and that her influence will help promote success in them. It is my hope that we remember Dr. Margo Prade for her life's accomplishments, not just for how she died; and that the very essence of her ***kindred spirit*** will live within the hearts of many forever.

* * *

Special thanks to the following City of Akron Police Detectives; without their tenacity and dedication to their profession, Dr. Margo Shamberger Prade's murder would have remained an unsolved mystery.

- *Detective Capt. Rick Mullins (Retired)*
- *Deputy Chief Craig Gilbride*
- *Deputy Chief Gus Hall*
- *Lt. Ed. Duvall (Retired)*
- *Capt. Beth Daugherty*
- *Detective Capt. Mary Myers Ph.D (Retired)*
- *Capt. Paul Calvaruso*
- *Detective Sgt. Ed. Moriarty (Retired)*
- *Detective Sgt. Sean Matheny (Retired)*
- *Detective Sgt. Larry White (Retired)*
- *Detective Rod Smith (Retired)*
- *Detective Russ McFarland*
- *Detective Steve Geiger*
- *Detective Rodney Tucker*
- *Detective Donald Gaines (Retired)*
- *Detective Washington Lacy (Retired)*
- *Detective Bertina King*
- *Detective Sgt. Gerald Miles*
- *Detective Amy Frame*
- *Detective Sue Hackbart*

"She shone on me.
Angels are those who lift our feet when our wings have trouble remembering how to fly."
—Maya Angelou

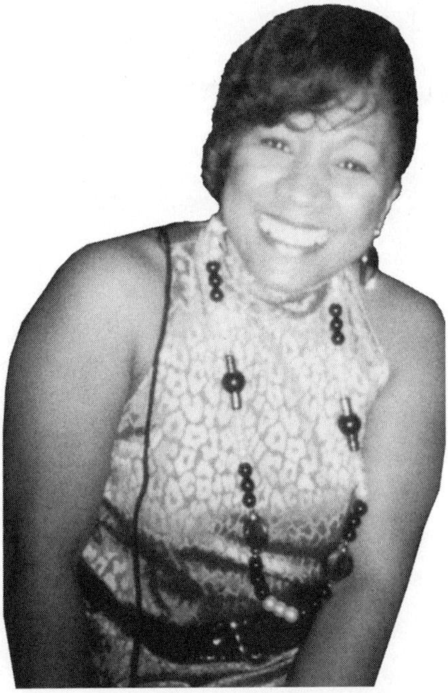

January 1987, B.L.E.O.A. ball
10 years and 11 months before her death
Rest in Peace

References

The *Akron Beacon Journal* (October 18, 1998) *Sunday Beacon* Magazine: *"Breaking the Prade Case."* Pgs. 6–17.

City of Akron Clerk of Courts. (September 1998). *Prade Case Court Testimony.*

City of Akron Law Department (November 26th 1997–September, 1998) *Report on Investigation.*

HBO Presents. (Date Unknown) *Autopsy 6: The Margo Prade Case.*

Mansfield, Eric. (Feburary 14, 1999). *The Doug Prade Case: A Community Torn.* Channel 3 News Report.

Prade, Douglas E. (1968–1997) *Personnel File.* City of Akron Police Department.

Murphy, Dennis and Pauly, Jane. (2000, present). *Interactive* Dateline Court TV Exclusive. Dateline MSNBC.

Arnold, Dayne (April, 2001). Personal Communication.

Duvall, Edward. (September 29, 2001). Personal Communication.

Edwards, Cranston (April, 2002). Personal Communication.

Farr, Layne. (October, 2003). Personal Communication/

Fedyna, Dina. (October 25, 2001). Personal Communication.

Foster, Joyce. (January 14, 2001). Personal Communication.

Foster, Pam. (July, 2001). Personal Communication.

Fowler, Tony (May 21, 2004) Personal Communication.

Fowler, Frances (April 2001) Personal Communication.

Freeman, Jane (April, 2000). Personal Communication.

Gilbride, Craig. (Feburary 6, 2002). Personal Communication.

Harper, Adolph Jr. M.D. (February 20, 2003). Personal Communication.

Hendricks, Lillie (April, 2002). Personal Communication.

Jackson, CeeJay (March, 2001). Personal Communication.

Malone, Aaron (October, 2000). Personal Communication.

McCarty, Alison (October 5, 2000). Personal Communication.

Poole, Jaquetta (July 19, 2002). Personal Communication.
Prade, Sahara (September 9, 2001). Personal Communication.
Shamberger, Edith (April, 2002). Personal Communication.
Taylor, Vickie (June 28, 2002). Personal Communication.

James Clerk Maxwell
and the Theory of the Electromagnetic Field

James Clerk Maxwell and the Theory of the Electromagnetic Field

John Hendry

Adam Hilger Ltd, Bristol and Boston

British Library Cataloguing in Publication Data

Hendry, John
James Clerk Maxwell and the theory of the electromagnetic field.
1. Maxwell, James Clerk——Contributions in electromagnetic theory 2. Electromagnetic theory
3. Electromagnetic fields
I. Title
530.1′41 QC665.E4

ISBN 0-85274-563-X

Consultant Editor: **Professor A J Meadows**
University of Leicester

Published by Adam Hilger Ltd
Techno House, Redcliffe Way, Bristol BS1 6NX, England
PO Box 230, Accord, MA 02018, USA

Typeset by Mathematical Composition Setters Ltd, Salisbury, UK
Printed in Great Britain by J W Arrowsmith Ltd, Bristol

To my wife

Contents

Preface and Acknowledgments

The origins of this book lie in a long-standing interest in the contrasting attitudes to physical science to be found in the early and middle nineteenth century. As my study evolved, I because increasingly aware of the importance of Maxwell, both as an active recipient of earlier traditions and as a moulder of those that were to follow. Maxwell was, as his biographers note, an 'heir to all ages'. He was also the classical physicist who, more than any other, addressed the problems whose resolution was to characterise the quantum mechanical revolution of the twentieth century. This book can indeed be seen as something of a prologue to my earlier work, *The Creation of Quantum Mechanics and the Bohr–Pauli Dialogue* (Reidel, 1984).

My aim in the present work has been to get to the heart of the intellectual activity in which Maxwell engaged and the intellectual movements of which he was a part. I have not attempted the far more ambitious task of setting this activity and these movements in their wider social context, which task would, for me at least, be premature. It is said that one may know a man by the company he keeps, but I should prefer to know the man himself first, and make the judgment after. I have also refrained from any great investigation of previously unpublished manuscript material, but not without looking far enough to satisfy myself that this would be unlikely to change my account in any significant way. Archival materials are the bread and butter of every professional historian but there comes a point, different for each subject and for each person, at which the law of diminishing returns sets in and additional material becomes a burden of little use rather than a source of significant fresh insight. In this case, thanks largely to the efforts of others, that point came fairly soon, and as the project was being pursued alongside another for which the archival demands were considerable I was indeed grateful. I can only hope that I was not misled by the circumstances into resting too content with the material already at my disposal.

As with any book that focuses upon one topic but touches upon many, my greatest debt is to my fellow scholars, who have done much of the surrounding groundwork for me. My specific debts in this respect are recorded in the footnotes and bibliography, but as I have been somewhat brief in my referencing I should like to make explicit here the extent to which some parts of my account in particular follow the work of others. In Chapter 2 I draw particularly heavily on the joint work of Peter Heimann and Ted McGuire (1971) as well as on their individual works. In Chapter 3 my discussions of Ampère and, to a lesser extent, Oersted are based on the work of Christine Blondel (1982). That of Faraday draws heavily on the biography by L Pearce Williams (1965) and the numerous papers by David Gooding, while that of Thomson is based on the work of Norton Wise (1981). In Chapter 5 the discussion of energy physics draws heavily on the work of Crosbie Smith (1978), while parts of Chapter 7 are indebted to a range of works by Russell McCormmach. I have not accepted any of these works uncritically: in all cases I have gone back to the published sources at least and adjusted my interpretation accordingly. But that does not lessen the debt and I am sincerely grateful to these scholars, most of whom are also personal acquaintances, as well as to others on whose work I have less obtrusively or less consciously drawn. Needless to say, they bear no responsibility for what I've made of their efforts, and if apologies rather than thanks are due I offer them!

Of those who gave their favours more willingly, I am grateful to those of my friends and colleagues, both historians and physicists, who were kind enough to read and criticise parts of the manuscript, including Bruce Brackenridge, David Cook, Jack Meadows, Simon Schaffer and Crosbie Smith. Not all their criticisms have been heeded, however, and the responsibility for what I have written is mine alone. The final word must go to Maxwell himself, whose writings have been a source of encouragement and guidance far transcending the limits of this book:

> He that would enjoy life and act with freedom must have the work of the day continually before his eyes. Not yesterday's work, lest he fall into despair, nor to-morrow's, lest he become a visionary,—not that which ends with the day, which is a worldly work, nor yet that only which remains to eternity, for by it he cannot shape his actions.
>
> Happy is the man who can recognise in the work of To-day a connected portion of the work of life, and an embodiment of the work of Eternity. The foundations of his confidence are unchangeable, for he has been made a partaker of Infinity. He strenuously works out his daily enterprises, because the present is given him for a possession.
>
> Thus ought Man to be an impersonation of the divine process of nature, and to show forth the union of the infinite with the finite, not slighting his temporal existence, remembering that in it only is individual action possible, nor yet shutting out from his view that which is eternal, knowing that Time is a mystery which man cannot endure to contemplate until eternal Truth enlighten it.

This philosophical fragment and the poems at the beginning and end of the book, all of which date from Maxwell's early twenties, are taken from the *Life* by Lewis Campbell and William Garnett (1884).

John Hendry
South Leigh, June 1985

A Student's Evening Hymn

Cambridge, April 25, 1853

I

Now no more the slanting rays
  With the mountain summits dally,
Now no more in crimson blaze
  Evening's fleecy cloudlets rally,
  Soon shall Night from off the valley
Sweep that bright yet earthly haze,
  And the stars most musically
Move in endless rounds of praise.

II

While the world is growing dim,
  And the Sun is slow descending
Past the far horizon's rim,
  Earth's low sky to heaven extending,
  Let my feeble earth-notes, blending
With the songs of cherubim,
  Through the same expanse ascending,
Thus renew my evening hymn.

III

Thou that fill'st our waiting eyes
  With the food of contemplation,
Setting in thy darkened skies
  Signs of infinite creation,
  Grant to nightly meditation
What the toilsome day denies—
  Teach me in this earthly station
Heavenly Truth to realise.

IV

Give me wisdom so to use
  These brief hours of thoughtful leisure,
That I may no instant lose
  In mere meditative pleasure,
  But with strictest justice measure
All the ends my life pursues,
  Lies to crush and truths to treasure,
Wrong to shun and Right to choose.

V

Then, when unexpected Sleep,
  O'er my long-closed eyelids stealing,
Opens up that lower deep
  Where Existence has no feeling,
  May sweet Calm, my languor healing,
Lend me strength at dawn to reap
  All that Shadows, world-concealing,
For the bold inquirer keep.

VI

Through the creatures Thou hast made
  Show the brightness of Thy glory,
Be eternal Truth displayed
  In their substance transitory,
  Till green Earth and Ocean hoary,
Massy rock and tender blade
  Tell the same unending story—
"We are Truth in Form arrayed."

VII

When to study I retire,
  And from books of ancient sages
Glean fresh sparks of buried fire
  Lurking in their ample pages—
  While the task my mind engages
Let old words new truths inspire—
  Truths that to all after-ages
Prompt the Thoughts that never tire.

VIII

Yet if, led by shadows fair,
  I have uttered words of folly,
Let the kind absorbing air
  Stifle every sound unholy.

So when Saints with Angels lowly
Join in heaven's unceasing prayer,
Mine as certainly, though slowly,
May ascend and mingle there.

Two stanzas omitted, the Author knows where, but not to be inserted till he knows how.

Teach me so Thy works to read
That my faith,—new strength accruing,—
May from world to world proceed,
Wisdom's fruitful search pursuing;
Till, thy truth my mind imbuing,
I proclaim the Eternal Creed,
Oft the glorious theme renewing
God our Lord is God indeed.

Give me love aright to trace
Thine to everything created,
Preaching to a ransomed race
By Thy mercy renovated,
Till with all thy fulness sated
I behold thee face to face
And with Ardour unabated
Sing the glories of thy grace.

James Clerk Maxwell

Notation and Symbols

As a general policy in this book I have sought to use Maxwell's own symbols wherever possible, so as to assist any reader wishing to return to the original publications. Since Maxwell's usage differs considerably from the modern one, however, this does introduce the possibility of confusion, especially where Maxwell uses symbols familiar from modern presentations of the theory for completely different variables. In order to minimise this confusion, while at the same time providing as much help as possible for the modern reader, I have translated Maxwell's equations as they are developed in the course of his work into modern symbols, but have always placed such translated forms in boxes. Unless specifically stated to the contrary any symbols occurring other than in these boxes are derived historically (occasionally with modifications) and are explicitly *not* to be confused with the modern usage. Throughout the book, however, I have taken the liberty of rewriting many of Maxwell's formulae, originally expressed in coordinate form, in modern vector notation. Since Maxwell himself introduced a vector notation to physics in his *Treatise,* and since he seems always to have thought, physically, in terms of vector concepts, this seems a justifiable aid to comprehension—though I have always indicated explicitly where I have done it. A final way in which Maxwell's expressions differ from their modern equivalents is in the absence from his work of any special symbol for partial differentiation. Where we would use ∂ he sticks to d, the partial operation being apparent from the context. This does not seem to lead to any confusion, and I have therefore retained Maxwell's own expressions when quoting these directly in coordinate form. In writing equations in vector form I have used bold type for vectors and have written $\boldsymbol{a} \cdot \boldsymbol{b}$, $\boldsymbol{a} \times \boldsymbol{b}$ for scalar and vector products respectively. I have used ∇, $\nabla\cdot$ and $\nabla\times$ for the differential operators *grad, div* and *curl* respectively.

Even in modern times notation is not completely standardised and I have used the boxed symbols below for the variables featuring in Maxwell's equations in their modern form. Symbols to the left of the box are the most prominent of Maxwell's equivalents, adapted to vector form.

$\boldsymbol{\alpha}_0$, $\boldsymbol{F} = (F, G, H)$	$\boldsymbol{A}$	vector potential
$\boldsymbol{a}_1, \mu\boldsymbol{\alpha}$	$\boldsymbol{B}$	magnetic flux density or magnetic induction
$f = (f, g, h)$	$\boldsymbol{D}$	electric flux density or electric displacement
$\boldsymbol{\alpha}_2, \boldsymbol{P} = (P, Q, R)$	$\boldsymbol{E}$	electric field strength or electromotive force at a point
	$\boldsymbol{F}$	mechanical force on a charged particle in the field
$\boldsymbol{\alpha}_1, \boldsymbol{\alpha}$	$\boldsymbol{H}$	magnetic field strength
$\boldsymbol{p}' = (p', q', r')$	$\boldsymbol{I}$	total current
$\boldsymbol{a}_2, \boldsymbol{p} = (p, q, v)$	$\boldsymbol{J}$	electric current density (conduction current)
	$\boldsymbol{M}$	magnetic polarisation
	$\boldsymbol{P}$	electric polarisation
	$\mathcal{E}$	electromotive force in a circuit
e	q	electric charge
	ρ	electric charge density
	ψ	electric potential.

Using the modern symbols, Maxwell's equations as we now know them may be written as follows, assuming no isolated magnetic poles:

$$\nabla \times \boldsymbol{E} = -\frac{\partial \boldsymbol{B}}{\partial t} \tag{0.1}$$

$$\nabla \times \boldsymbol{H} = \boldsymbol{I} \tag{0.2}$$

$$\boldsymbol{I} = \boldsymbol{J} + \frac{\partial \boldsymbol{D}}{\partial t} \tag{0.3}$$

$$\nabla \cdot \boldsymbol{B} = 0 \tag{0.4}$$

$$\nabla \cdot \boldsymbol{D} = \rho \tag{0.5}$$

$$\nabla \cdot \boldsymbol{J} = -\frac{\partial \rho}{\partial t} \tag{0.6}$$

$$\boldsymbol{J} = \sigma \boldsymbol{E} \tag{0.7}$$

$$\left.\begin{aligned} \boldsymbol{D} &= \epsilon_0 \boldsymbol{E} \quad (0.8) \\ \boldsymbol{B} &= \mu_0 \boldsymbol{H} \quad (0.9) \end{aligned}\right\} \text{in a vacuum}$$

$$\left.\begin{aligned} \boldsymbol{D} &= \epsilon \boldsymbol{E} = \epsilon_0 \boldsymbol{E} + \boldsymbol{P} \quad (0.10) \\ \boldsymbol{B} &= \mu \boldsymbol{H} = \mu_0 \boldsymbol{H} + \boldsymbol{M} \quad (0.11) \end{aligned}\right\} \text{in a medium}$$

$$\boldsymbol{B} = \nabla \times \boldsymbol{A} \tag{0.12}$$

$$E = -\frac{\partial \boldsymbol{A}}{\partial t} - \nabla \psi \tag{0.13}$$

$$\boldsymbol{F} = q\boldsymbol{E} + \boldsymbol{I} \times \boldsymbol{B}. \tag{0.14}$$

In the presence of isolated magnetic poles there would be additional terms on the right-hand sides of (0.4) and (0.14).

1

Introduction

If we were to draw up an all-time 'top ten' of physical scientists, there is a good chance that James Clerk Maxwell would not only feature in it but come pretty near to the top. Apart from a range of achievements in mathematics and engineering science he is remembered today as the prime author of the modern theory of colour vision, as the principal creator of statistical thermodynamics and, above all perhaps, as the author of the classical electromagnetic field theory, with its identification of light and electromagnetic waves. In view of these massive achievements there are remarkably few books on Maxwell and his work, and the definitive biography is still, after over a century, the *Life and Letters* compiled after Maxwell's death by his lifelong friend Lewis Campbell.[1] The main reason for this lack of attention is probably the fact that Maxwell is very much a 'physicists' physicist', and a mathematical one at that. Whereas the achievements of a Faraday or Rutherford can be presented dramatically (if distortedly) to a lay audience, the appreciation of the 'Maxwell distribution' or, even more, of 'Maxwell's equations' calls for more specialised tastes. In some ways, moreover, Maxwell does not fit the popular image of the scientist. He was, for example, no 'discoverer', and each of his major contributions to science rested heavily on the work of others.

If Maxwell did not make many discoveries, however, he did provide an almost unrivalled contribution to our understanding of the physical world, and to the formulation and articulation of this understanding.[2] And he was no narrow scientist. His interests and activities were catholic, encompassing literature, philosophy, social responsibility and religion as well as science. He was himself, as the examples given in this volume show, a poet of some ability. Most important of all, he fused his areas of interest and ability into a single whole. His life, of just 48 years, was a relatively short one, but it was both rich and instructive.

[1] Campbell and Garnett (1882, reprinted 1969, 1884).
[2] On discovery and understanding see Hendry (1983a).

Of all Maxwell's achievements, the electromagnetic theory is probably his most famous; it also has a special historical interest. For it consists of not just one paper or book, but a series of book-length monographs, covering a period of twenty years, in each of which the subject is treated from a different viewpoint. Through this series of studies we have an opportunity to study a scientist, a supreme scientist, working in his most characteristic fashion—not merely setting down a theory and passing on, but developing the theory continuously and arriving at each stage at new results and a new and deeper understanding. Furthermore, the period of development in this case covers a period of major changes in the physical sciences in general, including the advent of methods based on the principle of energy conservation and the beginnings of vector analysis. These changes are well reflected in Maxwell's work. His first major contribution to electromagnetic theory belongs to the era before the energy principle had been clearly expounded and applied. In his later writings, however, the new synthesis of Lagrangian dynamics and energy conservation played an increasingly important part, and in his famous *Treatise on Electricity and Magnetism* he himself pioneered the introduction of vector analysis. Thus besides providing an insight to the individual development of a scientific theory, Maxwell's work also provides an introduction to the wider changes that were taking place in the methodology of physics at the time, and that themselves constituted something of a scientific revolution.

Clearly the development of Maxwell's electromagnetic theory contains an historical story worth telling. The question is, though, how to tell it. From the viewpoint of the historian, there are many ways in which a subject such as this may be approached. We could focus, for example, on the scientist's personal biography, on his family life and on his response to such stimuli as love, marriage, illness and death. Or we could concentrate instead on the evolving language, customs and conventions of the society in which he lived, or the profession in which he practised. Yet again we could remain, so to speak, within the laboratory, and treat all matters external to the science itself as having only marginal significance. Ideally, we should like to cover all such angles, internal and external, social and psychological. But such is the complexity of real life that we can scarcely hope to encompass it within the confines of the written word, let alone within those of a single readable book. In practice we must therefore focus on a relatively narrow set of concerns, and the choice of approach, though partly a question of judgment as to what seems important in a particular case, is largely a matter of personal tastes and interests.

In this book I have chosen to tell the story of Maxwell's theory on just two interconnected levels, both of which are relatively internal to the physics. One is concerned with the technical details of physical theory, the other with considerations of scientific methodology. The resulting story is certainly not 'the whole' one, and I doubt if it is even self-contained. I could for example envisage another book treating of much of the same events but from the very different viewpoint of the development of physics as a selfconscious discipline and profession. Moreover, I should consider such an approach every bit as valid and as valuable, historically, as my own. Just at the moment, however, I should not find it so interesting. In short, I have adopted the viewpoint that I have simply because the questions it raises appear to me to be especially interesting ones, and I make no apology for having written this book rather than another!

Apart from this self-imposed limitation of approach the levels of analysis within the approach also carry their own intrinsic limitations, and these too should be noted. I shall be concentrating upon what may be called the technical level of the development of scientific theory: that is, on Maxwell's work as a physicist and mathematician, on the way in which he did his physics and on the ways in which his achievement contributed to the development of physics, interpreted in a fairly narrow sense. Despite this technical bias I have tried to write the story in a way that will be reasonably accessible to the non-mathematician, the non-physicist and even the perservering non-scientist. But I have also tried not to sacrifice the guts of the science simply for the sake of easy reading, and in some cases this latter consideration has had to take priority. Like almost all physicists since, and many before, Maxwell not only wrote but also reasoned in a highly technical, mathematical, language. This language can usually be paraphrased in ordinary everyday non-technical terms, but it cannot always be translated into such terms. The domain of mathematics in particular provides a range of mental experiences which, though they may find analogues in non-mathematical thought, do not seem to have any direct counterparts there. I have therefore retained most of the mathematical language (albeit sometimes in modern notations or symbols: see the prefatory 'note'), and although I have usually tried to explain what was going on in a non-technical manner as well, I have occasionally had to admit defeat.

The second level of analysis, which is deeper but also, since hidden from sight, rather more speculative, is a philosophical one. Besides being a physicist in the modern sense, (the word 'physicist' was in fact coined by Whewell in 1840, when Maxwell was a child), Maxwell was also a traditional natural philosopher, in the broadest possible sense of that phrase. Like many physical scientists of his own and earlier generations, and like at least a few of his great successors, he was acutely aware of the philosophical context within which his technical enterprise was located. Considerations of scientific method, and of the nature of scientific knowledge, were to him the foundation stones upon which theories must be built. They were not, as they sometimes are nowadays, mere ornamentations or appendices to be treated, if at all, only after a theory had been developed.

Uncovering the philosophical foundations of physics is always a tricky and at times a risky business. But when such foundations are known to exist as genuine historical elements, and not merely as part of a speculative logical reconstruction, the risks are surely worthwhile. Most working physicists now treat their science as philosophically non-problematical. So too did many of Maxwell's contemporaries. But both Maxwell and most of the earlier founders of classical electromagnetic theory, on whose work he built, took a different view. They saw the philosophical foundations of science as a genuine problem area, and to some extent at least they reasoned upwards from their purely philosophical conclusions to their more strictly physical ones. This is in itself, I believe, a point of sufficient historical importance to justify a study of the foundations they used, even though this use may not always have been rigorous, and even though the precise layout of the foundations, rarely discussed in public, may be unclear. Besides, this study also raises an interesting and important historiographical point concerning the philosophical realm that transcends the particular subject matter being treated. One of the most prominent features of the landscape of natural philosophical debate in the period immediately before Maxwell concerned something that was called the 'dynamical philosophy' and that was opposed to the more usual 'mechanical philosophy'. In some of its more visible and florid manifestations this dynamical philosophy featured as part of the movement known as Romanticism, a movement that was represented in England, for example, by the poetry of Wordsworth and by the paintings of Constable. The tendency among historians of science has been to treat the dynamical philosophy as confined to the Romantic movement, and as essentially antiscience, with the mechanical philosophy being the norm, at least in the development of science. I shall be arguing in contrast that mechanism and dynamism represent two approaches to science and philosophy both of which are always present, and the difference between which probably has more to do with individual psychological attitudes, whether innate or socially impressed, than with socially defined cultural movements—though culture itself may also be sympathetic to one attitude or the other, swinging between them like some slowly varying schizophrenic. Neither attitude, on the view adopted here, has a monopoly of scientific achievement; nor would either make any substantial and long-term progress in science without the provoking and tempering power of the other.

To comprehend the foundations of nineteenth-century physics in terms of philosophical dynamism and mechanism is relatively straightforward. But to describe them without introducing confusion is unfortunately less so, and some comment on the language I shall use is appropriate. As will be explained in detail in the next chapter, the use of the words 'dynamical' and 'mechanical' to describe philosophical attitudes or approaches often clashes with their technical use in mathematics and physics: a technically mechanical theory may well reflect a philosophically dynamical approach or vice versa. To complicate matters further there also grew up in Maxwell's time a tradition of 'dynamical' explanation in physics which, while carrying philosophical overtones, was nevertheless quite distinct from the 'dynamical philosophy' of the earlier part of the century. To abandon the use of the words 'dynamical' and 'mechanical' altogether in any of their historical meanings would be anachronistic, and since the meanings would still turn up in quotations it would probably not help matters much anyway. But in order to minimise the possible sources of confusion I have used the words in their philosophical sense *only* where the context removes all ambiguity. Wherever there is a chance of ambiguity, and wherever, indeed, it does not appear totally anachronistic to do so, I have adopted the alternative adjectives 'dynamistic' and 'mechanistic' to describe the philosophical approaches and reserved 'dynamical' and 'mechanical' for technical use.

The relationship between the two levels of analysis, the physical and the philosophical, is slightly ambivalent. In one sense it is a very close one. If we were to try to uncover the deepest workings of the creative mind, we should no doubt find that even epistemological foundations rested upon some deeper bedrock of spiritual or religious convictions. Maxwell, typical in this respect of his age, was a deeply religious man. If on the other hand we look in the opposite direction, beyond the level of physical argument and theory, there is also yet another level, corresponding to the laborious grinding of equations and the painstaking setting up of workable experiments. I should argue, however, that the focal point of Maxwell's achievements occurs neither in the inner realm of religion nor in the outer one of observation, experiment and calculation, but somewhere between the two. It occurs, namely, at the very point at which the two levels I have chosen to concentrate on come together, at the point at which fundamental concerns of scientific knowledge and method meet the main structure of scientific theory and technical problem-solving. At this focal point the two levels are thus bound intimately together.

At the same time, however, it is also apparent that while the creative point may lie at the junction between the two levels, the action takes place primarily within one of them and only secondarily within the other. Thus the principal discourse of science takes place within the technical problem-solving complex, at the level at which a well developed scientific language, working alongside a planned experimental exploration, makes possible the communication between scientists and the analysis and comparison of alternative theoretical structures. In this sense the philosophical level provides a background framework of reference and associations rather than a foreground thread of argument.

This distinction is reflected in the treatment given below, in which the greater attention is devoted to the physical rather than the philosophical level. It is however with the philosophical level, as providing the context and background, that we must of necessity start.

2

Mechanistic and Dynamistic Traditions in Nineteenth-century Physics

The existence of two fundamentally contrasting attitudes towards the world is a general phenomenon, not confined to physics, which has often been noted and has been much discussed. Samuel Taylor Coleridge, remembered today as a poet and critic, was also one of the leading philosophers and theologians of the early nineteenth century. Elaborating in his 1818 *Philosophical Lectures* on a distinction drawn by Goethe, he divided all self-consistent philosophers into Platonists and Aristotelians, a division that has been widely used in the history of ideas ever since.[1] Plato, he explained, 'began in meditations [and] thought deeply within himself of the goings-on of his own mind and of the powers that were in that mind', and progressed *from* there *to* the outside world:

> Now Plato argued that, as there was that power in the mind which thinks and images its thoughts, analogous to this was the power in nature which thought and imaged or embodied its thoughts, in consequence of which he resolved the ground of all things into the dynamic.
>
> Aristotle on the contrary, affirmed that all our knowledge had begun in experience, had begun through the senses, and that from the senses only we could take our knowledge of reality . . . .

Aristotle thus progressed *from* the outside world *to* that of the mind.

Around the turn of the twentieth century, the pragmatic philosopher and psychologist William James noted that 'the history of philosophy is, to a great extent, that of a certain clash of human temperaments',[2] and that,

[1] Coleridge (1949), especially pp. 186–7 from which the quotations are taken.
[2] James (1907) pp. 7–8.

moreover,

> [The temperament of a philosopher] really gives a stronger bias than any of his more strictly objective premises. It loads the evidence for him one way or another, making for a more sentimental or more hard-hearted view of the universe, just as this fact or that principle would. He trusts his temperament. Wanting a universe that suits it, he believes in any representation of the universe that does suit it. He feels men of opposite temper to be out of key with the world's character, and in his heart considers them incompetent and 'not in it', in the philosophical business, even though they may far excel him in dialectical ability.

Many other writers have drawn similar distinctions in different terms, some of them psychological, others sociological. But the best known categorisation is probably that of the psychologist Carl Gustav Jung. In 1921, in his classic work *Psychological Types*, Jung introduced and elaborated on the categories of 'introvert' and 'extravert', corresponding roughly to Coleridge's Platonist and Aristotelian.[3]

As Jung recognised, categories such as these are far from being absolute. They represent tendencies rather than constraints, both tendencies being present to a greater or lesser extent in any one individual, and with the imbalance between them compensated for by secondary characteristics of the personality. Moreover, the judgment as to which tendency dominates in an individual is apt to be strongly influenced by the commentator's own dominant tendency. Jung defined the introvert as one who tended to interpret the external world in terms of his inner mental experience, to reason from mind to nature; and the extravert as one who tended to reason in the reverse direction, from nature to mind. This definition of categories comes very close indeed to that used by Coleridge in the quotation given above. But whereas Jung saw the philosopher Kant as an introvert, for example, Coleridge tended to view him as an Aristotelian (or in Jungian terms extravert, or at least balanced), at least in respect of his moral and religious philosophy. When Coleridge himself, in his later years, grew disaffected with the romantic *Naturphilosophie* of Schelling, whom he had always admired and viewed as a Platonist, and when he began to strengthen his allegiance to Kant, he accommodated this change by recategorising Kant as a Platonist and moving Schelling to the realm of untenable philosophies beyond Platonism, rather than by admitting any change in his own stance. Again, whereas Coleridge, writing as a philosopher, restricted his categories to attitudes he considered philosophically consistent and tenable, Jung, writing as a psychologist, also incorporated the extremes of introversion

[3] Jung (1923). Jung did not explicitly discuss Coleridge's distinction, but he did open his work with a quote from Heine: 'Plato and Aristotle! These are not merely two systems; they are also types of two distinct human natures, which from immemorial time, under every sort of cloak, stand more or less inimically opposed.'

and extraversion, in which thought remained pathologically locked in the internal or external worlds, and so brought coherent Aristotelian and Platonist viewpoints towards the middle ground.

Applied universally, categories such as those used by Coleridge and Jung will always be problematic. Even in relation to a specific set of people and problems their use may lead to difficulties and inconsistencies. But despite this qualification the basic dichotomy remains, if used with care and subject to the provisos noted, an extremely useful one. Whether or not it accurately describes the spectrum of world views adopted it does provide a handle with which to grasp that spectrum and a framework in which to set the networks of ideas associated with rival approaches to a given problem. Of course, the dichotomy manifests itself in different terms in different periods and fields of thought. It would scarcely be appropriate to talk of nineteenth-century physics in terms of introversion and extraversion, Platonism and Aristotelianism, or even realism and nominalism, described by Jung as 'the opposites between which science has oscillated' from the earliest times to his own day, but historically more meaningful for the mediaeval than for the modern period.[4] It does, however, seem appropriate to describe the foundations of nineteenth-century science in terms of the categories of dynamical or dynamistic (very roughly speaking introverted) and mechanical or mechanistic (very roughly speaking extraverted) world views, a categorisation that has indeed been used very successfully for the realms of chemistry and matter theory by the historian Trevor Levere.[5] This categorisation, which may in fact be taken quite independently of the notion of psychological types, will be adopted here.[6]

The conflict between dynamistic and mechanistic attitudes appeared in different guises in different contexts. In general the dynamical philosophy tended to be suspicious of all hypotheses as to the structure of the natural world, but within the realm of science the well known mechanical philosophy, based on the hypotheses of atoms and their geometric configurations, also had a dynamistic counterpart in which systems of nature were built up akin to the mechanical systems but based on the philosophically dynamical hypotheses of active forces. In philosophy, the conflict between those who sought to explain the structure of mind in terms of matter and those who explained the perception of matter in terms of mind was rather sharper and more comprehensive. The most disputed areas tended to be the fundamental concepts of morals and, later, mathematics, which each group claimed to derive from its own starting point, but the conflict also covered the basic concepts of science and the forms of scientific laws.

[4] Jung (1923) pp. 48–9.

[5] Levere (1971), especially p. 5.

[6] Although I have chosen to introduce the dynamistic and mechanistic approaches as modes of thought characteristic of the individual they may be viewed equally well as social characteristics, or taken independent of any theoretical framework.

Finally, in the area of mathematical physics, the two debates merged into one. Each of these areas was important for the development of electromagnetic theory and for the formation of Maxwell's ideas on the subject, and we shall therefore treat them each in turn.

Mechanistic and dynamistic approaches to science in general

The Scientific Revolution of the seventeenth century is often portrayed as entailing the 'mechanisation of the world picture'[7]; and in many important respects it did. The revival of Greek atomism by Gassendi and others paved the way for the evolution of the mechanistic theories of atoms and the void that were to dominate the science of the Enlightenment.[8] In René Descartes's great theory of *The World* there was no void, but in all other respects this was the prototype of a mechanistic theory.[9] Descartes's world was made up of a plenum of hard impenetrable atoms interacting by contact actions only; the whole diversity of natural phenomena, organic as well as inorganic, was held to result from the combinations of and differences between the shapes, sizes and motions of the fundamental atoms.

Although Descartes's role in the Scientific Revolution was a pivotal one, however, his importance owed more to the enormous and profound advances he made in mathematics than to the physical philosophy we remember today.[10] Of his contemporary revolutionaries, moreover, at least one, Johannes Kepler, was a thorough-going Platonist and dynamical philosopher, investing the universe with living forces and design,[11] and although the two great scientific prophets of the period, Francis Bacon and Galileo Galilei, are generally classed as mechanical philosophers, this categorisation can be misleading. Certainly their outlooks were mechanical when compared with those of their Renaissance predecessors. Both, for example, were atomists. But they were not uncompromising mechanists in the sense of Descartes, Gassendi or Hobbes. Both embraced comprehensive

[7] See for example Dijksterhuis (1961). Many works have been written on the intellectual history of the Scientific Revolution. Some recent ones, emphasising different aspects, are Hall (1983), Webster (1983), Merchant (1980), Westfall (1977) and Debus (1978). Other classics include Hall (1962), which is more accessible than the recent rewrite cited above, Crombie (1959), Collingwood (1945), Boas (1952) and Harré (1964). References to more specialised works, and to works encompassing the social as well as the intellectual domain of science, may be found in the works cited.

[8] Gassendi (1972); Charleton (1966).

[9] Descartes (1664 and see also 1983).

[10] See for example Gaukroger (1980) and Clarke (1982).

[11] See for example Holton (1973) and Koyré (1973) It should be stressed that Kepler was also a very hard-headed scientist. Dynamism must not be confused with mysticism or spiritualism, nor mechanism with materialism.

visions of the development of science, and while Bacon drew on elements of Paracelsian dynamism Galileo espoused that positivism with respect to mechanical hypotheses, that we have already noted as being associated with the modern dynamistic tradition.[12]

A similar ambivalence is apparent in the attitudes of the two men whose writings acted as the foundation for the scientific philosophies of the eighteenth century, Isaac Newton and Gottfried Wilhelm Leibniz. It was of course Newton whose image dominated the Enlightenment, and the dominant image was that of a mechanical philosopher. But there was also something in his writings for the dynamists. A vast amount of historical scholarship in recent years has been devoted to Newton's thought and the picture that has emerged is a complex one, in which the most consistent elements are mathematical and theological rather than physical or philosophical.[13] Through his introduction of a mathematically precise concept of force, Newton changed the very terms in which the dynamical and mechanical approaches could be defined.[14] But he did not himself come out unequivocally in favour of either approach. With forces introduced to the technical vocabulary of physics the point at issue became whether these forces should be treated as simply inherent in active matter, the dynamical view, or as something superposed onto passive, inert matter as a further component in the mechanical machinery. If the latter approach were adopted, there was a further choice to be made between treating the forces as elemental, or treating them as being themselves subject to explanation in terms of some aetherial medium. If such a medium were introduced, the original issue returned: the aether could be treated as either dynamical, a matrix of forces, or mechanical, a material fluid.

Newton himself was not disposed towards mechanical hypotheses, and for most of the time he was careful to take a neutralist stance, keeping within the mathematical–theological domain in which he was most confident. In respect of the force of gravity he was reluctant to be drawn at all beyond the observation that such a force existed, and when pressed on its cause he attributed it directly to the Divine Presence. He was not, however, immune from the fascination of speculation. As with most scientists, indeed, speculation played a crucial heuristic role in his work. In some contexts, such as gravitation, his success enabled him to pass beyond the speculative stage. But in others, and especially in chemistry, to the study of which he devoted most of his working life, he was less successful. At times

[12] On Bacon, see for example Rossi (1968), Webster (1983) and Rees (1980). On Galileo see for example Drake (1978), Clavelin (1974), Shea (1972) and Koyré (1978). Galileo's own work is eminently readable—see especially Galileo (1974).

[13] See especially Westfall (1980), Cohen (1980) and Bechler (1982).

[14] In the language of the seventeenth and eighteenth centuries the word force could have many meanings. I shall use it in the modern sense of a force acting on a body to change its state in some way, and specifically not in the sense of the 'force' possessed by a body, or as we should say its energy or momentum.

when his chemical (in those days, and for Newton, alchemical) researches were dominant he speculated freely on aetherial media and the structure of light and matter. In successive editions of his *Opticks*, published in the early eighteenth century, he set down some of his speculations in print.[15] In essence, his conception of the aether seems to have been a dynamical one. He recognised that an aether composed of atoms and void would itself be subject to forces which would themselves have to be explained by recourse to an even finer aether, and so on *ad infinitum*, until all that remained in the limit were attractive and repulsive forces between point centres. At no time, moreover, did Newton either consider forces as being mechanical in the sense of being reducible to contact actions, or accept the principle of action at a distance. His conception was dynamical both in its rejection of mechanism and in its adherence to some concept of active principles—forces, or causes of forces, diffused throughout space and in some sense physical, but yet immaterial.[16]

So much, then, for Newton's own opinions. But his written speculations in the famous Queries of the *Opticks* were also open to a mechanical interpretation and it was this interpretation, reinforced by the philosophy of Locke, that acted as the foundation for Enlightenment science and the proclaimed 'Newtonian' natural philosophy of the eighteenth century. The mechanical philosophy in eighteenth-century science had three main strands. One was a continuation of Cartesianism. This was, however, of relatively little importance, and although its emphasis upon the plenum may have played a part in Leonhardi Euler's development in mid century of the mathematics of continuous media, with important consequences for the later development of field theory, it was a dying tradition.[17] The other two strands, traditionally represented by the theories of imponderable fluids such as those supposed to constitute electricity, and by theories incorporating systems of particles, void and interparticulate forces, were both derived largely from Newton and Locke.[18]

[15] Newton (1730 and 1952) and see also Westfall (1971), McGuire (1978) and McGuire and Tamny (1983).

[16] McGuire (1978), Heimann and McGuire (1971) and see also Levere (1971).

[17] See Hesse (1961) and Burckhardt *et al* (1983).

[18] Heimann and McGuire (1971) and McGuire (1978). The treatment given here rests very heavily upon these two papers, with which I have only one small quibble, namely that both authors tend to underplay the epistemological qualifications accompanying ontological statements. They thus make statements about nature (atoms etc) seem much more dogmatic than they were, and tend to treat statements about knowledge as mere apologia or superimposed justifications when they were intended to be taken rather more seriously. This is however a minor criticism for they, and especially McGuire, have done far more than any other recent scholars to bring out the philosophical complexities of the natural science of this period. For the distinction between the two mechanical Newtonian traditions, quite rightly played down by Heimann and McGuire, see Schofield (1970) and Thackray (1970).

Though a keen observer of the Scientific Revolution, John Locke was no scientific philosopher, and much of his argument on the status of what he called primary and secondary qualities was quickly rejected by Berkeley and Hume. But Locke's *Essay Concerning Human Understanding*, published in 1690, just a few years after Newton's *Principia*, was widely taken up as the philosophical companion of that work.[19] Together with Newton's *Opticks* these books became the gospels of the Enlightenment. Newton's work, particularly that on gravity in the *Principia*, constituted the great scientific achievement on which the values of the Age of Enlightenment were based. But although his *Principia* provided the prototype of a modern scientific theory, and although the Queries in the *Opticks* provided suggestions and speculations on which science could build, Newton's cautious and qualified dynamism did not provide a clear manifesto on method such as the new movement needed. Locke's *Essay* did, and his manifesto, which covered the whole range of philosophy, was an uncompromisingly mechanical one. Nature was to be viewed in terms of insensible corpuscles, characterised by the mechanical 'primary' qualities of extension, motion and solidity. All causal explanation was to be in terms of the geometrical relationships between the corpuscles, and all forms of action were to be reduced to impulse action. 'Secondary' qualities, such as colour or chemical behaviour, were to be treated as the effects of 'powers', arising simply from the dispositions of the corpuscles. These powers were not active powers, inherent in the bodies themselves, but passive powers, the mechanical consequences of relationships between bodies.

The combination of Locke's mechanist approach to nature with Newton's aetherial speculations and mathematical theory of gravitation formed the basis for what is generally, if misleadingly, called the Newtonian science of the eighteenth century. Depending largely on the level of discourse adopted, the scientific area of enquiry, and personal preferences, the so-called Newtonian scientists constructed their theories in terms of either imponderable fluids or systems of particles related by passive forces of attraction and repulsion.[20]

Although it constituted the scientific orthodoxy of the period, the Newtonian tradition was a relatively sterile one, and the eighteenth century was not an era of dramatic scientific advance. But the imponderable fluid concept did provide an invaluable conceptual tool for the exploration of electrical phenomena by scientists such as Benjamin Franklin.[21] Then, towards the end of the eighteenth century, the mechanistic approach achieved a belated but monumental success at the hands of two Frenchmen, Antoine-Laurent Lavoisier and Pierre Simon de Laplace. Lavoisier, apply-

[19] Locke (1979) and, for a concise presentation, McGuire (1968). See Rogers (1983) for the relationship between Locke and Newton.

[20] See Schofield (1970) and Thackray (1970).

[21] See the monumental studies by Cohen (1956) and Heilbron (1979).

ing a thoroughly mechanical perspective to the problems of chemistry and focusing entirely on the weights and densities of substances rather than on the apparent but mechanically intractable forces of chemical combination, succeeded in bringing chemistry wholly within the mechanical philosophy for the first time.[22] Early in the nineteenth century John Dalton, building on Lavoisier's work, put forward the atomic theory of the chemical elements on which modern chemistry is based.[23] Meanwhile, Laplace, in his *Exposition du Système du Monde* of 1796, had carried forward with remarkable success a programme of reducing the whole of physics to an analysis of the mechanistic force-and-corpuscle variety.[24] We shall return to Laplace's work in the specific context of mathematical physics later in this chapter, but since it constituted the epitome of the mechanistic approach to physics it may be worth noting here the elements of his approach. He took as the basis for his programme the hypothesis of finite molecules, never clearly defined but consisting apparently, and consistently with the chemical work of his colleague Lavoisier, of the smallest elements into which matter could be divided without losing its particular (chemical) nature. A physical explanation then consisted, in Laplace's view, of establishing a system, entirely hypothetical, of molecules, intermolecular forces and configurations, the mathematical analysis of which led to the observed phenomena.[25]

Lavoisier's work amounted to a chemical revolution. Laplace's, backed up by the tremendous authority he acquired as author of the *Mécanique Celeste*, the definitive analysis of Newtonian celestial mechanics, was almost equally impressive. In addition both men fathered continuing traditions of mechanistic science running through the nineteenth century. In comparison with these achievements, the dynamistic science of the eighteenth century had relatively little to offer, but it did encapsulate a current of ideas that were to become of increasing importance as the nineteenth century developed, especially in the realm of electromagnetic theory.

While the mechanical philosophy advanced apace in England and France under the joint influence of Newton and Locke, Scotland and Germany played hosts to the evolution of rival dynamical philosophies. These were based broadly on the dynamistic elements of Newton's work, the sceptical philosophy of Hume and the philosophy of Newton's arch-rival in the development of the calculus, Leibniz. Like most natural philosophers, Leibniz rejected out of hand Newton's suggestion that gravity might be sufficiently explained as a direct consequence of the Divine Presence and

[22] Lavoisier (1802) and see Guerlac (1975).

[23] Dalton (1808–10) and see Thackray (1972).

[24] Laplace (1809 and see also 1799).

[25] For Laplace himself see Gillispie (1978), volume 15, pp.273–402. The best treatments are, however, of the Laplacian tradition: Herivel (1966), Kargon (1969), Merz (1904–12), Fox (1974), Crosland (1967) and Arnold (1983).

demanded instead some physical cause. In his famous debate with Newton's selfstyled apologist, Samuel Clarke, he also rejected any mechanical approach in terms of atoms and the void. This debate focused on the consistency of Newton's arguments rather than on any alternative proposed by Leibniz, but in his *Monadology*, published posthumously in 1720, Leibniz did put forward a view of nature as a dynamical plenum, a continuum of forces in which the forces themselves gave rise to extension and the primary mechanical qualities rather than the other way around. Each point or 'monad' of Leibniz's universe contained within itself the whole universe, in the sense of a dynamic relationship between the part and the whole.[26]

Leibniz's rather strange and difficult metaphysic did not in itself provide an heuristically valuable approach to the physical world, but it did lead on to what was to be an important idea of the atom as a non-material force centre. Moreover, Leibniz's influence in the German-speaking world, as a renowned mathematician, philosopher, historian and politician, was immense.

In 1756, in his brief *Physical Monadology*, Immanuel Kant attempted to reconcile the natural philosophies of Newton and Leibniz by treating matter as composed of non-extended centres of attractive and repulsive forces.[27] Two years later, in his *Theoria Philosophiae Naturalis* of 1758, the Italian natural philosopher Roger Boscovich presented a similar theory.[28] Both theories were in some sense mechanistic, for the point-centres of which matter was supposed to be made up were not relegated, as they were by Leibniz, to mere consequences of the forces. The atoms remained the primary entities. But the theories were nevertheless dynamistic in the sense that the defining characteristics of matter were taken as the forces observed to be associated with it rather than any hypothetical mechanical qualities. The point-atoms had no extension and the other key mechanical quality, impenetrability, was treated as a consequence of the strong repulsive forces exerted by the atoms at close range.

Some years later Kant developed the critical philosophy for which he remains famous. His *Critique of Pure Reason* was first published in 1781 and five years later, in 1786, he also completed his *Metaphysical Foundations of Natural Science.*[29] In this latter work Kant presented what might be called the dynamical foundations of mechanics. Although matter remained the prime entity it was no longer viewed either as finite atoms or as point-atoms but rather as a visually undefined substratum, 'the moveable',

[26] Leibniz (1898). See Doran (1974), which has good references to other work on Leibniz, and Koyré and Cohen (1962).
[27] Kant (1902).
[28] Boscovich (1922). See also Heimann (1971a).
[29] Kant (1933 and 1883).

whose properties were derived from its active forces, which alone could be empirically known. Solidity, extension and impenetrability were the consequences of the observed 'moving forces' of attraction and repulsion, and the laws of mechanics, such as that of the conservation of matter, were deduced from those of dynamics.

So far as the late eighteenth and early nineteenth centuries are concerned, Kant's *Metaphysical Foundations* provides one of the clearest and most notable expressions of the dichotomy between the dynamistic and mechanistic approaches to physical science, and his discussion of matter theory in particular is worthy of quotation:[30]

> But as concerns the procedure in natural science in respect of the most important of all its problems, namely, the explanation of a possible *specific variety of matters* [extending] to infinity, one can only strike out two ways: the *mechanical*, by the union of the absolutely full with the absolutely empty, or a *dynamical* way, opposed to it, by explaining all varieties of matter through the mere variety in the combination of the original forces of repulsion and attraction. The first has, as the materials of its deduction, *atoms* and *the void*. An atom is a small portion of matter physically indivisible .... An atom, in so far as it is specifically distinguished from others by its figure, is called a *primal* body. A body whose moving force depends on its figure is called a *machine*. The mode of explanation of the specific variety of matters by the construction and composition of their smallest parts as machines is *mechanical natural philosophy*, but that which derives the specific variety of matter from matters not as machines, that is, mere tools of external moving forces, but from the moving forces of attraction and repulsion originally belonging to them, may be called *dynamical natural philosophy*.

Kant himself favoured

> a dynamical mode of explanation (which is far more suited and more advantageous to experimental philosophy, in as much as it leads directly to the discovery of the proper moving forces of matters and their laws, while it limits the freedom of assuming empty mediate spaces and fundamental bodies of definite figures, neither of which admit of definition or discovery by any experiments).

The dynamical philosophy was a many-headed beast, and Kant's version of it was only one of several variations. Within the physical sciences the atomism that Kant associated with the mechanical philosophy, and that he spent several pages following the above quotation attacking, was often retained by men whose attitudes were in other respects dynamical. In such cases the crucial distinction made was that whereas the mechanists built up their theories upon *specific* atomic *hypotheses*, the dynamists eschewed such

[30] Kant (1883), pp. 210–11.

hypotheses and drew only on the supposition that matter was in some *unspecified* way atomic. Within the life sciences this eschewal of hypotheses often gave way, as in *Naturphilosophie*, to an advocacy of vital forces and spirits, and to theoretical structures built upon metaphysical hypotheses such as that of dynamic polarity. In that context the tradition that built upon Kant's own works, sometimes called vital materialism or teleomechanism, represented a middle way between the mechanists and the vitalists.[31] Even in vitalism, though, there remained an element of positivism, and throughout the sciences of the eighteenth and nineteenth centuries the fundamental cornerstone of the dynamistic tradition may be considered the same: the outright rejection of detailed, experimentally unverifiable, mechanical hypotheses.

Ironically, one branch of the dynamistic tradition in science was developed from the work of a thorough-going mechanist, the dissenter and chemical philosopher Joseph Priestley. Priestley accepted in large measure the doctrines of Locke and argued strongly, in his *Disquisitions Relating to Matter and Spirit* (1777), that '[mind] is nothing more than a modification of [matter]'.[32] But in attempting to reduce mind to matter he afforded matter something of the dynamical quality of mind:[33]

> I therefore define [matter] to be a substance possessed of the properties of *extension*, and of *powers of attraction or repulsion*. And since it has never yet been asserted that the powers of *sensation* and *thought* are incompatible with these (*solidity*, or *impenetrability* only, having been thought to be repugnant to them) I therefore maintain, that we have no reason to suppose that there are in man two substances so distinct from each other, as have been represented.

Priestley divorced matter from the property of solidity and interpreted it as mere extension, together with the powers of attraction and repulsion. The traditional impenetrability of matter was explicitly denied, and the powers envisaged were not passive or relative as in the mechanical philosophy of Locke, but active. They were not the cause of extension, as they were for Kant, but they were not a consequence of it either: matter was extension plus powers, with the relationship between the two left essentially undefined.[34]

Priestley's theory of matter seems to have been shared by John Michell, and it was taken up in a slightly altered form by Robert Young in his *Essay*

[31] For a comprehensive treatment of the life sciences see Lenoir (1982). See also, for example, Benton (1974), Culotta (1973), Mendelsohn (1965), Brown (1974), Roll-Hansen (1976), Coleman (1977) and Lenoir (1980, 1981).
[32] Priestley (1817–31), volume 3, p. 220. For a full discussion of this whole tradition see Heimann and McGuire (1971).
[33] Priestley (1817–31), volume 3, p. 219.
[34] See Heimann and McGuire (1971).

on the Powers and Mechanisms of Nature of 1788. William Nicholson, in his *Introduction to Natural Philosophy* of 1782, went one stage further by arguing that the supposition of extended matter was itself an unnecessary hypothesis, the phenomena being quite adequately explained by a sphere of repulsive force. In the early nineteenth century the ideas of Priestley and Nicholson were again taken up by Thomas Exley, and they were also important for the work of Michael Faraday.[35]

Faraday's main contact with the dynamical philosophy was through his mentor Humphrey Davy, who advocated a Boscovichean type of point-atomism. Faraday himself also speculated on point-atoms, and in his 'Speculation touching electric induction and the nature of matter', an important paper to which we shall return in the next chapter, he proposed what he thought was a Boscovichean matter theory. (It was in fact the theory due to Priestley, the false attribution to Boscovich being derived from Priestley's own comments.) In an unpublished note of the same year, 1844, Faraday argued for pure force-atoms:[36]

> What real reason, then, is there for supposing that there is any ... nucleus in a particle of matter? That an atom of matter is an unchangeable amount of power, I believe; ... and that this power is grouped around & attached to a centre I believe, just as others suppose it associated with a nucleus; but what the nucleus is wanted for, or how it is recognised, or what it is independent of the power around & about it, I cannot imagine.
>
> ... Matter acts and is acted upon only by its forces, and the atoms of matter are to my imagination centres of force. What forces I know not; the nature of our existence gives us only to recognise and to estimate it by its effects.

This argument provides a particularly clear example of the developed dynamical theory of matter. Some notion of atomism is retained, but the materiality normally associated with that notion is not. From the empirical effects of matter we may, according to Faraday, deduce the existence of forces, but there is no empirical justification for specifying the precise nature of these forces, of for postulating any hypothetical material entities underlying them. A similar view to Faraday's was also taken at about the same time by the Irish mathematician William Rowan Hamilton, who saw the theory of force-atoms as 'having a subjective truth, and as being a fit medium between our understanding and certain phenomena.'[37]

A second branch of the dynamistic tradition in physical science may be seen in the work of a series of Scottish natural philosophers, beginning with James Hutton. Hutton's view of nature was closer to that of some of the

[35] These works are discussed in Heimann and McGuire (1971).
[36] See Levere (1968), quotation from p. 107. See also Heimann (1971a).
[37] See Graves (1882–9), volume 1, p. 593 and also Kargon (1965).

dynamical philosophers considered in the next section than to those of the dynamically oriented scientists we have considered so far, and Coleridge indeed described him as 'on the precincts of the Critical Philosophy with which and the previous treatises of Kant he appears to have had no acquaintance.'[38] But his was an idiosyncratic form of dynamism, resulting from a particularly pure form of empiricism. Whereas contemporary Scottish philosophers maintained, as we shall see, that all knowledge of the external world was relative to the mind, Hutton argued that it was relative to the conditions obtaining in the active powers of nature, through which, he asserted, we experience nature. In crude terms he took Locke's dictum of essential primary qualities, such as extension and impenetrability, and consequent passive powers, and inverted it, the powers becoming active and the mechanical qualities becoming conditional on them. As he wrote in his *Investigation of the Principles of Knowledge* (1794), 'power, the cause of our sensation, is to be considered as a first cause', and again, 'power properly denotes a thing, a real existence; for, this is all that is known of the external cause.'[39] Matter was for Hutton, as for others in the dynamical tradition, an undefined and undefinable substratum of which power was the known attribute.

Despite their opposite philosophical attitudes, Priestly and Hutton agreed on the effectively dynamical proposition that power, active power, was the essence of matter; and this view was absorbed by many of their contemporaries and followers, especially in Scotland. These included the common-sense philosopher Dugald Stewart (who, however, denied the notion that even the concept of power could be derived from experience), the natural philosopher Jon Robison and Hutton's biographer John Playfair, who wrote in his *Biographical Account of James Hutton*:[40]

> Thus it appears, that power is the essence of matter, and that none of our perceptions warrant us in considering even body as involving anything more than force, subject to various laws and combinations.

Playfair also stressed what was to become an important aspect of this view of nature in the nineteenth century, namely that it was incompatible with the usual notions of material interaction. With matter interpreted as force indefinitely extended throughout space, all concepts based on the supposition of spatially defined atoms interacting through either contact action or action at a distance became unintelligible.

The third manifestation of dynamism in science of relevance here was the

[38] Heimann and McGuire (1971), p. 284.

[39] Hutton (1794), volume 2, pp. 387, 385. Hutton's work and that of his successors is discussed in Heimann and McGuire (1971).

[40] Playfair (1822), volume 4, p. 85.

tradition deriving from Kant and built on the idea of polarity. Kant, replacing the mechanists' atomic foundations of the science of mechanics by dynamical foundations in terms of forces, had first introduced only a repulsive force, this being the force corresponding to the mechanical notion of penetrability that features in our immediate empirical experience. He had then introduced the force of attraction as a necessary consequence of that of repulsion. Picking up on this, both Friedrich von Schelling and Samuel Taylor Coleridge argued that, in Coleridge's words, 'every power in nature . . . must evolve an opposite, as the sole means and condition of its manifestation: and all opposition is a tendency to re-union.'[41]

The first extended treatment of the polarity concept was given by Schelling in his *Ideas Towards a Philosophy of Nature* of 1803, but it was Coleridge who introduced it to English readers.[42] Writing in 1818, in *The Friend*, he argued that the reason that electricity had proved more susceptible to theoretical analysis than magnetism lay in its more obvious manifestation in terms of polarity, 'or the manifestation of one power by opposite forces'. He applied the polarity concept to the explanation not only of electricity and magnetism but also of chemical binding, envisaged as a dynamic synthesis of the constituent chemical elements.[43] His *Hints Towards the Formation of a More Comprehensive Theory of Life*, published posthumously in 1848, was more or less an extended essay on the polarity concept in natural philosophy.[44]

The dynamical concept of polarity is rather metaphysical for our modern tastes. But in the early and middle nineteenth century it enjoyed a considerable vogue among dynamically-oriented scientists, in particular in chemistry, where it formed the basis of a research programme opposed to the mechanistic atomic theory of Dalton. Of course, the mechanistic view in this case prevailed, but the dynamists were not all scientific amateurs like Coleridge. The polarity concept also featured in the chemical writings of Humphrey Davy,[45] and, more significantly, in the chemical and electromagnetic writings of Michael Faraday and Hans Christian Oersted, to be treated in the next chapter. The enormously influential Cambridge mathematician and natural philosopher William Whewell, who was intimate with both the philosophical underpinnings of polarity in the writings of Kant and the practical application of the concept by Faraday, devoted a whole book of his *Philosophy of the Inductive Sciences* to 'the Idea of Polarity'. This idea, he explained, had 'only recently been applied, with any

[41] Coleridge (1818), volume 1, p. 155. For Coleridge and the scientific community see Levere (1981).
[42] Schelling (1956).
[43] Coleridge (1818).
[44] Coleridge (1848).
[45] For a good account of Davy see Levere (1971).

great degree of clearness, among physical philosophers; and is even yet probably entertained in an obscure and antiquarian manner by most experimental enquiries.'[46] But the application of the idea by Faraday, Oersted and Ampère in chemistry and electromagnetic theory had convinced him that it was the idea for the future, the fundamental concept upon which the next round of developments of natural science would be based.

Mechanistic and dynamistic attitudes in philosophy and the philosophy of science

The mechanical philosophy of the Enlightenment was not confined to science. Locke attributed all our ideas, whether of space and time, of number, or of good and bad, to an origin in our experience of the outside world:[47]

> Whence has [the mind] all the materials of reason and knowledge? To this I answer, in one word, from experience: in that all our knowledge is founded, and from that it ultimately derives itself.

The Frenchman Condillac developed Locke's philosophy, and throughout the eighteenth and early nineteenth centuries the mechanically-oriented 'sensationalism' of Locke and Condillac held centre stage in the philosophy of England and France. In the nineteenth century this same attitude was also apparent in the popular utilitarian philosophies, and especially in the work of John Stuart Mill, for whom, as for Locke, all material concepts derived from the perception of the external natural world.

The mechanists' application of material explanations to the properties of the mind could have little effect on the development of the natural sciences, but the opposing dynamistic tradition could be, and was, of the utmost significance for that development. The dynamical philosophy developed in two forms, one due to the German, Kant, and the other represented by the 'common-sense' tradition of Scottish moral philosophy. Both evolved as responses to the work of the Scottish philosopher, David Hume.

Hume was a sceptical philosopher, and in his two best known works, the *Treatise of Human Nature* (1739) and the *Enquiry Concerning Human Understanding*, this scepticism was directed against the claim that man could have objective knowledge, whether scientific, moral or religious.[48] In the scientific field this meant the claims of natural philosophers to have any objective knowledge of the natural world, and in particular any such

[46] Whewell (1967), volume 1, p. 374.
[47] Locke (1979), p. 42.
[48] Hume (1978 and 1975).

knowledge going beyond the evidence of the senses—though even these were suspect. As he explained,[49]

> Even mathematics, natural philosophy, and natural religion, are in some measure dependent on the science of man; since they lie under the cognizance of men, and are judged of by their powers and faculties. It is impossible to tell about changes and improvements we might make in these sciences, were we thoroughly acquainted with the extent and frame of human understanding, and could explain the nature of the ideas we employ, and of the operations we perform in our reasonings.

Hume criticised both the mechanical philosophies, and the distinction between primary and secondary qualities on which, in Locke's formulation, they rested; and the dynamical philosophies, in so far as they too rested upon metaphysical assumptions. The quotation given above carries an element of challenge: study the mind and you may improve your science. As we shall see, this challenge was taken up, most notably by Kant. But Hume's writings as a whole conveyed a far more pessimistic tone. Scientific systems based upon hypotheses, whether mechanical or dynamical, had for him no objective validity at all. They were in essence belief systems derived from the natures of the minds asserting them, rather than statements of knowledge concerning the physical world and derived as was claimed from reason and experience alone. More generally, whether the knowledge proclaimed by a man was of atoms or forces, morals or divinity, Hume asserted that it simply could not be derived purely from reason and experience.[50]

Applied specifically, Hume's criticisms were not particularly startling. Some philosophers did present their constructs of the world as having objective validity, but others clearly recognised their hypothetical nature and their dependence on an attitude of mind as well as upon more objective criteria. Applied generally, however, Hume's arguments had tremendous force, for they seemed to threaten both the Christian faith upon which the whole structure of society depended and, more significantly in the present context, the very ideal of an objective science that underlay the whole of the Scientific Revolution and Enlightenment. With a forceful argument and with consequences as far reaching as these, Hume's work provided the necessary starting point for any serious philosopher in the period that followed. In so doing, moreover, it also laid the foundation for the further development of the dynamical philosophy into something that could rival the established and highly popular mechanism of Hobbes, Locke and Condillac. For although the proclamation of a dynamical system of the world was as open to sceptical criticism as was that of a mechanical system, Hume's emphasis upon the primary role of the human mind, totally

[49] Hume (1978), p. 2.
[50] A recent treatment of Hume is that by Wright (1983).

antipathetic to the matter-orientation of mechanism, was basically in sympathy with the dynamistic approach. His scepticism can perhaps be compared with that of Socrates, and in much the same way as Plato developed his philosophy in terms of a counter-example to Socrates's assertion that he knew only that he knew nothing, so Kant and others responded to Hume.

We have already discussed Kant's *Metaphysical Foundations of Natural Science* as an attempt to reformulate Newtonian mechanics according to a consistent dynamical philosophy. More generally, though, it may also be seen as an attempt to defend that mechanics against the scepticism of Hume. Whereas the earlier tendency of Newton, Leibniz, Boscovich and Kant himself had been to start with the basic framework of the new mechanics and interpret it dynamically, Kant eventually broke away from that framework completely and built up the science anew on the basis of the directly perceived qualities of motion and force. At the same time, he also responded to Hume's challenge in respect of the fundamental concepts of the structure of scientific theories, such as space, time and the principle of cause and effect. The principle of cause and effect in particular had suffered the full force of Hume's scepticism, being condemned as a subjective belief with no foundation in the observed world. Kant's response was to accept the subjectivity, but to assert that this was not a problem. Space, time and the principle of cause and effect were among the forms and categories of thought, in terms of which man ordered his observations. They were indeed subjective in the sense that they rested in the mind of man rather than in the external world, but they were also objective to the extent that they were shared by all men.

Kant's emphasis upon the mental component of science was to be a key feature of the dynamical tradition as it developed over the next half century, and in his *Critique of Pure Reason* he indicated just how important this component was:[51]

> Even physics, therefore, owes the beneficial revolution in its point of view entirely to the happy thought, that while reason must seek in nature, not fictitiously ascribe to it, whatever as not being knowable through reason's own resources has to be learnt, if learnt at all, only from nature, it must adopt as its guide, in so seeking, that which it has itself put into nature.

In his *Prolegomena* he expressed himself more strongly still on the mental, *a priori*, content:[52]

> The highest legislation of nature must lie in ourselves, namely, in our understanding, and ... we must seek its universal laws, not in nature, by

[51] Kant (1933), p. 20.
[52] Kant (1883), p. 67.

> means of experience; but conversely, must seek nature, as to its universal regularity, solely in the conditions of the possibility of experience lying in our sensibility and understanding. ... *The understanding draws its lessons (a priori) not from nature, but prescribes them to it.*

For Kant, the regularity of our picture of nature, the necessity of the laws we ascribe to nature, the principle of cause and effect and the concepts of space and time in terms of which we frame these laws were all provided by the mind. In the early nineteenth century one of his principal successors, Samuel Taylor Coleridge, explained how this fitted in with the aims and characteristics of scientific enquiry:[53]

> The necessary tendency therefore of all natural philosophy is from nature to intelligence; and this, and no other, is the true ground and occasion of the instinctive striving to introduce theory into our views of natural phenomena. The highest perfection of natural philosophy would consist in the perfect spiritualization of all the laws of nature into laws of intuition and intellect. The phenomena (the material) must wholly disappear, and the laws alone (the formal) must remain. Thence it comes that in nature itself the more the principle of law breaks forth, the more does the husk drop off, the phaenomena themselves become more spiritual and at length cease altogether in our consciousness. The optical phaenomena are but a geometry, the lines of which are drawn by light, and the materiality of this light itself has already become a matter of doubt [i.e. in the wave theory]. In the appearance of magnetism all trace of matter is lost, and of the phaenomena of gravitation, which not a few amongst the most illustrious Newtonians have declared no otherwise comprehensible than as an immediate spiritual influence, there remains nothing but its law, the execution of which on a vast scale is the mechanism of the heavenly motions. The theory of natural philosophy would then be completed when all nature was demonstrated to be identical in essence with that which in its highest known power exists in man as intelligence and self-consciousness.

The aim of science was to derive laws, and these laws were representations of 'truths originating in the *mind*, and not abstracted or generalised from observation'.[54]

It is for his emphasis on the *a priori* that Kant is chiefly remembered. As we have already seen in our discussion of his *Metaphysical Foundations of Natural Science*, however, and as the above quotation from the *Critique of Pure Reason* also shows, he combined this with a belief in the reality of the physical world and argued strongly for the description of this world in terms of its empirically observed behaviour (which the mind then converted into laws in its own image), rather than in terms of mechanical hypotheses or

[53] Coleridge (1956), p. 146.

[54] Coleridge (1818), volume 3, p. 459. See also Coleridge (1949), chapter 12.

fictions. By explicitly identifying the traditional dynamical qualities with those of our most immediate empirical experience, and by identifying the traditional concepts of science with universal forms of thought, Kant set the dynamistic approach to physical science upon a new and much surer footing.

It is probably true to say that no other philosopher since Thomas Aquinas, Bacon perhaps excepted, has had such a deep and enduring influence on Western scientific thought as has Kant, and the impact of his critical philosophy was both strong and pervasive. His most immediately important contribution to physical science was probably his rescue of the principle of cause and effect from Hume's scepticism. But his work was also important in other ways. One concerned the problem of visualisation and the use of visual pictures in science. This was not a problem Kant tackled explicitly, but he did tackle the root problem, namely that of the limiting role of the human faculties in general. Writing of the expression of ideas of observed that:[55]

> The mind cannot always adequately represent in the concrete and transform into distinct images abstract notions derived from the pure intellect. But this contradiction, which is in itself merely subjective (i.e. an incapacity in the nature of man) too often passes for an incongruity or impossibility in the object (i.e. the notions themselves) and seduces the incautious to mistake the limitations of the human faculties for the limits of things as they really exist.

Kant's concern here was with those who treated as impossible intellectual notions that were merely irrepresentable. But the same could also be said in respect of irrepresentable properties of the physical world, and Coleridge used the argument against mechanically oriented scientists whose hypothetical models were based on the presumption, quite unwarranted in his view, that the natural world was structured in a way that was conformable to our visual senses. The problem, he explained, was that[56]

> Under that despotism of the eye ... this strong sensuous influence, we are restless because invisible things are not the objects of vision; and metaphysical systems, for the most part, become popular not for their truth but in proportion as they attribute to causes a susceptibility of being seen, if only our visual organs were sufficiently powerful.

Attacking the mechanists explicitly, Coleridge wrote:[57]

> According to the creed of our modern philosophers, nothing is deemed a clear

[55] Kant (1770), quoted in translation by Coleridge (1956), pp. 156–7.
[56] Coleridge (1956), p. 62.
[57] Coleridge (1956), pp. 156–7.

> conception but what is represented by a distinct image. Thus the conceivable is reduced within the bounds of the picturable.

Physics was not wholly to free itself from this constraint until the advent of general relativity theory and quantum mechanics.[58] Meanwhile, however, Coleridge's comments appeared in his widely read *Biographia Literaria* (editions in 1817 and 1847), and the problem was, as we shall see, one that seemed to trouble James Clerk Maxwell.

The representatives of the Kantian philosophy in Britain, though influential, were relatively few. In the work of William Whewell, however, and in that of the Scottish philosopher William Hamilton (not to be confused with the Irish mathematician William Rowan Hamilton, also a Kantian) the German Kantian tradition merged with another philosophical tradition that was native to Scotland. This was the tradition of 'common-sense' philosophy deriving from the work of Thomas Reid in the 1760s. Like Kant's philosophy it developed in response to the scepticism of Hume, and like that philosophy too it had a distinctly dynamical flavour.

For Reid, Hume was both teacher and antagonist. He accepted much of Hume's scepticism, and discussing the development of science he argued that it should be a 'fundamental principle ... that no regard is due to the conjectures or hypotheses of philosophers, however ancient, however generally received'.[59] This was, he recognised, no easy matter. Scientists were by nature inventive of hypotheses, and the public receptive towards them. Talking of Descartes's mechanism, he explained that[60]

> The invention of a hypothesis, founded on some slight probability, which accounts for many appearances of nature, has been considered as the highest attainment of a philosopher. If the hypothesis hangs well together, is embellished by a lively imagination, and seems to account for common appearances, it is considered by many as having all the qualities that should be recommended to our belief, and all that ought to be required in a philosophical system.

But Reid emphasised repeatedly that natural science should be concerned only with empirical laws and not with efficient causes, which must ever remain hidden from man:[61]

> In natural philosophy, ..., we seek only the general law, according to which nature works, and these we call the causes of what is done according to them. But such laws cannot be the efficient causes of anything. ... Efficient causes,

[58] See Hendry (1984b) and Miller (1978 and 1985).
[59] Reid (1858), p. 236.
[60] Reid (1858), p. 235.
[61] Reid (1858), pp. 57–8.

> properly so called, are not within the sphere of natural philosophy. Its business is, from particular facts in the material world, to collect, by just induction, the laws that are general, and from these the more general, as far as we can go. And when this is done, natural philosophy has no more to do.

Reid's archetype was Newton's law of gravitation. 'Natural philosophy informs us', he observed, 'that matter gravitates according to a certain law; and it says no more. Whether matter be active or passive in gravitation, cannot be determined by any experiment I can think of.'[62]

So far as science was concerned, Reid's main emphasis was thus on a strict empiricism. But just as Kant introduced the forms and categories of thought to provide a framework for scientific theory, so Reid responded to Hume's scepticism by introducing 'common-sense' principles, which 'the constitution of our nature leads us to believe, and which we are under a necessity to take for granted in the common consensus of life.'[63] As in Kant's work the image of objective science that had been torn apart by Hume was replaced by an image of effectively objective science, founded on the human mind rather than the natural world and in that sense subjective, but founded on elements common to all human minds, and so universally shared. But Reid's solution was rather different from Kant's. Whereas Kant made space and time, for example, *a priori*, purely intellectual forms of thought, Reid preserved them as features of the natural world, cognised *a posteriori*, but recognised, so to speak, by the mind, and valid as scientific concepts only on the grounds of that common recognition. So too with the principle of cause and effect. Whereas the mechanical philosophers assumed that the world was innately causal and was therefore automatically perceived as such, and whereas Kant asserted that one could not legitimately attribute causality to the world but rather perceived the world as causal on account of the nature of the human mind, Reid suggested that because of this nature one was able to perceive the causality, which must therefore exist in the world itself.

Reid's main concern was with moral philosophy and with the re-establishment of the religious and moral beliefs that had been threatened by Hume. Reid was Professor of Moral Philosophy at the University of Edinburgh, and his followers in the common-sense tradition both shared his priorities and succeeded to his chair. Indeed, his first two successors, Dugald Stewart and Thomas Brown, were both less interested in and more critical of science than he was. The next in line, however, occupying the Edinburgh chair for much of the first half of the nineteenth century, was William Hamilton, and through his work, and through that of the Englishman William Whewell, the common-sense philosophy acquired a relevance for science in general and for the young Maxwell in particular.

62 Reid (1858), p. 59.

63 Reid (1858), p. 108. See Olson (1975).

The dynamistic syntheses of Hamilton and Whewell

William Hamilton and William Whewell were the two teachers whose ideas Maxwell most esteemed. Both were dynamical philosophers and both drew on both the Kantian and the common-sense traditions.

Hamilton's main interests were in logic and moral philosophy rather than natural science, but like Reid before him he also applied his philosophy to questions of scientific knowledge and method and, of particular interest here, to the method of analogy. The use of analogies had been a general concern of the common-sense philosophers since Reid, but their attitude had generally been one of mistrust. Reid himself had recognised that[64]

> It is natural to men to judge of things less known, by some similitude they observe, or think they observe, between them and things more familiar and better known. In many cases we have no better way of judging. And, where the things concerned have really a great similitude in their nature, when there is reason to think that they are subject to the same laws, there may be a considerable degree of probability in conclusions drawn from analogy.

In some areas of enquiry, indeed, analogy might be the only means of progress, as for example, in religion where one could only study the creator through his creations. But having once introduced the analogical method Reid immediately drew attention to and concentrated on its dangers. Men tended, he pointed out, to see similarities even when they weren't there and to draw analogies between quite disparate entities. Even at its best, moreover, '[analogical] reasoning can afford only probable evidence', and could not be certain.

Dugald Stewart who gave, in his *Elements of the Philosophy of the Human Mind*, a systematic treatment of analogy, was also critical of its use in science and especially of the application of mathematical ways of thinking to physics and vice versa.[65] Thomas Brown was similarly mistrustful. But with William Hamilton a new and more positive perspective emerged. Hamilton was still critical, as Reid had been, of those who attributed too great a certainty to arguments based on analogy. He criticised Whewell, for example, for supposing 'as a logical canon, that a presumption from analogy affords a criterion of truth, subjectively necessary and objectively certain.'[66] The value of analogy for Hamilton was as a guide towards theory, not as a guarantee of its truth. But it was nevertheless the only guide. He had accepted Reid's common-sense principles and reinterpreted much of Kant's analysis in terms of them. He was, however, acutely aware of the limitations of human intelligence and of the absence of any objective

[64] Reid (1858), pp. 236–7.
[65] Stewart (1858), volume 2, and see Olson (1975).
[66] Olson (1975), p. 149.

or absolute knowledge, something he framed in terms of a 'principle of relativity':[67]

> All our knowledge of mind and matter is merely relative. We know, and can know, nothing absolutely and in itself: all that we know is existence in certain special forms or modes, and these, likewise, only in so far as they may be analogous to our faculties.

Hamilton also pointed out that 'it does not follow that all relative existence is relative to *us*, that all that can be known, even by a limited intelligence, is actually cognisable by us.'[68] Even relative knowledge was limited. But such knowledge as could be derived was analogical: it consisted of an awareness of similarity and, moreover, of formal similarities between relations rather than of material analogies between the things related. The aim of science was to discover these similar relations, and the method by which the appropriate relations could be highlighted and singled out from the substratum of observations, physical and mental, was the method of analogy. For Hamilton the analogical method was thus *the* method of natural science and also, historically, the method that had directed the genius of scientific invention. Discussing Newton's general law of gravitation, he even conceded that in this case and in some others 'the principle of analogy . . . is too forcible and too extensive in its sway to admit of much dispute.'[69]

William Hamilton's contribution to science consisted solely of his advocacy and analysis of the analogical method, and was effectively communicated only to his students. William Whewell's contribution in contrast was a broad and pervasive one. Whewell's philosophy had none of the rigour of the Scottish and German systems it developed. It did, however, have an unequalled relevance to the work of physical scientists. Whewell was himself a prominent man of science, in correspondence with many of the leading scientists of his day. In particular he maintained an active correspondence with Faraday, following his work and discussing with him the questions of method it raised. He had an excellent command of both current and past scientific theory and of the way in which that theory had actually been developed. And he was widely accepted within British science as the prime authority on matters philosophical.

Whewell based his *Philosophy of the Inductive Sciences* upon the proposition that 'in all human knowledge both Thoughts and Things are concerned',[70] and he was strongly critical both of Locke and other mechanical philosophers, who sought to reduce thoughts to things, and of the French positivist philosopher Comte, who treated both thoughts and

[67] W Hamilton (1865), volume 1, p. 153.
[68] W Hamilton (1865), volume 1, p. 140.
[69] W Hamilton (1865), volume 2, p. 525.
[70] Whewell (1967), part 1, p. 17.

things as hypothetical fictions. In line with both the Scottish and the German dynamical philosophers, whose views he outlined and compared in his book, Whewell took the view that things did exist in the natural world but that our knowledge of them was also a function of mind, and in particular of a range of fundamental ideas:[71]

> The *Senses* place before us the *Characters* of the Book of Nature; but these convey no knowledge to us, till we have discovered the Alphabet by which they are to be read. . . .
>
> The *Alphabet*, by means of which we interpret phenomena, consists of the *Ideas* existing in our own minds; for these give to the phenomena that coherence and significance which is not an object of sense.

In other words the substance of scientific laws was derived empirically from our perceptions of nature, but the form or structure of those laws was imposed *a priori*, by the structure of the mind.

Whewell explained that according to Kant fundamental concepts such as past and future or cause and effect were imposed on nature by the mind, while according to the Scottish philosophers they existed independently and were only recognised and connected by the mind; but he was not prepared to come down on either side himself. Indeed, having once established the relevance of both mind and matter to scientific knowledge he tended to take a practical rather than a philosophical view of how the two elements combined. He recognised for example the importance of psychological attitudes in the shaping of philosophies:[72]

> The combination of the two elements, the subjective or ideal, and the objective or observed, is necessary, in order to give us any insight into the laws of nature. But different persons, according to their mental habits or constitution, may be inclined to dwell by preference upon the one or the other of these two elements.

He further argued that it was not always possible to say whether something was a subjective theory or an objective fact, the distinction being in effect a socially rather than a philosophically determined one:[73]

> A true Theory is a Fact; a Fact is a familiar Theory. . . . The most recondite theories when firmly established are facts: the simplest facts involve something of the nature of Theory

The only distinction one could make was in terms of familiarity and the consciousness or otherwise of the mental component, largely a function of social convention.

[71] Whewell (1967), part 2, p. 443.
[72] Whewell (1967), part 1, p. 30.
[73] Whewell (1967), part 1, p. 40.

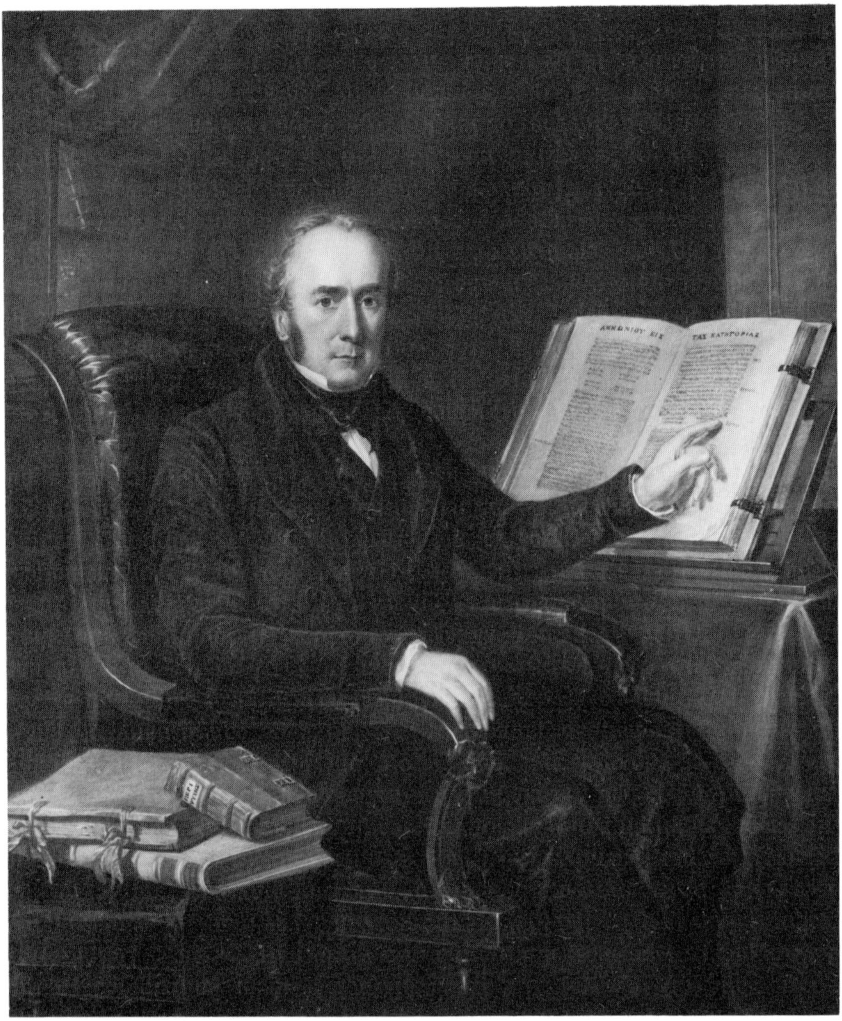

William Whewell. Reproduced by kind permission of The Master and Fellows of Trinity College, Cambridge.

This practical approach, in which the foundations of the dynamical philosophy were interpreted in the context of actual science, was also apparent in Whewell's discussion of hypotheses. In keeping with his philosophical stance he saw no truth value in hypothetical systems, whether these were composed of mechanical or of dynamical elements. Both systems composed ot solid atoms and systems based on force atoms were 'merely modes of representing mechanical laws of nature; and cannot, either of them, be asserted as possessing any evident truth or peremptory authority to the exclusion of the other.'[74] In a discussion rather reminiscent of Reid's, he insisted that science was concerned with laws rather than with efficient causes. But he also stressed what Reid had merely noted, that hypotheses were heuristically valuable. On one hand he emphasised the dangers of hypothesis. The scientist was, he observed, typically ingenious and fertile in the invention of hypotheses and had to take great care to place truth in first place, to abandon hypotheses as well as inventing them, and not to fall 'in love with his own fancies':[75]

> It has often happened that those who have undertaken to instruct mankind have not possessed this pure love of truth and comparative indifference to the maintenance of their own inventions.

On the other hand, he also emphasised that science could not progress without hypotheses and criticised Comte in particular for asserting that it should. It was in Whewell's view impossible to contain the 'irrepressible speculative powers of the human mind', and wrong-headed to try:[76]

> To debar science from enquiries [involving hypotheses], on the ground that it is her business to inquire into facts, and not to speculate upon causes, is a curious example of that barren caution which hopes for truth without daring to venture upon the quest for it.

Such a course was fruitless and it was also dangerous, for the hypotheses would still inevitably appear, only without being recognised as such. Giving yet another argument in favour of the limited and careful use of hypotheses, Whewell also observed that while a scientific law might ultimately be independent of hypotheses there were likely to be many cases in which it could not be adequately communicated and understood, or even expressed in the first place, without the illustrative use of hypotheses:[77]

> The laws of phenomena, in many cases, cannot be even expressed or understood without some hypotheses respecting their mode of production.

Mechanistic and dynamistic attitudes in mathematical physics

In discussing the mechanistic and dynamistic traditions so far, we have not yet touched upon their manifestation in what is for us the most relevant

[74] Whewell (1967), part 1, p. 260.
[75] Whewell (1967), part 2, p. 58.
[76] Whewell (1967), part 2, pp. 104–5.
[77] Whewell (1967), part 2, p. 103.

field of mathematical physics. In some ways this is the most confusing part of the philosophical background to Maxwell's work, if only because the words 'mechanics' and 'dynamics' carry technical meanings therein which are largely unrelated to the issue at hand. To illustrate this confusion, the classic treatment of dynamics, in both the scientific and the philosophical senses, is in Lagrange's work entitled *Analytical Mechanics*; the most prominent dynamical theory of modern times is similarly called quantum mechanics. In each case the qualifying adjective (analytical, quantum) indicates that the theory is not an ordinary mechanics, but in neither case does this prepare us for the dynamical and dynamistic attitude represented. A further source of confusion lies in the fact that mathematical techniques originating within one philosophical tradition or one branch of mathematical physics were freely employed within the other. In order to make any headway at all we therefore have to look to the form of a theory and specifically not to the nomenclature it contains. Once this is recognised, however, the distinction between the two attitudes is if anything clearer and more precise in mathematical physics than in the other areas of science and philosophy we have considered. And of course, the different approaches to mathematical physics constitute a subject of particular interest for our understanding of Maxwell's work in electromagnetic theory.

For much of the eighteenth century the contrast between mechanistic and dynamistic systems of science did not feature explicitly in the mathematical context. Attempts to extend Newton's explanatory framework from gravitational to electrical, magnetical and chemical phenomena remained essentially qualitative and non-mathematical, while those problems that were mathematically treated were predominantly in the macroscopic domain, requiring no physical assumptions on the debated microscopic level. Problems of planetary systems, pulley systems or springs and weights did not lend themselves to rival treatments along the lines we have been discussing. The behaviours of fluids and elastic solids were more sensitive, but it was only in the nineteenth century that the mathematical analyses in these areas became subject to physical scrutiny and criticism.

The mathematical physics of the eighteenth century did however witness a marked tendency towards increasing abstraction and generality, manifest in the work of the French mathematician Jean d'Alembert and culminating in the work of the Italian, Joseph Louis Lagrange. The focus of attention in this context was upon the foundations of Newtonian dynamics and the status of Newton's laws of motion. Whereas from the mechanistic viewpoint, espoused for example by some of Newton's British disciples, the laws of motion were based firmly on experience, d'Alembert treated Newton's theory as an abstract mathematical system based on axioms that were obviously and self-evidently true, demonstrable by pure reason and independent of any empirical verification. In his opinion Newton's first law (of action and reaction) already satisfied the requirement of a purely rational axiom and he was able to reformulate the third (force) law so as also to satisfy, in his opinion, this rational criterion.[78]

Lagrange's early researches, incorporating his development of the variational method, were set in the context of Leonhardi Euler's work. But in the early 1760s he broke away from this context and drew on d'Alembert's achievement and his own principle of virtual velocities in developing a purely analytic or rational mechanics.[79] In the *Mécanique Analytique*, published in 1787, by which time he was living in Paris, he set out the principles of mathematical physics as he saw them.[80] Lagrange's method was totally analytic, a system being defined in terms of arbitrary 'generalised' coordinates, and divorced from any visual, geometrical or mechanical representations or constructions. Instead of setting up specific models and equations of motion for each system treated, he proposed a completely general set of equations, known since as the Lagrangian equations of motion, applicable to any system and expressed in terms of small changes in what we now know as the kinetic energy of the system in response to the applied forces rather than in terms of a complete description of that system.

Lagrange's approach to mathematical physics was a dynamistic one, in two senses: in his rational claim that the laws of dynamics were rooted in the mind rather than in nature and in his analytic approach to the solution of physical problems. As a dynamistic approach to the problems of mathematical physics his work represented a triumphant achievement. It required no mechanical hypotheses, eliminated all postulated internal forces of constraint and, starting with only the observed behaviour of a system, treated everything in terms of applied forces and responses. But to the French mathematician Pierre Simon de Laplace, whose pre-eminence in the mechanistic tradition we have already noted, Lagrange's approach went quite against the spirit of Newtonian physics and barely deserved to be called physics at all. Laplace was just 13 years Lagrange's junior. In 1796, in his *Exposition du Système du Monde*, he put forward and illustrated the alternative approach and methodology of the mechanical philosophy: to hypothesise the existence of unobservable molecules and intermolecular forces, work out mathematically the consequences of the hypothetical mechanism and check these with experiment.[81] If the observed behaviour was correctly predicted, then the hypotheses were confirmed. In terms of the mathematics Laplace used an integral formulation, in which the whole hypothetical mechanico-molecular system was precisely described, in contrast to Lagrange's differential formulation which treated only of small

[78] d'Alembert (1921 and 1929). See also Hankins (1970).
[79] See Fraser (1983).
[80] Lagrange (1788).
[81] Laplace (1809).

changes in a system described only by its overall energy. Whereas Lagrange took the fundamental axioms of mechanics as deduced *a priori*, from pure reason, Laplace interpreted them as deduced from empirical observation of the physical world. In contrast with the dynamistic tenor of Lagrange's approach, Laplace's was thus a purely mechanistic attitude. It was also, and this, though not essential to the mechanistic world view, was to be important, an action-at-a-distance attitude:[82]

> I have wanted to establish that the phenomena of nature reduce in the final analysis to action *ad distans* from molecule to molecule, and that the consideration of these actions ought to serve as the basis of the mathematical theory of these phenomena.

Geniuses have a habit of appearing in complementary pairs. Lagrange and Laplace were two of the great mathematical physicists of all time, and despite their contrasting attitudes they remained personally on friendly terms, each respecting the achievements of the other and each secure in his own ability. But their work, polarised as it was in terms of the fundamental and well-established philosophical dichotomy of dynamism and mechanism, could not but spawn rival traditions. If the dynamism–mechanism debate had not been strongly apparent in the realm of mathematical physics before the publication of their respective masterpieces it was present with a vengeance afterwards. For the first forty years of the nineteenth century the development of mathematical physics in France and French-speaking Europe was polarised into two rival schools of thought. The Laplacian school was represented by Laplace himself, until his death in 1827, by Biot, Navier, Cauchy and, above all, Poisson. Their rivals, pursuing the analytic Lagrangian approach, included Fresnel, Fourier, Ohm and Ampère.

As these names themselves suggest, the rivalry between the two schools was to be a prominent feature of the history of electromagnetic theory and we shall return to it in that context in the next chapter. Its clearest and most visible and influential manifestation was however in the context of the theory of heat.

The early-nineteenth-century debate on the theory of heat centred on the work of Joseph Fourier, who based his theory on the model of Lagrange's rational mechanics.[83] Such work as had been done on heat theory had been within the mechanistic tradition of Laplace, But in line with the dynamistic traditions we have discussed Fourier declared that 'primary causes are unknown to us', and that physics should not be based, as it was by the

[82] Laplace (1878–1912), volume 12, p. 295.

[83] Fourier's work is treated in Herivel (1975), Wise (1981) and Kargon (1969), and see also Grattan–Guinness with Ravetz (1972).

mechanists, on untestable hypotheses. In the place of such hypotheses he proposed to substitute 'simple and constant laws, which may be discovered by observation', and thus to 'reduce all physical researches on the propagation of heat to problems of the integral calculus whose elements are given by experiment.'[84]

In practice, Fourier's approach entailed a complete reversal of the more usual mechanical procedure. The established mechanical view of heat transfer was in terms of atoms of heat (or 'caloric') supposed to be radiated from sources within each individual molecule. To establish the laws of heat transfer in a solid, which was the problem to which Fourier addressed himself, the mechanists would have had first to consider the interaction at a distance between two radiating molecules and then to integrate over all the interacting molecules to be considered in the body, this leading to the macroscopic law. Fourier, in contrast, started from the macroscopic behaviour, and from the empirical observation that the rate of heat transfer from a hot body to the surrounding cooler air appeared to be roughly proportional to the temperature difference between the body and the air, but independent of their absolute temperatures. To convert this empirical law into a basis for mathematical analysis he considered the case of heat flowing across a finitely thick prism or, in order to eliminate boundary problems, across a finitely thick but infinitely extended plate, each side of which was maintained at constant temperature.[85] He then made the crucial assumption that instead of each molecule in the body interacting at a distance with other molecules, as in the mechanical image, 'the layers in contact are the only ones which communicate their heat directly ... There is no direct action except between points extremely near.'[86]

This assumption was empirically based, for experiments showed that radiant heat incident on a solid did not penetrate beyond its boundaries. But whereas the experiments applied to macroscopical behaviour, and to the failure of heat to penetrate more than very small distances, Fourier applied the assumption to microscopic behaviour and assumed that the heat could not penetrate more than infinitely small distances. This ensured that his first empirical law, for the rate of heat transfer from a solid body to the medium, could also be applied to the rate of heat transfer from any one part of a solid body to another. Assuming that each side of the plate remained in equilibrium, that the total heat was conserved, and that in accordance with the empirical law the heat flow between any two points was directly proportional to their temperature difference, Fourier reasoned that the temperature gradient through the plate must be constant. Considering a

[84] Fourier 1955), pp. 1, 14.

[85] The structure of my analysis here follows that of Wise (1981), to which I am greatly indebted, but there are differences between our assessments.

[86] Fourier (1955), p. 460.

plane surface within the plate and parallel to its two faces, he could then apply the empirical heat transfer law to the heat transfer across this surface, the temperature difference being expressed in the microscopic limit as a temperature gradient and the law taking the form

$$\text{Flux} = -k\,\partial V/\partial n \tag{2.1}$$

or in modern vector notation

$$\mathbf{Flux} = -k\nabla V \tag{2.2}$$

with **Flux** the heat flux, V the temperature and $\partial V/\partial n$ the temperature gradient at right angles to the surface. The constant could depend only on the material concerned, and was defined as the thermal conductivity of the body. A second formula, for the boundary between a hot solid and cooler air,

$$h(V - V_0) = -k\,\partial V/\partial n \tag{2.3}$$

with V the temperature of the body, V_0 that of the air and h the 'external conductibility', was similarly derived, as was the general equation for heat conduction in a body,

$$-CD\frac{\partial V}{\partial t} = \frac{\partial \text{Flux}_x}{\partial x} + \frac{\partial \text{Flux}_y}{\partial y} + \frac{\partial \text{Flux}_z}{\partial z} = \nabla\cdot\,\mathbf{Flux} \tag{2.4}$$

$\nabla\cdot\mathbf{Flux}$ being the net heat flux from an infinitesimal volume element, D the density and C the heat capacity per unit mass of the body.

Fourier's laws could still be expressed in terms of the usual mechanical models, and he himself expressed the first law, for example, as:[87]

> If two molecules of the same body are extremely near, and are at unequal temperatures, that which is most heated communicates directly to the other during a certain interval a certain quantity of heat; which quantity is proportional to the extremely small difference of the temperatures.

But the theory departed from these models in four different ways. First, it did not depend upon them:[88]

> The knowledge of the mathematical laws to which [the effects of heat] are subject is independent of all hypotheses; it requires only an attentive examination of the chief facts which common observations have indicated, and which have been confirmed by exact experiments.

In particular,[89]

> The fundamental equations are demonstrated in the most clear and most rigorous manner without it being necessary to examine if the propagation is

[87] Fourier (1955), pp. 456–7.
[88] Fourier (1955), p. 26.
[89] Quoted by Herivel (1975), p. 225.

> carried out by way of radiation in the interior of the solids, whether or not it consists in the emission of a special matter that the molecules interchange with each other, or if it results, like sound, from vibrations of an elastic medium. *It is always preferable to restrict oneself to the enunciation of the general fact indicated by observation, which is no other than the preceeding principle.* One shows thus that the mathematical theory of heat is independent of all physical hypotheses; and in effect the laws to which the propagation is subject are admitted by all physicists in spite of the extreme diversity of their sentiments on the nature and the mode of its action.

The theory was essentially analytical, in Lagrange's sense, with no room for geometrical or mechanical constructions or hypotheses.

Secondly, and somewhat rashly, Fourier denied the basic premise of the mechanical philosophy, namely that all physical phenomena could be given a mechanical explanation:[90]

> Mechanical theories ... do not apply to the effects of heat. These [effects] make up a special order of phenomena which cannot be explained by the principles of movement and equilibrium.

Thirdly, so far as the theory could be physically interpreted at all it entailed a rejection of action at a distance, which was fundamental to Laplacian mechanism. Finally, the theory was precisely valid only in the limit in which both matter and heat were treated as continuous and in which the actions known to take place at small distances were treated as taking place at infinitely small ones. Again, so far as this implied a physical theory, it was one fundamentally opposed to the mechanical theories, which were based on discrete atomic hypotheses. More important than this, however, and even more opposed to mechanism, was the fact that it was not meant to imply such a physical theory at all. Fourier did not actually reject the molecular hypothesis. He treated it as an hypothesis rather than as a fact, but he expressed his results in molecular terms and never suggested that the molecular picture of matter should be replaced by a continuum one. This meant that his laws had to be interpreted as providing an approximate description of the behaviour of heat, valid for all practical purposes but not intended to provide a real description, and therefore physically neutral at the microscopic level. The theory went not so much against the particular mechanical hypotheses generally adopted as against the whole ideal of mechanism: it was thoroughly dynamistic.

The reception of Fourier's theory in France was cool.[91] It was first put

[90] Quoted by Herivel (1975), p. 224.

[91] The positivist philospher Comte was delighted with the theory and dedicated a volume of his published lectures to Fourier: see Comte (1830–42). But this enthusiasm, which probably did Fourier more harm than good, was based on something of a misunderstanding as to how the theory had been developed. Fourier's use of both hypotheses and ideas was actually far freer than Comte would have permitted.

forward (in a slightly different form from that outlined above) in a monograph presented to the Institut de France in 1807, but it was not published for many years after as the committee appointed to report on it, which included among its members both Lagrange and Laplace, simply did not report. To what extent this may have reflected deliberate delaying tactics and to what extent mere disagreement is not clear.[92] Lagrange was presumably sympathetic to the physics but he was critical of what he saw as a lack of rigour in the mathematics, in which functions were represented by what we now term Fourier series. Laplace shared this mathematical criticism and was also unhappy with the physical approach which he criticised in a paper completed in 1808.[93] There was as yet no mechanical counterpart to Fourier's theory. Laplace had not tried to develop one himself and his principal disciples were much younger men than Fourier. But Laplace now laid out the lines upon which a valid theory of heat would have, in his view, to be established. Instead of starting with the macroscopic behaviour and leaping from there to differential equations, a procedure that was in his view both unjustified and perverse, one should start by analysing a layer of molecules and the heat radiated between that layer and all other layers, at all distances from the original layer. From this analysis one would establish a set of integral equations describing the true behaviour of the solid. Fourier's equations could then be derived by differentiation, but they would feature explicitly as approximations to the precise integral equations for small distances and would thus have no intrinsic value.

Despite his criticisms Laplace does not seem to have shown any hostility towards Fourier. He appears, indeed, to have recognised the value of Fourier's theory even though he did not agree with it. His disciples were, however, less temperate, and in 1809 Jean Baptiste Biot, one of whose own papers on heat seems to have acted as a stimulus for Fourier's work, published further criticisms of this work.[94] Some years later, in 1815 and 1816, Biot and Siméon Poisson both published attempted mechanical derivations of Fourier's heat laws.[95] Meanwhile the Institut de France had made the properties of heat conduction in solid bodies the subject of their 1811 prize, which Fourier had naturally won. But the prize committee, dominated by Laplace, were still critical of his work and once again they delayed their approval, so that by the time the analyses of Biot and Poisson appeared it had still not been published. As Fourier wrote rather angrily, and quite understandably, to Laplace about the credit that Biot and Poisson were claiming for themselves,[96]

> One does not extend the bounds of science by presenting in a form said to be

[92] See Herivel (1975), pp. 100*ff.*
[93] Laplace (1878–1912), volume 12, p. 295.
[94] Biot (1809 and see also 1804).
[95] Biot (1816) and Poisson (1815).
[96] Quoted by Herivel (1975), p. 127.

> different results which one has not found oneself and, above all, by forestalling the true author in publication.

The criticism was further justified, as Laplace himself realised, by the fact that the mechanical treatments contained several relatively obvious mistakes.

Fourier's theory was eventually published, in the form of his prize essay, between 1819 and 1821, well over a decade after it had first been put forward in the monograph. In 1822 it was published in revised form in his *Theory of Heat.*[97] Only after Fourier's death did Poisson publish, in 1835, his own thoroughly mechanical *Mathematical Theory of Heat*, based on Laplace's prescription.[98] Poisson's treatment was in one sense more up to date than Fourier's, for it allowed for the non-linearity of temperature change according to the Dulong–Petit law of 1817. But Fourier had recognised that the empirical law he used might be only an approximation and had shown that his theory could be just as well based on the new law, or indeed on any other law that might follow. That was indeed one of the great advantages of the empirical approach he adopted.

As we shall see, Fourier's theory of heat was to play a central role in the development of the mathematical physics with which the young Maxwell grew up. The same conflict as that which developed in heat theory was also apparent, though less clearly defined, in the theories of light and elastic solids. Following Thomas Young's demonstration of the interference of light in 1801, the wave theory of light developed by Augustin Fresnel between 1814 and 1821 may be seen as a dynamistic theory, put forward in explicit opposition to the mechanistic corpuscular theory of light developed by Laplace and his followers.[99] Whereas the mechanists treated light, much as they did heat, as an atomic substance radiated by matter, Fresnel treated it as a waveform in a luminiferous aether. This aether was itself analysed as an elastic solid, but as one whose properties were defined empirically by the observed phenomena of light and not according to the mechanics of a true elastic solid. Just as in Fourier's theory of heat, a hypothetical mechanical treatment was replaced by an analytic empirical one bearing all the hallmarks of the dynamistic approach. In 1830 Augustin Cauchy, who was, like Poisson, a disciple of Laplace, and who had already contributed to the general mechanical theory of elastic solids, tried to replace Fresnel's empirically defined medium with a true mechanically defined one, but the attempt was unsuccessful.[100]

From a modern point of view, it is easy to invert chronologically the

[97] Fourier (1955).
[98] Poisson (1835).
[99] Fresnel (1819 and 1866–70) and Young (1807). For the development of aether theories see Whittaker (1951), Schaffner (1972), Silliman (1974), Doran (1974) and Cantor and Hodge (1981). For a good account of Young's work see Cantor (1983).
[100] Cauchy (1830).

representatives of the two traditions of mathematical physics. Lagrange seems more modern than Laplace, but was thirteen years older. Fourier seems much more modern than Poisson, but was nearly twenty years older. This illusion reflects the fact that the Laplacian tradition, though it continued to dominate French mathematical physics, was something of a blind alley for the history of physics as a whole.[101] In France, and indeed on the continent of Europe as a whole, the dominant tradition throughout much of the nineteenth century remained the Laplacian one of molecular hypotheses, action at a distance, and derived integral formulations. The theories of Fourier and Fresnel were not without their supporters, and, as we shall see, some of these supporters were to play a significant role in the development of physics in general and electromagnetic theory in particular. But the environment was generally hostile to such dynamically oriented approaches. Away from the Continent in Britain, however, things developed rather differently, and it was Britain that was to be the principal location of the next phase in the development of physics.

As a result of numerous factors, including for example a patriotic devotion to Newtonian fluxional analysis rather than the continental Leibnizian differential analysis, but including also such external features as the Napoleonic wars, a general malaise in British science and particular problems affecting such institutions as the Royal Society and retarding the development of the conservative universities of Oxford and Cambridge, the British were largely isolated from the development of continental mathematical physics in the late eighteenth and early nineteenth centuries.[102] The work of Laplace did make a belated impact but that of Lagrange was largely unknown in Britain well into the nineteenth century. Even when French mathematicial physics was imported it was in the context of the Cambridge mathematical tripos and of concerns, to do with the foundations of calculus and definitions of derivatives and integrals, that, although controversial, produced rather different divisions from those we have discussed here.[103] Lagrange and Laplace, arch-rivals in respect of their physical methodologies, were allies in the pure mathematical context, both featuring in a rigorous 'algebraic' tradition that was opposed to a 'geometric' tradition within which were classed Fourier (with his use of trigonometric series approximations) and Fresnel.

Some of the issues of mathematical physics had, however, been picked up in Britain. The Scotsmen John Playfair and Jon Robison, for example,

[101] See Fox (1974).

[102] In terms of general science, Scotland, where there was a flourishing scientific tradition with close links with the Continent, was less isolated than England. But in mathematics, as opposed to chemistry or medicine, the isolation did extend to Scotland as well.

[103] See Becher (1980).

had argued in support of the purely rational origins of the laws of dynamics.[104] There was also the strong if technically unsophisticated native tradition of 'force physics' to which we have already referred. By the nineteenth century this was more or less a Scottish tradition, represented by, among others, Playfair and Robison, but by then too Scottish physics was overwhelmingly dominant in Britain. This ensured that so far as the British did choose between the mechanistic and the dynamistic traditions, they tended to be predisposed towards the latter. The situation in the context of mathematical physics, which was to be of the utmost importance for the development of electromagnetic theory, is perhaps best described in terms of the views adopted by some of the more prominent individual British mathematicians and physicists.

The isolation of Britian from the Continent seems to have been less severe in the case of Ireland than in those of England and Scotland. One mathematician who was fully aware of continental developments was the Astronomer Royal of Ireland, William Rowan Hamilton. Hamilton is often treated as an oddball, and he was certainly unusual. Several nineteenth-century scientists were competent poets, but no other had Wordsworth for a tutor. Few scientists of any period based their work on such an explicitly metaphysical approach as he did. But Hamilton also created the quaternion analysis from which modern vector analysis evolved and developed generalised dynamics in the form in which it has proved to be best adapted for advanced physical problems; and these achievements cannot be neglected.[105] In the present context Hamilton's significance lies in the second of these achievements, in his development of a generalised dynamics based on a characteristic function and law of varying action and applicable equally to mechanical and optical problems. The new dynamics, which was developed in the context of the continuum wave theory of light, was not used to any great extent until the twentieth century, when it turned out to be the natural formulation for problems in quantum mechanics. But the ideas underlying it were to be of more immediate importance, largely through the mediacy of Whewell. These ideas were unequivocally dynamistic. Hamilton's philosophy was, as he discovered from Coleridge at about the time he started working on his dynamics, extremely close to the dynamical philosophies of Kant and Coleridge himself. He saw dynamics as composed of two distinct but united sciences, one purely physical and *a posteriori* and the other purely metaphysical and developed *a priori*. Whereas others sought to derive its axioms either from the physical world or from rational first principles Hamilton argued that they could be derived equally well from either starting point, and that this was possible because of the uniting of the mental and physical in God. He thus combined the

[104] See for example Playfair (1814).
[105] See Hankins (1980) and Graves (1882–9).

dynamistic concept of a rational dynamics with a dynamistic attitude towards empirical physics. The physical dynamics, a science of 'Power acting by Law in Space and Time', was purely empirical, 'discernible by observation and generalisation of facts or phenomena.'[106] The mental dynamics was purely analytical and a natural extension of what Hamilton called the 'scientific poem' of Lagrange.

Like Hamilton, William Whewell did not feature in the mainstream of developments in mathematical physics; but he was nevertheless one of the leading mathematical authorities in Britain and his contemporary influence was enormous. He was also, like Hamilton, a Kantian, with a strongly dynamistic attitude towards his subject matter. Whewell's early textbooks on mechanics were written before he had met Hamilton but his important and influential *History of the Inductive Sciences* (1837) and *Philosophy of the Inductive Sciences* (1840, second edition 1847) were written after they had met in 1832 and found in each other stimulating and sympathetic company.[107] In these works, Whewell adopted a view of mathematical physics similar to Hamilton's with dynamics being marked by both *a priori* and *a posteriori* elements, the latter firmly rooted in experience. As in his treatment of science in general, however, he adopted a very flexible and practical approach to the relation between the two sets of elements. Having discussed the arguments of d'Alembert and Playfair on the necessary rational origins of the laws of motion he returned an open verdict:[108]

> Whether the laws of motion, as we now know them, can be rigorously traced to an absolute necessity in the nature of things, we have not ventured absolutely to pronounce.

But he continued to observe that:[109]

> Some of the most acute and profound mathematicians have believed that, for these laws of motion, or some of them, there was such a demonstrable necessity compelling them to be such as they are and no other.

He himself, he admitted, tended to agree. At the same time, however, he insisted that 'no-one can doubt that, as historical fact, the laws were collected from experience.'[110] For Whewell, then, the laws of motion were physical interpretations of rational ideas, derived from experience, but

[106] Quoted by Hankins (1980), pp. 175, 178.
[107] Whewell (1837, 1840, 1847 and 1967).
[108] Whewell (1967), part 1, p. 246. The key word in this and the following quotations is 'necessity', which for Whewell as for Kant could only be inferred *a priori*, all *a posteriori* knowledge being merely probable or contingent.
[109] Whewell (1967), part 1, p. 246.
[110] Whewell (1967), part 1, p. 247.

shaped by the mind into the form of its own ideas:[111]

> The laws of motion borrow their *form* from the Idea of Causation, though their matter may be given by experience: and hence they possess a universality which experience cannot give.

In respect of the derivation of the first law, for example, 'action and reaction must be equal; but much thought and some trial were needed to show what *action* and *reaction* are.'[112]

Whewell also indicated, both in his *Philosophy* and in a keynote 'Report' to the recently formed British Association for the Advancement of Science in 1835, his attitude to the debate on the theory of heat. He was very critical of Comte's interpretation of Fourier's work, but as we might expect he praised Fourier's theory itself and criticised the Laplacian approach adopted in Poisson's rival work:[113]

> That ... by suitably assuming the forces which these particles exert on each other, we may represent their mechanical condition, and trace its consequences, is undoubtedly true. But it would be to go too far, to assert, on this account alone, that the only true conception of the physical structure of bodies is that which represents them as so constituted. This would be to mistake the use of the differential calculus for the evidence of physical truth.

Whewell, as we have noted, was relatively approving of hypotheses, but whereas atomism 'as a convenience' was acceptable, Poisson went too far:[114]

> In exploring the properties of matter as we find them in nature, the assumption of solid, hard, indestructible particles is of no use or value.

In respect of mathematical physics, Whewell was essentially a teacher and establishment authority rather than an active participant. It is notable, however, that the three most significant practitioners of the science in this period in Britain all shared something of his dynamistic approach and in particular his approval of Fourier's theory. They were George Green, George Gabriel Stokes and William Thomson, later Lord Kelvin.

George Green's most famous work, his *Essay on the Application of Mathematical Analysis to the Theories of Electricity and Magnetism* of 1828, was privately published and distributed; it was, however, extremely important for the development of the subject, and it was partly inspired by

[111] Whewell (1967), part 1, p. 250.
[112] Whewell (1967), part 1, p. 248.
[113] Whewell (1835), p. 22.
[114] Whewell (1967), part 1, p. 438.

Fourier's theory of heat.[115] Following Cauchy's attempt to model the luminiferous aether on a true mechanical elastic solid, Green also attempted, in 1837, to build a theory of light, and in particular of reflection and refraction, on a more analytic basis.[116] Arguing that physicists were in reality 'perfectly ignorant of the mode of action of the elements of the luminiferous aether on each other', and that it was scarcely sound to 'assume certain modes of action, which, after all, may be widely different from the mechanism employed by nature', he rejected Cauchy's molecular hypothesis. Instead he built up the mathematics of a strained elastic solid as an exercise in pure mathematics, independent of the body's structure, and then used this to provide a mathematical rather than a physical model of the aether.[117] The replacement of Cauchy's mechanical theory by a purely analytical dynamical one did not get him very far in practice and the discrepancy between the observed phenomena of light and those reproducible on a mechanically consistent elastic solid aether basis remained. But Green's work did provide an important model for others to follow in pursuit of a dynamical theory of physics. A similar approach was also taken at about the same time by the Irishman James MacCullagh.[118]

In 1845 George Stokes, like Whewell a prominent teacher at Cambridge, took Green's approach a step further. Although Green had rejected molecular models and mechanical methods he had built up an analytical model of an elastic solid aether of a particular mechanical type. Stokes derived instead the equations for a perfectly general continuous medium.[119] Stokes was essentially a mathematician with an eye to the possible physical applications of his work; to compare this work in terms of physical methodology with that of Fourier or Poisson would thus be to treat it out of context. But so far as he prepared the mathematical ground for others his work stood, like Green's, firmly in the dynamical tradition of Lagrange and Fourier. The emphasis was entirely on analytic generality as opposed to mechanical specificity, and the media under investigation were treated as continuous, with continuous pressures and stresses, in approximation to their macroscopic behaviour—not as discrete, as in the mechanical theories.

The third key figure of British mathematical physics of the period, and the most important in our present context, was William Thomson. Unlike those of his contemporaries we have so far considered Thomson was more of a physicist than a mathematician and he was very much concerned with problems of physical method. As we shall see when we review his work on electromagnetic theory in the next chapter, his viewpoint, developed in the

[115] Green (1828) and see Wise (1981), p. 47.
[116] Green (1839) reprinted in Green (1871).
[117] Green (1839), p. 1.
[118] MacCullagh (1840).
[119] Stokes (1849).

context of British rather than French mathematical physics, cannot be expressed simply in terms of the Fourier–Poisson divide. Whereas both Frenchmen had built up their mathematical structures on the basis of physical assumptions, whether of microscopic molecular hypotheses or macroscopic empirical laws, Thomson, in line with both Stokes and Green, tended to build up his mathematical structures independently of any physical context and only afterwards to consider the question of a physical interpretation. Like Whewell, and like his fellow Scottish natural philosophers of the period, he was also very conscious of the heuristic value of mechanical models, as distinguished from mechanical theories. But like the other British mathematicians we have considered, his starting point was the work of the French analytical–dynamical school, and in particular that of Fourier. Thomson's earliest published papers, written in 1841 when he was only 17, were devoted to a defence of Fourier's methodology and an extension of this methodology from the realm of heat to that of electricity.[120] With these and the papers that followed during the next few years he laid the ground for an empirically founded dynamistic treatment (soon to be called field theory) of a range of phenomena that had previously been treated only mechanistically, in terms of molecular hypotheses and action at a distance.[121]

We shall consider the work of Green, Stokes and Thomson in much more detail in the next chapter. Even from the brief glance given here, however, it is clear that while several of the most prominent British physicists had a strong respect for the utility of the mechanistic approach to their subject, their work also had very strong roots in the opposed, dynamistic, approach.

Unification, analogy and mechanical models

We have already discussed in the previous sections some of the manifestations of the dynamistic and mechanistic attitudes in terms of scientific methodology, both generally and in the particular case of analogical method. In setting the scene for Maxwell's work, three aspects of this issue deserve more explicit attention: the principle of the unity of physics and the search for unified theories; the formulation of the method of analogy; and the use and justification of mechanical models.

The ideal of unification has always occupied a prominent place in the development of science, whether associated with a dynamistic or with a mechanistic attitude towards the physical world. Within the mechanical philosophy it appeared in the form of a hypothesis to the effect that all physical phenomena may be reduced to the same basic mechanical

[120] Thomson (1841a and 1841b).
[121] See for example Wise (1981) and Buchwald (1977).

elements—for the Laplacians, for example, to molecules and action at a distance, or for Dalton to the motions of fluids. Unification acquired particular importance, however, within the framework of the dynamical philosophy. This was largely because it appeared in that context as an epistemological necessity, and so acquired a status it never had within the mechanical tradition. If we ask why there should be unity, the mechanists of the eighteenth and nineteenth centuries could offer only one convincing answer or explanation, namely that the world in all its aspects shared the same creator, God. But while this might act as a perfectly reasonable explanation, especially if backed up, as it often was, by a sophisticated theology, it had obvious weaknesses and limitations. Assuming there was a measure of unity, how could mere mortals know what form it took within God's creation? And why, in particular, should it be mechanical? How, given these doubts, could it be applied as a guiding principle to the realm of earthly physics? Questions such as these were not necessarily unanswerable, but they were not easy to answer. If, however, one adopted a dynamistic attitude, both the foundations and the implications of unity became much clearer.

As we have seen, one of the key characteristics of the dynamistic tradition in the eighteenth century, whether in its Scottish or in its Germanic form, was the acceptance of Hume's criticism to the effect that scientific knowledge could not in fact be deduced as objective knowledge from reason and observation alone, but also had a necessary subjective component, imposed by the nature of the 'knowing' mind. None of the philosphers who followed Hume in the eighteenth and nineteenth centuries were able to argue round his scepticism on this point. They were, however, able to turn it to positive use. For although it opened the way for the possibility of conflicting systems of scientific knowledge, objectively incommensurable since derived from different states of mind, it also raised the possibility of an effectively objective science based on that which was common to all human minds. It was this latter possibility that the dynamically inclined philosophers exploited and it provided the foundation for an epistemologically based principle of unity. All scientific laws were, on this view, derived from the common properties of the human mind, and this unity of origin could not but be reflected in a unity of form. William Hamilton, in his *Lectures*, argued further that the desire for unity in science was itself a product of the mind, so that in his view the unification of scientific theory had a two-fold psychological origin.[122]

At the most basic level this enforced unification appeared in manifestations that were not even questioned by the mechanical philosophers: the unification through the forms of space and time and through the principle of cause and effect. At another level the unification was imposed through

[122] W Hamilton (1865) and see Olson (1975).

ideas such as that of polarity, or through intellectually derived structures such as that of rational dynamics.

The epistemological justification of the unity of science was not always explicit in the works of the dynamic scientists themselves, but it was often strongly implicit, as we shall see, in their use of analogical method, and it was no accident that the strongest advocates of the unification of science in the early and middle nineteenth century were all inclined towards the dynamical philosophy. Oersted, for example, who demonstrated the unity of electricity and magnetism, was a Kantian philosopher. Faraday, perhaps the most ardent unifier of all, also adhered to many of the key tenets of the dynamistic tradition.

Inseparable from the concept of a psychologically determined unification of science was that of analogy, both the analogy between sciences and, more fundamentally, the analogy between nature and the mind. The dynamical philosophers saw no justification for assuming, as their mechanical opponents seemed to, that whatever existed in nature was necessarily representable in terms of mechanical constructions. As Coleridge realised, however, the very fact that physical science was possible, that laws could be derived which, like the law of gravitation, described perfectly the phenomena observed in nature, could only be accounted for in terms of the 'remarkable fact . . . that the material world is found to obey the same laws as had been deduced independently from the reason.'[123] This fact was for Coleridge 'a mystery which of itself should suffice to make us religious',[124] and in developing a theory of natural philosophy as the study of the science and language of symbols (a symbol being something which, in contrast to a metaphor or analogy, partook of the reality it rendered intelligible)[125] he carried the discussion of analogy into a discourse more closely allied with religion than with science. As we have already seen, however, a theory of analogical method was also developed in a more scientific context by William Hamilton.

That the pursuit of analogies between different aspects of nature could be fruitful had been demonstrated by a number of scientists, not least by Newton in his theory of universal gravitation, and was widely recognised. Two examples are, however, worth noting specifically. One concerns James Forbes, a Scottish scientist who was Professor of Natural Philosophy at Edinburgh, alongside William Hamilton as Professor of Moral Philosophy, when Maxwell was a student there. Forbes was himself educated within the Scottish common-sense tradition of philosophy, and he learnt much of his science by correspondence with Whewell. He was thus well ensconced in the dynamical tradition and in his work the use of analogy took on a special

[123] Coleridge (1818), volume 3, p. 462.
[124] Coleridge (1972), p. 79.
[125] Coleridge (1972), p. 30.

importance.[126] Exploring the similarity between light and radiant heat, proposed by Macedonio Melloni in 1833, he asserted that:[127]

> The importance of analogies in science has not, perhaps, been sufficiently insisted upon by writers on the method of philosophizing. A clear perception of *connexion* has been by far the most fertile source of discovery. That of gravitation itself was only an extended analogy. ... The penetrating sagacity of M. Fresnel, in his prosecution of the undulatory theory of light, has led him to draw from mechanical and mathematical analogies, accurate representations of laws which no strict reasoning could have enabled him to arrive at.

Forbes himself demonstrated that heat could be polarised and was subject to total internal reflection, just like light, and that all the results achieved by the undulatory theory of light were also applicable to radiant heat. In a completely different subject area he was also the first to use the visual analogies between glaciers and rivers to derive a theory of glacier motion.

The second example of an analogising scientist is Michael Faraday, whose quest for the unification of physics manifested itself in an ardent search for analogies between the entire range of phenomena to be unified: light, heat, electricity, magnetism, gravity and chemical effects. For Faraday, indeed, analogy was the principal guide in the exploration of the unknown, and his series of *Researches* bore eloquent witness to the faith he placed in that guide and to the degree in which such faith was justified.[128]

In the realm of non-mathematical science the concepts of unification and analogy presented were often implicit or imprecise. In the realm of mathematical physics, however, they were both explicit and precise, the central theme being the *a priori* content of dynamics.

As dynamics had been abstracted more and more from physical structure during the eighteenth century, so it had come to be seen more and more as a product of the human mind. In nineteenth-century Britain it was interpreted in this way by, among others, Robison and Playfair, who were Forbes's predecessors in the Edinburgh chair of natural philosophy, and, with slight qualifications, by Whewell. In the view of these scientists, as stated explicitly by Playfair, the laws of dynamics, being mental in origin, were equally applicable to all aspects of the physical world and so served to unify physical science. In this way the belief in the epistemological necessity of unification was encapsulated in hard physics and a unifying agent, mathematical dynamics, was identified.

Robison and Playfair, though out of sympathy with Laplace's natural

[126] See Olson (1975).

[127] Forbes (1835), p. 147.

[128] Faraday (1821–57, 1965 and see also 1932–6). See Williams (1965) and Gooding (1982).

philosophy, took Laplace's mathematics as their model of dynamics. The exploitation of the unifying force of dynamics they had identified was, however, to rest on the work of Lagrange. His was the purer, more abstract form of dynamics, and being based on the overall energetic properties of a system rather than on its internal structure it was intrinsically independent of the particular types of physical action being treated. Its full value in this respect did not become apparent until after the establishment of the conservation of energy had served to emphasise the unifying effect of the energy principle. But its utility was well recognised by Fourier, for whom Lagrangian analysis was a powerful unifying force. This analysis was, he declared,[129]

> as extensive as nature itself; it defines all perceptible relations, measures times, spaces, temperatures. ... Its chief attribute is clearness; it has no words to express confused rules. It brings together phenomena the most diverse, and discovers the hidden analogies which unite them.

Moreover, he declared,

> [Mathematical analysis] seems to be a faculty of the human mind destined to supplement the shortness of life and the imperfection of the senses; and what is still more remarkable, it follows the same course in the study of all phenomena; it interprets them by the same language, as if to attest the unity and simplicity of the plan of the universe, and to make still more evident that unchangeable order which presides over all natural causes.

Fourier's emphasis on the use of mathematical dynamics as a tool with which to lay bare the analogies between different phenomena was reflected in its use for precisely that purpose by people like Green, Thomson and William Rowan Hamilton. Hamilton's dynamics was based on the use of a principle of action and defining characteristic function, both of which were completely independent of the type of physical phenomenon being treated. It was accompanied by his enunciation of the famous optical–mechanical analogy that was eventually put to dramatically successful use by Schrödinger in 1926. Besides exploiting dynamics for the exploration of analogies between physical phenomena, moreover, Hamilton also emphasised the manifestation in dynamics of the analogy between mind and nature. Writing to Whewell, he explained that[130]

> The opinion which I think I tried to express when I had the pleasure of talking the thing over with you, and which I have not since reflected on enough to alter it, was in substance this; that there are, or may be imagined, two

[129] Fourier (1955), pp. 7–8.
[130] Quoted by Hankins (1980), p. 175.

> dynamical sciences: one subjective, *a priori*, metaphysical, deducible from meditation on our ideas of Power, Space, Time; the other objective, *a posteori*, physical, discoverable by observation and generalization of facts or phenomena: that these two sciences are distinct in kind, but intimately and wonderfully connected, in consequence of the ultimate union of the subjective and objective in God, or, to speak less technically and more religiously, by virtue of the manifestation which he has been pleased to make of himself in the universe to the intellect of man; so that the two sciences are never wholly separate, but may and ought to advance together, and use many common expressions, and each possess an analogon to many if not to all of the results and theorems of the other.

If Hamilton's religious metaphysics were not widely shared among the community of mathematical physicists, they nevertheless serve as an elegant illustration of the high romantic end of the dynamical philosophy expressed by one who was also an unrivalled exponent of that philosophy at the technical mathematical level. The fruitful analogical uses of dynamics in the hands of the less metaphysical Green and Thomson were more typical of the mathematical tradition that emerged in the wake of Fourier's work, but since they played important roles in the development of electromagnetic theory before Maxwell their consideration is more appropriate to the next chapter than to this.

One important if rather bizarre consequence of the use of analogy in the dynamical tradition was that it opened the way for the use of mechanical models. So long as mechanical constructions were presented as objectively valid 'true' representations of nature they were of course rejected completely by dynamically oriented philosophers and scientists. But for those prepared to consider the heuristic use of hypotheses, as for example was Whewell, the emphasis on analogy afforded the very same constructions a new validity as models. Since it was claimed that man could do no more than model nature in terms of the forms afforded by the intellect, the careful use of mechanical models might indeed prove to be the most appropriate way of going about physical science; the models themselves might well act, to borrow William Rowan Hamilton's phrase, as fit media between nature and the human mind.

This justification for the use of mechanical models was obviously of the utmost importance, for without it the dynamical tradition would in certain respects have been hamstrung as compared with the mechanical view. As it was, however, the heuristic of mechanical models was common to both approaches and it was indeed the mechanical philosophers who were the more restricted, for their models had to conform strictly to mechanically possible behaviours, while those of the dynamical scientists, serving only as illustrations and guides, did not. Within the dynamical view indeed, a model could be just as valuable through failing to produce the observed results as through succeeding, and often more so. The dynamists had in effect the best of both worlds.

In exploring the characteristics of the dynamistic and mechanistic attitudes in this chapter, we have tended to focus predominantly on the dynamistic. This is partly because the dynamistic attitude was less straightforward than the mechanistic attitude and partly because the dynamical tradition is rather less familiar than its mechanical counterpart. It is also apparent, however, that the dynamical tradition is peculiarly relevant to the context of Maxwell's work. This is not to say that the mechanical tradition is irrelevant: on the contrary. But whether we look at the teachers whom Maxwell most respected—William Hamilton, Forbes, Whewell and Stokes—or the scientists upon whose own electromagnetic researches he built—Oersted, Ampère, Faraday and Thomson—there is no escaping the dominance of a dynamistic attitude. All eight philosophers and scientists were indeed clearly associated with aspects of the dynamical tradition and the two British philosophers, Hamilton and Whewell, were two of the most prominent spokesmen for that tradition. We should not jump from this observation to any conclusions concerning Maxwell himelf. He could have acted against, or independently of, this background. The concept of influence as applied from individual to individual is historically very suspect. But given that Maxwell was sympathetic to aspects of the dynamical attitude, and we shall see that he was, its prominence in the background to his work suggests strongly that we should take it as the starting point for our discussion and as defining, in effect, not one pole of the prevailing context but rather the mid-point, from which deviations in either direction may be noted. As we shall see in the next chapter there was indeed a strong sense in which the dynamistic attitude, in the practical empirical formulation of Whewell, and with the addition of a mechanical heuristic, had by the middle of the century captured the middle ground in physics (though not of course in chemistry, where dynamism seems to have failed completely), usurping the mechanism dominant in the early part of the century.

3

Electromagnetism before Maxwell

Introduction

By the middle of the nineteenth century the phenomena of electromagnetism had already been studied for several hundred years. But for our purposes the theories of electricity, magnetism and electromagnetism are most conveniently picked up in about 1820, just thirty years, or one generation, before Maxwell entered the field.

At the beginning of 1820, before Oersted had undertaken his famous experiments on the mutual influence of electricity and magnetism, there were in effect three separate sciences of electromagnetic phenomena, those of electrostatics, magnetism and galvanism. The most advanced of these was the science of electrostatics, the dominant theory of which was due to Coulomb, Laplace and Poisson. Following the pioneering work of Franklin in the middle of the eighteenth century, Charles Augustin Coulomb had, in the 1780s, established the inverse square law for the repulsion between like electric charges and the attraction between opposite ones.[1] In 1812 Siméon Denis Poisson, whose championing of the mechanical approach to physics was noted in the last chapter, had published his classic memoir on the distribution of electricity on the surface of conductors, a mathematical treatment of electrostatics based on Laplacian mechanico-molecular principles.[2] By 1820 Poisson's theory had become widely accepted as the standard treatment of the subject and it was indeed still so thirty years later, both in France and in Britain.[3]

Opinions as to the physical nature of electricity differed somewhat between the English- and the French-speaking worlds. The English, following Henry Cavendish, tended to treat electricity as a single imponderable fluid. But the dominant hypothesis, adopted by Coulomb and his French suc-

[1] Coulomb (1884). See Gillmor (1971) and Heilbron (1979), chapter 2.

[2] Poisson (1812). See Fox (1974) and Arnold (1983).

[3] See Buchwald (1977).

cessors, was that of two imponderable fluids corresponding to the two types of electricity, positive and negative. If the two fluids were also assumed to be mechanically incompressible a theory could be developed using attractive forces only and this tied in well with the strict self-proclaimed Newtonianism of the Laplacian programme. As we noted in the last chapter, the relationship between mechanism and mathematics was a complex one and Poisson's theory of electrostatics was built, as indeed was Laplace's own mechanics, upon the concept of a potential introduced (though not named) by the dynamistically oriented mathematician Lagrange. Laplace had introduced a gravitational potential V, defined so that the gravitational force $\mathbf{G}$ was given by $\mathbf{G} = -\nabla V$, or $G_x = -\partial V/\partial x$, in order to simplify his analysis. In the presence of a gravitating spheroid of density ρ at distance r, the potential took the form

$$V = \iiint \frac{\rho \, d\omega^3}{r} \tag{3.1}$$

and in empty space

$$\nabla^2 V = \frac{\partial^2 V}{\partial x^2} + \frac{\partial^2 V}{\partial y^2} + \frac{\partial^2 V}{\partial z^2} = 0. \tag{3.2}$$

In order to establish a corresponding theory of electrostatics, Poisson introduced an analogous electrostatic potential V_e. The potential due to a conducting spheroid of charge density ρ_e at distance r, was given by

$$V_e = \iiint \frac{\rho_e \, d\omega^3}{r} \tag{3.3}$$

and the fundamental equation of electrostatics then took the form

$$\nabla^2 V \propto -\rho_e \tag{3.4}$$

for the potential V at a point at which the charge density was ρ_e. (Neither Laplace nor Poisson used the word 'potential', which was introduced later by Green.) The experimental results of Coulomb on the electrical behaviour of variously shaped charged bodies were derived by Poisson from a hypothetical structure of material and electrical molecules with attractive forces acting at a distance between them. The success of the theory in reproducing the observed results was then taken as confirmation of the physical hypotheses. In 1816 Jean Baptiste Biot, like Poisson one of Laplace's disciples, had asserted in one of the leading Laplacian textbooks that Poisson's theory 'gives the highest degree of probability, not to say complete certainty, to the real existence of the two fluids'.[4]

The theory of magnetism was less well developed than that of electricity, and there was indeed far less certainty about the empirical behaviour of

[4] Biot (1816), volume 2, p. 312. See Frankel (1977).

magnets than about that of electrical conductors. But the inverse square law had again been established by Coulomb and in 1824 Poisson would complete a theory of magnetism parallel to that which he had already provided of electrostatics.[5] Because of the experimental uncertainty it was not possible to draw the physical conclusions, for example as to the existence of imponderable magnetic fluids, with as much assurance as it had been in the electrical case. But the approach was fundamentally the same, and Poisson, Biot and their fellow Laplacians adopted a two-fluid theory of magnetism—austral and boreal—analogous to their theory of electricity.

The third area of electromagnetic theory, that of galvanism, presented a rather different picture. 'Animal electricity', as it was at first known, had been demonstrated by Luigi Galvani in the late eighteenth century,[6] and had been brought into the realm of the physical sciences as a result of Allessandro Volta's demonstrations of the electrical action of the 'Voltaic pile' in the 1790s and the publication of his experiments in 1800.[7] The electrical properties of this pile or battery had quickly been identified with those demonstrated by Galvani, and experimental work using voltaic piles had been developed rapidly. But in 1820 galvanic electricity was still something of a mystery. Volta himself had argued that the electricity produced by the pile was substantially the same as that manifest in electrostatic phenomena and this view had soon become generally accepted. An isolated pile behaved as a conductor in terms of its electrostatic attraction and repulsion of other conductors. A pile could also be used to produce a discharge that seemed to be similar to, though much more feeble than, that of an electrostatic Leyden jar. Behind these similarities, however, there were also marked differences which could not be ignored. Whereas electrostatic discharge was a discrete phenomenon, galvanic discharge was a continuous one. Static electricity was, as the name suggests, static, whereas galvanic electricity had more of a dynamic quality. In 1820 these contradictions were still unresolved, and there was as yet no mathematical theory of galvanism.

There were, however, a number of rival theories of the voltaic pile, and while these were not central to the development of electromagnetic theory they were of some relevance.[8] Volta himself favoured a contact theory according to which the contact between the metallic layers of the pile, copper and zinc, provided in some unspecified way for the build-up of positive and negative electric fluids on the two sides of the metal–metal junction. According to this theory the third component of the pile, the liquid-impregnated cardboard between the pairs of metal plates, acted only as a

[5] Coulomb (1884) and Poisson (1826).
[6] Galvani (1791).
[7] Volta (1800). See T Brown (1969).
[8] See Blondel (1982) and T Brown (1969).

conductor. Volta's theory was supported by Laplace and Poisson and was developed by Biot, whose treatment of the subject became the prevailing orthodoxy of the day. Its chief rival was a chemical theory due to the British scientists Wollaston and Davy, according to which the crucial junctions were not those between the two metals but those between metal and liquid, at which a chemically produced polarisation of electricity was supposed to take place. A third theory, of particular relevance in our present context but virtually unknown at the time, was published in 1806, after the two main theories had already become established, by the Danish philosopher Oersted.[9]

Oersted

It would be hard to think of anyone less in sympathy with the dominant French mechanico-molecular tradition of Laplace, Poisson and Biot than Hans Christian Oersted. For Oersted was a thoroughly dynamical philosopher.[10] As a young man he had first trained as a pharmacist (his father's profession) and had then completed a doctoral thesis in philosophy. The subject of this thesis was a study of Kant's *Metaphysical Foundations of Natural Science,* which was, as we saw in the last chapter, one of the key works in the establishment of the dynamical tradition in physical science. Oersted studied under one of Kant's successors, Fichte, and was friendly with another, Schlegel. His own philosophy was based explicitly on Kant's, and he was also very sympathetic with aspects of Schelling's *Naturphilosophie.* In tune with the dynamical outlook that he espoused he rejected all specific mechanical hypotheses and laid emphasis instead upon pure empirical observations and upon the *a priori* input of the human mind through which such observations were transformed into scientific laws. The *a priori* content of natural laws provided for Oersted, as for Schelling, Coleridge and other dynamical philosophers, the basis for a unification of science through the concept of polarity, this polarity being manifest in nature in the form of fundamental and opposing polar forces:[11]

> There are two opposing forces which exist in all bodies and which can never be completely removed from them. Each of these forces has an expansive and repulsive action in the volume which it dominates; but each attracts and produces a contraction when it acts on the other.

In terms of his philosophical attitude, Oersted was in complete sympathy with Kant, Schelling, Coleridge and the other prominent representatives of

[9] Oersted (1806).
[10] See Blondel (1982), Stauffer (1957), Dibner (1961) and Williams (1965).
[11] Williams (1965), p. 138.

the dynamical philosophy discussed in the last chapter. Where he differed from most of these people, however, was in his bringing his philosophy of science to bear on science itself. His active interest in the physical sciences, and in particular in those of electricity and magnetism, seems to have been stimulated by his friendship with the German Wilhelm Ritter, who was also a pharmacist, even more of a *Naturphilosoph,* and a keen electrical exprimenter. Oersted worked with Ritter on the study of galvanism and in 1803 he communicated some of Ritter's theories and results in Paris, then the centre of the scientific world. The experimental results were at first well received but the theories, which were based on a unification of galvanism with magnetism, were too tainted with the stain of romantic *Naturphilosophie* to go down well in a city dominated by the mechanical spirit of Laplace. Oersted's own interest in electricity and magnetism was, however, established, and three years later he put forward his theory of the voltaic pile.

According to Oersted's theory, galvanic electricity was 'a kind of dynamic oscillation', or polarising wave motion:[12]

> We know that the force being transmitted attracts its opposite, whereas it repels the force of the same kind. When the attracted force has reached a certain intensity, it combines with a portion of the attracting force, leaving the repelled force in an even more perfect state of liberty. This force produces a new distribution by its attractive and repulsive faculty and, a moment later, a new equilibrium is achieved like the first and so on.

He also declared, moreover, that[13]

> Everything that has been said so far about electricity must apply equally to magnetism. The action of a magnet begins in a polarisation, and must consequently communicate itself *as a wave motion* [*undulatoirement*] like electricity.

The previous year Oersted had written to Ritter proposing that the implied unification of electricity and magnetism be extended to chemistry, and indeed that all natural phenomena should be seen as produced by the same polarising power:[14]

> What else are the chemical forces but the opposite electricities? . . . The same forces manifest themselves in magnetism as in electricity. . . . All forces in Nature may be reduced to these two.

He now suggested that 'this mechanism of the action of wave propagation

[12] Williams (1965), p. 138.
[13] Oersted (1806), p. 370.
[14] Oersted (1920), p. xlv.

is without doubt general throughout nature', though he admitted at the same time that this was 'very difficult to demonstrate'.[15]

Despite Ritter's attempts, the identity of galvanic and magnetic forces could not yet be proved experimentally; but the search for a unification of the forces of nature continued to dominate Oersted's scientific work. In 1813 he published his *Researches on the Identity of the Chemical and Electrical Forces* and in this context he again discussed the relationship between electrical and magnetic forces.[16] He noted that if one described them in terms of the violence of their effects the three known electric and magnetic forces could be ranked in order as static electricity (the most violent), then galvanism and then magnetism. He suggested that while the difference in this respect between static electricity and magnetism might make it rather difficult to discover the true relationship between them, one might fare rather better by looking at magnetism and galvanism, the 'most latent' form of electricity: 'It is necessary to test whether electricity in its most latent state has any action upon a magnet as such.'[17]

Oersted and Ritter were not the only ones to suggest a unification of electricity and magnetism. Nor were the concepts of unification and analogy the sole preserve of their dynamistic approach. Volta's work had itself had a unifying effect, suggesting the analogy between galvanism and ordinary electricity. The mechanistic, Laplacian, approach to the subject also entailed a kind of unification through the reduction of all phenomena to the action of mechanical forces acting at a distance between molecules. Biot himself drew attention in 1819 to 'the most complete, the most perfect, and the most ultimate analogy between the laws of the two magnetic principles and those of the two electrical principles.'[18] But for Biot the unification of these forces could only come about through purely mechanical explanations, such, for example, as that he used to explain the known effect of an electrical discharge on a magnetic wire or needle:[19]

> ... it is proved that every piece of iron which has suffered any friction becomes magnetic, and ... an electrical discharge, *acting like a blow,* develops magnetism in iron wires through which it is made to pass. From the same cause, lightning produces a similar effect upon the mariner's needle, and sometimes even reverses its poles.

Biot would probably have been delighted to see all magnetic and electric phenomena reduced to 'blows' describable in terms of ordinary particle mechanics. He had, however, no time whatsoever for any form of unification other than through such mechanisms, and certainly not for the vague,

[15] Oersted (1806), p. 370.
[16] Oersted (1812 and 1813).
[17] Oersted (1813), p. 238.
[18] Biot (1819), p. 277.
[19] Biot (1819), p. 250.

metaphysically inspired and mathematically and mechanically unrigorous assertions that characterised Oersted's work. Together with his fellow Laplacians he was completely out of sympathy with Oersted's programme.

Anyone waiting for further developments of electrical science in 1820 would naturally have looked to Biot and the other Parisian physicists, but on this occasion, quite unexpectedly, it was the dynamistic approach that was to bear fruit. In 1820 Oersted took up his electrical researches again, and this time, according to his own accounts, he looked specifically for a lateral action exerted by a galvanic conductor on a magnet. As he explained later, talking of himself in the third person, this idea was based on an analogy between the proposed magnetic effect of a galvanic current and its known heating and lighting effects:[20]

> As the luminous and heating effect of an electrical current goes out in all directions from a conductor, which transmits a great quantity of electricity; so he thought it possible that the magnetical effect could likewise eradiate.

From Oersted's notebooks (figure 3.1) it would appear that he first placed the magnetic needle perpendicular to the galvanic conductor, or current-carrying wire, and that having gone through all the possible dispositions of this type he next placed it parallel to and above the wire.[21] The deflection of the needle he obtained with the new arrangement was at first too weak for him to take it as conclusive evidence. But it was real enough, and in July, using a stronger current, he repeated the experiments to his satisfaction, observing a clear deflection of the needle (figure 3.2) and the dependence of the effect on the relative orientation of current (+ and −) and needle (N and S), on which was placed above the other, on the distance between them and on the strength of the current. He also noted the independence of the effect, in contrast with the effects of static electricity, of any non-conducting medium placed in between the current and the needle. The science of electromagnetism was born.[22]

The immediate response to Oersted's claims of the interaction between galvanic and magnetic phenomena, which were broadcast in a memoir sent to the leading physicists of Europe, was one of disbelief.[23] His early advocacy of unification and the *Naturphilosophie* context of that advocacy were not forgotten and, as the physicist Dulong wrote from Paris, the news was received 'very coldly'.[24] It was seen, he reported, as 'just another

[20] Oersted (1830), p. 575.
[21] Oersted (1920), p. lxxiv.
[22] For an English translation of the memoir, originally in Latin, see Oersted (1928) and Tricker (1965).
[23] Blondel (1982) and Snelders (1975).
[24] Dulong to Berzelius, 2 October 1820, quoted by Blondel (1982), p. 44.

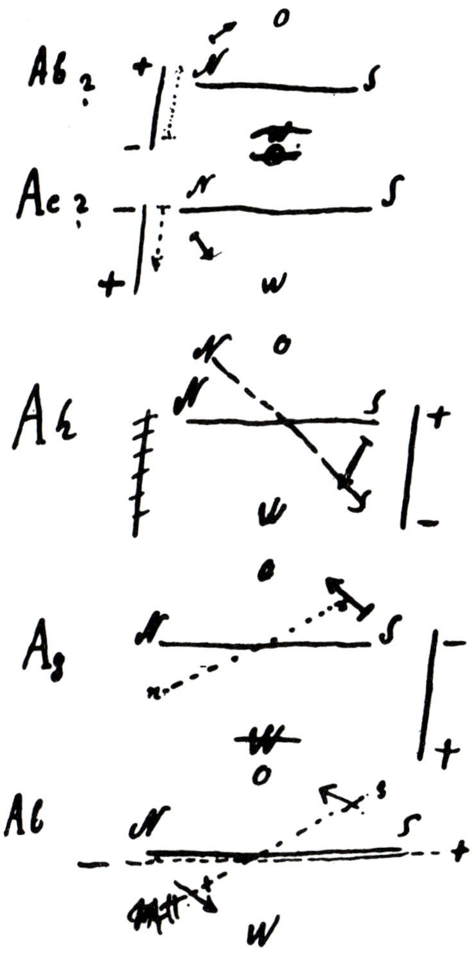

Figure 3.1 Oersted's record of his experiments with a magnetic needle and current-carrying wire. From Oersted (1920). p. lxxiv.

German dream', a figment of the Romantic imagination.[25] Oersted's experiment was, however, eminently reproducible. François Arago, who was reported as not believing a word of Oersted's claims when they were first announced,[26] soon obtained the same results himself, first in Geneva and then in front of an audience of eminent sceptics at the Academy of Sciences in Paris.[27]

Once the results of the experiments were accepted, attention turned

[25] Dulong to Berzelius, 2 October 1820, quoted by Blondel (1982), p. 44.

[26] Blondel (1982), p. 44.

[27] Blondel (1982), p. 44.

towards their interpretation. Oersted himself treated the experiments as confirming his belief in an underlying unity of forces, with magnetism now established as the most latent form of electricity and galvanism standing between it and static electricity. Elaborating on his wave propagation concept of galvanic electricity he envisaged the current as flowing in two spirals along the conducting wire, one carrying positive electricity in a dynamical wave motion in one direction, the other carrying negative electricity, similarly propagated, in the opposite direction. He suggested that if the voltaic pile driving the current were sufficiently powerful the wave propagation in the wire might not be fast enough to carry the whole current produced, so that some of the electricity would also have to be transmitted, as he had originally envisaged, in a lateral direction. This weak lateral electricity then manifested itself, on this interpretation, as a magnetic force on the iron needle, the positive electricity acting on the south pole and the negative electricity on the north pole of the magnet.[28]

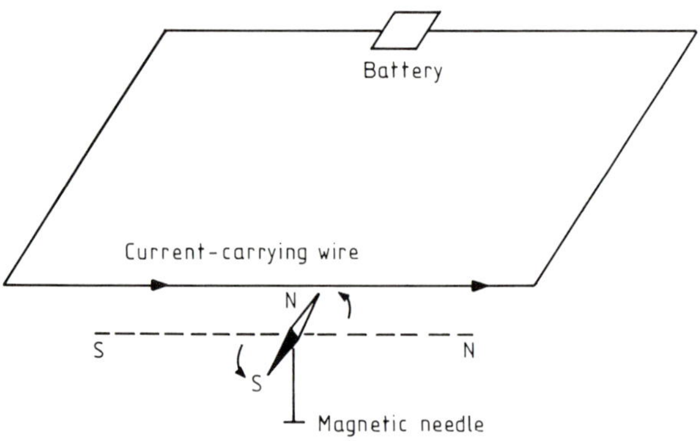

Figure 3.2 Oersted's experiment.

Resting as it did on Oersted's rather idiosyncratic picture of electric current, this explanation seems to have found few if any adherents. The most popular alternative hypothesis was that of a temporarily induced magnetism in the conducting wire. One of the first responses to Oersted's work was a suggestion made by Jöns Jacob Berzelius and repeated by Humphrey Davy to the effect that Oersted's results indicated a magnetic property of the current-carrying wire.[29] As Oersted himself pointed out, the particular magnetic disposition they proposed did not in fact accord with the symmetry of the experimental result.[30] But J Prechtl soon put forward an alternative hypothesis according to which the circumference of the wire was envisaged as forming a unipolar magnet, with the sense of which the

[28] Oersted (1928 and 1821a).

[29] Berzelius (1821) and Davy (1821).

[30] Oersted (1821b and 1823).

magnetic needle aligned itself.[31] Prechtl's explanation of this 'transverse magnetism' was hardly convincing, but the general idea of treating the phenomenon as a purely magnetic one was firmly established by the work of Biot, who was of course already responsible for the standard interpretation of the pile itself.[32]

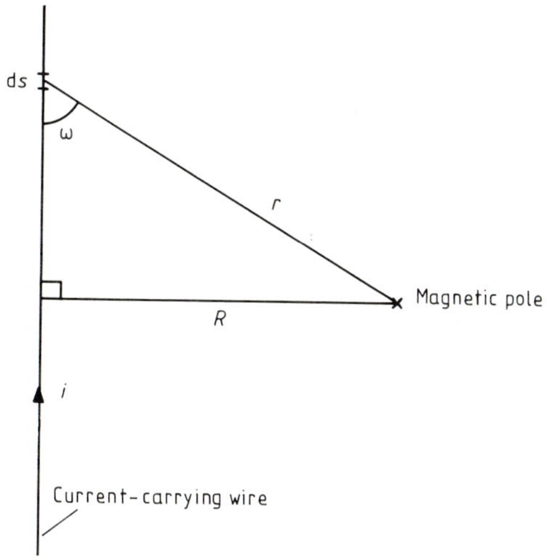

Figure 3.3

Biot wisely refrained from hypotheses as to the precise magnetic distribution within the wire. But he expressed his conviction that the action was a purely magnetic one owing to a 'genuine molecular magnetisation communicated to the particles of the metallic body'.[33] He set out to derive the experimental results mathematically on this basis by integrating the Coulomb forces between elements of the conductor and the poles of the magnet; and although he failed in the attempt he did establish, on the basis of some experiments conducted with Felix Savart, a law, the Biot–Savart law, for such elemental forces. This stated that the force $\mathscr{B}$ exerted by an infinitesimal transverse current element (a slice of the conducting wire) on a magnetic pole was given by

$$\mathscr{B} \propto \frac{i ds \sin \omega}{r^2} \tag{3.5}$$

with i the current and r and ω as in figure 3.3.[34]

[31] Prechtl (1822).

[32] Biot (1820) and see also (1821a and 1821b).

[33] Biot (1824), volume 2, p. 773.

[34] Biot first established for the force due to the whole wire (an infinite straight current), $\mathscr{F} \propto 1/R$, and the basic form for the force due to an infinitesimal element, $\mathscr{B} \propto f(\omega)/r^2$, was formally due to Laplace. Experiments by Biot and Savart using bent wires then gave the dependence on sin ω, at least approximately. See Blondel (1982), pp. 55–7.

Ampère

Contrasting strongly with the mechanistic magnetic theory of Biot, and closer in spirit to Oersted's own dynamistic interpretation, was the electrical interpretation of André Marie Ampère. It was Ampère who, in the course of the next few years, transformed Oersted's empirical demonstration of electromagnetism into a fully fledged mathematical theory of electrodynamics.

If Oersted was representative of the full-blooded dynamistic attitude that we saw associated in the last chapter with such philosophers as Coleridge and Schelling, and if Biot and Poisson represented the traditional mechanistic attitude, then Ampère's approach may be characterised by the same sort of down-to-earth dynamism as we saw in Whewell. In his early career, around the beginning of the nineteenth century, Ampère had adopted a rather mechanistic outlook on physics, seeking to incorporate electric and magnetic phenomena in a mechanical theory of fluids. But this effort was motivated by concerns that, while perfectly consistent with a mechanistic approach, were nevertheless to become characteristic of the dynamistic opposition to this approach in the 1820s and 1830s. Thus Ampère rejected the supposition of action at a distance that was central to the theories of Coulomb and Laplace, and he also rejected Coulomb's hypothesis of two electric fluids and the consequent dependence of the electrical phenomena upon a variety of different attractive or attractive and repulsive forces. As yet these concerns, though distinguishing his position clearly from that of the Laplacians, did not estrange him from the mechanical approach itself, for a theory such as he sought, based on a single Newtonian attraction with the force propagated by contact action through a medium, could only be described as mechanical. But as Ampère's interests, which had already included botany as well as physics, chemistry and mathematics, broadened still further to include psychology and philosophy, he developed a more dynamical perspective. He read and admired the works of Kant and he adopted Kant's force theory of matter, in which atoms were reduced to point centres of attractive and repulsive forces. He came to regard metaphysics as the 'only really important science', prior to all others,[35] and he adopted Kant's characteristic dynamical position of a belief in a real noumenal world allied to a rejection of the possibility of objective knowledge beyond the phenomenal realm. He came into contact with Davy, Faraday and Oersted on their visits to Paris and was greatly impressed by their dynamical approach to science.[36]

[35] Ampère to Roux, 11 March 1814, quoted in Levere (1971), p. 114.

[36] The best account of Ampère's work at the time of writing is Blondel (1982), on which much of this section is based. Also valuable are Tricker (1965) and especially Caneva (1978 and 1980) and Williams (1970, 1983 and 1965). Further important work from both Caneva and Williams is also imminent.

Perhaps because of the existence of a vacancy in the Academy after Lagrange's death, to which he was indeed duly elected, Ampère decided to stick to mathematics as a career, but he continued to 'dream alternately of chemistry and psychology'[37] and to keep abreast of developments in physics. In the late 1810s, having previously adopted the mechanical emissionist theory of light, he was won over by Fresnel to the wave theory of light and the concept of a luminiferous aether, and in the years that followed he associated closely with Fresnel and Arago in their opposition to Biot and the Laplacian school.

Like Fresnel, Fourier, and the other dynamistically oriented physicists of this period, Ampère centred his main objection to the mechanistic approach on its abuse of hypotheses. The correct approach to physics was not in his view to impose hypotheses upon nature, as the mechanists seemed to him to do, but[38]

> to observe first the facts, varying the conditions as much as possible, to accompany this with precise measurement, in order to deduce general laws based solely on experience, and to deduce therefrom, independently of all hypotheses regarding the nature of the forces which produce the phenomena, the mathematical value of these forces, that is to say, to derive the formula which represents them.

This could have been Fourier speaking, or Reid or Whewell, and like the latter philosophers Ampère attributed his approach to Newton. His own work on electrodynamics was, he claimed, 'guided by Newton's philosophy' and, of course, free from all hypotheses.[39]

It has long been recognised by historians that Ampère's work was not in fact free from hypotheses and was not quite the model of inductive reasoning his programmatic statements led some to believe. It has been noted, for example, that his description of experiments tended to be in the future tense; but this does not mean he was deluding either himself or his readers, for his use of hypotheses was not only masterly in terms of its results but also controlled in a way that the use of mechanical hypotheses had not generally been, and in a way that lends some justification to his claims.

Oersted's experiments had demonstrated an effect of a current-carrying wire upon a magnet, but although both Oersted himself and others sought physical explanations of this effect, and although Biot and his colleagues tried to express the result mathematically, none of them subjected the effect itself to a really thorough analysis. Ampère did, and within a few months of Oersted's announcement, in the course of a series of memoirs read to

[37] Ampère to Bredin, February 1815, quoted by Blondel (1982), p. 65.
[38] Quoted in Tricker (1965), p. 156.
[39] Tricker (1965), p. 157.

the Academy of Sciences between September and December 1820, he had already been able to show substantial progress.[40]

A large part of Ampère's first memoir was devoted to the distinction between electric current and potential difference. At the time of Oersted's experiments the distinction between a conducting wire, a static conductor and a voltaic pile was not at all clear, and there was as yet no concept of a closed electric circuit. As we noted in our discussion of Oersted's work, galvanism was in his view a weak form of static electricity. Ampère himself did not reach the concept of the closed circuit straight away, but he did use Oersted's experiments to elaborate on the distinction between what he called electric tension—the potential difference existing between two conductors or two poles of a battery—and electric current, which he interpreted conventionally as being composed of the two electricities flowing in opposite directions. He demonstrated experimentally that the magnetic effect observed by Oersted could be caused by an electric current but not by a state of electric tension, either in a battery (with the poles unconnected) or between two conductors; and he showed that one could use the experimental effect to measure the strength of an electric current in terms of the amount of deflection of a magnetic needle. He coined the name galvanoscope, later changed to galvanometer, to describe this new instrument.[41]

Having divided the types of electrical phenomena (battery, conductor, galvanic current) into two classes, Ampère proceeded in October 1820 to elaborate on the distinction between the electrostatic or tensional and electrodynamic or galvanic effects.[42] He showed that whereas conductors of opposite charge attracted, while those of similar charge repelled, parallel conducting wires in which currents flowed in the same sense attracted, while those in which they flowed in opposite senses repelled. He also showed that whereas attracting static conductors lost their attraction on contact, attracting conducting wires did not, and he suggested that while static conductors did not attract or repel each other in a void, conducting wires did. (His experiments on the latter effect were not, however, conclusive.) By December 1820, experiments proposed by Laplace on the reproduction of Oersted's effect using a portion of conducting wire a long way removed from the battery had indicated to Ampère that the electrical current was present undiminished throughout the length of the wire, which could not

[40] Ampère's results were given in full in Ampère (1826). His early memoirs to the Academy of 1821–2 were published in the *Annales de Chimie et de Physique,* the *Annales Générales des Sciences Physiques* and the *Journal de Physique* and in Ampère (1822). Blondel (1982) goes through these in some detail, memoir by memoir, and some English extracts from the memoirs covering the period 1820–5 are also given by Tricker (1965). All the memoirs are collected in Ampère (1885–7).

[41] Blondel (1982), p. 73.

[42] Blondel (1982), p. 79.

therefore be seen just as forming extensions to the poles of the battery, meeting at some neutral point. This suggested to Ampère the concept of a closed electrical circuit, a concept that was eventually clarified and elaborated by Georg Ohm in 1826.[43]

By 1822 Ampère had developed a picture in which the two electricities, conventionally regarded as fluids, were seen as making up between them the luminiferous aether, 'in which they mutually saturate one another'.[44] On this picture the transmission of electric current could be seen as a process of successive composition and decomposition of the aether round the circuit. This would result in the net motion of the two electricities in opposite directions round the circuit and also in the transmission of vibrations through the aether, through which attraction and repulsion between current elements could be effected.[45]

Ampère's analysis of electric current did much to clarify the relationship between static and galvanic electricity but until Ohm's work distinguished clearly between potential difference and current that relationship remained essentially confused. Far more successful was Ampère's analysis of the interactions between electric currents and magnets. Central to this analysis was his interpretation of magnetism as being in essence an effect of electric currents. To Ampère's detractors this was of course a completely unjustified hypothesis but it seems to have been intended by Ampère himself rather more as an analogy. In sympathy with the dynamical tradition he placed great stress upon the use of analogical method, arguing that while the real world and even the phenomenal world in an absolute sense were beyond the realm of human knowledge, one could hope to discover something of the relationships between real entities through studying those between phenomena—an argument close to that we have already seen expressed by the philosopher William Hamilton, for whom it also underlay a stress on analogy.[46]

Ampère's first response to Oersted's experiments seems to have been to compare the effect of an electric current in realigning an iron needle with that of the earth's magnetic influence in aligning it in the first place. The orthodox interpretation in terms of some temporarily induced magnetism in the current-carrying wire did not strike him as satisfactory, for it reduced everything to magnetism, which was a largely unquantifiable and apparently static phenomenon. Heuristically, he saw little hope of advancement in this way. The electric current, in contrast, was dynamic rather than static and, as a result of the new effect, accurately measurable, and it seemed to offer a much more promising line of attack. Ampère therefore reasoned

[43] Blondel (1982), pp. 81–2. Ohm (1826).
[44] Ampère (1885–7), volume 1, p. 216, quoted in Williams (1965), p. 149.
[45] Ampère (1885–7), volume 1, p. 249, and see Williams (1965), p. 149.
[46] See Blondel (1982), p. 117.

that if both an electric current and the earth's magnetic force acted so as to align a magnetic needle, the earth's magnetic force should by analogy be describable in terms of electric currents. Extending the analogy the same should be true for any other magnet. This reasoning also suggested, as Biot's hypothesis of induced magnets did not, that magnetic effects in general and the Oersted effect in particular should be reproducible as interactions between two electric currents as well as between two magnets or a magnet and an electric current. In his experiments Ampère therefore sought to demonstrate the 'magnetic' attraction between a magnet and a current-carrying conductor, between the earth's magnetic influence and a current-carrying conductor and between two current-carrying conductors.

Ampère's experiments, many of them conducted jointly with Fresnel, were rather more successful than unsuccessful. He demonstrated that the rotation of a magnetic needle by a current was independent of the earth's magnetic influence, and by hanging a magnet vertically he also demonstrated its attraction and repulsion by a current, independent of the rotation.[47] With Fresnel he also demonstrated the attraction and repulsion between magnetic poles and current-carrying spirals, acting in this respect as single magnetic poles, and the attraction and repulsion between pairs of spirals (figure 3.4). He succeeded in getting helical coils to behave as whole magnets in terms of their effects upon each other, though not in getting them to respond to the earth's magnetic influence.[48] In one investigation of the forces acting between two current-carrying helices he was surprised to find the helices attracting each other, as if they were straight wires, rather than repelling each other as he had expected from the analogy with similarly aligned magnets. This led him, however, to analyse the helical current into two components, one straight along the axis of the helix and the other circular, and thus lent weight to the assumption he had already made that the forces between current elements were simply additive (by what we should call vector addition) and pointed to the need for careful consideration of the degrees of freedom in any experiment. When the constraints of the helices in the expriment he was conducting were taken into account the results in fact tied in with those of his other experiments.[49]

Although Ampère's experiments lent very strong support to his suggested unification of galvanic and magnetic properties, and although their results could not be predicted either by Oersted's own theory of his effect or by that of Biot, they did not succeed in winning over the majority of physicists to Ampère's position. For most people the reduction of magnetism to an electrical effect was simply unthinkable. In Paris, in particular, Ampère could rely on the support only of his close colleagues, Arago and Fresnel, with

[47] Blondel (1982), p. 72.
[48] Blondel (1982), pp. 75–6.
[49] Blondel (1982), pp. 87–8.

the Laplacian majority wholly opposed.[50] Nor did the experiments adequately prove, even to his own satisfaction, the contention that was to be central to his theory, namely that all electrical and magnetic effects could be deduced from the law that parallel currents in the same sense attracted while those in opposite senses repelled each other. Against this, however, Ampère's ideas were somewhat more favourably received in Britain, where they were supported by Herschel and Babbage, and the experiments did afford sufficient support for these ideas to encourage him to pursue them. After all, if they were to be valid then the way would be open for a complete mathematical theory of electricity and magnetism based on the interaction of current elements and this was a goal well worth seeking.

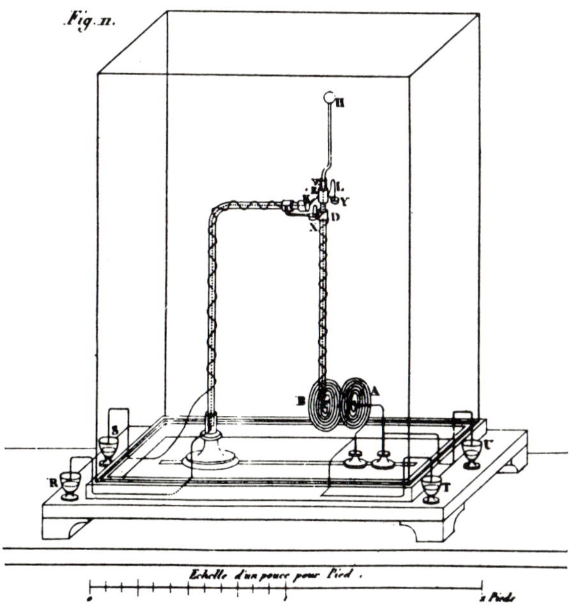

Figure 3.4 Ampere's experiment on the forces between two current-carrying spirals. From *Ann. Chim. Phys.* **15** 352 (1822).

The problem, which had already been encountered by Biot, was how to define the force between infinitesimal current elements when electricity was a line or surface phenomenon rather than a volume phenomenon. Fourier's path of proceeding by strict analogy with the macroscopic behaviour did not seem to be open in this case and Ampère's first step was simply to guess a law, based loosely on the behaviour he had observed experimentally, but not rigorously derived from that behaviour. In a memoir of early October

[50] See Blondel (1982), p. 79, and Levere (1971), pp. 113–22.

1820 he proposed as the simplest possible hypothesis that the force between two current elements should be given by

$$\mathscr{F} \propto \frac{\cos\gamma \sin\alpha \sin\beta}{r^2} \tag{3.6}$$

with α, β, γ and r as in figure 3.5. This gave the required attraction and repulsion for parallel currents and seemed eminently reasonable.[51] Having reached this formulation he then tried to test it experimentally, but this was not easy and in December 1820 he returned to the mathematical analysis. He assumed first that the force between two current elements was, in contrast with that proposed by Biot and Savart between a current element and a magnetic pole, a central one, with no couple or rotational component. This conformed to his preference for simplicity and it also ensured the retention of Newton's principle of action and reaction, which the Biot–Savart law, which had been derived for the influence of a current on a magnet only and not vice versa, did not. He also assumed a probable inverse square dependence on the distance between the two elements, from which he deduced the inverse distance law of Biot for the force exerted by an infinite straight current. He assumed that the force elements were additive, that the force was proportional to the product of the current intensities, that it was a maximum when the elements were parallel and thus, from considerations of symmetry, zero when they were perpendicular. Including, as he had not before, a possible interaction between collinear components of the current elements, and leaving open the relative strength of this reaction compared to that between components orthogonal to the line joining the elements, he deduced a more general formula than before,[52]

$$\mathscr{F} \propto \frac{i_1 i_2 \, \mathrm{d}s_1 \, \mathrm{d}s_2}{r^n} (\sin\alpha \sin\beta \cos\gamma + k \cos\alpha \cos\beta). \tag{3.7}$$

He still thought that the collinear component might be zero ($k = 0$) and the formula, with $n = 2$, reduce to his original suggestion, but despite a series of further experiments he could not establish this empirically to his satisfaction.

Although Ampère continued to work on the electrical theory of magnetism he was unable to develop the basic mathematical theory further for some months. Then in the autumn of 1821 Michael Faraday demonstrated the continual rotation of a magnet under the influence of a current-carrying conductor and vice versa, and this served both to support Ampère's theory against that of Biot and to stimulate Ampère himself to further investigations.[53] Ampère first repeated Faraday's experiments and

[51] Blondel (1982), pp. 83–4.
[52] Blondel (1982), p. 94.
[53] Faraday (1821) and see Williams (1965), p. 156

extended them to cover the electrically induced rotation of a magnet about its own axis.[54] He could not, however, obtain the effect for two magnets, and this suggested that the basic effect could not be a purely magnetic one as Biot's theory would seem to require. As Ampère explained in a public session of the Academy the following year, there were in his view two types of hypothesis. One was a kind devised specifically to fit an original phenomenon, and tended to get harder and harder to maintain as new phenomena continued to be demonstrated. Such was Biot's magnetic hypothesis. The other type were not strictly hypotheses at all, but rather 'expressions of the true relations between the facts they explain', and they tended accordingly to be confirmed by each successive discovery. Such, he claimed, was his own repesentation of magnetic phenomena in terms of electricity.[55] This distinction was of course drawn largely for polemical reasons, but even apart from the heuristic value of starting from a measurable quantity such as electricity, Ampère's method was distinguishable from Biot's and there was some degree of justification for his statement.

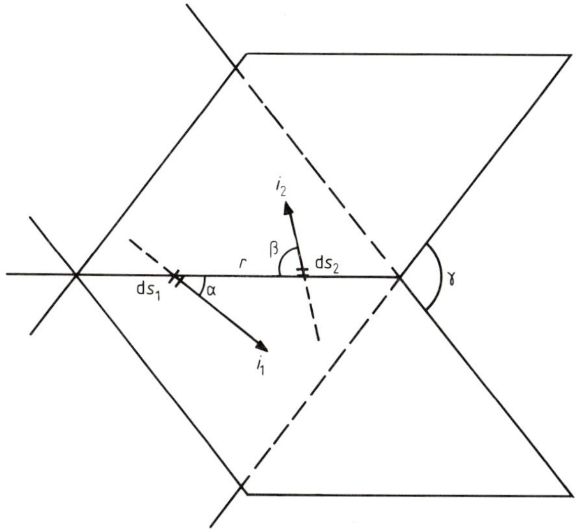

Figure 3.5

Following the impetus afforded by Faraday's work, Ampère continued to develop his theory of magnetism. He had at first attributed magnetism to coaxial currents in the masses of magnets, but following some experiments by Fresnel which went against this hypothesis he accepted Fresnel's own

[54] Blondel (1982), pp. 110–11.
[55] Blondel (1982), p. 117.

suggestion that magnetism might derive from molecular currents and elaborated this into an electrodynamic theory of matter. According to this theory each material molecule (a molecule for Ampère consisted of a number of point atoms in a characteristic arrangement) acted 'as a little voltaic pile in which the currents, entering by one extremity of the molecule and leaving by the opposite end, come together across the space around the first of these two extremities, thus forming a closed solenoid which ... cannot exert any action since all these currents are of the same intensity and equidistant before the molecule is magnetised.'[56] Magnetism itself then occurred in those materials in which the electrodynamical molecules (effectively the currents rather than the matter) were free to align themselves, and was a result of their taking up parallel alignments.

Ampère also reached a new deduction, arising from further attempts to determine the force between two current elements empirically. These further experiments led him to the conclusions that the force exerted by a closed circuit or magnet upon a current element must be perpendicular to the current in that element and that the force between two collinear elements must be repulsive. These two results between them allowed him to fix the arbitrary constants in his general expression for the force between two elements. Using the notation of equation (3.7) they gave $2k + n = 1$ and since there could be little doubt that n was in fact equal to 2 this gave $k = -\frac{1}{2}$ and

$$\mathscr{F} \propto \frac{i_1 i_2 \, \mathrm{d}s_1 \, \mathrm{d}s_2}{r^2} \left(\sin\alpha \sin\beta \cos\gamma - \tfrac{1}{2}\cos\alpha \cos\beta\right). \tag{3.8}$$

This new expression, reached in 1822, then acted as the fundamental formula of Ampère's electrodynamic theory, which he wrote up at length in 1826 and from which the whole of electromagnetic theory as it was then known could be deduced.[57]

Ampère's work was a masterly combination of theory and experiment, and his electrodynamics marked, in effect, the establishment of an electromagnetic theory for steady currents. It also constituted another demonstration, alongside Fourier's theory of heat, of the power of a liberally interpreted dynamistic approach based on the rejection of detailed mechanical hypotheses combined with the acceptance of heuristic (and sometimes no less mechanical) analogies—an approach, essentially, in which hypotheses did feature, but as the means rather than as the end. Ampère himself compared his achievement explicitly with Fourier's and with Newton's before them:[58]

> The expression for universal attraction from the laws of Kepler is completely

[56] Ampère (1885–7), volume 1, p. 404, quoted in Williams (1965), pp. 149–50.
[57] Blondel (1982), pp. 127–8.
[58] Tricker (1965), pp. 157–8.

> independent of the hypotheses which some writers have advanced to justify the mechanical cause to which they would ascribe it. The theory of heat is founded on general facts which have been obtained by direct observation; the equations deduced from the facts, being confirmed by the agreement between the results of calculation and of experiment, must be equally accepted as representative of the true laws of heat propagation by those who attribute it to the radiation of calorific molecules as by those who take the view that the phenomenon is caused by the vibration of a diffuse fluid in space ....
>
> It is the same with the formula by which I represented electrodynamic action. Whatever the physical cause to which the phenomena produced by this action might be ascribed, the formula which I have obtained will always remain the true statement of the facts.

The electrodynamic theory of magnetic phenomena and the mathematical theory with which it was bound up remained very uncertain, and in this respect Ampère's fundamental analogies or hypotheses remained unproven. Faraday noted in a letter of 1821 that while Ampère's experiments were excellent and his theory ingenious the experiments were few and 'theory makes up the great part of what Ampère has published, and theory in a great many points unsupported by experiments when they ought to have been adduced.'[59] This was a sound judgment, and for all Ampère's care over the use of hypotheses they do seem to have held a somewhat greater hold over him than his own scientific philosophy would permit. This was, however, of secondary importance compared with the mathematical formulation of electrodynamics to which they had led and with the experimental demonstrations of electromagnetic phenomena by which this formulation was supported. Even the molecular theory of magnetism, viewed with justifiable scepticism by many practising physicists, found strong support from a dynamical philospher such as Whewell, who wrote in his *Philosophy of the Inductive Sciences* that[60]

> Ampère, by framing his hypotheses of the action of voltaic currents and the constitution of magnets, reduced all [the] technical rules to rigorous deductions from one general principle. And thus the vague and obscure persuasion that there *must* be *some* connexion between electricity and magnetism, so long an idle and barren conjecture, was unfolded into a complete theory, according to which magnetic and electromotive actions are only two different manifestations of the same forces; and all the above-mentioned complex relations of polarities are reduced to one single polarity, that of the electro-dynamic current.

[59] Faraday to de la Rive, 12 September 1821, in Faraday (1971), volume 1, pp. 122–5.
[60] Whewell (1967), part 1, pp. 360–1.

Faraday

Ampère's theory of electrodynamics constituted a complete theory of steady currents and when Maxwell turned to electromagnetism in the 1850s this theory still provided part of the basis from which he had to work. There were in the meantime other developments, however, and of particular importance both for Maxwell's work and for the development of physics in general were those due to Michael Faraday.

Faraday's contribution to the science of electromagnetism was of course enormous and we can scarcely do justice to it in this short introduction, but we can pick out some of the key elements of his work. We have already noted in the last chapter that Faraday's scientific ideas were strongly characteristic of the dynamistic attitude. He adopted a dynamical theory of matter and he came in the course of his electrical researches to attribute a fundamental role to the idea of polarity. He was, throughout his work, quite condemnatory of the use of mechanical hypotheses. He believed that primary causes were in essence unknowable, and the hallmarks of the dynamistic approach to physics, the search for unification and the method of analogy, were also the dominant themes of his own research. William Whewell, who was, philosophically speaking, one of Faraday's closest scientific colleagues, took his electrochemical researches as the archetypal example of the dynamical philosophy in practice.[61] Despite all this, however, it would be in some sense misleading to characterise Faraday as a dynamistic natural philosopher. He was not, indeed, a philosopher at all in the sense that Whewell, Oersted or even Ampère were, and his dynamistic sympathies were derived from a pure, even naive, form of empiricism rather than from any more sophisticated philosophy of science. As we shall see, this difference was particularly apparent in his relationship with Ampère, for although their views of electromagnetic phenomena came far closer to each other's than to those of any of their rivals, and although they were in considerable agreement on such fundamental issues as the nature of matter, the importance of polarity and the unity of forces, and united too in their opposition to the mechanical theories, they yet approached the subject from completely different starting points and clearly had some difficulty in appreciating each other's positions.

Faraday began to look at electromagnetic phenomena in the summer of 1821. Following Oersted's demonstration of the electromagnetic effect the previous year, the extensive investigations of Ampère through the ensuing autumn and winter and a host of further experimental investigations and theoretical propositions by others, there was by then a clear need for a

[61] Whewell (1967). For historical accounts of Faraday's dynamical leanings see Williams (1965), Levere (1971), Gooding (1978, 1980a, 1980b, 1981 and 1982), and H B Jones (1870). This section is based largely on the work of Williams, corrected and augmented by that of Gooding.

review of the recent developments. Faraday, who had himself found these developments very confusing, accepted with pleasure a request that he write a review for the *Annals of Philosophy* and he set out, characteristically, to repeat all the reported experiments for himself.[62] As yet his concern was predominantly experimental, and although he reviewed the theories that had been put forward it was with a highly sceptical attitude. He was, however, impressed by Ampère's theory. He did not consider it proven and did not indeed fully understand it. Ampère's mathematics, being largely concerned with deductions from the theory rather than with the deduction of it, do not seem to have posed a significant problem, but his use of the conventional mechanical terminology of electric fluids seems to have misled Faraday into associating the theory with the traditional mechanical fluid theories of electricity. Faraday himself was not yet prepared to replace these theories with any definite alternative, but he was prepared to reject them as unwarranted mechanical hypotheses and to note that an electrical current might just as well be 'the induction of a particular state' as the passage of substance. He does not seem to have realised at this stage that Ampère was in agreement with him on this, and that even so far as he was prepared to hypothesise electrical fluids heuristically it was as components or aspects of the luminiferous aether.[63]

Within a few weeks of beginning his experiments Faraday reached his first experimental discovery in electromagnetism, that of the continual rotation effect. The idea that some sort of continual rotation of a current-carrying conductor might occur had already been put forward by Wollaston on the basis of his own theory of Oersted's effect, but Faraday's discovery was independent of this suggestion and concerned a rather different effect from that predicted. In September 1821 he began to notice a number of odd effects occurring when he varied the degrees of freedom of the conducting wire in the basic Oersted experiment, and he soon established that the electromagnetic force on a conducting wire tended to drive it in a circular motion round each pole of the magnet: 'the effect of the wire is always to pass off at a right angle from the pole, indeed to go in a circle around it.'[64] To test this effect he suspended a wire over a vertical magnetic pole (figure 3.6), its lower end in a bowl of mercury. When a current was passed through the wire it revolved around the pole continuously until the current was switched off. In a similar experiment he was also able to get a magnet to rotate around a conductor.[65]

This result, which was reached independently of any theory by the simple method of varying the experimental conditions as widely as possible, was

[62] Williams (1965), pp. 153*ff*.

[63] Williams (1965), p. 154.

[64] Faraday (1932–6), volume 1, p. 50. See Williams (1965), p. 156.

[65] Faraday (1965), volume 2, p. 147, and Faraday (1821). See Williams (1965), p. 156.

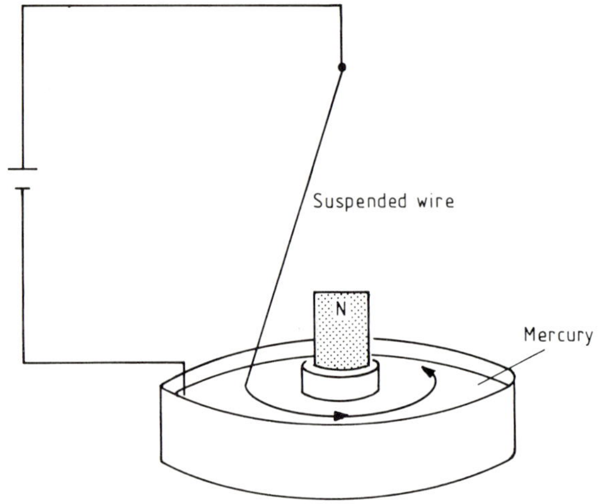

Figure 3.6 Faraday's experiment on the rotation of a current-carrying wire round a magnetic pole.

of the utmost importance for Faraday. By providing a demonstration of the continual conversion of electricity into mechanical work it gave the strongest support yet to his belief in the unity of the forces of nature. More significantly in our present context, it also offered him a way into electromagnetic theory, and it was here that the contrast between his approach and that of Ampère became manifest. For Ampère, theory had acted largely as a heuristic device, in conformity with certain principles (such as the principle of action and reaction and a fundamental principle of simplicity), but in the first instance at least as a way of proceeding towards a mathematical description of phenomena. In accordance with this approach he had based his electrodynamic theory upon an expression for the attraction and repulsion between current elements, along the line joining them. To Faraday, however, arguing simply from experiment, and without any concern as to mathematical synthesis, it seemed that it was the rotating rather than the linear force that was primary. Given sufficient freedom, a single conducting wire and magnet rotated around each other. Only when they were constrained, as for example in Oersted's experiment, did the force manifest itself in terms of attraction and repulsion. Faraday therefore took as the basis of his own theory the proposition that the force emanating from a magnet or current was a circular one and set out to show how such a circular force could result in linear attraction and repulsion when the wire was bent into a circle, spiral or helix, with the circular forces due to currents moving in opposite directions combining as linear forces inside and perpendicular to the coils. Responding to this theory, Ampère took the view that neither the circular nor the linear effect could be taken as primary in a physical sense, since both involved complex bodies made up of large numbers or even infinities of points. (Neither Ampère nor Faraday, we may recall, accepted the mechanical hypothesis of elementary finite material molecules.) The linear effect, however, permitted the phenomena to be reduced to mathematical analysis, which the circular effect did not.[66] For Faraday, in contrast, the circular effect was that which experiment revealed to be the simpler on the observable, macroscopic, level, while the linear effect was at this level a derived one.[67]

Corresponding regularly if not frequently, Faraday and Ampère continued to differ in a friendly way, as Faraday found himself in agreement with Ampère on most things and yet out of sympathy with and mistrustful of his method. Thus, for example, Faraday's own experiments with a helical current led him to agree with Ampère on the resemblance between such a current and a permanent magnet but not on their identity. The status of magnetism with respect to electricity also featured in the development of Faraday's own ideas on the nature of electricity and magnetism, and one experiment he tried was to get a magnet or wire to rotate about its own axis. In due course Ampère succeeded in this for a magnet, but neither of them was successful with a wire, and Faraday came to the tentative conclusion that the electromagnetic force must be associated with the current rather than with the wire, so that while magnetism could not apparently act independently of matter electricity could. In his experimental comparison of a magnet and a helical current Faraday also introduced the image of lines of magnetic action, as he conducted the comparison in terms of actions of the two 'magnets' on a magnetic pole in their vicinity, demonstrated through the medium of scattered iron filings.[68]

The next significant development in electromagnetic science occurred in 1825, when Arago and others demonstrated what they took to be the induction of magnetism in metals as a consequence of the mere rotation of the metals. In Arago's experiment a copper disc was free to rotate around its axis with a magnetic needle suspended above it. When the disc was rotated the magentic needle rotated as well.[69] In response to this phenomenon, Biot suggested that it demonstrated the separation of the two magnetic fluids by centrifugal force, thus disproving Ampère's theory of the electrodynamic origins of magnetism.[70] In England, however, John Herschel and Charles Babbage set out to explore the effect in detail and to explain it according to Ampère's mathematical theory. The theoretical attempt failed, as they were unable to explain satisfactorily the dependence

[66] Ampère (1885–7), volume 1, p. 184.
[67] Williams (1965), pp. 161–8.
[68] Williams (1965), pp. 161–8.
[69] Arago (1826) and see Williams (1965), p. 170.
[70] Biot to Babbage, 11 November 1825, quoted in Williams (1965), p. 170

of the effect on motion, but the experimental enquiry, using discs suspended above a large rotating magnet so that the rotation of the magnet induced that of the discs, was exhaustive and illuminating. They ranked different metals in order of their apparent magnetic susceptibility and found that the effect was destroyed altogether if a slit was made in the metal disc.[71] Faraday himself responded by testing the equivalence between electricity and magnetism, searching for similar electrically induced effects. At this stage, however, looking for a continuous steady-state effect, he was unsuccessful.

Had Faraday looked for transient rather than steady effects he might well have demonstrated electromagnetic induction at this stage. As it was, however, this demonstration was delayed for several years and took place only after he had picked up his electromagnetic researches again in 1831. In the interim, his thoughts on physics in general developed considerably. In the late 1820s, at a time when Faraday was pursuing researches on the nature of light, a non-mathematical survey of Fresnel's work on the wave theory of light was published in English translation and this prompted Faraday to give more precise expression to his notion that electric current, while clearly a dynamic rather than a static property, should somehow be thought of as a state rather than as the motion of a fluid.[72] That wave propagation might provide an approach to the unification of forces, the ideal that above all dominated Faraday's researches, was also emphasised by Herschel's stress, in his *Preliminary Discourse on the Study of Natural Philosophy* of 1830, on the analogy between light and sound as vibrating motions.[73] Faraday was strongly impressed by the possibilities inherent in wave motion, and in 1831 he undertook an investigation of these possibilities through an analysis of acoustical figures in different media, a context in which he was able to 'see' the effects of a sound wave passing through a variety of different media.[74] In the course of this work he noted the presence of regular stationary crispations in vibrating liquid media and these suggested a way in which a static arrangement or state might result from a dynamic wave motion. At about the same time Faraday's friend Gerritt Moll in Holland observed the almost instantaneous reversal of the polarity of an electromagnet upon reversal of the current passing through it and drew attention to the high intensity of magnetic force that could be produced in a large electromagnet.

Faraday thus turned back to his electromagnetic researches in August 1831 disposed to think of electric and magnetic force in terms of wave motions and to investigate the possible existence and effects of such mo-

[71] Babbage and Herschel (1825) and see Williams (1965), pp. 170–1.
[72] Williams (1965), pp. 176–7.
[73] Herschel (1830) and see Williams (1965), pp. 178–9.
[74] Williams (1965), pp. 179*ff*.

tions. He was disposed also to look for these effects through those of an electromagnet, and to concentrate in particular on the transient effect produced on the reversal of current, rather than on the steady effects that had previously dominated his attention. If, he reasoned, a long helical coil were to be wound round a soft iron core and the current then switched on, the setting up of a state of magnetism in the core should be accompanied by a wave motion. If the core were extended into a closed ring, this wave motion might then be detectable through a further long coil attached to a galvanometer on the other side of the ring as in figure 3.7. Testing this hypothesis he found that a transient current was indeed generated in the secondary coil, both when the primary current was switched on and when it was switched off. The effect, he suggested, must be due to 'a wave of electricity' generated at moments of breaking and completing the contacts in the primary circuit.[75]

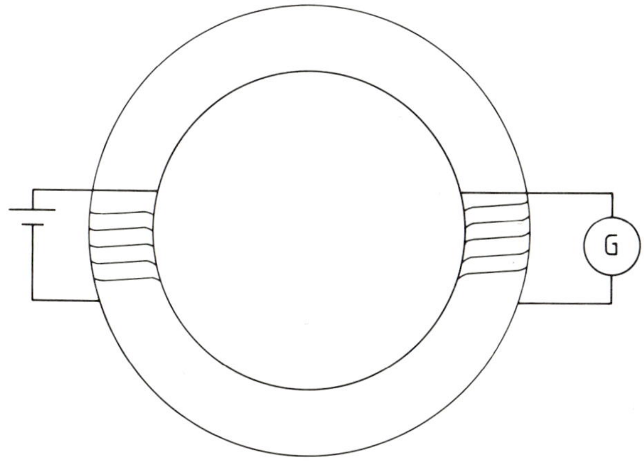

Figure 3.7 Faraday's experiment on electromagnetic induction.

Having demonstrated the effect of electromagnetic induction, Faraday immediately tried varying the conditions and looking for similar effects in other situations. In October 1831 he tried the experiment using a permanent magnet instead of an electromagnet and observed a transient current whenever a magnet was moved sharply into or out of a helical circuit. Adapting the experiment for rotating rather than reciprocating motion, he demonstrated the electric dynamo. He also explained the apparent magnetic induction of Arago's wheel in terms of an induced electrical current, dependent on the electrical conductivity of the wheel and therefore absent when the wheel was split.[76] Encouraged by his success with these

[75] Faraday (1932–6), volume 1, pp. 367–9, and see Williams (1965), pp. 181–3.
[76] Faraday (1965), first series. Williams (1965), pp. 191*ff*.

experiments he also put forward in public one of the ideas that had guided them, that of the 'electro-tonic state'.[77] Of precisely what the state consisted he did not know, nor could he as yet detect its presence directly. But the induction experiments suggested clearly to his mind that there was some change in the state of a conductor when it was placed under a magnetic influence, and again when that influence ceased:[78]

> When the wire is subject to either volta-electric or magneto-electric induction, it appears to be in a peculiar state; for it resists the formation of an electrical current in it, whereas, if in its common condition, such a current would be produced; and when left uninfluenced it has the power of originating a current, a power which the wire does not possess under common circumstances.

Progressing from the induction ring experiment to the phenomenon of magneto-electric induction due to moving magnets, the concept of the electrotonic state then suggested to Faraday a picture of electric current as a rapid building up and breaking down of the electrotonic state, or, in conformity with his guiding ideas, as a wave of strain. Moreover, the magneto-electric induction experiments also suggested that the force inducing the electrotonic state, whatever it was, must extend beyond the particles of the magnet, and this brought him back to the importance of the lines of magnetic force. Analysing the experiments in terms of these lines he determined that the direction and strength of the induced current corresponded to the direction in which and speed with which the conducting wire passed across the lines of magnetic force.[79] This approach gained additional significance when, a few years later, Faraday demonstrated the induction of a current by a magnet rotating on its own axis, the magnet resting in a pool of mercury and itself forming part of the conducting circuit (figure 3.8). Faraday reasoned that since a current was induced in this case the magnetic lines of force must be being crossed, which meant that they must be independent of the material mass of the magnet: they did not rotate with it. He was also able to explain the induction effects, using the concept of lines of force, in terms of the expansion and contraction of the lines.[80]

At about the same time as he conducted the last series of experiments referred to, Faraday also endeavoured to prove that, as he and Ampère had assumed, all forms of electricity, whether galvanic, static or induced, were fundamentally the same.[81] In due course he succeeded in establishing this beyond reasonable doubt and he then turned his attention to electro-

[77] Williams (1965), pp. 198–9.
[78] Faraday (1965), volume 1, p. 60, and see Williams (1965), p. 198.
[79] Williams (1965), pp. 198–200.
[80] Williams (1965), pp. 203–4.
[81] Faraday (1965), third series, and see Williams (1965), pp. 211*ff.*

chemistry before returning to electricity itself, and to electromagnetism, in 1835.

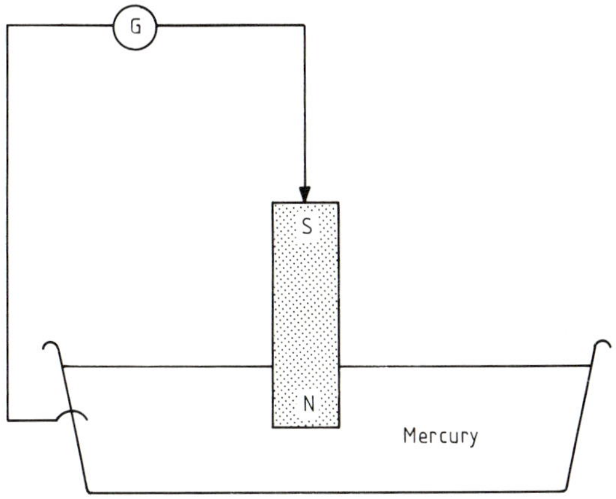

Figure 3.8 Faraday's experiment on the induction of a current by a rotating magnet.

At this point, despite his enormous experimental success, Faraday's theoretical ideas were still rather vague. They certainly did not constitute a developed theory such as that of Ampère. Writing to Whewell, he admitted that 'I accept Ampère's theory as the best present representation of the facts.' But he was still unhappy with it: 'I hold it with a little reserve. This reserve is more a general feeling than anything founded on distinct objections to it.' And he still hoped for a development of his own theoretical ideas concerning the lines of magnetic force and the electrotonic state. These are sometimes presented as having been rival theories for Faraday and his work discussed in terms of the giving up of one in favour of the other and vice versa, but they were far more complementary viewpoints. Although the image of magnetic lines of force was already in some sense a physical hypothesis, and took on a significance as such in, for example, Faraday's claim that the lines were independent of the material of a magnet, it was also important quite independently of such connotations as a way of visualising and describing phenomenally the effects of magnetism. Similarly with the electrotonic state. Faraday explained to Whewell that he had 'given up this electrotonic state for the time as an experimental effect (. . .) because I could find no fact to prove it'. But, he insisted, 'I cling to it in fancy or hypothesis.' Whether the hypothesis were proven or not it remained useful, and it had already led, indeed, to the laws of electrochemistry.[82]

[82] Faraday to Whewell, 19 September 1835, in Faraday (1971), volume 1, pp. 294–6, and see Williams (1965), pp. 285–7.

Faraday's new series of researches, which extended over several years, were prompted by some analogies he had derived between electrochemical and electrostatic actions. Since the notion of the electrotonic state had served him so well in electrochemistry, his first aim was to test the theory of electricity as a power or wave propagation against the orthodox theory of the two electric fluids. He was able to determine to his satisfaction that electricity could not be separated from matter, and that the two supposed electricities could not be separated from each other. Carrying out an exhaustive series of experiments on static induction he also developed a theory of specific inductive capacitance, introducing the notion of dielectrics, and showed, through one single but powerful experiment, that static induction took place along curved rather than straight lines.[83]

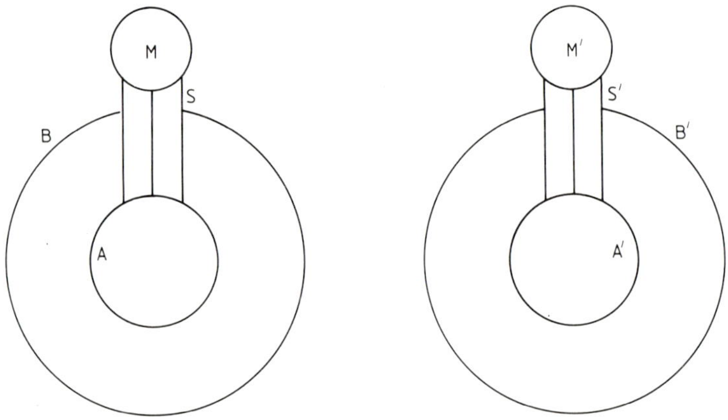

Figure 3.9 Faraday's apparatus for measuring specific inductive capacity. Shellac insulation S separates interior sphere A (linked electrically to M) from exterior sphere B. The substance being investigated occupies the space between A and B.

A key experiment on specific inductive capacitance is shown in figure 3.9. The two identical systems shown were filled, one (B′) with air and the other (B) with a dielectric, which could be solid (in which case it would not, of course, be filled completely), liquid or gas. One metal sphere M′ was charged, and the surface charge density induced on the external container B′ was measured. The two spheres M′ and M were then connected and disconnected, and the charge density on B measured. If B were filled with air, or indeed any gas, the final surface charge density on B was just half that originally measured on B′; but with other media introduced the charge on B varied and the ratio between the two measurements provided a

[83] Faraday (1965), volume 1, paragraphs 1186–317. See Williams (1965), pp. 288–99.

measure of the inductive capacity k ($=1$ for air) of the medium. For all solids Faraday found that the inductive capacity, or ability to transmit induction, was greater than for air, $k > 1$.

The experiment indicating that induction took place in curved lines is shown in figure 3.10. Placing a metal sphere or disc upon a statically charged shellac column as in the figure, Faraday tested the space around and above the sphere with an electrometer. Had the action proceeded in straight lines only, the sphere would have acted as a shield and there would have been no inductive effect within its shadow. As Faraday observed, however, there was such an effect. Illustrating the effect in terms of lines of inductive force ('a temporary conventional mode of expressing the direction of the power in cases of induction'), these lines were curved.

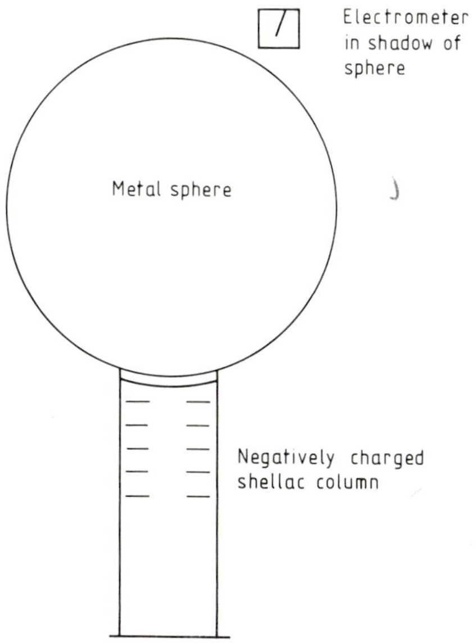

Figure 3.10 Faraday's experiment showing induction in curved lines.

The demonstration that induction took place along curved lines was an important result for Faraday, for whom induction was the 'essential principle of the development of electricity'.[84] On the basis of this and his other recent results he at last felt confident in June 1838 to put forward some specific theoretical proposals. The new theory assumed[85]

> ... that all the *particles,* whether of insulating or conducting matter, are as wholes conductors. That not being polar in their normal state, they can

[84] Faraday (1932–6), volume 2, paragraph 2768.
[85] Faraday (1965), volume 1, paragraphs 1669–78, quoted in Williams (1965), pp. 312–13.

> become so by the influence of neighbouring charged particles, the polar state being developed at the instant, exactly as in an insulated conducting *mass* consisting of many particles. That the particles when polarized are in a forced state, and tend to return to their normal or natural condition. That being as wholes conductors, they can readily be charged, either *bodily* or *polarly.* That particles which being contiguous are also in the line of inductive action can communicate or transfer their polar forces one to another *more or less* readily [conductors or insulators]. That those doing so less readily require the polar forces to be raised to a higher degree before this transference or communication takes place.

This theory of induction was not the consequence of a single theoretical idea so much as of an intersupporting mesh of related ideas derived both from electrical experiments and from analogies with other forces of nature. The key features of the theory were that electricity was a state of strain, and specifically of polarity, rather than a mechanical fluid or fluids, with electrostatic induction operating by communication of this polarity; and that the communication was one of contiguous action rather than action at a distance. The demonstrated existence of varying specific inductive capacities indicated that conductivity was a continuously varying property, which in turn indicated a state of strain of some kind rather than a substance. Induction in curved lines suggested a contiguous theory rather than a distance theory, with transmission appearing as some kind of wave motion, and this tied in with the notion of strain. The supposition of a wave motion allowed in addition, as Faraday had earlier realised, for the convertibility of electrical with other forces. The theory could also be related to both his working images of the past years, the electrotonic state, reflected in the image of electricity as a state of strain, and the lines of force, reflected in the pattern of communication of that strain.[86]

Faraday's concept of contiguous action has caused some trouble, as he insisted that this action could take place between particles separated by as much as half an inch, which sounds suspiciously like action at a distance. He was, however, quite clear what he meant. A contiguous particle was defined as 'the next existing particle',[87] and the point was that the action was communicated between one particle and those next to it, whether or not space intervened, but could not be communicated across intervening particles. Such an action could proceed in curved as well as in straight lines, as the experiments indicated it was.

The notion of microscopic polarity remained hypothetical, but besides the status of polarity within the dynamical philosophy (which probably mattered little to Faraday) it did correspond to the nature of the observed phenomena. Thus Faraday wrote that 'electricity appears to exist only

[86] See Gooding (1980b), pp. 96–7.

[87] Faraday (1965), volume 1, paragraph 1616.

in polarity, as in air, glass, electrolytes, etc. ...',[88] and to extend this macroscopic observation by analogy to the microscopic level, in line with the method adopted by Fourier and others, was natural to Faraday. Macroscopic observations were indeed on his view the sole legitimate source of theoretical principles. Moreover, Faraday was increasingly seeing polarity as characteristic not only of electric and magnetic phenomena, but also of those of light and, especially, of chemistry. It had, he declared, 'in reality the character of a first, essential, and fundamental principle.'[89]

Because Faraday tended to be critical of all theory, and hypercritical of his own, while being at the same time an irrepressible theoriser, his research notes exhibit an extraordinary theoretical heterogeneity. Sometimes he would push Ampère's molecular electrodynamics as the best worked out theory available, while at others he would try out a host of notions or fancies of his own. But through all this a coherent picture was emerging based on his opposition to mechanical hypotheses and on his treatment of the empirical phenomena as theoretically fundamental. He had always inclined towards a dynamical theory of matter in which the forces manifest took precedence over the entities supposed to produce them, and in January 1844, in a 'Speculation touching electric conduction and the nature of matter', he put forward publicly the idea that matter should be treated as a plenum of forces filling space rather than as discrete atoms.[90] Theories of matter seem to have been of secondary rather than primary interest for Faraday, but his tendency to take the observed phenomena rather than their supposed causes as the primal theoretic entities was apparent throughout his work. As we have noted, electricity was expressed in terms of an observed polarity rather than in terms of a supposed unobservable fluid. In magnetism too, Faraday had distinguished the effects, expressed in terms of lines of force, from the material of the magnets producing them, and emphasised the importance of the former as opposed to the latter. Also underlying Faraday's theoretical work was another, closely related, principle, namely that of the unity, and especially the convertibility, of forces. The two principles together provided the foundation for his expression of electrical and other effects as wave-like actions, a convertibility between which was to be expected, rather than as material phenomena, which interpretation would have emphasised their distinction rather than their unification. In the course of his work on electrostatics he had drawn analogies between electrostatic phenomena and those of light and sound, and the theory of the phenomena he had reached was related explicity to that of

[88] Faraday (1932–6), volume 2, paragraph 2768.
[89] Faraday (1965), volume 1, paragraph 1162, and see also Gooding (1978), pp. 132–4.
[90] Faraday (1865), volume 2, pp. 284*ff*. See also Levere (1968) and Heimann (1971a).

heat, electrostatic induction and specific inductive capacity corresponding to heat conduction and conductivity.[91]

Following his electrostatic researches, Faraday's outstanding problem had been to bring magnetism into his analogical framework. He had already suggested that electricity and magnetism appeared to be differently directed components of a single power, but all attempts at this time to extend the notion of the specific inductive capacity of a dielectric to magnetism had failed.[92] The breakthrough in this respect came in 1845, after he received a letter from the young William Thomson. Thomson had been trying to mathematise Faraday's theory of electrostatics and had come up with a number of predicted phenomena that had not to his knowledge been observed. He wrote to Faraday enquiring about these phenomena and Faraday promptly turned his attention to them, and in particular to an investigation proposed by Thomson into 'the action of a transparent dielectric on polarised light'. It was known, observed Thomson, that mechanical strains in glass affected the polarisation of light passing through the glass. If Faraday's theory were to be correct then it seemed probable that electrically induced strains should have a similar effect.[93] This possibility had not in fact been lost on Faraday, and in the course of his repeated attempts to detect his proposed electrotonic state he had tried several times to obtain the effect proposed by Thomson, but without success. Thomson's letter now prompted him, however, to take up the subject afresh. Despite a further prolonged attempt he still failed to find any effect (it was not in fact demonstrated until 1875), but this time his strong conviction in the connection between electricity, magnetism and light led him to persevere and, the experiment having failed with an electrically induced state, to try it with a magnetic strain induced by an electromagnet. Then, using a strong electromagnet and a piece of dense optical glass with a high refractive index, he got an effect. When the apparatus was arranged so that the polarised light passed through the glass parallel to the lines of magnetic force, the activation of the electromagnet produced a clearly observable change in the plane of polarisation of the light.[94] Further experiments established that the amount by which the plane of polarisation was rotated was proportional both to the distance travelled by the light in the medium and, so far as it could be measured, to the intensity of the magnetic force. Having once obtained the effect he was also able to demonstrate it, to differing degrees, for a variety of media.[95]

[91] Gooding (1980b), pp. 96–7.
[92] Gooding (1981), p. 235.
[93] Thomson to Faraday, 6 August 1845, in Faraday (1971), volume 1, pp. 458–60. See also Williams (1965), pp. 383–4.
[94] Faraday (1932–6), volume 4, paragraphs 7498*ff*, and Faraday (1965), volume 3, paragraphs 2151*ff*.
[95] Faraday (1965), volume 3, paragraphs 2146–242, and Faraday (1846a). See Williams (1965), pp. 286–7, and Gooding (1981), pp. 234–5.

Faraday's demonstration of the magneto-optic effect provided further evidence of the equivalence of forces and, most significantly, the first evidence of the existence of a magnetic analogue to dielectrics: the bodies and liquids in which the effect could be observed included many in which neither permanent nor even induced magnetism was experienced. The experiment also served to emphasise once again to Faraday the significance of the lines of force, for using this effect they could actually be observed, in the sense that their direction could be visibly determined. There were still problems to be solved, however. The properties of 'dimagnetics', as Faraday first called those media in which the magneto-optic effect could be observed (the classification eventually adopted of diamagnetic, paramagentic and ferromagnetic was suggested slightly later by Whewell) had still to be determined. And one peculiarity of the magneto-optic effect had still to be explained before diamagnetic induction could be accorded the status of its electrical analogue: despite observing the effect for a wide variety of media, Faraday was unable to observe it for any gases, and unable to explain why this should be so.

The key property of diamagnetic media to be investigated was the nature of their direct interaction with magnets. Analogy with electrostatic induction suggested that materials in which a magnetic strain was induced should themselves act as magnets and be attracted or repelled by the poles of the primary magnet. At first Faraday was unable to observe such an effect, but again he was persistent and in early November 1845, just a couple of months after beginning the new series of investigations, he succeeded in demonstrating an interaction between a powerful electromagnet and a bar of heavy glass suspended between its poles. If placed skew to the line of magnetic force, the bar would move so as to set across them, as in figure 3.11.[96] This effect had in fact been observed by others before, but without the concept of diamagnetism nothing had come of their observations.[97]

Pursuing the analogy with electrostatics, Faraday at once tried interpreting the new experiment in terms of a difference between the magnetic susceptibilities of the glass bar and the surrounding air. He knew that magnetic bodies tended to set along the lines of magnetic force, and the new observation that a diamagnetic body set across them suggested that the medium, air, was in some sense more magnetic than the diamagnetic material itself and so pushed it out of the preferred magnetic position. Had the air been the less magnetic of the two, he reasoned, the bar would have set like a magnet, along the force lines, as in figure 3.12.

As Faraday's experiments proceeded, however, he came across further effects not predicted by this simple theory. Suspending a small bar of bismuth in the region of what he now began to call the magnetic field, or

[96] Faraday (1932–6), volume 4, paragraphs 7902*ff*. See Williams (1965), pp. 392*ff* and Gooding (1981), pp. 236*ff*.

[97] Williams (1965), p. 393.

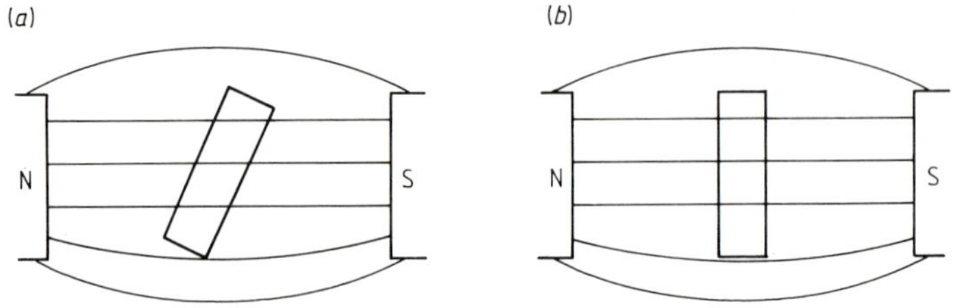

Figure 3.11 Faraday's experiment on diamagnetic set: a diamagnetic bar placed skew to the lines of force (*a*) appeared to set across them (*b*).

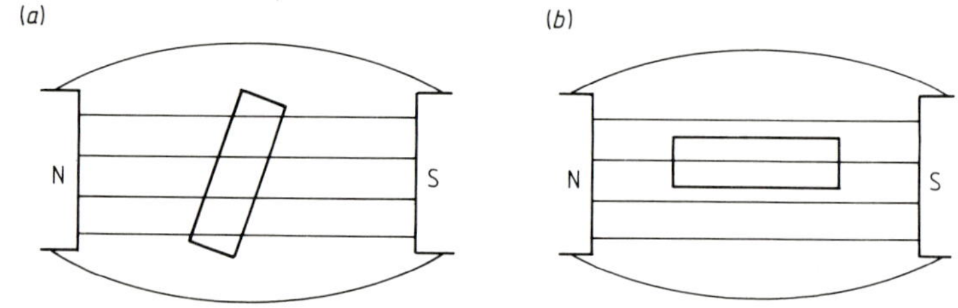

Figure 3.12 Faraday's experiment on magnetic set: a magnetic bar placed skew to the lines of force (*a*) set along them (*b*).

the area within which a magnetic force acted, he found that so long as the magnet was switched on the bismuth tended to be repelled away from the axis joining the magnetic poles (figure 3.13). Then, when the magnet was switched off again, the bismuth returned to its original position. Whereas magnetic bodies travelled along the lines of magnetic force, diamagnetic bodies seemed to move in a completely different way, away from an area of strong force and towards one of weaker force. There were still other puzzles too. Despite the role he had attributed to the medium in the diamagnetic set experiments, Faraday still could not produce any observable magnetic effect in air or other gases. Nor could he detect any polarity in the diamagnetic materials, a result which sat uncomfortably with the electrostatic analogy he was pursuing.[98]

Over the next few years Faraday continued to explore diamagnetic effects both theoretically, through, for example, Ampère's electrodynamical theory of magnetism, and experimentally, testing for the magnetic properties of gases and, so far as he could, the vacuum. In the course of this work his own ideas continued to develop in much the same direction as they had done already. In particular, the absence of polarity in diamagnetic substances and the relative magnetic behaviour of the vacuum both served to increase the significance of the image of the lines of force. The absence of polarity in diamagnetic materials suggested that magnetic polarity must

[98] Gooding (1981), pp. 238*ff*.

be essentially a property of the lines of force rather than of the materials through which they passed, a conclusion that was also supported by the magneto-optical experiments. The role of the vacuum was of critical importance. In experiments on diamagnetic set, Faraday could not yet determine with complete confidence whether the vacuum ranked in the middle of the magnetic hierarchy, more susceptible to the magnetic force than diamagnets but less so than paramagnets, or whether it ranked at the bottom of the list, with no magnetic susceptibility at all. And he still could not produce magnetic effects directly in either a vacuum or a gas. But the transmission of magnetic force across a vacuum and his original interpretation of diamagnetic set both inclined him towards the former option, and this again emphasised the primacy of the lines of force, especially as they were able to curve in a vacuum.[99]

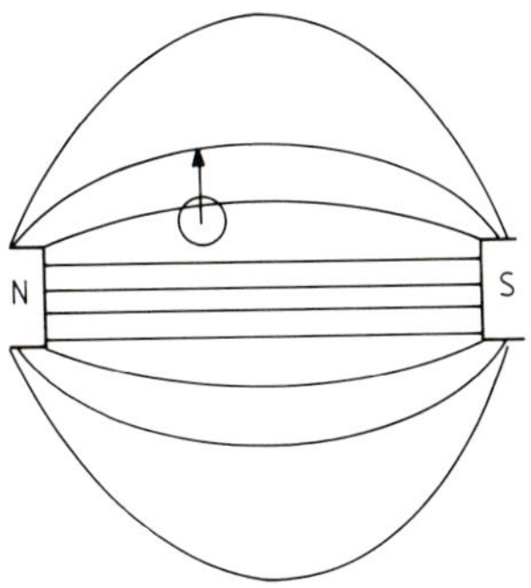

Figure 3.13 Faraday's experiment on the motion of diamagnetic bodies. A bar of bismuth suspended in a magnetic field was repelled away from the strong part of the field towards the weaker part.

Considerations drawn from matter theory also came into play. To many physicists of the period the vacuum was not a vacuum at all but an imponderable aether. The notion of an aether was based closely on the model of substantial matter and it was therefore quite alien to Faraday's conception in which the observed forces took precedence over the supposed material substratum. For Faraday, matter was interpreted as composed solely of forces or active powers, and the vacuum, the absence of matter, was consequently interpreted as the absence of such forces. Yet the vacuum seemed to be a magnetic conductor. In 1846, in his famous 'Thoughts on ray vibrations', he used the recently established interaction of magnetism and light in the magneto-optic effect, an interaction that implied for him that the two phenomena were two different but interconvertible aspects of the same fundamental force, to propose a way out of the apparent

[99] Gooding (1980 and 1981) and Williams (1965), pp. 428*ff*.

contradiction.[100] We may recall that Ampère, pursuing a rather different approach, had already hypothesised a luminiferous aether made up of purely electrical components. Faraday now proposed that the vibrations of light waves might be none other than vibrations in the magnetic lines of force.

This seems, even now, a bold hypothesis, but since the existence of magnetic force lines was the one property Faraday could ascribe to empty space, through which of course the light waves passed, the hypothesis was, in the context of his ideas, a very reasonable one. For other physicists light was a vibration in the aether, but for Faraday, whose vacuum was characterised by a magnetic conductivity rather than by any pseudo-material properties, it had to be a magnetic vibration.

The increasing importance of the magnetic lines of force for Faraday's theoretical conceptualisation in this period was also apparent in his description of the repulsion of the small bismuth bar away from the axis of a magnet:[101]

> All the phenomena resolve themselves into this, that a portion of [diamagnetic] matter, when under magnetic action, tends to move from stronger to weaker places or points of force. When the substance is surrounded by lines of magnetic force of equal power on all sides, it does not tend to move.

Before, the magnetic lines had been purely directional. Now the phenomena were explicable rather in terms of a variation in force from point to point and the variation could only be attributed in Faraday's current perspective to a variation in the strength of the lines of force, which themselves acquired a new type of physical reality.

In his theoretical ideas of this period Faraday already had the elements of what we now term a field theory, but there was still much to be clarified. In June 1848 Thomson removed one complication by pointing out that a diamagnetic could in fact set *either* along *or* at right angles to the axis between the magnetic poles, but that the latter position, treated by Faraday as characteristic, was actually unstable. Faraday had noted the alternative direction of set before, but he had thought nothing of it, and had not noticed the instability of the orthogonal set. Now, however, the new information served to emphasise the primacy of the move from a stronger to a weaker area of the field, as opposed to the directed set, and the latter ceased to play an important part in his theoretical analysis.[102] That same summer the experiments of Julius Plücker on diamagnetic crystals prompted further investigations by Faraday, leading, through an analogy with optical axes

[100] Faraday (1846b) and Faraday (1965), volume 3, pp. 447–52.
[101] Faraday (1965), volume 3, paragraph 2418, and see Williams (1965), pp. 435–6.
[102] Thomson to Faraday, 27 June 1848, in Faraday (1971), volume 1, pp. 523–4. See Gooding (1981), p. 254.

and light rays, to an expression of the results on diamagnetism in terms of which the motion of a body from stronger to weaker parts of the field was replaced by a strain due to the deformation of the lines of force from their normal position of least resistance or maximum conductivity.[103]

Despite an analogy with the deforming effect of soft iron, which concentrated the magnetic force lines, the idea of diamagnetic bodies diffusing them was only slowly reached. The absence of diamagnetic polarity prevented the analogy from going through smoothly, as did the failure of diamagnetic crystals to have any diverging effect on light.[104] There was as yet, moreover, no direct evidence of the diverging action of the bismuth. But if the theory of diamagnetism in terms of a magnetic susceptibility analogous to electrical conductivity were to be upheld, there was no escaping the conclusion that diamagnets, as poor magnetic conductors, should cause the force lines to diverge, just as magnets, as good conductors, caused them to concentrate or converge. In June 1849 Thomson, developing Faraday's own ideas, wrote to him suggesting that the lines of force could be taken as representing the effect of the magnetic conductivity of matter in the region of a magnet.[105] This emphasised again the disturbing effects magnets and diamagnets had on the lines of force. By the end of the decade Faraday had come to see the value of the divergence analogy.[106]

The experiments prompted by Plücker's work also led Faraday to confirm the status of the vacuum as a neutral magnetic conductor, acting neither to converge nor to diverge the magnetic force lines, and in the process to resolve the problem of the magnetic susceptibility of gases. The only remaining obstacle to his putting forward his theoretical ideas, now reasonably well developed, as a coherent theory of magnetism was the existence of rival theories such as that due to Ampère and, in particular, the development of Ampère's theory put forward by Wilhelm Eduard Weber.[107] (Other theories based on Ampère's, due to E P Becquerel and Auguste de la Rive, were less impressive than Weber's.)[108] In 1849 Faraday accordingly set out to disprove Weber's theory.

Weber's theory had been built on Faraday's own earlier discussion of the possible extension of Ampère's theory to diamagnetism. Faraday had suggested that diamagnetism might be due to a reverse polarity induced in materials by the primary magnet. Weber had expressed this idea in terms of Ampère's electrodynamic molecules and had developed on this basis a complete if somewhat artificial theory of diamagnetism. He had also supported this theory experimentally by demonstrating, or so he claimed, the

[103] Plücker (1852). See Gooding (1981), pp. 253*ff*.
[104] Gooding (1981), p. 262.
[105] Thomson to Faraday, 19 June 1849, in Faraday (1971), volume 2, pp. 559–61.
[106] Gooding (1981), pp. 262–6.
[107] See Weber (1846, 1852a,b,c and 1853).
[108] See Williams (1965), pp. 420*ff*.

existence of reverse polarity. The absence of any observable polarity in diamagnets had at first troubled Faraday, spoiling as it did the analogy with electrostatics. But once he had developed the idea of the physical primacy of the lines of force, and the presence of polarity as a property of these lines rather than of the media through which they passed, the absence of diamagnetic polarity caused him no problems. It would, however, cause problems for Weber, and Faraday therefore set out to demonstrate that the reverse polarity claimed by Weber was spurious and that diamagnets were not in fact polarised.[109] Having succeeded in this, he then put forward explicitly, in 1850, his own theory of magnetism.[110]

According to Faraday's theory, the behaviour of matter in a magnetic field was explained in terms of its disturbing effect on the lines of force, this effect depending on the magnetic conductibility of the matter. Diamagnets, being poor conductors, diverted the lines of force so that fewer of them, or less force, passed through them than through the surrounding, more conducting, medium. Paramagnets, being good conductors, converged the lines of force, so that more force passed through them than through the surrounding, less conducting, medium. The vacuum, and gaseous media, had specific magnetic conductibilities between those of diamagnets and paramagnets, with the vacuum characterised by the absence of any power to influence the lines of force at all. The observed dynamical effects of magnets were explained by a tendency for material bodies to move so as to cause the least possible disturbance of the lines of force from their normal positions, according to a principle of least constraint. As indicated in figure 3.14, a diamagnetic body, tending to diverge the force lines, would move towards a region of maximum divergence, away from the magnet, while a paramagnetic body would do the opposite.[111]

Faraday's explanation could be taken either as a phenomenal description or as a physical theory, depending on what type of reality was attributed to the lines of force. Over the next couple of years he developed the concept of physical lines of force, or lines of force as a 'physical mode of transmission of force', expressed in his 1852 paper 'On the physical character of the lines of force'.[112] This was the direction in which his thoughts had been developing for many years and constituted the natural expression of his conception of force as a primary entity propagated by wave motion and manifest in states of tension. (After all these years, and despite the emphasis upon lines of force, the electrotonic state was still very much present in his thoughts.) A wave propagation of magnetic force required a magnetic medium, which role could only be filled on Faraday's view by the lines of

[109] Gooding (1981), pp. 263*ff*, and Williams (1965), pp. 431*ff*.
[110] Faraday (1965), volume 3, pp. 169–268, especially paragraphs 2718–96; Faraday (1851).
[111] See Gooding (1981), p. 273.
[112] Faraday (1965), volume 3, paragraphs 3243–99. See Gooding (1980), pp. 105*ff*.

magnetic force. The role of matter was then as the manifestation of force, whether magnetic or otherwise, in terms of a resistance offered to its free conduction, or a disturbance of the equilibrium state. The physical conception of the lines of force raised the status of Faraday's explanation to that of a physical theory, but even if it were rejected the explanation still held good as a description, in which case the magnetic lines of force acted only to specify the strength and the direction, now clearly brought together, of the magnetic force at all points in the field of the magnet. The theory in this sense can fairly be called a field theory.

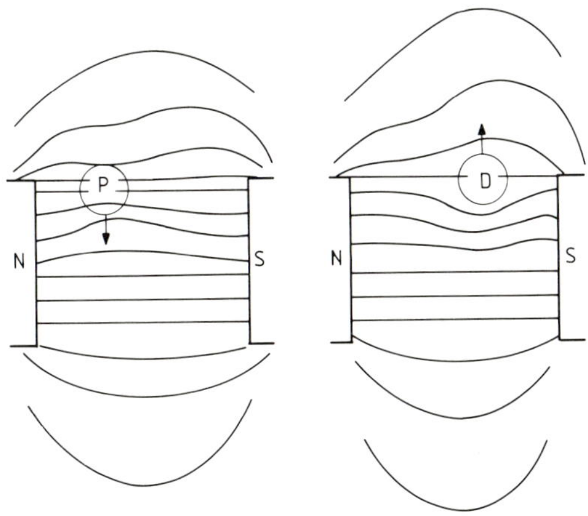

Figure 3.14 Faraday's experiments on the motion of paramagnetic and diamagnetic bodies. A paramagnetic body (left) concentrated the lines of force and moved towards an area of concentration. A diamagnetic body (right) diverged the lines of force and moved towards an area of divergence.

Thomson

We have already noted some connections between the work of Faraday and that of William Thomson, and these connections reflect one of the most remarkable collaborations in the history of science. Between 1845 and 1850 Faraday and Thomson met and corresponded regularly. Faraday was then in his middle and late fifties, a man with profound physical insight but no mathematics. Thomson, in his twenties, was an applied mathematician. Their approaches to the problems of electromagnetism were totally different, but their work developed in such close harmony that historians still have difficulty in separating out their respective contributions.

Thomson's early interest in electricity was to some extent accidental, in that it arose from a study of mathematical techniques rather than from a study of physics *per se.* As a student at Glasgow University, Thomson would probably have learnt his electrostatics according to the Laplacian theory of Poisson, which was incorporated in an English textbook written by Murphy.[113] Murphy's book also included a mechanical treatment of heat transfer, but besides this Thomson had also studied Fourier's *Analytical Theory of Heat,* and Fourier's treatment had impressed him considerably. He was, he recalled, 'filled with the utmost admiration for the splendour and poetry of Fourier.'[114] Within a year of first reading Fourier's work, and while still a student at Glasgow, he had written two papers defending Fourier's mathematical methods, in particular his use of infinite trigonometric series approximations, against attacks by the Edinburgh mathematician Phillip Kelland.[115] Then in 1841, by when he had moved to Cambridge but was still only 17 and an undergraduate there, Thomson wrote a paper in which he drew attention to a mathematical analogy between Fourier's theory of heat conduction and Poisson's theory of electrostatics.[116] Fourier, we may recall, had based his theory on an expression for the heat conduction through an isothermal surface. Poisson's theory was concerned with the behaviour of a uniformly charged conducting surface. Despite the very different approaches of the two theories there was, Thomson noted, a close analogy between the mathematical expressions they used.

According to Fourier's theory of heat (see Chapter 2), the heat flux across an isothermal surface of temperature v in a medium of conductivity k was given, in modern terminology, by

$$\mathbf{Flux} = -k\,\nabla v \tag{3.9}$$

with

$$\nabla^2 v = 0$$

in the steady state. On Poisson's electrostatic theory the attractive force of a charged spheroid on a point outside it was given by

$$\mathbf{Force} = -\,\nabla V \tag{3.10}$$

with V, which had been named a potential by George Green, given by

$$V = \iiint \frac{\rho}{r}\,\mathrm{d}\omega^3 \tag{3.11}$$

113 Murphy (1832), and see Buchwald (1977).
114 Thompson (1910), volume 1, p. 14, quoted in Wise (1981), p. 32. On Thomson see Wise (1979 and 1981), Knudsen (1972 and 1976), Siegel (1981), Buchwald (1976 and 1977) and Smith (1976a and 1980). Of these Buchwald (1977) gives a detailed treatment of Thomson's early work. My analysis throughout this section draws particularly heavily on Wise (1981).
115 Thomson (1841a and 1841b).
116 Thomson (1842).

ρ being the electrical density, r the distance from the point and $d\omega^3$ a volume element, and with

$$\begin{aligned} &\nabla^2 V = 0 && \text{outside the spheroid} \\ &\nabla^2 V = -4\pi\rho && \text{inside the spheroid.} \end{aligned} \qquad (3.12)$$

This analogy and others similar to it had already been noticed by Laplace and Poisson, but from their strictly mechanistic viewpoints such mathematical analogies were seen primarily as sources of potentially dangerous confusion in the physics, and they had not therefore developed them. Thomson, however, whose interest at this stage was largely in the mathematics, did develop them. Considering an electrical conductor in which all the charge was distributed over the (closed) surface, he observed that the equation for the attractive force on an external point (3.10) could be written (again using modern terminology) as

$$\mathbf{Force} = -\nabla \iint \frac{\rho}{r} d\omega^2 \qquad (3.13)$$

with ρ again the electrical density and $d\omega^2$ a surface element. Considering the effect of a volume of heat sources enclosed by an isothermal surface on a point outside that surface, he reasoned that the temperature at this point could be also given by the form

$$\nu = \iint \frac{\rho_1}{r_1} d\omega_1^2 \qquad (3.14)$$

with ρ_1 this time representing the intensity of the heat sources on the surface that would be equivalent, in their effect outside it, to those within it. Taking the conductivity of the medium as unity or absorbing it into the definition of ρ_1, he could then write an equation for heat flux equivalent to

$$\mathbf{Flux} = -\nabla \iint \frac{\rho_1}{r_1} d\omega_1^2 \qquad (3.15)$$

in perfect analogy with that for electrical force.

The value of this analogy was twofold. First, Thomson made it possible to draw on the very considerable mathematical apparatus developed in the context of action-at-a-distance electrostatics and apply it to the treatment of heat phenomena. Secondly, he could also carry across the idea of equivalent surfaces developed in heat theory to electrostatics. In the context of Fourier's theory of heat flow as depending only on the temperature gradient and not on the sources producing it, he could argue that 'it is obvious that the temperature of any point without a given isothermal surface, depends merely on the form and temperature of the surface, being independent of the actual sources of heat by which this temperature is produced, provided there are no sources without the surface.'[117] Having established

[117] Thomson (1872), p. 2.

a precise mathematical analogy he could carry this idea over into electrostatics and argue that any distribution of electricity could also be replaced by an equipotential surface. Thus for example, considering a closed isothermal surface with no heat source within it, Fourier's theory indicated that the total heat flux across such a surface must be zero and that, by consideration of adjacent surfaces, the temperature within such a surface must be constant. Carrying the analogy over to electrostatics, this implied that the attractive force of a charged body (the charge being located on the surface of the body) on a point within its surface must be zero, in analogy with the gradient of the temperature. From this Thomson could deduce as the condition of equilibrium of electricity distributed over the surface of a body 'that it must be so distributed that the attraction on a point at the surface, oppositely electrified, may be perpendicular to the surface.'[118] This approach also led Thomson towards a geometrical picture of electrostatics that was to be of particular significance in the context of Faraday's work a few years later. Since in equilibrium the heat flux or attractive force was always perpendicular to an isothermal or equipotential surface, the direction of flow or attraction could be represented as a series of lines orthogonal to a family of isothermal or equipotential surfaces (figure 3.15)—a representation that corresponded to Faraday's own use of lines of force.

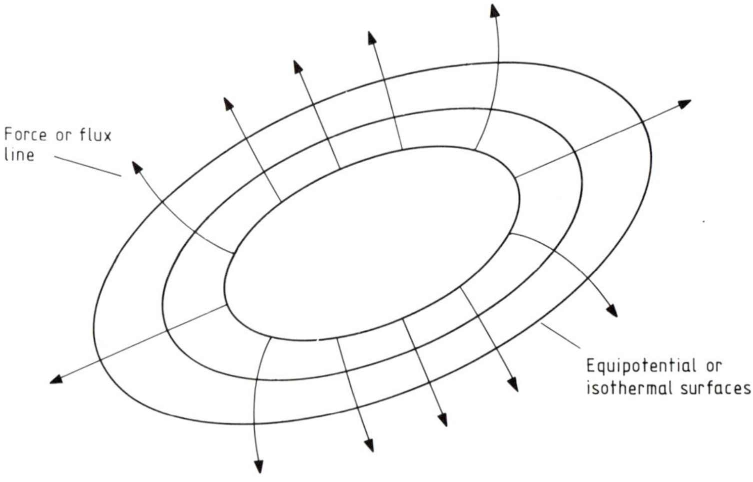

Figure 3.15 Diagram based on Thomson's description of the representation of the direction of heat flow or attraction as a family of curves orthogonal to a family of isothermal or equipotential surfaces.

Although Thomson's analogical approach was novel, the mathematics that resulted from it was not because, as he soon discovered, a theory of

[118] Thomson (1872), p. 4.

equivalent surfaces had already been developed and applied to electrostatics by George Green and, more recently, by Carl Friedrich Gauss.[119] Green's work, which was published privately in 1828 but which Thomson did not read until early 1845, was of the utmost importance, for although it was essentially a development of Poisson's theory of electricity and magnetism the method adopted was much closer in spirit to that of Fourier. Moreover, although Green did not draw any specific analogies with Fourier's work in the way that Thomson did, he did note the general similarity of method and indicated his own sympathy with Fourier's approach.[120] Whereas Poisson had built up his theory in terms of the attractions and repulsions between molecules of electric fluids, Green based his treatment on the potential function V, defined in terms of the macroscopic, empirically observed, polarisation. Poisson had proceeded by integration of hypothetical microscopic actions. Green used differential equations, just as Fourier had done, and assumed in effect that a description based on macroscopic observations could also be applied at the microscopic and indeed infinitesimal level.

In Fourier's theory of heat the approach adopted had been based on an explicit methodological and epistemological view of physics. As we saw in Chapter 2, Fourier had rejected outright the detailed molecular hypotheses characteristic of the mechanical approach to nature and had sought to base physical theory solely on observed physical behaviour, without recourse to hypotheses. His work was more than any other characteristic of the dynamistic approach to mathematical physics. Green's theory of electricity and magnetism shared completely the methodology of Fourier's theory, but was not put forward as a physical theory in the same way. From the point of view of a mechanical philosopher such as Poisson, both Fourier's theory and Green's were approximate theories in the sense that they were based on infinitesimal laws that could hold only as continuous approximations to the real microscopic laws, which, it was commonly agreed, would depend on discrete atomic or molecular behaviour. In Green's theory this approximate character was particularly apparent in the treatment of a conductor, for whereas according to the molecular theory of Poisson the surface charge distribution on a conductor took the form of a finitely thick layer of electric charge (necessarily so, since the electric fluid took up a finite volume), in Green's theory such a surface was treated as a mathematical surface, of infinitesimal thickness. Fourier had accepted that his theory might entail approximations at the microscopic level, but had rejected the claim that the true behaviour at such a level could be known anyway. All that could be done legitimately was to develop, as he had done, a mathematical theory of the phenomena. It is tempting to ascribe a similar attitude to Green, but

[119] Green (1828) and Gauss (1843).
[120] Green (1828), preface.

this cannot be done. Green did not discuss the nature of approximation used, not did he discuss the electric layer. He did not raise the issue of molecular hypotheses. The importance of his work was presented as resting solely on its utility in providing a mathematical method by which the laborious calculations necessary if an analysis were to be based on detailed systems of molecular forces could be replaced by a very simple analysis based on a potential distribution. His remembrance in terms of 'Green's theorem' for the relationship he derived between surface and volume integrals is an appropriate reflection on what he himself apparently considered important.

Thomson's attitude in respect of this question seems to have been closer to Green's than to Fourier's. His analysis depended, as had Green's, on the treatment of a charged surface as being infinitesimally thin, and this assumption was in fact critical to his theorem on the equilibrium conditions for such a surface. But like Green also he did not discuss this, even though he must have been well aware—as Green may not have been—of the importance attached to the finitely thick electric layer by Poisson and Murphy.[121] Moreover, although we may with hindsight be tempted to read Thomson's paper as being concerned with the application of Fourier's hypothesis-free treatment to electrostatics, Thomson seems to have been more concerned at this stage with the utility of mathematical methods than with any physical considerations. His other early publications indicate a willingness to use any method, including that of Poisson, if this led to a simpler deduction of results.[122] Associated with this catholicity, however, was an increasingly apparent concern that different methods of mathematically describing the same or similar phenomena should be shown to be equivalent, and this growing emphasis on the phenomena rather than on the theory does reveal a sympathy with the dynamistic attitude of Fourier. Moreover, although his early papers did concern mathematical methods rather than physical hypotheses, Thomson was far from being uninterested in the status of such hypotheses. In 1841 he had not mentioned the problem of the finite electric layer. But in the winter of 1844–5 he discovered a theorem by Samuel Earnshaw which seemed to cast doubt upon the existence of such a finite layer, and he promptly rederived Earnshaw's result and extended it to show that a finite electric layer could only be in stable equilibrium if all the electrical particles within it were in contact with the external bounding surface (other equilibrium positions were possible but they were not stable):[123]

> If a mechanical theory be adopted, *electricity* will actually be a number of material points without weight, which repel one another according to the inverse square of the distance. Thus the result we have arrived at is, that there

[121] See Buchwald (1977).
[122] Thomson (1842–3 and 1843)
[123] Thomson (1845a). Quotation from reprint in Thomson (1872), p. 102.

> can be permanently no free electricity in the interior of a conducting body under any circumstances whatever. ...
>
> Since every particle is on the surface, the whole *medium* ... will be an indefinitely thin stratum, the thickness being in fact the ultimate breadth of an atom or material point. If we suppose these atoms to be merely centres of force, the thickness will therefore be absolutely nothing ...

For Thomson, this result had two implications. On one hand the concept of the electric layer defended by Poisson and Murphy was seriously challenged, as indeed was the concept of an electric fluid: Thomson used the word 'medium', but he also asked in parentheses whether a surface a single atom thick could properly be called a medium.[124] On the other hand, however, Thomson also used the result as a confirmation of the mechanical theory of electricity, freed from the hypothesis of an extended fluid. If the electrical atoms were treated as force atoms then Poisson's theory of electrostatics, based on the inverse square attraction and repulsion between the atoms, led to a conclusion as to the nature of the surface layer that was in complete conformity with experiments, which 'confirm the fact that there is no electricity in the interior of conducting bodies, or that the stratum has absolutely no thickness.'[125] Rather than challenging the fundamental action-at-a-distance mechanism of the traditional theory of electrostatics, Thomson actually provided very strong support for the mathematical development of this theory along the lines of Green's, Gauss's and his own work.

Thomson's paper on the electric layer was dated 16 January 1845. Just eight days later, on 24 January, he received from William Hopkins, the famous Cambridge mathematical tutor, a copy of Green's *Essay*. By then his mathematical education at Cambridge was complete (he was second wrangler and first Smith's prizeman) and by March he was in Paris, gaining some experience of experimental physics in the laboratory of Regnault. While there he was asked by Liouville, editor of the *Journal de Mathematique Pure et Appliqué*, to write a short paper on Faraday's electrostatic results of the 1830s and their relationship to the established theory of electricity.[126] Faraday, we may recall, had used his experiments on electrostatic induction to support the theory of the propagation of electricity by an induction of polarity by contiguous action. This clearly clashed with the established mechanical theory based on action at a distance and electric fluids, but as the relationship between Faraday's experimental results and his theory was, as we saw, a symbiotic one rather than one of direct deduction, it was still an open question as to how far the experiments themselves

[124] Thomson (1872), p. 103, and see Buchwald (1977).

[125] Thomson (1872), p. 103.

[126] Thomson to James Thomson, 30 March 1845, in Thompson (1910), volume 1, p. 128.

challenged the mechanical theory. Thomson's response to Liouville was that he had always taken Faraday's experiments to be actually confirmatory of the established theory and in his paper, a first draft of which was written in May 1845 with an extended version being completed in November, he set out to demonstrate this.[127]

Already in Thomson's immediate response to Liouville, and even more clearly in the paper that resulted, his developing attitude towards physical theory is strikingly apparent. To most people the accepted mathematical theory of electricity was still Poisson's, complete with its mechanico-molecular hypotheses. From Thomson's point of view, however, Poisson's theory taken as a physical theory was simply irrelevant. Thomson's aim was to reconcile the experimental results of Faraday (principally the transmission of induction in curved lines and its dependence upon the dielectric medium) with Coulomb's theory of electrostatics, based on action at a distance according to the inverse square law but *excluding* the hypothesis of the electric fluids, and its mathematical development by Poisson, Green and others. It was of course Coulomb who had introduced the two-fluid theory of electricity in the first place, but in doing this he had also noted something that had become forgotten in the later development of the mechanical theory, namely that 'in the supposition of the two electric fluids, I had no other intention than to present the results of calculation and experiment with as few elements as possible, and not to indicate the true cases of electricity.'[128] Quoting this, Thomson interpreted Coulomb's theory as being based empirically on the observed law of attraction and repulsion between distant charged conductors, and 'independent of any hypothesis'. He then treated the theory of Poisson, so far as he accepted it, and that of Green as mathematical developments of the same empirically based theory.[129] Since the mechanical action-at-a-distance theory thus interpreted was derived from experience he argued that experience could not be in contradiction with it and that Faraday's results should therefore be conformable to it.

Thomson's analysis of Faraday's results fell into two parts. In the first part he drew on the mathematical analogy between action-at-a-distance electrostatics and Fourier's heat theory to reconcile the curved lines of induction and the concept of a dielectric medium with the action-at-a-distance theory. In the second part he drew on Poisson's mathematical theory of magnetism to give an action-at-a-distance formulation of Faraday's critical experiment on the specific inductive capacity (figure 3.9 above). The first part was a simple extension of his former analysis, for if

[127] Thomson (1845b). See Thompson (1910), volume 1, pp. 220–1, and Wise (1981), p. 41.

[128] Coulomb's note, from *Histoire de l'Académie,* 1788, p. 673, is quoted in French by Thomson (1872), p. 15.

[129] Thomson (1872), p. 15.

a dielectric medium was assumed to fill the space between two conductors, then the specific inductive capacity would be constant in that region, corresponding on the heat analogy to a constant thermal conductivity k. The analogy between the formulae for heat flux and electric force then went through as before, k being set to unity or absorbed into the definition of the equivalent heat source density ρ_1. Moreover the curved lines of induction could be seen to correspond to the flux lines orthogonal to isothermal or equipotential surfaces to which he had drawn attention in his earlier paper, and Faraday's results could be expressed in terms of a geometrical projection of a surface along the flux lines from one conductor to another.

In Faraday's experiments on specific inductive capacity the dielectric did not (e.g. for a solid) fill the space between the two conductors, and the analogy could not therefore be carried through with constant k. An analogy could however be drawn with the laws of magnetic induction worked out by Poisson. On this analogy the specific inductive capacity of a homogeneous dielectric between the two conductors could be represented by an imaginary density of electricity induced on the surface of the dielectric and related to the force and potential in the same way that a real source would be. If $\mathcal{F}_n^{\mathrm{i}}$ and $\mathcal{F}_n^{\mathrm{o}}$ were the normal components of the polarising force inside and outside a surface of the dielectric, the usual boundary conditions gave

$$\mathcal{F}_n^{\mathrm{o}} - \mathcal{F}_n^{\mathrm{i}} = 4\pi\rho \tag{3.16}$$

with ρ the charge density, or rather the imaginary charge density, on the surface, corresponding to the normal component of polarisation at the surface. But ρ and $\mathcal{F}_n^{\mathrm{i}}$ were also related, treating ρ as the component of polarisation at the surface, by

$$\rho = k_0 \mathcal{F}_n^{\mathrm{i}} \tag{3.17}$$

with k_0 representing the polarisability of the dielectric medium. Defining $k = 1 + 4\pi k_0$ this gave

$$\frac{\mathcal{F}_n^{\mathrm{i}}}{\mathcal{F}_n^{\mathrm{o}}} = \frac{1}{k} \tag{3.18}$$

k being equivalent to Faraday's definition of inductive capacity (unity in a gas or the vacuum where the polarisability was zero). From this result Thomson could calculate the apparent charge density on the surface of the dielectric and thus, using Green's work, the change in potential produced by the insertion of the dielectric. The experiment, with Faraday's definition of specific inductive capacity, could thus be brought into the realm of the established mathematical theory.

Thomson's analysis was impressive—and impressively simple. But there was one source of confusion. In the first part of his analysis Thomson wrote that 'the *resultant flux of heat* replaces the *resultant attraction* of the electrified bodies, in direction and magnitude.'[130] This was consistent with an analogy between force and temperature gradient, but not with that between force and flux explicitly enunciated earlier in the paper. This confusion may be related to the distinction in Faraday's work between the quantity of electric force summed across all the lines of electric force joining two conductors, and analogous to the total heat flux between two surfaces, and the intensity or tension of the force measured along the lines of induction and analogous to the temperature gradient. Thomson's concern, however, was not to mathematise Faraday's theory. It was, rather, to defend the empirically interpreted mathematical theory of Coulomb, based on, but not in his view physically requiring, action at a distance; and to demonstrate the equivalence of this theory with one based on propagation by contiguous action and adopting the mathematical approach of Fourier:[131]

> Now the laws of motion for heat which Fourier lays down in his *Théorie Analytique de la Chaleur,* are of that simple elementary kind which constitute a mathematical theory properly so called; and therefore, when we find corresponding laws to be true for the phenomena presented by electrified bodies, we may make them the foundation of the mathematical theory of electricity: and this may be done if we consider them merely as actual truths, without adopting any physical hypothesis, although the idea they naturally suggest is that of the propagation of some effect by means of the mutual action of contiguous particles; just as Coulomb, although his laws naturally suggest the idea of material particles attracting or repelling one another at a distance, most carefully avoids making this a *physical hypothesis,* and confines himself to the consideration of the mechanical effects which he observes and their necessary consequences.

Faraday's theory led in Thomson's view to Fourier's method of establishing the mathematical theory. But the dynamistically orientated preference for a theory based on empirical phenomena and empirically defined mathematical terms that Thomson shared with Fourier left him completely neutral in respect of the competing physical theories, and Faraday's theory was no more sanctioned by his treatment than was Poisson's. Starting from this almost anti-physical perspective, Thomson did not note either the distinction between a flux-like and a force-like quantity in Faraday's work or that between the two contrasting analogies he used.[132]

Despite his attitude to physical theory, however, Thomson was far from indifferent to Faraday's ideas, which, he noted, had been 'illustrated or

[130] Thomson (1872), pp. 28–9.
[131] Thomson (1872), p. 29.
[132] This important observation is due to Wise (1981), who discusses the subject in much greater detail than is possible here.

demonstrated by experiment', and which had led Faraday directly to a 'knowledge of some of the most important of the general theorems, which, from their nature, seemed destined never to be perceived except as mathematical truths.'[133] The basic results on specific inductive capacity could be incorporated into the existing mathematical framework, but it was clear that further results might well lead to further significant developments of the mathematics, especially if Faraday's ideas on the unity of forces should be experimentally supported. Despite his defence of Coulomb's theory, moreover, Thomson seems already to have been aware, at least by November 1845 when he wrote the final version of his paper, that Faraday's theoretical ideas represented a simpler and more natural approach to the more complex electrical phenomena now being investigated. He was clearly impressed too that the development of the mathematical theory of electricity as a theory of potentials and surfaces rather than of charged particles was bringing it much closer, conceptually, to the continuous wave-propagation way of looking at things.

Before leaving Cambridge, Thomson had attended the lectures of James Challis, who was seeking the unification of physics in terms of the luminiferous aether. He had indeed come across Earnshaw's result in a paper on the aether and was also thoroughly familiar with the work George Stokes was doing in Cambridge on the same subject. The idea that light and electricity might be different manifestations of the same fundamental force had also been suggested independent of the aether-theory context by both Faraday and Whewell. And it was soon after his return to England in the summer of 1845, and after he had met Faraday for the first time at a meeting of the British Association, at which he presented his own mathematical results, that Thomson put to Faraday the question as to the effect of a dielectric on polarised light that was to lead to the demonstration of the magneto-optic effect.[134] Faraday's results on the magneto-optic effect and on diamagnetic behaviour provided the strongest evidence yet in support of his ideas on the continuous propagation of polarising action and on the connection between electrical and optical phenomena, and they reinforced his belief, no doubt communicated to Thomson, that experiment could distinguish his own theory from those based on action at a distance. Whether this should be so or not, Thomson was by this time convinced of the need for a mathematical formulation of Faraday's theory going beyond that provided by the heat analogy. That analogy had proved useful for the treatment of simple phenomena involving a single manifestation of force as electricity, but could be of no use for those in which electric, magnetic and optical effects interacted. Moreover, such phenomena would also stretch the Coulomb theory, developed on the basis of simple actions, beyond its

[133] Thomson (1872), pp. 29–30.

[134] See Wise (1981), pp. 40 and 51–2.

range of natural application. The existence of interference effects between different phenomena, and in particular the now established interference effect between electromagnetism and light, pointed clearly towards a mathematical theory of wave propagation as their most natural expression, and by the time Faraday wrote up his 'Thoughts on ray vibrations' in 1846 Thomson was well embarked on the development of a mathematical wave representation of electricity and magnetism.[135]

The first stage of Thomson's new programme consisted simply of the construction of a third mathematical analogy alongside those he had already explored, and this was a move he may well have been tempted to make quite independent of his interaction with Faraday. Mathematical physics in the 1840s could in effect be characterised by three approaches: the inverse square law action-at-a-distance approach that had dominated gravitational and electromagnetic theory; the flow approach introduced by Fourier for heat theory; and the elastic solid approach that had been developed in the context of the wave theory of light. This last approach, according to which optical effects were either represented mathematically by, or attributed physically to, the mechanical vibrational behaviour of an elastic solid luminiferous aether, was being actively pursued in Cambridge and had already attracted Thomson's attention. It was natural that he should seek to incorporate it into his analogical framework, and it was also the natural choice of mathematical representation for Faraday's ideas. The first step for Thomson, however, was not to use it for the representation of Faraday's work but to establish an analogy with Coulomb's expression of the basic laws of electric and magnetic attraction and repulsion. From Thomson's point of view these laws were still identified with the basic empirical facts of the subject matter and it would have been idle to pursue any mathematical analogy without first establishing its ability to conform to them.

Thomson's task was simplified considerably by the work of the mathematician George Gabriel Stokes, with whom he had built up a friendship in Cambridge. (Stokes took his degree roughly when Thomson matriculated, but stayed in Cambridge, as did Thomson later, as a Fellow.) The French mathematician and physicist Augustin Louis Cauchy had developed the theory of the luminiferous aether as a truly mechanical theory, the properties invested in the aether being those of a real physical molecularly constituted substance. In Britain, however, Green and McCullagh had adopted the more dynamistically orientated procedure manifest in Green's work on electricity and magnetism, developing the theory as a mathematical one consistent with the observed properties of light but regardless of and indeed inconsistent with any hypothetical mechanical properties.[136] Stokes's approach was even further removed

[135] Wise (1981), p. 52.

[136] See Chapter 2 above.

from physical specificity, for he developed the theory of elastic media in its most general possible form, but his attitude towards mechanical hypotheses was much the same. Starting from the properties of the observed phenomena rather than those of a hypothetical medium he treated the medium as a continuum, the properties of which could be chosen to correspond with whatever behaviour was observed, regardless of the implications of this behaviour for a physical theory.[137] Stokes's analysis was completed in 1845, while Thomson was in France. In November 1846, Thomson completed his own paper describing the analogy he required between the mathematical representation of states of strain in an elastic solid and that of elementary electric and magnetic forces acting at a distance.[138] Electric force was represented by a displacement of the medium, the magnitude of which followed the inverse square law, while magnetic and electromagnetic forces were represented, in conformity with Faraday's ideas, by rotational components of displacements.

This much was relatively straightforward, and it was also a source of encouragement. Thomson had been able to reach it by treating the aether as perfectly homogeneous, isotropic and incompressible, and he was therefore left with considerable freedom of manoeuvre in seeking to incorporate further effects and interactions in the elastic solid analogy. But what he had completed so far was only the merest beginning and it was far from clear exactly how to proceed. In June 1847 he sent a copy of his paper to Faraday under the following cover:[139]

> I enclose the paper which I mentioned to you as giving an analogy for the electric and magnetic forces by means of the *strain,* propagated through an elastic solid. What I have written is merely a sketch of the mathematical analogy. I did not venture even to hint at the possibility of making it the foundation of a physical theory of the propagation of electric and magnetic forces, which, if established at all, would express as a necessary result the connection between electrical and magnetic forces, and would show how the purely statical phenomena of magnetism may originate either from electricity in motion, or from an inert mass such as a magnet. If such a theory could be discovered, it would also, when taken in connection with the undulatory theory of light, in all probability explain the effect of magnetism on polarized light.

Thomson wrote to Faraday using the language of physical theory, but it was also true that any complete mathematical representation of electricity and magnetism, or as Thomson would term it a true mathematical theory, would have to incorporate the effects and phenomena he mentioned.

To attempt to develop the elastic solid analogy, appropriate as it seemed,

[137] Stokes (1849).
[138] Thomson (1847a).
[139] Thomson to Faraday, 11 June 1847, in Thompson (1910), volume 1, pp. 203–4, also quoted by Wise (1981), p. 52.

into a complete mathematical representation of electromagnetism would have been an exceedingly ambitious task, and although it was one to which he was often to return Thomson does not seem to have pursued it, at least with any success, at this stage. He turned instead, motivated perhaps by Faraday's recent researches into the motions of diamagnetic bodies, to the general question of the motions of bodies under static electric or magnetic forces, which had 'not been made the subject of a special investigation by any writer, so far as I am aware.'[140] For this he drew again on the mathematics of Poisson's theory of magnetism. Considering a small iron sphere of magnetic capacity i in the region of a magnet, the resultant magnetic force at the centre of the sphere, R, was related to the intensity of the induced magnetism there, k, by

$$k = \frac{3i}{4\pi} R. \tag{3.19}$$

By considering the variation of the force over the sphere he deduced, as Poisson had done, the formula for the total resultant force over the whole sphere, and showed that this was given by

$$\mathcal{F}_x = \left(\frac{3i}{4\pi}\right) \sigma R \frac{\mathrm{d}R}{\mathrm{d}x} \tag{3.20a}$$

or in modern terminology

$$\mathcal{F} = \nabla \left(\frac{3i}{8\pi} \sigma R^2\right) \tag{3.20b}$$

with σ the volume of the sphere, so that, in conformity with Faraday's experiments, 'a sphere of soft iron is urged in the direction in which the magnetizing force increases most rapidly'.[141] For diamagnets, i could be taken as negative, and Faraday's conclusion that such substances tended 'to move from stronger to weaker places or points of force' was also represented.

Thomson concluded his analysis by considering the positions of equilibrium of magnetic and diamagnetic bodies in the region of a magnet, and it was his result here that led Faraday to concentrate on the motion of bodies in the field rather than on the misleading directional set. For Thomson himself, the analysis pointed towards a generalisation of potential theory to include the movements of diamagnetic and, by analogy, dielectric bodies. In his analysis he had been concerned only with the motion of a body of constant magnetic capacity in a medium that was assumed to be unaffected by any magnetic force. The whole thrust of Faraday's work was, however, away from the idea of bodies acting in a neutral medium and

140 W Thomson (1847b). Quotation from reprint in Thomson (1872), p. 494.
141 Thomson (1872), p. 496.

towards that of a magnetic force propagating and acting throughout the field of a magnet. In his electrostatics too his emphasis was on the properties of media rather than on those of bodies moving in neutral media. This suggested to Thomson a generalisation of his latest result from the effect of a magnet on a small magnetic body to the total effect on the entire, non-homogeneous magnetic (or electric) field, giving the new equation

$$\mathcal{F} \propto \nabla \iiint iR^2 \, d\omega^3 \tag{3.21}$$

and the requirement that $\iiint R^2 \, d\omega^3$ be an extremum. But this expression was already familiar from the potential theory of electrostatics, where it could be related to the potential V and charge density ρ by

$$\iiint R^2 \, d\omega^3 = 4\pi \iiint \rho V \, d\omega^3 \tag{3.22}$$

and where the condition that the latter integral be a minimum was the condition established by Gauss for the uniqueness of solutions to the continuity equation

$$\nabla^2 V = 4\pi\rho$$

for the surface of a conductor. For the general case of inhomogeneous media now being considered by Thomson, the continuity equation itself had to be generalised to

$$(\nabla \cdot \alpha^2 \nabla V) = -4\pi\rho \tag{3.23}$$

where α^2 represented the inductive capacity of the medium (electric or magnetic). In a paper completed in October 1847, Thomson gave the uniqueness and existence proofs for this new equation.[142]

Besides this generalisation, the identity of Gauss's condition with that on the force integral also suggested a new physical basis for the whole of potential theory, for in Thomson's analysis of diamagnetic behaviour the force integral, the gradient of which was the ponderomotive force acting, provided a measure of the total work expended in the motion of a body. Taking the integral over all space it was precisely the work necessary to assemble the system from infinity, named by Thomson the 'mechanical effect' or 'mechanical value', effectively the total potential, of the system. The equilibrium of the system, whether it be a magnetic, electric or any other system represented by a potential, could be determined by the requirement that its mechanical effect be a minimum. Any force acting in a system not in equilibrium would act so as to minimise the mechanical effect.

[142] Thomson (1848a). The modern notation used here was not of course available to Thomson, who expressed everything in terms of the cartesian coordinate components.

Thomson's articulation of this new perspective was not altogether clear, for his published papers took the form of either pure mathematical propositions or discussions of specific effects, and the general theory was never laid out explicitly. But it could be extracted from the various papers on electricity and magnetism he wrote around 1848–51, and it provided the first mathematical representation of the electromagnetic properties of materials that had been demonstrated by Faraday.[143] Ironically, it did so in the form of a potential theory whose origins still lay in action-at-a-distance mathematics, and through a *mechanical* representation of electrical and magnetic forces. But with the analogy of flow established for the static case, and indeed extended by Thomson to the dynamic case in which the *vis viva* (we would now say kinetic energy) was minimised, the relationship between the mathematical theory and the physical assumptions from which it had been developed was becoming increasingly remote and less and less a matter for concern. Although the analogy was *mechanical*, the approach was *dynamical,* and to that extent Thomson's programme of establishing the mathematical theory independent of physical hypotheses was succeeding. His work also had important implications for the unification of physics, for the mechanical effect provided a measure common to any force whose effects could be measured in dynamical terms. As early as 1848, indeed, he proposed the conservation of mechanical effect as the basis for an interpretation of Faraday's laws of electromagnetic induction.[144] A full understanding of the conservation of energy and its implications was to follow a few years later, after he had turned his own attention to the theory of heat.

[143] These papers are reprinted in Thomson (1872), pp. 341–513.
[144] Thomson (1848b). See Wise (1981), p. 61.

4

Maxwell's Apprenticeship: Analogy and Lines of Force

By 1850 physical science was in the midst of a revolution. The modern concepts of energy conservation (discussed in Chapter 5 below) and the field were clearly emerging, and the unification of physics so eagerly sought by men such as Oersted, Ampère and Faraday was becoming a realistic possibility. The phenomena of electricity, magnetism, light and radiant heat could all be experimentally related, and several of these relations also involved mechanical work. In a separate set of advances the interchangeability of heat and mechanical work was also being established. Only gravitational force remained outside the emerging synthesis, as although Faraday repeatedly sought evidence of its effects in terms of the other forces he remained unable to find any.[1] Mathematically, the exclusion of gravitation was inevitably in some sense a hindrance, as gravitational theory remained the model of a well developed mathematical theory. For the continuing adherents to a strict mechanical philosophy, the inability to closely relate the more complex forces to that of gravity was a serious if not insurmountable barrier to the development of a unified physics. But within the emerging middle ground of a heuristically liberal form of the dynamistic approach the situation was distinctly promising. Thomson's emphasis on the analogy between rival physical theories and on their equivalence at the empirical level, following the success of the empirically based theories of Fourier, Fresnel and Ampère, had opened up the possibility of a universal and unifying dynamics acting as the basis for the experimentally revealed synthesis. This synthesis was not, however, complete, and its completion required not only hard work but further incisive insight and a still firmer control of method than had yet been developed. The man who, more than anyone, was to provide these contributions was of course James Clerk Maxwell, still, in 1850, an undergraduate.

[1] See Faraday (1932–6), *passim*.

The young Maxwell

James Clerk Maxwell was born in Edinburgh in June 1831, and spent his early years at his parents' country seat, Glenlair, in the Maxwell estate of Middlebie.[2] His father John Clerk, who inherited both the name and the estate of Maxwell as a younger son while his brother succeeded to the Clerk estate, was a lawyer by profession but a society man and scientific enthusiast by practice. The account given of him by Maxwell's intimate friend and biographer Lewis Campbell brings to mind a kindly, benevolent and comfortable man, combining imagination and enthusiasm with a degree of plodding care and caution amounting almost to laziness. He was no real scientist or engineer, but he clearly revelled in the scientific environment of Edinburgh, which in the early nineteenth century was still one of the leading scientific centres of the world. In his youth he was something of an amateur inventor, and he remained an enthusiast for all things technical, a keen visitor of factories and works, and an addict to the meetings of scientific societies. His favourite entertainment was not a ball or a dinner but a meeting of the Royal Society of Edinburgh or the Edinburgh Society of Arts. His interests and enthusiasm are perhaps best portrayed by a letter he wrote to James in 1853, when the latter was to visit some friends in Birmingham:[3]

> Ask Gedge to get you instructions to Brummagem workshops. View, if you can, armourers, gunmaking and gunproving—swordmaking and proving—*Papier-mâché* and japanning—silver-plating by cementation and rolling—ditto, electrotype, Elkington's works—Brazier's works, by founding and by striking up in dies—turning—spinning teapot bodies in white metal, etc.—making buttons of sorts, steel pins, needles, pins, and any sorts of small articles which are curiously done by subdivision of labour and by ingenious tools—glass of sorts is among the works of the place, and all kinds of foundry work—engine-making—tools and instruments (optical and philosophical) both coarse and fine. If you have had enough of the town lots of Birmingham, you could vary the recreation by viewing Kenilworth, Warwick, Leamington, Stratford-on-Avon, or suchlike.

He was only visiting for a few days!

Fortunately for Maxwell he did share his father's interest in such things and needed little encouragement to explore the fruits of the industrial revolution. He seems to have been one of those children who are always into things, trying to find out how they work, and what *else* they can be used for. From an early age he was also a keen maker of things. Needless to say

[2] The estate was on Urr Water, just south of Corsock about 15 miles west of Dumfries. Campbell and Garnett (1882 and 1884) remains by far the best biography of Maxwell.

[3] Campbell and Garnett (1884), pp. 131–2.

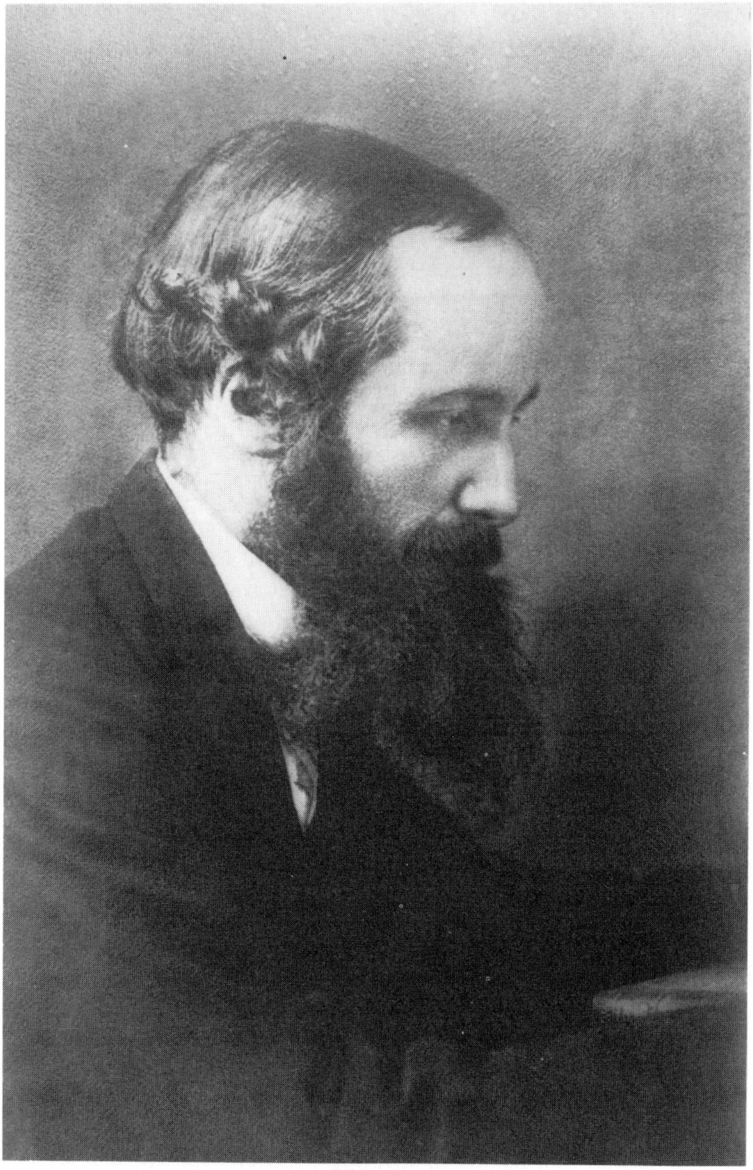

James Clerk Maxwell. Courtesy the Cavendish Laboratory, University of Cambridge.

he was given every encouragement to indulge in such activities. His father must have been delighted and was indeed so pleased with his son's development that he planned to have him educated at home before sending him to the university, perhaps when he reached about 13. As things turned out, however, his education was conducted at rather a leisurely pace.

Although John Clerk Maxwell continued to spend as much time as he could in Edinburgh throughout his life, he had decided in his late thirties to settle down, had married Frances Kay, the sister of a close friend, and had set about building a family house on the Maxwell estate. By the time of James's childhood the house was substantially complete and the greater part of the year was spent there, with visits to Edinburgh. Education at home, by a private tutor, seemed a natural course. But in 1839 Frances died at the age of 47, leaving her husband, then 52, to bring up the eight year old James. So in 1841 James was sent to Edinburgh to live with his father's sister, herself a widow, and to attend the Edinburgh Academy. The holidays were spent in the country, of course, and his father spent as much of the term as he could in Edinburgh.

Maxwell's early school years seem to have been relatively undistinguished, but in 1845 he shared almost all the prizes and medals going at the Academy with his friend Lewis Campbell, and in 1846, aged 14, he had his first original mathematical paper read at the Royal Society of Edinburgh.[4] The paper was not a deep one—it concerned a new way of drawing ovals—but its existence and background tell us a lot about Maxwell's education at this time. The formal education he received at the Academy was still very elementary, but his father was now taking him regularly to the meetings of the Society of Arts and Royal Society, and he was clearly benefiting from them. The project of drawing ovals came out of a lecture at the Society of Arts by D R Hay, a decorative painter. Moreover, the young Maxwell's introduction to the learned society of Edinburgh did not stop at lectures. Once he had drawn his new ovals his father took him first to meet Mr Hay, and then to meet James Forbes, the Professor of Natural Philosophy at the University. Forbes not only gave time to listen to the boy, but communicated the result to the Royal Society and began to take a personal interest in Maxwell's development. John Clerk Maxwell's contribution to his son's projects thus went far beyond mere encouragement.

Despite this early success, Maxwell was not sent up to Edinburgh University until 1847, and having gone there he remained a full three years before matriculating at Cambridge in 1850. By contrast Peter Guthrie Tait, his friend and fellow mathematical prodigy (their friendship was apparently based on the exchange of mathematical propositions), who was a year below him at the Academy, went to the University at the same time and to Cambridge two years earlier, in 1848. But Maxwell's interests were much

[4] Maxwell (1846). Campbell and Garnett (1884), pp. 54–7.

wider than Tait's and his leisurely course gave him time to indulge not only in mathematics but also in his own extra-curricular experiments in physics, as well as in poetry, classics and philosophy, in all of which he excelled. His father's decision to keep him at Edinburgh would appear to have had more to do with a reluctance to be parted from him than to more strictly educational reasons, and the parting when it came was perhaps even more traumatic than it would have been if made earlier, but in every other respect Maxwell seems to have gained rather than lost by the decision.

Edinburgh University in the late 1840s was in a period of transition. The traditional ideals of Scottish education, with the aim of producing a 'man o' parts' and the emphasis on moral philosophy as the core discipline, were still being upheld by Sir William Hamilton, the last in the great tradition of Scottish common-sense philosophers. But James Forbes had already been advancing a rival set of ideals, based on those of the Cambridge mathematical tripos, for some years.[5] Maxwell, who had the most catholic of academic tastes, benefited from the best of both worlds, combining the study of natural philosophy and mathematics under Forbes and Kelland with that of logic and moral philosophy under Hamilton and C N Wilson. He also attended classes in chemistry and practical chemistry, and appears to have struck up a close friendship with George Wilson, the Professor of Technology. He also kept up his own scientific researches, as well as a heavy programme of reading which covered everything from the latest scientific articles to the classic Greek and Latin authors and the full range of contemporary poetry, philosophy and fiction.

Maxwell's responses to his teachers were mixed. His own mathematical inclinations were towards geometrical representations, with their clear connection with physical manifestations, but Kelland's preference was for algebraic analysis, and this must have helped balance his studies.[6] Forbes of course he already knew. He recalled later that he had loved him, and while Forbes encouraged Maxwell's own investigations Maxwell in turn took an interest in those of the Professor. It is doubtful if he ever learnt anything significant from Forbes directly, but he certainly became familiar with his scientific style and methodology. Through Forbes he was also introduced to probability theory, and in particular to the work of George Boole, whose mathematical treatment of logic as the laws of thought, presented in his books on *The Mathematical Analysis of Logic* (1847) and *The Laws of Thought* (1854) combined the dynamistic attitude of Sir William Hamilton with a mathematical approach quite alien to Hamilton.[7]

[5] See Davie (1964) and Olson (1975), especially pp. 235–6.

[6] See Smith (1976a) and Becher (1980).

[7] Boole (1847 and 1854, and see also 1851) and see Heimann (1970a). In 1849 Forbes took centre stage in a debate on the use of probabilistic arguments in the analysis of double stars, a debate which was resolved by Boole.

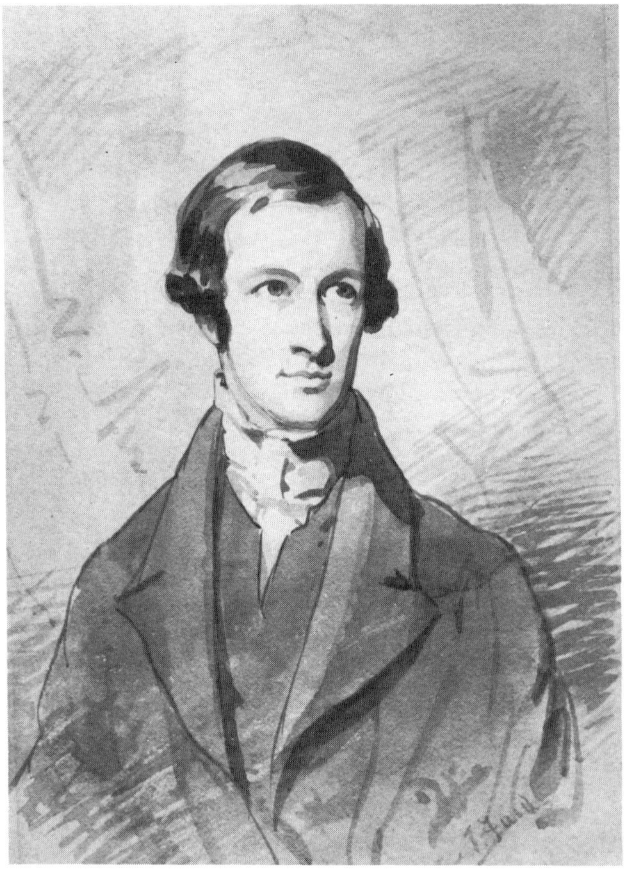

J D Forbes. Courtesy the National Galleries of Scotland.

On the philosophical side, Maxwell was deeply inspired by Hamilton, whose lectures on logic and metaphysics were clearly the highlights of his formal education, and with whose dynamistic synthesis he was sympathetic. As we shall see, Maxwell's own philosophy was rather closer to Whewell's than to Hamilton's, but Hamilton's lectures were his first introduction to a deeply thought out metaphysics and epistemology. As Lewis Campbell, who remained Maxwell's principal confidant on matters of non-scientific philosophy, noted,[8]

> However strange it may appear that a born mathematician should have been thus influenced by an enemy of mathematics [as Hamilton, in his theory of

[8] Campbell and Garnett (1884), p. 66. For Hamilton's opposition to mathematics, manifest in debates with the mathematician de Morgan, see for example Laita (1979).

> Logic, was], the fact is indisputable that in his frequent excursions into the region of speculative thought, the ideas received from Sir William Hamilton were his habitual vantage-ground

Ironically, the lectures on moral philosophy, which still constituted the core of the system Hamilton was trying to defend but which were now given by Christopher North Wilson, were the least impressive of all. 'Wilson', Maxwell reported to Campbell, 'after having explained his own opinions, has proceeded to those of other great men ... '. He had misunderstood Plato, and garbled Aristotle. His lectures did 'not improve on reconsideration', and he clearly earned no respect at all from Maxwell, who responded, however, quite typically, by reading up on the subject himself and attempting, over the next few years, to develop his own coherent system of morals.[9]

Turning from public to private education—and this was Maxwell's own distinction—Maxwell's experimental investigations in this period seem to have been concerned mainly with electrochemistry, electromagnetism and the patterns produced by polarised light passing through solids. His mathematical investigations seem to have focused first on rolling curves and then, in 1849, on the properties of elastic solids, and he wrote up papers on both subjects. His paper on the equilibrium of elastic solids, written in the spring of 1850, is of particular interest.[10] The subject had of course received considerable attention on account of its importance for the wave theory of light, and George Stokes had given a very general theory. But Stokes had not tried to apply this theory to the behaviour of real elastic solids; and the earlier theories of Navier, Poisson, Cauchy and others, though claiming to treat of real solids, were in fact at variance with a number of experimental results. They clashed in particular with measurements obtained by Oersted and others for the cubical compressibility of liquids. The particular interest of the subject for Maxwell at this time was that the most effective way of observing the effects of strains in elastic solids was in terms of the patterns created by the passage of polarised light through strained transparent elastic solids such as gutta-percha or isinglass jellies. The subject was thus a natural continuation of Maxwell's own experiments on the patterns produced by polarised light in unannealed glass, and it was also one of the many to which Forbes had turned his attention: Maxwell indeed cited one of Forbes's experiments in his paper.

In this paper, Maxwell began by re-deriving the equations of Stokes's theory. Stokes's analysis had a been purely mathematical one, based on the equations of fluid motion, and it had the advantage that it incorporated more degrees of freedom, including separate coefficients for linear and cubical elasticity, than had the earlier mechanical theories. Maxwell was however interested at this stage in the physical properties of observed elastic

[9] Campbell and Garnett (1884), pp. 83–5, 98–9, 346–7, and see also 109–11.
[10] Maxwell (1850).

solids rather than in the mathematical description of an ideal solid or hypothetical luminiferous aether, and he therefore re-derived Stokes's equations from physical axioms. He then applied the equations to a range of physical circumstances and used both the published experimental investigations of others and a number of his own experiments to confirm the mathematical predictions. In contrast with the work of Stokes, or even with the early work of Thomson, Maxwell's account was uncompromisingly physical. The equations were derived from physical axioms and interpreted physically at all stages. But the axioms did not take the form of mechanical hypotheses such as those adopted by the earlier French workers in the field. They were instead simply physical expressions of the equations linking the components of pressure and compression and defining, in effect, the coefficients of cubical and linear elasticity.

One final event of interest, occurring just before Maxwell left Edinburgh, in September 1850, was a meeting there of the British Association for the Advancement of Science. Maxwell not only attended this meeting but spoke at it, criticising an aspect of Brewster's colour theory. He was also introduced there to William Thomson, who, learning of his interest in making things, asked him to make up some magnecrystallic preparations for experiments on the magnetocrystallic effect.

In October 1850 Maxwell moved to Cambridge to read for the mathematical tripos, starting at Peterhouse and moving after about a term to Trinity. For the next three and a quarter years his formal education, apart from some classics in which he revelled, was directed towards the tripos from which he emerged in January 1854 as second wrangler and equal first Smith's prizeman. Both the Cambridge educational system in general and the mathematical tripos in particular had undergone substantial changes over the previous decades. The most recent change, following the Grace of 1846, had been the introduction of the Natural Sciences tripos in 1848, to be followed by the Moral Sciences tripos in 1851, but it was to be some time before these made any significant impact.[11] The nature of the mathematical tripos itself had oscillated, as a successful attempt by Whewell, Peacock and Babbage to introduce continental algebraic analysis alongside the traditional fluxional approach with its emphasis on geometrical and physical illustration had been followed by second thoughts and back-tracking on the part of Whewell. A Grace of 1848 had set up a new Mathematical Board of Studies and in Maxwell's time the syllabus was well balanced, with the examination questions being divided roughly equally between pure and applied mathematics and between algebraic and geometric approaches.

[11] See Becher (1980). Completion of part of the mathematical tripos was still required before entering any of the non-mathematical triposes, Classics, introduced in 1827, being the third of these.

For someone of Maxwell's ability, however, the tripos was merely a cram—a question of how quickly the problems could be solved rather than of how to solve them. He worked in the elite group of the successful tutor Hopkins, and a fellow pupil from that group recalled[12]

> how, when I had been working the night before and all the morning at Hopkins's problems with little or no result, Maxwell would come in for a gossip, and talk on while I was wishing him far away, till at last, about half an hour or so before our meeting at Hopkins's, he would say—"Well, I must go to old Hop's problems;" and by the time we met there they were all done.

As before, the real education took place outside the formal system. Maxwell arrived in Cambridge with personal introductions to the geologist, Sedgwick, and to Stokes, and he was quickly befriended by the latter. If his mathematical self-education needed any guidance, it was Stokes who provided it. William Whewell, a true polymath, was by this time Professor of Moral Philosophy, and although he was also Master of Trinity College there is no evidence of his having entered into any personal relationship with Maxwell. But Maxwell did read his book on *Morality* in 1851 and was encouraged in his own efforts to develop a moral system: 'Whewell's *Morality* is worth reading, if only to see that there *may* be such a thing as a system of ethics.'[13] He also read the important *History* and *Philosophy of the Inductive Sciences*, and he seems to have been very sympathetic to Whewell's notion of guiding ideas, and indeed to his philosophy in general.[14]

It would be presumptuous to claim that Maxwell was influenced by any specific tenets of Hamilton or Forbes, Whewell or Stokes, or even his father, for the views he developed in science and philosophy were essentially his own. But given that he was attracted to the dynamistic view of nature, and to the synthesis of this view with the concerns of the practical scientist, he could scarcely have grown up in a more sympathetic environment. He had studied under the two most prominent exponents of the dynamical philosophy in Britain, Hamilton and Whewell, and through Hamilton he had also been introduced to the works of Kant and the Scottish common-sense philosophers. In the teachings of Whewell he would have found a ready-made adaptation of the characteristic features of the dynamical philosophies of Germany and Scotland to the requirements of the working physicist. As we saw in Chapter 2, the works of both Stokes and Forbes may also be related to the dynamistic tradition. Forbes was, besides, well up with everything going on in the world of physics, while Stokes was equally so in

[12] Campbell and Garnett (1884), p. 123.

[13] Campbell and Garnett (1884), p. 110. Whewell (1845).

[14] Maxwell (1890 and 1965), volume 2, pp. 528–32; Campbell and Garnett (1884), pp. 156–7.

mathematics, and under their care the young Maxwell must have received the best possible introduction to recent and current works in these subjects. His own scientific creativity, both mathematical and experimental, was also fostered and given every encouragement, first by his father, then by Forbes, and later by Thomson and Stokes.

There can be no doubt that Maxwell was extremely lucky to have the parents and teachers he did, and to grow up in an environment that assisted rather than hindered him in his scientific development. At the same time, however, the picture we get of the young Maxwell from his letters and from the stories told of him is of a fiercely independent character.[15] He was considerate to others and acutely aware of their consideration towards himself. He was also rather shy. But he went his own way. As a child he seems to have been in remarkable control of himself, while at times quite out of the control of his parents and aunt, and a similar observation applies to his intellectual life as a youth. He took, and was extremely grateful for, everything his teachers could give, but he does not seem to have been directed by them. He read both voraciously and omnivorously, not only in science and mathematics but also in poetry, literature, theology and metaphysics, and in everything he read—as in everyone he met—he both sought out the best and at the same time remained politely critical. He could extract something of value even from the writings of those with whom he was quite out of sympathy, and could find fault even with those whose sympathies lay closest to his own. For all his shyness he was also an incurable talker, making a point of putting up his own fancies to be criticised and shot down. His philosophy on this point was quite explicit: man develops by intercourse with other men, and the wider his experience in this respect, both personal and intellectual, the greater the opportunities for self-improvement.[16] In March 1852 he wrote to Campbell of his 'great plan':[17]

> Now, my great plan, which was conceived of old, and quickens and kicks periodically, and is continually making itself more obtrusive, is a plan of *Search* and *Recovery*, or Revision and Correction, or Inquisition and Execution, etc. The Rule of the Plan is to let nothing be wilfully left unexamined. Nothing is to be *holy ground* consecrated to Stationary Faith, whether positive or negative. All fallow land is to be ploughed up, and a regular system of rotations followed. All creatures as agents or as patients are to be pressed into the service, which is never to be willingly suspended till nothing more remains to be done; i.e. till A.D. $+\infty$. The part of the rule which respects self-improvement by means of others is:— Never hide anything, be it weed or no, nor seem to wish it hidden. So shall all men passing by pluck up the weeds

[15] The following character sketch is based on the information in Campbell and Garnett (1882 and 1884). It is inevitably, however, a personal appraisal, and is certainly not to be taken as dogma.

[16] See for example Campbell and Garnett (1884), pp. 101 and 112.

[17] Campbell and Garnett (1884), p. 126.

> and brandish them in your face, or at least display them for you inspection.... Again I assert the Right of Trespass on any plot of Holy Ground which any man has set apart ... to the power of Darkness.

With what attitudes to science and philosophy did Maxwell emerge from his education? We have already noted the practicality of his approach in the context of his work on elastic solids and this aspect was evident in other contexts too. His was of course a practical age. Britain, and especially Scotland, were at the forefront of the industrial revolution, and in Maxwell's case the interests of his father and of his teachers had had a strong technological bias. His father, writing to inform him of the forthcoming Great Exhibition in the Crystal Palace in 1851, observed that splendid though this would be there was unlikely to be anything there that Maxwell had not already seen.[18] Many of the British physical scientists of his own and his father's generations were actively involved in the advancement of technology, and it is noticeable too that William Rankine, who had himself studied a few years before Maxwell under Forbes, Kelland and George Wilson, shared with Maxwell a characteristic fusion of the interests of the scientist and the engineer. In later life Maxwell was to write several papers directed specifically at engineering problems. Meanwhile, his practical interest was already apparent, not only in his science but even throughout his philosophical discourse. Having noted the way in which Hamilton's ideas remained Maxwell's common vantage point in his excursions into speculative thinking, Campbell adds that[19]

> the great difference [was] that while Sir William remained for the most part within the sphere of Abstract Logic, Maxwell ever sought to bring each 'concept' to the test of fact.

Reading the work of the positivist philosopher Comte in this period, Maxwell noted that 'Comte has good ideas about method, but no notion of what is meant by a person'.[20] Something of what he meant by this may be gleaned from a discussion of logic in the course of a long letter to Campbell on the subject of moral philosophy, written while he was still at Edinburgh:[21]

> [Philosophers] say that Understanding ought to work by the rules of right reason. These rules are, or ought to be, contained in Logic; but the actual science of Logic is conversant at present only with things either certain, impossible, or *entirely* doubtful, none of which (fortunately) we have to reason

18 Campbell and Garnett (1884), p. 106.
19 Campbell and Garnett (1884), p. 66.
20 Campbell and Garnett (1884), p. 148.
21 Campbell and Garnett (1884), p. 97.

> on. Therefore the true Logic for this world is the Calculus of Probabilities, which takes account of the magnitude of the probability (which is, or which ought to be in a reasonable man's mind). This branch of Math., which is generally thought to favour gambling, dicing, and wagering, and therefore highly immoral, is the only "Mathematics for Practical Men", as we ought to be.

The sequel is also worth quoting:

> Now, as human knowledge comes by the senses in such a way that the existence of things external is only inferred from the harmonious (not similar) testimony of the different senses, Understanding, acting by the laws of right reason, will assign to different truths (or facts, or testimonies, or what shall I call them) different degrees of probability. Now, as the senses give new testimonies continually, and as no one ever detected in them any real inconsistency, it follows that the probability and *credibility* of their testimony is increasing day by day, and the more a man uses them the more he believes them. What is believing? When the probability (there is no better word found) in a man's mind of a certain proposition being true is greater than that of its being false, he believes it with a proportion of faith corresponding to the probability, and this probability may be increased or diminished by new facts. This is faith in general. When a man thinks he has enough of evidence for some notion of his he sometimes refuses to listen to any additional evidence *pro* or *con*, saying, "It is a settled question, *probatis probata*; it needs no evidence; it is certain." This is knowledge as distinguished from faith. He says, "I do not believe; I know." "If any man thinketh that he knoweth, he knoweth yet nothing as he ought to know."

Maxwell's discussion of the calculus of probabilities as the basis for the rules of reason was probably inspired by his recent reading, for there are resonances with contemporary writings by Boole, Herschel and Whewell, with all of which he was almost certainly familiar, But his expression of the ideas nevertheless seems characteristically original. At any rate Maxwell appears to have been moving, by his own route, in a very similar direction to Whewell, who also treated fact and opinion as essentially relative and subjective. Just as Whewell had been concerned that a philosophy of science should have some relation to the way in which scientists behaved, so Maxwell was concerned that logic should be related to the way in which the mind actually functioned.

The quotations given above demonstrate forcefully and eloquently that Maxwell's practical attitude, though it permeated his philosophy, did not in any sense lead him away from philosophy. On the contrary, as Campbell records, he was extremely fond of metaphysics, in which he adopted a thoroughly dynamical attitude. He wrote to Campbell in 1856 that[22]

> I find I get fonder of metaphysics and less of calculation continually, and my

[22] Campbell and Garnett (1884), p. 178.

> metaphysics are fast settling into the rigid high style, that is about ten times as far *above* Whewell as Mill is *below* him, or Comte or Macaulay *below* Mill, using above and below conventionally, like *up* and *down* in Bradshaw [the railway timetable].

Campbell also notes Maxwell's keen interest in theology, and although any Victorian *Life and Letters* may be expected to over-emphasise the religiosity of its subject—especially, perhaps, when its author was like Campbell an ordained member of the church—there can be no doubting the truth of this impression. At the time Maxwell was in Cambridge, Anglican theology was going through a period of intense and often bitter debate, and it is clear that Maxwell not only read both widely and deeply but actually disputed too.[23] He did not, however, associate with any particular school or sect. His own upbringing had been divided between the Presbyterian (protestant) and Episcopal (Anglican) churches and he was, to quote Campbell 'too much the heir of all the ages'; as he himself expressed it, his faith was 'too deep to be in bondage to any set of opinions'.[24]

More significant by far than any single aspect of Maxwell's study, be it science, philosophy or religion, was the way in which these were blended together and treated by him as a whole. Having asserted as part of his great plan for self-improvement, quoted above, that no plot of holy ground should be allowed to be set apart to the power of darkness, he continued to argue in a way reminiscent of Coleridge that[25]

> No one but a Christian can actually purge his land of these holy spots. Any one may profess that he has none, but something will soon occur to every one to show him that part of his ground is not open to the public. . . . Christianity . . . is the only scheme or form of belief which disavows any possessions on such a tenure. Here alone all is free. You may fly to the ends of the world and find no God but the Author of Salvation. You may search the Scriptures and not find a text to stop you in your explorations.

Perhaps the most eloquent expressions both of his faith and of the way in which this related intimately to his scientific work and study are the two poems given at the beginning and end of this volume, the first written in 1853, at a time of happiness, the second shortly after his father's death in 1856. The way in which religion and philosophy came together not only to enrich his science but actually to direct it may be seen from a remarkable letter to Campbell of 1851. This was Maxwell's creed:[26]

> I believe, with the Westminster Divines and their predecessors *ad infinitum* that "Man's chief end is to glorify God and to enjoy him forever."

[23] Campbell and Garnett (1884), p. 114.
[24] Campbell and Garnett (1884), p. 119.
[25] Campbell and Garnett (1884), p. 126.
[26] Campbell and Garnett (1884), pp. 110–11.

That for this end to every man has been given a progressively increasing power of communication with other creatures. That with his powers his susceptibilities increase.

That happiness is indissolubly connected with the full exercise of these powers in their intended direction. That Happiness and Misery must inevitably increase with increasing Power and Knowledge. That the translation from the one course to the other is essentially *miraculous*, while the progress is natural. But the subject is too high. I will not, however, stop short, but proceed to Intellectual Pursuits.

It is natural to suppose that the soul, if not clothed with a body, would run on in an unprogressive circle of barren meditation. In order to advance the soul must converse with things external to itself.

In every branch of knowledge the progress is proportional to the amount of facts on which to build, and therefore to the facility of obtaining data. In the Mathematics this is easy. Do you want a quantity? Take x; there it is!—got without trouble, and as good a quantity as one would wish to have. And so in other sciences,—the more abstract the subject, the better it is known. Space, time, and force come first in certainty. These are the subjects in Mechanics.

Then the active powers, Light, Heat, Electricity, etc. = Physics.

Then the differences and relations of Matter = Chemistry, and so on.

Here the order of advancement is just that of abstractedness and inapplicability to the actual. What poor blind things we Maths. think ourselves! But see the Chemists! Chemistry is a pack of cards, which the labour of hundreds is slowly arranging; and one or two tricks,—faint imitations of Nature,—have been played. Yet Chemistry is far before all the Natural History sciences; all these before Medicine; Medicine before Metaphysics, Law, and Ethics; and these I think before Pneumatology and Theology.

Now each of these makes up in interest what it wants in advancement.

There is no doubt that of all earthly creatures Man is the most important to us, yet we know less of him than any other. His history is more interesting than natural history; but nat. history, though obscure, is much more intelligible than man's history, which is a tale half told, and which, even when this world's course is run, and when, as some think, man may compare notes with other rational beings, will still be a great mystery, of which the beginning and the end are all that can be known to us while the intermediate parts are perpetually filled up.

So now pray excuse me if I think that the more grovelling and materialistic sciences of matter are not to be despised in comparison with the lofty studies of Minds and Spirits. Our own and our neighbours' minds are known but very imperfectly, and no new facts will be found till we come in contact with some minds other than human to elicit them by counterposition. But of this more anon.

Maxwell's description of light, heat and electricity in terms of active powers, and of mechanics as composed of space, time and force rather than space, time and matter, were of course in tune with the dynamistic approach of scientists such as Faraday, and no doubt reflected the standard teaching at Edinburgh, with which Campbell would have been familiar. More interesting are his emphasis upon the value of science as a medium for the development of the individual soul and his harmonising of a practical and empirical attitude with a dynamistic and metaphysical overview. Both were to be continuing features of his work in physics.

Mathematics of the magnetic field

After graduating, Maxwell stayed on at Trinity, first as a Bachelor Scholar and then as a Fellow. While he had been a student he had published a number of papers on mathematics, but once free from the tripos he turned his attention back to literature, philosophy and physics, and in particular to the theory of colour vision and the theories of electricity and magnetism. Of these two project areas the study of colour vision at first dominated, as Maxwell sought to develop and substantiate a set of ideas dating back to his Edinburgh days. Very briefly, the traditional theory of colour vision, which was still defended in Edinburgh, for example, by Brewster, was based on the hypothesis of three kinds of corpuscular light (red, blue and yellow), distributed in varying proportions throughout the spectrum. A rival theory based on three different receptors in the eye had been put forward at the turn of the century by Thomas Young, in the context of a wave theory of light, but had been neither proven nor, it would appear, taken very seriously. Following the success of Fresnel's wave theory of light, however, a number of scientists including Maxwell had independently revived the receptor theory in the 1840s. Maxwell and Forbes, working together, had been able to demonstrate that the primary colours were red, blue and green rather than red, blue and yellow, the apparent primary nature of yellow being a secondary absorption effect in pigments. Maxwell had also begun to test the receptor theory experimentally, constructing a 'colour top' with which to test the effect on different individuals of different colour combinations. Returning to the subject in 1854 he quickly built up a corpus of personal colour equations, demonstrating the dependence of colour vision upon the individual, showing in particular that colour blindness ('Daltonism' after a famous colour blind scientist, John Dalton) resulted from a defect in one or more of the receptors, and developing for a typical or average fully-sighted person a full set of exact colour equations. In effect, Maxwell did nothing less than develop the modern theory of colour vision. Typically, he also looked into the general philosophy of perception, reading for example Berkeley and Mill, and began to investigate the physiology of the problem, devising an instrument with which to see through the pupil into the eye.[27]

[27] For a detailed treatment of this work see Sherman (1981), and for a briefer survey Everitt (1975).

Maxwell was to continue his experiments on vision throughout the greater part of his life, but once he had sufficiently demonstrated and written up the receptor theory, and even, indeed, before that, the main focus of his research shifted to the science of electricity and magnetism. This was again a subject he had pursued in Edinburgh. Like Thomson a few years earlier he had studied and been dissatisifed with Murphy's Poissonian textbook, and he had also become familiar, though not yet perhaps intimate, with the work of Faraday. He had not, however, immersed himself thoroughly in the subject, and he was still somewhat cautious of it. Writing to Thomson in February 1854, soon after graduating, he asked his advice on how to approach it systematically.[28]

> Suppose a man to have a popular knowledge of electrical show experiments and a little antipathy to Murphy's Electricity, how ought he to proceed in reading & working so as to get a little insight into the subject wh may be of use in further reading?
>
> If he wished to read Ampere Faraday &c how should they be arranged, and at what stage & in what order might he read your articles in the Cambridge Journal?

Thomson's reply has not survived, but we know it took the form of a 'long letter about electricity',[29] and some years later, in the preface to his *Treatise on Electricity and Magnetism* (*Treatise* for short), Maxwell recalled that, following Thomson's guidance, he had begun his research with a study of Faraday's work.[30]

> Before I began the study of electricity I resolved to read no mathematics on the subject till I had first read through Faraday's *Experimental Researches in Electricity*. I was aware that there was supposed to be a difference between Faraday's way of conceiving phenomena and that of the mathematicians, so that neither he nor they were satisfied with each other's language. I had also the conviction that this discrepancy did not arise from either party being wrong. I was first convinced of this by Sir William Thomson ...

From Maxwell's subsequent correspondence with Thomson it would appear that he combined the study of Faraday's work with that of Thomson's own papers, pursuing this thread of research alongside his optical work through 1854. Only in 1855 did he take up the serious study of the 'heavy German writers'—principally Weber and Neumann—and of Poisson.[31] By then he had already developed his own perspective on the

[28] Maxwell to Thomson, 20 February 1854, in Larmor (1937), p. 3.

[29] Maxwell to Thomson, 13 November 1854, in Larmor (1937), p. 7.

[30] Maxwell (1954), volume 1, p. viii.

[31] Maxwell to Thomson, 13 November 1854, 15 May 1855 and 13 September 1855, in Larmor (1937), pp. 7–19; Maxwell to his father, 5 May 1855 and 5 October 1855, in Campbell and Garnett (1884), pp. 154,158.

subject, substantially the same as that he published in his famous paper on 'Faraday's lines of force', which he wrote up in the winter of 1855–6.[32]

Maxwell's paper on 'Faraday's lines of force' has been much discussed but much misunderstood by historians of science. The basic form of the paper was not so much that of an original contribution as that of a constructive review, of a similar type to those in which Niels Bohr would specialise in the twentieth century. Maxwell's personal aims in this respect were clearly expressed in a letter to Thomson of 13 September 1855, a few weeks before he wrote the paper itself, in which he also noted the dependence of his work on the writings of Thomson himself and Faraday.[33]

> I have got a good deal out of you on electrical subjects, both directly & through the printer & publisher & I have also read other helps and read Faraday's three volumes of researches. My object in doing so was of course to learn what had been done in electrical science, mathematical & experimental, and to try to comprehend the same in a rational manner by the aid of any notions I could screw into my head.

A venture such as that described by Maxwell is normally a preliminary to original research rather than the subject of a publication, but in this case the topic was so difficult, and the existing investigations were so disconnected, that the establishment of a coherent view of the existing knowledge and ideas itself constituted a significant advance. Opening his published paper, Maxwell explained that electrical science as it stood was a hodgepodge of unconnected or incompletely connected areas, some of which lacked even the most basic empirical data while others were the subject of masses of difficult mathematics. Any major development of the theory would have to incorporate connections between the different parts, and to do so in such a way as to tie in with all the existing laws. To do this, he suggested, the student would have to 'make himself familiar with a considerable body of most intricate mathematics, the mere retention of which in the memory materially interferes with further progress.'[34] In these circumstances, he argued, the first requirement was for the simplification and clarification of the existing knowledge, which was what he proposed to provide:[35]

> The first process therefore in the effectual study of [electrical] science, must be one of simplification and reduction of the results of previous investigations to a form in which the mind can grasp them.

Absolutely central to the process of Maxwell's review, and, as we shall

[32] Maxwell (1856).
[33] Maxwell to Thomson, 13 September 1855, in Larmor (1937), p. 17.
[34] Maxwell (1890 and 1965), volume 1, p. 155.
[35] Maxwell (1890 and 1965), volume 1, p. 155.

see, to his whole approach to physical science, was the principle implied in the above quotations that the known results should be expressed in 'a form in which the mind can grasp them' or, to return to his earlier and more personal expression, 'by the aid of any notions I could screw into my head'. While working on the investigation in June 1855 he wrote to his friend R B Litchfield that he was hard at work 'grinding out "appropriate ideas", as Whewell calls them', and in the paper on 'Faraday's lines of force' he talked again of the importance of 'exciting appropriate mathematical ideas'.[36] In the paper this approach was described in terms of a 'method of physical analogy', and we shall come back shortly to precisely what Maxwell meant by that, and to how the method he advocated tied in with what he actually did. First, though, we must consider the outcome of Maxwell's investigations as recorded in his letters to Thomson and in the published paper.

In simple scientific terms Maxwell's achievement was to mathematise the work of Faraday. As we saw in the last chapter this was a process which had been begun by Thomson, but whereas Thomson had concentrated on reconciling Faraday's results with the action-at-a-distance mathematics of traditional electrical theory, Maxwell's procedure was to start with Faraday's work, including his theoretical notions as well as his experimental results, to extract therefrom the key 'appropriate ideas', and then to seek a natural mathematical formulation of these. The initial attraction of Faraday's work for Maxwell's purposes was obvious, for the *Experimental Researches in Electricity*' constituted a detailed survey of all that was known experimentally about electricity and magnetism, and one that could be taken as effectively theory-free. Once into Faraday's work, however, Maxwell found much more than the empirical information he sought, and something of the excitement he must have felt is conveyed by the advice he gave to others in the *Treatise*. Having recommended that every student should read Ampère's work as an example of 'scientific style in the statement of a discovery', he urged that:[37]

> He should also study Faraday for the cultivation of a scientific spirit, by means of the action and reaction which will take place between the newly discovered facts as introduced to him by Faraday and the nascent ideas in his own mind.

Evidently Maxwell himself had experienced something of such an action and reaction, for elsewhere in the same work he urged his readers 'to read

[36] Maxwell to Litchfield, 6 June 1855, in Campbell and Garnett (1884), p. 156; Maxwell (1890 and 1965), volume 1, p. 157.

[37] Maxwell (1954), volume 2, p. 176. See also Campbell and Garnett (1882), p. 302, where Faraday's work is described by Maxwell as 'the nucleus of everything electric since 1830'.

carefully Faraday's *Experimental Researches in Electricity'*, and declared that:[38]

> If by anything I have here written I may assist any student in understanding Faraday's modes of thought and expression, I shall regard it as the accomplishment of one of my principal aims—to communicate to others the same delight which I have found myself in reading Faraday's *Researches*.

What Maxwell found in particular in Faraday's work were an attitude with which he was in strong sympathy and a set of guiding ideas that seemed to lend themselves quite naturally to mathematical expression. The attitude was a dynamical one, incorporating a search for unity and an emphasis upon observed behaviour rather than the mechanists' use of hypothesis. The guiding ideas, which represented different but interrelated physical ways of looking at things, were those of the electrotonic state, magnetic lines of force existing throughout space and independent of the matter of the magnet, and media characterised by polarity and strain. Within this complex of ideas, the magnetic lines were dominant in Faraday's more recent work, but the idea of polarity also had a special status as a 'first, essential, and fundamental principle', to which all the other conceptions used were related.[39] The 'Idea of polarity', besides having a long pedigree in the dynamical tradition, had also been treated by Whewell as the key appropriate idea for the next phase of the development of physical science, and it seems to have been the first of Faraday's ideas to be extracted by Maxwell for further consideration.

The results of the first stage of Maxwell's investigation are given in a letter to Thomson of November 1854, from which it would appear that Maxwell had already had some success in translating Faraday's researches into mathematical language. He had of course been helped significantly in this by being able to draw on Thomson's own past work, but he had also found that, quite generally, Faraday's work lent itself remarkably well to mathematical expression. Later he would describe Faraday as having been 'in reality a mathematician of a very high order',[40] not in the normal sense of someone adept at technical mathematics, which Faraday was not, but in the sense of someone who used physical ideas in much the same way as a mathematician would use mathematical concepts, 'by means of which we form a mental representation of the facts, sufficiently general, on the one hand, to stand for any particular case, and sufficiently exact, on the other, to warrant the deductions we may draw from them by the application of mathematical reasoning.'[41] In his letter to Thomson, Maxwell first thanked

[38] Maxwell (1954), volume 1, p. xi.
[39] Faraday (1965), volume 1, paragraph 1162.
[40] Maxwell (1890 and 1965), volume 2, p. 360.
[41] Maxwell (1890 and 1965), volume 2, p. 360.

him for the long letter on electricity that Thomson had sent in response to his earlier request and reported that, after involving himself in the subject, he had 'been rewarded of late by finding the whole mass of confusion beginning to clear up under the influence of a few simple ideas'.[42] Using Thomson's own work on the heat analogy of electrostatics, Maxwell had encountered no difficulties with that subject; but electrodynamics had proved more difficult. He had read and admired Ampère's works, but suspected shrewdly that Ampère's presentation 'must have been got up, after Ampère had convinced himself, in order to suit his views of philosphical inquiry, and as an example of what it ought to be.' He did not disbelieve Ampère's claims, but he had some trouble relating the theory to its empirical foundations, and was 'not satisfied with the form of the theory which treats of elementary currents & their reciprocal actions, & I did not see how any general theory was to be formed from it.'[43] He was, however, able to build something on Faraday's ideas, and in particular, though he was principally concerned with electricity, on the ideas of magnetic polarity and the magnetic field.[44]

> Now I have heard you speak of "magnetic lines of force" & Faraday seems to make great use of them . . . Now I thought that as every current generated magnetic lines & was acted on in a manner determined by the lines thro wh: it passed that something might be done by considering "magnetic polarization" as a property of a "magnetic field" or space and developing the geometrical ideas according to this view. I use the word "polarization" to express the fact that at a point of space the south pole of a small magnet is attracted in a certain direction with a certain force. "Polarity" is a property of magnets &c to produce pol^{n}.

Polarisation, it should be noted, was a vector quantity, indicating a direction as well as a force.

Although Maxwell implied that he was setting down ideas that Thomson must already have explored, and although he was, and was to remain, indebted to Thomson for the bulk of his mathematics, their approaches to Faraday's work were completely different. Thomson had recognised the importance of this work, but being unsympathetic with the speculative element in Faraday's physical approach he had started from the mathematical formulae and sought to incorporate elements of Faraday's work in them. Maxwell, in contrast, had gone right to the heart of Faraday's physical attitude, and by developing a geometry or visual calculus of magnetic polarisation akin to that of flow lines and surfaces in the heat analogy he was already able to make some headway. His analysis, which he sketched

[42] Maxwell to Thomson, 13 November 1854, in Larmor (1937), p. 7.
[43] Maxwell to Thomson, 13 November 1854, in Larmor (1937), p. 8.
[44] Maxwell to Thomson, 13 November 1854, in Larmor (1937), p. 8.

out in the letter to Thomson, is worth quoting at length. He began with two definitions that were explicitly provisional and subject to modification.[45]

> (1) The pol^n of a curve in space is the integral of the pol^n at any point resolved along it mult: into the element of the curve.
>
> (2) The pol^n of a surface is the integral of the pol^n resolved in the normal into the element of surface.
>
> The pol^n of a curve or surface arising from several sources is the algebraic sum of the effects taken separately.

Maxwell then introduced the relationship between a helical current and its magnetic effect as demonstrated by Ampère and drew some elementary conclusions.[46]

> It appears from experiment that the mag: effect of a current forming a helix of small uniform section at any point may be reduced to two forces of opposite kinds directed to the extremities and $\propto 1/d^2$.
>
> Whence it is easy to find the effect of a small circular current on a point at some distance from it. When forces act centrally according to the law of inverse square the pol^n of any closed curve is zero & that of any closed surface not passing thro the magnetic substance is zero.

Next he considered a magnetic surface, viewed, as by Ampère, as a surface of small electrical circuits, and deduced two theorems on the relationship between currents and polarisation.[47]

> Now let a number of little circuits be disposed so as to cover a given portion of a surface then the effect of any external point will be the same as that of a uniformly magnetized lamina (see your paper) and if we remove one of the circuits & draw a closed curve so as not to pass thro any one, its pol^n will be zero. But if we replace the circuit the pol^n will depend entirely on the strength of the circuit wh: thus is linked into the closed curve & will measure the intensity of the current as may be easily shown.
>
> But in this case we may suppose that all the contiguous currents of the small circuits destroy each other, leaving the current round the boundary. Hence these theorems
>
> (1) The pol^n of any closed curve is measured by the sum of the intensities of all the currents which pass thro' it.
>
> (2) The pol^n of any surface, round the boundary of wh: a current passes, is measured by the intensity of that current.

Maxwell did not express these theorems mathematically, and it is not clear precisely what he meant by the intensity of a current. He may not have been

[45] Maxwell to Thomson, 13 November 1854, in Larmor (1937), p. 8.
[46] Maxwell to Thomson, 13 November 1854, in Larmor (1937), p. 8.
[47] Maxwell to Thomson, 13 November 1854, in Larmor (1937), pp. 8–9.

entirely clear himself. But it may be helpful to translate the theorems at least partially into mathematical form, taking $\mathcal{M}$ as the magnetic polarisation, $\mathcal{M}_\lambda$ and $\mathcal{M}_n$ its components along a line of element $d\lambda$ and perpendicular to a surface of element $d\sigma$ respectively:

$$\oint \mathcal{M}_\lambda \, d\lambda = \iint_{\substack{\text{any surface bounded} \\ \text{by closed curve}}} \text{('Intensities of currents' passing through surface)} \tag{4.1}$$

$$\iint \mathcal{M}_n \, d\sigma = \text{'Intensity of current' in circuit bounding surface.} \tag{4.2}$$

In approaching electromagnetic theory in this way Maxwell had gone straight to the central feature in Faraday's work of the unity and partial symmetry between the electrical and magnetic forces. He also seems to have adopted from Faraday the image of interlocking closed lines of electric and magnetic force, and it is tempting to see his theorems as an attempt to construct some sort of symmetrical foundation for the science of electricity and magnetism based on this image. If in particular we treat what Maxwell calls the intensity of the current as the potential gradient at a point in the circuit, so that the right-hand sides of equations (4.1) and (4.2) become surface and line integrals respectively, the equations may be written symmetrically in terms of the magnetic polarisation and potential gradient. Maxwell did not do this, however.

In the next stage of his analysis, Maxwell re-derived an expression for the magnetic polarisation in terms of lines of force and the surfaces of equal potential (on the heat flow analogy) perpendicular to them. He quantified the lines of force by dividing the surfaces into elements of equal surface polarisation, and by taking a family of surfaces dividing the whole of space into cells of equal polarisation and 'potential difference'. In this way he was able to return to Faraday's relations between electric currents and numbers of lines and surfaces, but with the numbers exactly defined:[48]

> On any of the "equipotential surfaces" (or surfaces perp to the lines of force) draw two systems of curves so as to divide the surface into small elements, the pol^n of each of wh: is the same. Let lines of force move so as to pass thro' these curves so as to generate what I call ("surfaces of no pol^n") then these surfaces will intersect other equipotential surfaces forming elements of the same amount of pol^n as before. Finally let a series of equipotential surfaces be drawn so that the diff. of potential is the same between each.
>
> All space is now cut up into elements. Call the intersections of the surfaces of no pol^n "lines of no pol^n" then
>
> (1) The pol^n of a surface is expressed by the *number* of lines wh cut it.
>
> (2) The pol^n of a line is expressed by the number of equip^l surfaces wh: it cuts.

[48] Maxwell to Thomson, 13 November 1854, in Larmor (1937), p. 9.

> The work done by any displacement of two circuits is measured by the increase of the number of lines of pol^{n} wh pass thro both circuits.

Having developed a geometry of magnetic polarisation, Maxwell next turned to the theory of currents and indicated how a similar structure could be built upon the concept of electric motion, with definitions of the electric motion of a line and of a surface:[49]

> Let u, v, w be the vel^{ies} of a current in xyz that is, the quantity of electricity wh passes across unit section in unit time. XYZ electromotive forces, k coeff^{t} of resistance p electric tension at any point
>
> $$\mathrm{d}p = (X - ku)\,\mathrm{d}x + (Y - kv)\,\mathrm{d}y + (Z - kw)\,\mathrm{d}z$$
>
> also
>
> $$\frac{\mathrm{d}u}{\mathrm{d}x} + \frac{\mathrm{d}v}{\mathrm{d}y} + \frac{\mathrm{d}w}{\mathrm{d}z}\ [=0]$$
>
> From these notions we get the following which correspond to what we had in magnetism. Surfaces of equal tension cutting lines of electric motion at right angles. Electric motion along any curve made up of the sums of electric motions along its elements. Electric motion thro a surface made up of electric motion thro each element. When the surface is closed the whole electric motion is zero.

Again it is unclear what is meant by the electrical parameter used, now 'electric motion'. The suggested symmetry with the magnetic case points towards the gradient of the electric potential, or gradient of electric tension, but the phrase 'electric motion' and the closed surface equation point towards electric flux or velocity. This aspect of the analysis was, anyway, taken no further. Instead Maxwell returned to the magnetic imagery for the expression of electromotive force.[50]

> The electromotive force along any line is measured by the number of lines of pol^{n} wh that line cuts in unit of time. Hence the electromotive force round a given circuit depends on the decrease of the number of lines wh: pass thro it in unit of time, that is, on the decrease of the whole pol^{n} of any surface bounded by the circuit.

As with his other conclusions this was not mathematically expressed, but this time it may easily be so:

$$\oint \boldsymbol{X} \cdot \mathrm{d}\boldsymbol{\lambda} = -\frac{\partial}{\partial t} \iint \mathcal{M} \cdot \mathrm{d}\boldsymbol{\sigma} \qquad (4.3)$$

with $\boldsymbol{X}$ the electromotive force at a point.

[49] Maxwell to Thomson, 13 November 1854, in Larmor (1937), p. 9.
[50] Maxwell to Thomson, 13 November 1854, in Larmor (1937), p. 9.

Finally, Maxwell noted an attempted application of his approach on which he had been working, discussed briefly its implications for the theory of magnetic induction, and put to Thomson a number of questions: had he published any general theory relating to his work on the existence and uniqueness of the potential function for inhomogeneous media; where could Weber's theory be read; and might electrostatic phenomena be considered as extreme cases of electric conduction with high tension and high resistance.

Maxwell's analysis in this letter was neither rigorous nor even, it would appear, entirely coherent. But he did not claim that it was so. As he explained to Thomson, he was simply putting the 'electronic state of my mind before you that you may see how I am trying to make everything cohere, perhaps prematurely, and that you may know the kind of answers I want to my enquiries.'[51] He was clearly proceeding by guesswork and physical intuition as much as by mathematical analysis, and was still at the stage of sketching out the form that a geometrisation of Faraday's work might take, rather than at that of attempting even a first draft of a formal analysis. He had taken some very important steps. He had partially overcome Thomson's confusion between the quantity and the intensity of the magnetic field (flux and force analogies). Whereas Thomson in his mathematical treatment of magnetism had adopted functions corresponding roughly to Maxwell's line and surface polarisations as alternative representations of magnetic force, Maxwell saw the need for including both aspects. Again, Maxwell had begun to bring together the formulations of electricity and magnetism within a unified framework. In doing so he had captured something of Faraday's notion of symmetric systems of lines of electric and magnetic force, and of his image of interlocking closed lines, both of which were to prove valuable guides as his work progressed. But still it was all very incomplete. In particular, the combined problem of the symmetric representation of electricity and magnetism and the selection of appropriate functions of quantity and intensity was still causing confusion. Indeed the quantity–intensity distinction itself, which was to be crucial to the formulation of his representation of Faraday's work, may not yet have been consciously made.[52] But he had made a good start.

Over the next year Maxwell broadened his reading on electromagnetic theory to cover all the main continental contributions to the subject but without coming across anything that might cause him to change his own approach. The most significant of the continental works so far as his own pro-

[51] Maxwell to Thomson, 13 November 1854, in Larmor (1937), p. 9.

[52] Wise (1979) seems to have interpreted the letter in terms of a clear distinction between quantity and intensity and a clear image of Faraday's 'mutually embracing' lines of electric and magnetic force. While this interpretation is an attractive one, however, it cannot in my view be made without some distortion of what Maxwell wrote and is, I think, reading in too much.

gramme was concerned was the theory of Weber, for built upon the foundations of Ampère's electrodynamics this was a complete action-at-a-distance theory of electromagnetic phenomena. But Maxwell wrote to Thomson in May 1855 that 'I confess I like it not at first'. In order to build up a mathematical theory able to cover all the known laws of electricity and magnetism Weber had had to assume that the force acting between two current elements was not of the simple form upon which Ampère had insisted, but was dependent on the relative velocity and acceleration of the elements as well as upon their relative position. Maxwell found this artificial, and when he wrote to Thomson again in September it was to confirm his first impression. Weber's theory was one 'which ought to be compared with others and certainly gives many true results', but these results were 'at the expense of several startling assumptions', and the whole 'a mathematical speculation which I do not believe.'[53] For completeness and comparison he included a brief sketch of the theory in his paper on 'Faraday's lines of force', but he made no secret of his dissatisfaction with it.[54] One reason Maxwell gave for his position was that the principle of conservation of energy as expounded by Helmholtz ten years earlier required that the force between two particles should be along the line joining them, and should depend on their distance apart only, not on their relative velocity or acceleration. This argument, which had been put forward by Helmholtz himself, was not wholly sound and was eventually refuted by Weber.[55] It was not, however, Maxwell's main objection, which was more fundamental, and was the traditional dynamical objection to molecular–mechanical hypotheses. From Maxwell's viewpoint Weber's theory did not contribute any physical understanding of the phenomena to be explained. More serious still, by representing the phenomena in terms of what appeared from the physical viewpoint to be an arbitrary hypothesis it actually hindered such an understanding. As he explained in the paper,[56]

> I do not think that we have any right at present to understand the action of electricity, and I hold that the chief merit of a temporary theory [i.e. Maxwell's own] is, that it shall guide experiment, without impeding the progress of the true theory when it appears.

Later, in the *Treatise*, he explained that 'these physical hypotheses . . . are entirely alien from the way of looking at things which I adopt.'[57]

If Maxwell gained relatively little from his study of the continental writers he was nevertheless able to make significant progress in the course of 1855

[53] Maxwell to Thomson, 15 May 1855 and 13 September 1855, in Larmor (1937), pp. 11 and 17.
[54] Maxwell (1890 and 1965), volume 1, pp. 207*ff*.
[55] See for example Everitt (1974), p. 205.
[56] Maxwell (1890 and 1965), volume 1, p. 208.
[57] Maxwell (1954), volume 1, p. x.

with the development of his own view. One of the questions he had asked Thomson in the November letter had concerned Thomson's discussion of the continuity equation for the case of inhomogeneous media (equation (3.23)), and by May 1855 he had developed his physical concepts sufficiently to attempt a representation of electromagnetism in terms of a generalisation of Thomson's heat analogy to the mathematics of fluid motion in inhomogeneous media, based on the mathematical work of Thomson himself and of Stokes:[58]

> I am trying to construct two theories, mathematically identical, in one of which the elementary conceptions shall be about fluid particles attracting at a distance while in the other nothing (mathematical) is considered but various states of polarization tension &c at various parts of space. The result will resemble your analogy of the steady motion of heat. Have you patented that notion with all its applications? for I intend to borrow it for a season, without mentioning anything about heat (except of course historically) but applying it in a somewhat different way to a more general case to which the laws of heat will not apply.

By September Maxwell had embarked on the writing of 'Faraday's lines of force', and was asking Thomson 'whether you have not the whole draught of the thing lying in loose papers', and neglected until he had time to pursue it.[59] He had, he said, begun his project 'for the sake of acquiring knowledge sufficient to guide me in devising experiments', but he was now able to envisage the possibility that he might 'be satisifed that the theory would stick together all through, and that I could put it into a form not too abstrusely mathematical, but still exact and leading to numerical results.'[60] There could be no doubt, as Maxwell pointed out, that Thomson must have the mathematical part of the theory, since it was from his writings that Maxwell had gleaned it. There was also enough in Thomson's writings to suggest that he might already have framed a general theory of electricity and magnetism based on the heat and elastic solid analogies, without having published it explicitly. If so, then Maxwell urged him to publish it. If not, he implied, he would publish his own treatment:[61]

> I do not know the Game-laws & Patent-laws of science. Perhaps the Association may do something to fix them but I certainly intend to poach among your electrical images, and as for the hints you have dropped about the 'higher' electricity, I intend to take them.

[58] Maxwell to Thomson, 15 May 1855, in Larmor (1937), p. 11.
[59] Maxwell to Thomson, 13 September 1855, in Larmor (1937), p. 18.
[60] Maxwell to Thomson, 13 September 1855, in Larmor (1937), p. 18. 'The Association' was the British Association for the Advancement of Science.
[61] Maxwell to Thomson, 13 September 1855, in Larmor (1937), pp. 18–19.

Maxwell's plan was still the same as that he had outlined in his May letter, to draw up two theories, one essentially geometrical and independent of the phenomena to be treated and the other mathematically identical but incorporating the laws of electricity and magnetism. His approach was also substantially the same as that he had adopted in his original analysis of November 1854; only having worked out the appropriate mathematical framework and physical correspondences he could now discard the guiding notion of polarity in favour of the geometrical image of the lines of force:[62]

> Now I have been planning and partly executing a system of propositions about lines of force &c which may be *afterwards* applied to Electricity, Heat or Magnetism or Galvanism, but which is in itself a collection of purely geometrical truths embodied in geometrical conceptions of lines, surfaces &c.
>
> The first part of my design is to prove by popular, that is not professedly symbolic, reasoning, the most important propositions about V [the potential function] and about the solution of the equation in the last page [equation (3.23)] and to trace the lines of force and surfaces of equal V.
>
> The second part would be nothing else than a collection of examples of your "Electrical Images" worked out by the method of lines of force & equipotential surfaces, for cases of spheres of various conducting powers and for the case of a sphere of a "magnecrystallic" substance in a uniform field.
>
> The third part would be the theory of the connections of the three divisions of the subject, the passage of statical into current electricity and the magnetic properties of closed currents with the laws of induced current.
>
> I intend next to apply to these facts Faraday's notion of an *electronic* [*sic*] state. I have worked a good deal of mathematical material out of this vein and I believe I have got hold of several truths which will find a mathematical expression in the electrotonic state.
>
> One thing at least it succeeds in, it reduces to one principle not only the attraction of currents & the induction of currents but also the attraction of electrified bodies without any new assumption.

With some slight change in order, this programme was duly fulfilled.

Faraday's lines of force

The paper on 'Faraday's lines of force', which was completed over the next few weeks, was composed of two parts read to the Cambridge Philosophical Society in December 1855 and February 1856. The first part opened with a methodological introduction, to which we shall return in the next section. Maxwell then gave an outline of the theory of the motion of an incompressible fluid expressed geometrically, and for the most part without any mathematical equations, in terms of tubes of flow, or 'tubes of fluid

[62] Maxwell to Thomson, 13 September 1855, in Larmor (1937), pp. 17–18.

motion'. Taking lines of fluid motions as representations of the direction of flow, any tube generated by these lines had, since there could be no flow across its walls, a constant flux across any section. A system of unit tubes could therefore be defined so that the flux across any section in any tube was the same. Such a system filling the whole volume of the fluid constituted a complete geometrical description of the motion, with sinks and sources where the tubes met a bounding surface.[63] For the motion of an imponderable incompressible fluid through a resisting medium, surfaces of equal pressure could be defined perpendicular to the tubes of fluid motion, and these could be taken so as to divide the tubes into unit cells, with the ratio of cross section to length being proportional to the resistance of the medium. For a given resistance, knowledge of the surfaces of equal pressure was then sufficient to determine the fluid velocity at any point, and thus the sources and sinks present in the system. Conversely, a knowledge of the sources and sinks could be used to determine the pressure throughout the system. Mathematically, the pressure corresponded to the potential function of the system, and as in the heat analogy a distribution of sources on one side of a closed surface could be represented in its effect on the other side by an equivalent distribution on the surface. Using the technique of equivalent surfaces, and sticking to a purely visual description in terms of tubes of fluid motion, Maxwell next considered the flow across a surface joining two media of different resistances and that across a gradual change in resistance. Only when he generalised still further, to the case in which the resistance was not the same for different directions of motion, did he have to resort to an explicitly mathematical analysis in order to derive the generalised equation of continuity.

Having established the geometry of fluid motion in terms of tubes of force, and having derived a few general propositions, Maxwell turned to electricity and magnetism, and 'to shew how the idea of lines of fluid motion as described above may be modified so as to be applicable to the sciences of statical electricity, permanent magnetism, magnetism of induction, and uniform galvanic currents, reserving the laws of electromagnetism for special consideration.'[64] The analogy for electrostatics had already been derived by Thomson and was straightforward. Charged particles corresponded to sources and sinks, the negative of the electric potential to pressure, and electric force to the negative gradient of pressure, or to the product of the fluid velocity and the coefficient of resistance. The total potential of a system was proportional to the product of the coefficient of resistance (a constant) and the work done by the fluid in overcoming the resistance. Faraday's lines of electric force corresponded to the lines of fluid

[63] This analogy was later taken up by J J Thomson in his attempt to quantise the aether, in the early days of quantum theory. See Hendry (1983b).

[64] Maxwell (1890 and 1965), volume 1, p. 175.

motion and his concept of dielectrics with different specific inductive capacities could be represented by media with different coefficients of resistance.

For magnetism the same analogy could be employed. The poles of magnets were represented as sources and sinks and paramagnetic bodies were represented by media of lower resistance, and diamagnetic bodies by media of higher resistance, than that of the surrounding medium. The lines of force again corresponded to lines of fluid motion, and Faraday's results on diamagnetism could be obtained by consideration of equivalent surfaces or, as by Thomson, by consideration of the total potential or mechanical effect of the system. Maxwell pointed out here that the phenomena of magnetism could actually be visualised in three different ways: through the lines of force, through a field of induced polarisation, the elements of which he briefly outlined, or through the notion of imaginary magnetic matter suggested by the image of equivalent surfaces. There was nothing empirically to distinguish between these, but[65]

> As the theory of lines of force admits of the most precise, and at the same time least theoretic statement, we shall allow it to stand for the present.

Whereas the lines of force presented a geometric image that could be comprehended independent of any physical hypotheses, the alternative images, since they were less vivid geometrically, seemed to require some physical hypothetical notions in order to be readily comprehended. The analogy of lines of force also provided a straightforward representation of the laws of magnecrystallic induction, for which, Maxwell suggested, the alternative images were less directly adapted.

Maxwell next turned to the theory of electric currents, to which the fluid analogy was directly applicable, and to the relationship between this theory and that of electrostatics. In the flow analogy representation of the theory of currents, the resistance of the circuit corresponded to the resistance of a medium and the electric tension to a pressure, and this suggested the identification of electric tension with the (negative) electrostatic potential, and of the resistance of a circuit with the specific inductive capacity of a dielectric. The process of electrostatic induction could be understood as one of electric conduction, but with 'the quantity conducted ... insensible owing to the great resistance of the dielectrics'.[66] The electromotive force driving a continual circulation of current round a closed circuit was then expressed in terms of the difference in electric tension, or potential difference, that it maintained between the poles of the battery.

Maxwell's identification of electrostatic and electrodynamic or galvanic variables is not often commented upon. Perhaps this is because it seems

[65] Maxwell (1890 and 1965), volume 1, p. 180.
[66] Maxwell (1890 and 1965), volume 1, p. 181.

dwarfed by his later union of electricity, magnetism and light, or perhaps it is because we think automatically of the 'potential difference' in a circuit. But for Maxwell the connection was clearly an important one. One of his early questions to Thomson had been concerned with the possibility of making the connection, and his problem in seeing it through. 'I have not made it out yet', he had written in his letter of November 1854, 'or been able to see why there sh[d] be strong attraction along the lines of almost no conduction.'[67] Ten months later, when beginning to write up the published paper, he had seen the establishment of the connection as the 'one thing at least' in which he had succeeded. That the two forms of electricity were fundamentally related had of course been recognised well before Maxwell. Ampère's theory, for example, claimed to derive the laws of electrodynamics from the relations of action-at-a-distance attraction and repulsion between electric particles established for the static case. The notion of a continuous range of dielectric materials ranging from perfect insulators at one end to perfect conductors at the other had also been introduced by Faraday. But no exact connection had been made between the two sets of phenomena. Current electricity was measured in terms of its magnetic effect rather than in the units of electrostatics, and there was as yet no theoretical relationship, nor even any precise experimental relationship, between the two sets of quantities. From Maxwell's viewpoint this was a major bar to a unified theory, and one that it was essential to overcome. In the immediate context of the flow analogy, it was also important to establish a relationship between electrostatics and electrodynamics in order to bring the former fully within the analogy, for so long as electrostatic phenomena could not be envisaged in terms of flow the analogy was of little practical use. Finally, the relationship also served to clarify the problem as to which functions to take from the electrical side in attempting to build up a symmetric foundation for electromagnetic theory.

Following his discussion of electrical circuits and the electromotive forces driving them, Maxwell turned explicitly to the subject of electromotive forces and introduced explicitly for the first time Faraday's distinction between quantities and intensities. In the context of an electric circuit this distinction had already been established by Ohm, the electromotive force, $\mathscr{E}$, and the quantity of current transmitted in unit time or current velocity, U, being related as

$$\mathscr{E} = kU \tag{4.4}$$

with k denoting the resistance of the circuit. It had not, however, been made explicit as a distinction between a quantity (U) and an intensity ($\mathscr{E}$). Explicitly following Faraday, Maxwell now drew attention to this distinction as an important one, and indicated how it could also be applied

[67] Maxwell to Thomson, 13 November 1854, in Larmor (1937), p. 10.

to magnetism, and in particular to a solenoidal circuit. As in his earlier analysis, the magnetic intensity and quantity were represented by line and surface integrals respectively, these being expressed in terms of numbers of lines of force. Combining this discussion with those he had already given of electrostatics and the relationship between electrostatics and galvanic electricity, we may immediately set down a series of quantity–intensity relationships. For a complete circuit, he had for the electromotive force $\mathscr{E}$,

$$\mathscr{E} = kU = p - p' = V - V' \tag{4.5}$$

p being the pressure on the fluid analogy and V the electrostatic potential. At any point within the circuit this gave for the electromotive force at that point, X,

$$X = \nabla p = \nabla V = ku \tag{4.6}$$

u being the velocity of the fluid on the flow analogy and a quantity, the force X being an intensity. The galvanic and electrostatic theories having been connected, this relationship could also be carried over to the electrostatic state, X now being the electrostatic force in the direction of the line of force at a point in a dielectric medium. The total force between two conductors was given by the total potential, and was a quantity. For magnetism, Maxwell considered a surface section or small lamina of magnetic material, the force Y on which was related to the cross section s, magnetic resistance k' and quantity of magnetisation in the surface U' by

$$Y = U' \frac{k'}{s} \tag{4.7}$$

giving the magnetic force for a complete solenoidal circuit,

$$\mathscr{F} = k' U' \tag{4.8}$$

U' being represented by the number of magnetic lines passing through any section of the solenoid.

Finally, Maxwell closed part I of his paper by discussing the magnetic interactions of small electrical circuits and the production of currents by electromagnetic induction in terms of the flow analogy. In the course of this discussion he introduced Faraday's notion of the electrotonic state, but he deferred a proper analysis of this notion and the electromagnetic phenomena it was introduced to describe until the second part of the paper.

In the first half of the paper, Maxwell had concentrated entirely on the representation of electromagnetic phenomena in terms of the geometrical analogy of lines of flow. Despite his attempts over the previous two years, however, he had not been able to incorporate the laws of electromagnetic induction or the notion of an electrotonic state in this analogy. Explaining the effect of electromagnetic induction in terms of a change in the number of lines of magnetic force passing through an electric circuit he had suggested that it seemed natural to think of the induced electromagnetic force in terms of some change in state measured by the number of lines. In this context, he had suggested, Faraday's notion of an electrotonic state might be useful as 'a new idea by which our mathematical concepts may be rendered clearer'. But he had had to admit that he had not been able to derive a clearly visualisable physical analogy for the electrotonic state. It had 'not yet presented itself to my mind in such a form that its nature and properties may be clearly explained without reference to mere symbols.' He therefore proposed to follow Thomson in abandoning the simple fluid flow analogy in favour of the more complex mathematics of elastic solids and viscous fluid motion, in the hope of 'discovering a method of forming a mechanical conception of this electro-tonic state adapted to general reasoning'.[68]

In order to establish a mathematical representation of Faraday's idea of an electrotonic state in the second part of his paper, Maxwell began by returning to the distinction between quantities and intensities, and by establishing explicitly a full set of quantities and intensities for both electricity and magnetism.[69] The quantity of electric current was defined at a given point and in a given direction according to the flow across a small unit area perpendicular to that direction, and was denoted by the cartesian components (a_2, b_2, c_2). Taking p_2 as the electric tension at the point, and (X_2, Y_2, Z_2) as the externally applied electromotive force, then the total electromotive force at the point, $(\alpha_2, \beta_2, \gamma_2)$, was given by

$$\begin{aligned}\alpha_2 &= X_2 - \mathrm{d}p_2/\mathrm{d}x\\ \beta_2 &= Y_2 - \mathrm{d}p_2/\mathrm{d}y\\ \gamma_2 &= Z_2 - \mathrm{d}p_2/\mathrm{d}z\end{aligned} \tag{4.9}$$

and this was defined as the intensity of electric action at the point. For a medium of uniform resistance k_2

$$\begin{aligned}\alpha_2 &= k_2 a_2\\ \beta_2 &= k_2 b_2\\ \gamma_2 &= k_2 c_2.\end{aligned} \tag{4.10}$$

The line integral of the electric intensity was then defined, and shown to be equal for a closed curve to that due to the external electromotive force. The surface integral of electric quantity was also defined, and shown to be equal for a closed surface to the volume integral of the quantity gradient. Switching for convenience to modern vector notation, Maxwell thus had for

[68] Maxwell (1890 and 1965), volume 1, p. 188.
[69] Maxwell (1890 and 1965), volume 1, pp. 191–2.

a closed curve, line element $d\boldsymbol{\lambda}$,

$$\oint \boldsymbol{\alpha}_2 \cdot d\boldsymbol{\lambda} = \oint X_2 \cdot d\boldsymbol{\lambda} \tag{4.11}$$

and for a closed surface, element $d\omega_1\, d\omega_2$,

$$\begin{aligned}\oiint \boldsymbol{a}_2 \cdot (d\boldsymbol{\omega}_1 \times d\boldsymbol{\omega}_2) &= \iiint \nabla \cdot \boldsymbol{a}_2 \, dx\, dy\, dz \\ &= \iiint \left(\frac{da_2}{dx} + \frac{db_2}{dy} + \frac{dc_2}{dz}\right)\Bigg)\Bigg) \, dx\, dy\, dz \\ &= 4\pi \iiint \rho \, dx\, dy\, dz\end{aligned} \tag{4.12}$$

for a suitably defined electric density ρ.

Next, Maxwell indicated how a completely analogous set of quantities and intensities subject to precisely the same equations could be derived for magnetism. To emphasise the symmetry of the situation, he denoted the magnetic quantity (quantity of induction) by (a_1, b_1, c_1) and the magnetic intensity (equivalent to his earlier magnetic polarisation) by $(\alpha_1, \beta_1, \gamma_1)$, with k_1 for the magnetic resistance and p_1 for the magnetic potential or tension. The choice of subscripts suggests that as in his November 1854 letter to Thomson, Maxwell had actually started out with the magnetic case rather than the electric, and from the sequel it would appear that his discussion was in fact based on a clarified version of that in the early letter. Introducing the laws of attraction and repulsion between electric currents as demonstrated by Ampère, he again considered a magnetic surface composed of small electrical circuits. Referring explicitly now to Faraday's image of 'mutually embracing curves', or interlocking lines of electric and magnetic force, he derived results corresponding to his two earlier theorems. This time, however, the theorems were more carefully stated. The theorem relating the surface integral of magnetic polarisation to the current running round its boundary was now expressed as the magnetic effect of a uniformly magnetised shell being equivalent to that of a current round the edge of the shell. The theorem relating the closed magnetic line integral to currents passing through the surface bounded by it was now expressed as a relationship between the magnetic *intensity* of a closed curve and the electric *quantity* of a closed current passing through it:

$$a_2 = \frac{d\beta_1}{dz}\frac{d\gamma_1}{dy} \qquad b_2 = \frac{d\gamma_1}{dx}\frac{d\alpha_1}{dz} \qquad c_2 = \frac{d\alpha_1}{dy}\frac{d\beta_1}{dx} \tag{4.13}$$

or in modern vector notation

$$\boldsymbol{a}_2 = \boldsymbol{\nabla} \times \boldsymbol{\alpha}_1 \tag{4.14}$$

from which, for closed electric currents,

$$\frac{\mathrm{d}a_2}{\mathrm{d}x}+\frac{\mathrm{d}b_2}{\mathrm{d}y}+\frac{\mathrm{d}c_2}{\mathrm{d}z}=\boldsymbol{\nabla}\cdot\boldsymbol{a}_2=0 \tag{4.15}$$

and in the absence of an electric current

$$\alpha_1\,\mathrm{d}x+\beta_1\,\mathrm{d}y+\gamma_1\,\mathrm{d}z=\mathrm{d}p_1 \tag{4.16}$$

or

$$\boldsymbol{\alpha}_1=\boldsymbol{\nabla}p_1$$

for some p_1, defined as the magnetic tension or potential in analogy with the electric tension p_2. The total potential of a magnetic system was then given by

$$Q=\iiint\rho_1 p_1\,\mathrm{d}x\,\mathrm{d}y\,\mathrm{d}z \tag{4.17}$$

with ρ_1 being a magnetic density,

$$\rho_1=\frac{1}{4\pi}\left(\frac{\mathrm{d}a_1}{\mathrm{d}x}+\frac{\mathrm{d}b_1}{\mathrm{d}y}+\frac{\mathrm{d}c_1}{\mathrm{d}z}\right)=\frac{1}{4\pi}\,\boldsymbol{\nabla}\cdot\boldsymbol{a}_1 \tag{4.18}$$

so that

$$Q=\frac{1}{4\pi}\iiint\left(\frac{\mathrm{d}a_1}{\mathrm{d}x}+\frac{\mathrm{d}b_1}{\mathrm{d}y}+\frac{\mathrm{d}c_1}{\mathrm{d}z}\right)p_1\,\mathrm{d}x\,\mathrm{d}y\,\mathrm{d}z. \tag{4.19}$$

So far, the analysis was straightforward. But to develop it further Maxwell had to draw on the mathematical results of potential theory as developed by Green and Thomson. He therefore set down and indicated the proofs of a series of seven theorems based on the existence of a unique potential V such that $\nabla^2 V=-4\pi\rho$ for any finite function of position ρ. As a consequence of these theorems he was able to show that any equation in the form of (4.19) could generally be expressed in the form

$$Q=\iiint p_1\rho_1-\frac{1}{4\pi}\left(\alpha_0 a_2+\beta_0 b_2+\gamma_0 c_2\right)\,\mathrm{d}x\,\mathrm{d}y\,\mathrm{d}z \tag{4.20}$$

with α_0, β_0 and γ_0 determined from a_1, b_1 and c_1, and with a_2, b_2 and c_2 identifiable as the quantities of electric current. This suggested that equation (4.19) for the total potential of a purely magnetic system be generalised for an electromagnetic system in which currents were present to equation (4.20), the contribution of the currents being given by the second term in the integral. Maxwell now had an expression for the electromagnetic induction of a circuit which instead of depending on the quantity of magnetic induction passing through the circuit was expressed in terms of the functions (α_0, β_0, γ_0) 'existing in the same space with the current itself'.[70] Since

[70] Maxwell (1890 and 1965), volume 1, p. 203.

a change in the total potential gave a measure of the work done in any displacement of the system (Thomson's mechanical effect), Maxwell could also analyse changes in the electrotonic state by means of the conservation of energy, for which he drew on Helmholtz's classic paper of the previous decade.[71] Supposing that an external source of electricity generated in some medium currents represented by the quantities (a_2, b_2, c_2) and intensities (α_2, β_2, γ_2), then the total work due to this source in a time interval dt could be expressed as the sum of two components, one of which,

$$\mathrm{d}t \iiint (a_2\alpha_2 + b_2\beta_2 + c_2\gamma_2)\, \mathrm{d}x\, \mathrm{d}y\, \mathrm{d}z$$

represented the resistance overcome while the other,

$$\mathrm{d}t\left(\frac{1}{4\pi}\frac{\mathrm{d}}{\mathrm{d}t}\iiint (a_2\alpha_0 + b_2\beta_0 + c_2\gamma_0)\right) \mathrm{d}x\, \mathrm{d}y\, \mathrm{d}z$$

represented the work done mechanically by the electromagnetic action. In the absence of any external source, or taking the medium as over all space, the sum of these components must vanish, giving

$$a_2\alpha_2 + b_2\beta_2 + c_2\gamma_2 = -\frac{1}{4\pi}\frac{\mathrm{d}}{\mathrm{d}t}(a_2\alpha_0 + b_2\beta_0 + c_2\gamma_0) \tag{4.21}$$

or

$$\boldsymbol{a}_2 \cdot \boldsymbol{\alpha}_2 = -\frac{1}{4\pi}\frac{\mathrm{d}}{\mathrm{d}t}\left(\boldsymbol{a}_2 \cdot \boldsymbol{\alpha}_0\right)$$

for every point in the medium. Taking the quantity of electricity as constant, and the variation in the total potential as due to variations in the electrotonic state,

$$a_2\left(\alpha_2 + \frac{1}{4\pi}\frac{\mathrm{d}\alpha_0}{\mathrm{d}t}\right) + b_2\left(\beta_2 + \frac{1}{4\pi}\frac{\mathrm{d}\beta_0}{\mathrm{d}t}\right) + c_2\left(\gamma_2 + \frac{1}{4\pi}\frac{\mathrm{d}\gamma_0}{\mathrm{d}t}\right) = 0 \tag{4.22}$$

giving, since a_2, b_2, c_2, were independent,

$$\alpha_2 = -\frac{1}{4\pi}\frac{\mathrm{d}\alpha_0}{\mathrm{d}t} \qquad \beta_2 = -\frac{1}{4\pi}\frac{\mathrm{d}\beta_0}{\mathrm{d}t} \qquad \gamma_2 = -\frac{1}{4\pi}\frac{\mathrm{d}\gamma_0}{\mathrm{d}t}. \tag{4.23}$$

Drawing his analysis together, Maxwell finally summarised his theory of the electrotonic state in the form of six laws, all expressed non-mathematically.[72]

> LAW I. *The entire electro-tonic intensity round the boundary of an element of surface measures the quantity of magnetic induction which passes through that surface, or, in other words, the number of lines of magnetic force which pass through that surface.*

[71] Helmholtz (1847 and 1853).
[72] Maxwell (1890 and 1965), volume 1, pp. 206–7.

> LAW II. *The magnetic intensity at any point is connected with the quantity of magnetic induction by a set of linear equations, called the equations of conduction.*
> LAW III. *The entire magnetic intensity round the boundary of any surface measures the quantity of electric current which passes through that surface.*
> LAW IV. *The quantity and intensity of electric currents are connected by a system of equations of conduction.*
> LAW V. *The total electro-magnetic potential of a closed current is measured by the product of the quantity of the current multiplied by the entire electro-tonic intensity estimated in the same direction round the circuit.*
> LAW VI. *The electro-motive force on any element of a conductor is measured by the instantaneous rate of change of the electro-tonic intensity on that element, whether in magnitude or direction.*

Mathematically expressed, and using modern vector notation, we may write:

Law I $\oint \boldsymbol{\alpha}_0 \cdot \mathrm{d}\boldsymbol{\lambda} = \iint \boldsymbol{a}_1 \cdot (\mathrm{d}\boldsymbol{\omega}_1 \times \mathrm{d}\boldsymbol{\omega}_2)$ or $\boldsymbol{\nabla} \times \boldsymbol{\alpha}_0 = \boldsymbol{a}_1$

Law II $\boldsymbol{\alpha}_1 = k_1 \boldsymbol{a}_1$ (for uniform media)

Law III $\oint \boldsymbol{\alpha}_1 \cdot \mathrm{d}\boldsymbol{\lambda} = \iint \boldsymbol{a}_2 \cdot (\mathrm{d}\boldsymbol{\omega}_1 \times \mathrm{d}\boldsymbol{\omega}_2)$ or $\boldsymbol{\nabla} \times \boldsymbol{\alpha}_1 = \boldsymbol{a}_2$

Law IV $\boldsymbol{\alpha}_2 = k_2 \boldsymbol{a}_2$ (for uniform media)

Law V $Q = \oint \boldsymbol{a}_2 \cdot \boldsymbol{\alpha}_0 \, \mathrm{d}\lambda$

Law VI $\boldsymbol{\alpha}_2 = -\dfrac{1}{4\pi} \dfrac{\mathrm{d}\boldsymbol{\alpha}_0}{\mathrm{d}t}$ giving with Law III $\boldsymbol{\nabla} \times \boldsymbol{\alpha}_1 = \dfrac{1}{k_2} \dfrac{\mathrm{d}\boldsymbol{\alpha}_0}{\mathrm{d}t}.$

In addition, Laws I and III gave

$$\boldsymbol{\nabla} \cdot \boldsymbol{a}_2 = \boldsymbol{\nabla} \cdot \boldsymbol{a}_1 = 0.$$

For media in which the magnetic or electric resistance varied with direction, Laws II and IV took a more general linear form, k_1 or k_2 acting as a tensor quantity and the vector quantity and intensity no longer being parallel. It is interesting to observe that while Maxwell used the language of integrals over curves and surfaces, and made use of the existing theory of such integrals, the mathematical expressions he gave of his final laws were in differential form (effectively partial differential equations, though he never used the partial symbols), derived from the consideration of infinitesimal surface areas. This corresponded of course to his use of Faraday's continuous field concepts in preference to the discrete action-at-a-distance concepts of Weber. And it also shows up clearly the relationship between Faraday's non-mathematical approach and the mathematical approach of Fourier, who had also used a differential as opposed to an integral formulation.

Physical analogies

From the viewpoint of modern physics it is fascinating to see the gradual emergence of what we now know as Maxwell's equations of the electromagnetic field. But how should we assess Maxwell's contributions in contemporary terms? The first thing to do is perhaps to remind ourselves of precisely what he did. Then, having established this, we can look at his own methodological analysis and at what he saw himself—or at least proclaimed himself—as trying to do.

In the first part of his paper, Maxwell described the law of fluid motion in terms of the geometry of lines of flow and indicated how, using Faraday's image of lines of force, these laws could be used to represent 'some of the less complicated phenomena of electricity, magnetism and galvanism'.[73] The representation was put across in purely geometrical terms, and explicitly not as implying any physical explanation. In pursuit of the representation Maxwell took as basic certain elements of electricity and magnetism, distinguished as quantities and intensities of electric current and magnetic induction, but he did not claim any special physical significance for these elements. In the second part of the paper he indicated how the mathematical analogy of the first part might be extended to cover the phenomena of electromagnetic induction. He gave a more precise definition of quantities and intensities of electricity and magnetism at any point, and introduced a further set of fundamental intensities related to Faraday's notion of an electrotonic state. The mathematical framework of the extended representation was however too complicated to be captured in the visual geometric analogy of lines of flow, and in particular the elements of the electrotonic state lacked any clear visualisation. As with the other fundamental elements, these were not attributed any necessary physical significance.

It is instructive at this stage to compare Maxwell's contribution with those of Thomson and Weber. Maxwell depended heavily on Thomson's work for his mathematics. His own work may be seen in one sense as a continuation of the process of the mathematical representation of electromagnetic phenomena undertaken by Thomson, in which the distinction between quantities and intensities was introduced and the representation carried over to include the phenomena of electromagnetic induction. In this sense Maxwell's contribution may be seen as making a distinct advance beyond Thomson's, but along lines already laid down for him. In another sense, however, Thomson's contribution had been quite different from Maxwell's. Thomson had developed mathematical representations in terms of which the elementary phenomena of electricity and magnetism (but not electromagnetism) could be described, but the representations he had sought had been mechanical rather than geometric, and he had explicitly

[73] Maxwell (1890 and 1965), p. 159.

not included anything that could not be mechanically pictured and represented. Nor had he incorporated in his analogies any of Faraday's theoretical notions, such as the lines of force, magnetic polarity or electrotonic state, on which Maxwell's analogies were based. Only empirically established elements were included.

The differences between the approaches of Thomson and Maxwell indicate well the limitations of the mechanistic–dynamistic dichotomy we have been taking as a guideline, for although Thomson's approach was dynamistic in terms of the early nineteenth century it may actually be viewed as mechanistic in the more sophisticated terms of the second half of the century. In the 1840s, the qualities of his work that stand out are his opposition to molecular–mechanical hypotheses as to the nature of the physical world and his preference for a mathematical approach of which the foundations were purely empirical. As we shall see, this approach was to lead him towards a methodology based on general Lagrangian dynamics through which he was to contribute substantially to the armoury of the dynamistic approach. But following the establishment of a new orthodoxy, for which he was partly responsible, in which dynamical principles were linked with a mechanical heuristic, he himself was unable to accept the very free-wheeling use of mechanical models and other hypothetical notions that resulted, and that characterised Maxwell's work in particular. Whereas Maxwell, following Whewell or indeed Faraday, felt justified in giving free reign to his imagination by a fairly sophisticated philosophy of analogy, Thomson continued to insist on the dual foundations of direct empirical reference and consistent mechanical visualisation. Although he remained very friendly with Maxwell, he grew increasingly critical of the latter's approach to electromagnetic theory. If we were to consider the pendulum of history as moving between the mechanistic and the dynamistic, we might say that it passed Thomson *en route* from Laplace to Maxwell, but quickly returned to meet him again, and indeed to stay with him, as a representative of a new and more cautious mechanism, until swinging back to the more dynamistic outlooks of the founders of quantum mechanics in the twentieth century.

We shall return to this wider historical process at the end of the book. For the moment, the point is to emphasise the difference between Thomson's and Maxwell's approaches to electromagnetic theory while at the same time keeping sight of the strong thread by which they were united. Between Maxwell and Weber, the other contributor to electromagnetic theory with whom he may be directly compared, there was no such thread. We have already noted that Maxwell was totally out of sympathy with Weber's mechanistic approach to physics and that he had some grounds, or thought he had some grounds, for doubting Weber's theory from the principle of energy conservation. He had no grounds for dismissing the theory altogether, though, and since it offered an already existing complete explanation of the principal electromagnetic phenomena, while his own work was presented only as a small step towards such an explanation, he had to deal with it somehow in his paper.

Maxwell himself expressed his problem here in no uncertain terms. Weber's theory, which incorporated the results of Ampère, Neumann and others, was [74]

> A really physical theory, satisfying the required condition better perhaps than any yet invented, and put forth by a philosopher whose experimental researches form an ample foundation for his mathematical investigations. What is the use then of imagining an electro-tonic state of which we have no distinctly physical conception, instead of a formula of attraction which we can readily understand?

His answer, partly quoted already, was, [75]

> that it is a good thing to have two ways of looking at a subject, and to admit that there *are* two ways of looking at it. Besides, I do not think that we have any right at present to understand the action of electricity, and I hold that the chief merit of a temporary theory is, that it shall guide experiment, without impeding the progress of the true theory when it appears.

Elsewhere in the paper Maxwell readily admitted that his own contribution consisted of 'the results of mere speculation' offered to others as an aid in arranging and interpreting their experimental results, and in suggesting what experimental questions should be put. [76] It is clear, however, that to Maxwell it was not really 'mere' speculation. His stated aim, or 'design', was: [77]

> to shew how, by a strict application of the ideas and methods of Faraday, the connexion of the very different orders of phenomena which he has discovered may be clearly placed before the mathematical mind.

And the principal justification of this aim was that: [78]

> The conjecture of a philosopher so familiar with nature [as Faraday] may sometimes be more pregnant with truth than the best established experimental law discovered by empirical inquirers, and though not bound to admit it as a physical truth, we may accept it as a new idea by which our mathematical conceptions may be rendered clearer.

[74] Maxwell (1890 and 1965), volume 1, p. 208.
[75] Maxwell (1890 and 1965), volume 1, p. 208.
[76] Maxwell (1890 and 1965), volume 1, p. 159.
[77] Maxwell (1890 and 1965), volume 1, pp. 157–8.
[78] Maxwell (1890 and 1965), volume 1, p. 187.

Whereas Thomson approached physics in terms of empirical laws expressed through mechanical visualisations, and Weber approached it in terms of hypothetical laws of action at a distance between molecules, Maxwell approached it in terms of appropriate ideas, mathematically expressed so as to be physically comprehensible. The specific methodology of this approach, to which he devoted considerable attention, was that of the method of physical analogy.

There has been considerable confusion in the past over what exactly Maxwell meant by physical analogies and how they were to be related to what he referred to as 'true physical theories'. And both questions are important if we are to understand the place of his paper on 'Faraday's lines of force' in his electromagnetic researches as a whole. The nature of physical analogy itself was described by Maxwell in his paper, significant parts of which were concerned explicitly with methodology. But he also discussed the underlying epistemology in two other writings of this period: an essay on analogies that he read to the Apostles Club in Cambridge in February 1856, the same month in which he read the second part of 'Faraday's lines of force' to the Philosophical Society there;[79] and an inaugural lecture as Professor of Natural Philosophy at Aberdeen, delivered soon after he had taken up this post, in November 1856.[80]

The talk to the Apostles was entitled 'Are there real analogies in nature'. There were, Maxwell noted, apparent analogies in nature. But there were also apparent analogies between nature and the mind,[81]

> For, not to mention all the things in external nature which men have seen as the projections of things in their own minds, the whole framework of science, up to the very pinnacle of philosophy, seems sometimes a dissected model of nature, and sometimes a natural growth on the inner surface of the mind.

The question, then, was whether the analogies perceived in nature were real analogies in nature, or merely apparent ones, imposed by the mind:[82]

> Are we to conclude that these various departments of nature in which analogous laws exist, have a real inter-dependence; or that their relation is only apparent and owing to the necessary conditions of human thought?

This question is itself a revealing one, for in asking it Maxwell went straight to the heart of the epistemological issues that had been characteristic of the dynamical philosophy. The discussion that followed was diffuse, to say the least, and ranged from our knowledge of mathematics and the exact

[79] Campbell and Garnett (1884), pp. 347–55.
[80] R V Jones (1973).
[81] Campbell and Garnett (1884), p. 348.
[82] Campbell and Garnett (1884), p. 348.

sciences to that of moral law and human behaviour. It was also stylised, with substantial doses of wit and exaggerated complexity. The principal arguments were, however, clearly stated.

On one hand, Maxwell argued that the role of mind in forming our knowledge of nature was undeniable. Both space and time could be founded on the laws of human thought, and even 'the very first notion of number implies a previous act of intelligence.'[83] Nature itself was described as having 'a certain horror of partition', as a consequence of which the choice of unit could only be imposed through 'the focussing glass of theory'.[84] The other fundamental elements of scientific theory, causes, were also deemed by Maxwell to be mentally derived. Causes were 'reasons, analogically referred to objects instead of thoughts', and mechanical forces, principles and moral rules were all similarly related to reason.[85]

On the other hand, however, Maxwell also asserted that these elements of knowledge were not simply imposed by the mind, not, in his words, 'mere projections of our mental machinery', but that there was something in nature corresponding to them. Taking the concept of space, for example, he argued that:[86]

> When we say that space has three dimensions, we not only express the impossibility of conceiving a fourth dimension, co-ordinate with the three known ones, but assert the objective truth that points may differ in position by the independent variation of three variables. Here, therefore, we have a *real* analogy between the constitution of the intellect and that of the external world.

This belief in a real analogy between nature and the mind was of course characteristic of both Hamilton and Whewell, and it suggested a partial answer to Maxwell's question. If different aspects of nature were analogous to the same aspects of mind, then they might also be analogous to each other. But as Maxwell pointed out, they were not necessarily so. The appearance of space and time throughout nature was due to an identity, not an analogy, and the independent existence even of the qualities in nature corresponding to reason was not easily demonstrated. It could be on one hand that beyond the categories of space and time all knowledge of nature was in fact derived from the abstract laws of thought, in which case all the apparent analogies of nature 'become merely repetitions by reflexion of certain necessary modes of action to which our minds are subject'.[87] On the other hand, it could also be argued that the laws of thought, treated now

[83] Campbell and Garnett (1884), p. 348.
[84] Campbell and Garnett (1884), p. 349.
[85] Campbell and Garnett (1884), pp. 350–351.
[86] Campbell and Garnett (1884), pp. 349–50.
[87] Campbell and Garnett (1884), p. 353.

as organic, physiological, laws, were themselves laws of nature, in which case all the apparent analogies between nature and mind and between nature and herself would become identities.

Maxwell applied this dichotomy of derivations specifically to the case of the foundations of physical science, whether mechanical or dynamical, in his period, and to:[88]

> the opinion, that all the phenomena of nature, being varieties of motion, can only differ in complexity, and therefore the only way of studying nature, is to master the fundamental laws of motion first, and then examine what kinds of complications of these laws must be studied in order to obtain true views of the universe.

His temptation was to reject both derivations, or 'hypotheses', on the grounds that neither of them 'can account for the existence of one set of laws of which the supremacy is necessary, but to the operation, contingent.'[89] These were the laws of right reason and moral action, both necessary in the sense that they were independent of nature, but contingent in the sense that their operation could be perturbed by natural events. In a discussion of the concept of necessary retribution, however, he came round towards the view that any apparent discrepancy between the laws of nature and those of the mind might well be a consequence of the limitations of our knowledge. We might not be able to see it, 'but still we suspect that the two orders of things will eventually dissolve into one.'[90]

Finally in this talk, Maxwell put the problem of limited knowledge into a scientific context, in which he echoed again some of the views of Hamilton and Whewell. For Maxwell as for Hamilton, scientific knowledge was concerned with relations and with analogies between relations, not between the things related. Such analogies could be immensely useful in advancing knowledge, but they could also be very dangerous if not carefully controlled, in that they could lead to the erroneous identification of quite disparate phenomena:[91]

> Whenever [men] see a relation between two things they know well, and think they see there must be a similar relation between things less known, they reason from the one to the other. This supposes that although pairs of things may differ widely from each other, the *relation* in the one pair may be the same as that in the other. Now, as in a scientific point of view the *relation* is the most important thing to know, a knowledge of the one thing leads us a long way towards a knowledge of the other. If all that we know is *relation*,

[88] Campbell and Garnett (1884), p. 352.
[89] Campbell and Garnett (1884), p. 353.
[90] Campbell and Garnett (1884), p. 354.
[91] Campbell and Garnett (1884), p. 354.

> and if all the relations of one pair of things correspond to those of another pair, it will be difficult to distinguish the one pair from the other, although not presenting a single point of resemblance, unless we have some difference of relation to something else, whereby to distinguish them. Such mistakes can hardly occur except in mathematical and physical analogies, but if we are going to study the constitution of the individual mental man, and draw all our arguments from the laws of society on the one hand, or those of the nervous tissue on the other, we may chance to convert useful helps into Wills-of-the-wisp.

When it came down to it Maxwell believed that the apparent analogies of nature were ultimately derivable from identities, and that the worlds of mind and of matter were ultimately one. He closed his talk by stating with obvious conviction 'the great doctrine that the only laws of matter are those which our minds must fabricate, and the only laws of mind are fabricated for it by matter.'[92] Throughout the talk, however, it was the need for caution that prevailed, for the nature of the true identities was not apparent, and it was with merely apparent analogies that scientific knowledge was concerned. Such analogies might ultimately be traceable back to identities, but there were no grounds for assuming that they were themselves identities, or even real analogies.

Maxwell's essay on analogies left open two significant issues. First, although it ranged widely and combined arguments taken from science with others from ethics, it did not deal explicitly with religious belief, which we have already seen was central to Maxwell's philosophy. Secondly, while advocating in broad terms a cautious use of analogies in science, it stated but left unanswered an important question as to the degree of confidence that could in general be placed in the analogical method:[93]

> Perhaps the 'book', as it has been called, of nature is regularly paged; if so, no doubt the introductory parts will explain those that follow, and the methods taught in the first chapters will be taken for granted and used as illustrations in the more advanced parts of the course; but if it is not a 'book' at all, but a *magazine*, nothing is more foolish than to suppose that one part can throw light on another.

As we might suspect, these two issues were clearly linked, and they were in fact treated together in an address delivered by Maxwell just nine months after his Apostles talk. At the beginning of 1856 the professorship of natural philosophy at Marischal College, Aberdeen, had become vacant. Maxwell was attracted by the possibility of being closer to his father and being able to spend the whole summer at Glenlair, which he could not do while at Cambridge. He duly applied, and although his father died before

[92] Campbell and Garnett (1884), p. 355.
[93] Campbell and Garnett (1884), p. 354.

the appointment was finally made this in itself increased the time needed to manage affairs at Glenlair and so did nothing to remove the attraction of the position. He was appointed to the chair in the spring and took it from the autumn, delivering his inaugural lecture in November.

Maxwell's Aberdeen lecture was no less stylised than his talk to the Apostles had been, only this time the conventional qualities were seriousness and pious solemnity rather than wit and extravagant complexity. The requirement was for 'a solemn address and manifesto', and it took a good supply of coffee and anchovies and a roaring hot fire to give him the strength 'to make it all natural'.[94] Even then, what he wrote in the end was scarcely solemn—but it was utterly serious. Maxwell's manifesto was for an approach to physical science that was at once experimental and metaphysical. He admitted that metaphysicians were notorious for disagreeing with each other, and that it was natural to view modern science, stemming from the discoveries of the scientific revolution, as having grown beyond the errors of metaphysical systems:[95]

> You will perhaps be inclined to think that the root of the matter must lie somewhere among the discoveries of Galileo, Kepler or Descartes and that the great practical conclusion is "that once we were in error, and now we understand, and therefore let us be content."

But he urged his audience most strongly not to fall prey to this contentment, and to 'remember that the men to whom we owe the greatest discoveries in mathematics and physics were metaphysicians.'[96] If metaphysics were needed to guide thought and method and to upturn cherished notions and invade the 'holy ground' whose existence Maxwell had condemned as a youth, however, the second root of physical science, experiment, was equally essential. There was, he declared, no reason to believe that the intellect could weave a system of physics out of its own resources, without recourse to the phenomena of nature. And in a phrase that stands out from the studied tone of the lecture surrounding it he declared that the attempt to weave such a system usually led 'to a self-contradictory mass of rubbish'.[97] Again we are reminded of his youthful creed, of his insistence that the mind needed to communicate and compare in order to develop, and of his idea of physical science as providing the communication with nature through which development was possible.

A second thread of the Aberdeen lecture concerned the relationship between science and religion, and offered the answer to Maxwell's earlier question about the book or magazine of nature. It was apparent even from

[94] Maxwell to Monro, 14 October 1856, in Campbell and Garnett (1884), p. 179.
[95] R V Jones (1973), p. 73.
[96] R V Jones (1973), p. 73.
[97] Maxwell (1973), p. 76.

his talk to the Apostles that while he left both options open he personally believed in nature as not only a book but a very carefully written one, and he now made this view explicit:[98]

> But as physical science advances we see more and more that the laws of nature are *not* mere arbitrary and unconnected decisions of Omnipotence, but that they are essential parts of one universal system in which infinite Power serves only to reveal unreachable Wisdom and eternal Truth. . . . We see before us distinct physical truths to be discovered, and we are confident that these mysteries are an inheritance of knowledge, not revealed at once, lest we should become proud in knowledge, and despise patient enquiry, but so arranged that, as each new truth is unravelled it becomes a clear, well-established addition to science, quite free from the mystery which must still remain, to show that every atom of creation is *unfathomable* in its perfection. While we look down with awe into these unreachable depths and treasure up with care what with our little line and plummet we can reach, we ought to admire the wisdom of Him who has so arranged these mysteries that we find first that which we can *understand* at first and the rest in order so that it is possible for us to have an ever increasing stock of *known* truth concerning things whose nature is absolutely incomprehensible.

This declaration also indicated the value to be attached to analogies. There was nothing to suggest any change from Maxwell's view that analogies could be misleading and should be used only with the utmost caution. The underlying reality of nature was not only unknowable but absolutely incomprehensible. But if the revelation of the truths of nature took place in a definite order as suggested, then, to paraphrase his Cambridge talk, the introductory parts would explain the parts that followed and the methods taught in the early readings from the book of nature could be used as illustrations and guidelines in the more advanced parts. Cautious as one must be, analogical method, and in particular the exploration of analogies between natural phenomena or relations, was the appropriate method for understanding the natural world.

The methodology that emerges from Maxwell's talk to the Apostles Club in Cambridge and his inaugural lecture in Aberdeen is one based on the programme of understanding nature through the illustration of the more complex phenomena by analogy with simpler and better understood ones; and it was just such a use of analogy that he described in his paper on 'Faraday's lines of force'. In the introduction to this paper he suggested that the science of electricity and magnetism had reached a stage where the prime need was for simplification. Such a simplification might, he suggested, take the form of purely mathematical formulae. But to do this would be to lose sight of the physical phenomena to be explained and to limit oneself to a narrow view of 'the connexions of the subject'.[99] Since the whole point of

[98] Maxwell (1973), p. 77.
[99] Maxwell (1890 and 1965), volume 1, p. 155.

physics for Maxwell was to communicate with nature and so extend the range of one's understanding and knowledge, he would have found it perverse to restrict attention only to that aspect of the phenomena that could be captured in and expressed by abstract mathematical analysis, which could in itself add little that was not already clearly apparent to the mind. Completely different phenomena could be expressed by the same mathematical formulae and these formulae in themselves could neither express the full nature of the phenomena nor indicate how they might in reality be connected.

A second approach to simplification might be through physical hypotheses. But this approach was even more dangerous, for such hypotheses were both restrictive, in that they allowed the phenomena to be viewed only through the medium of the hypotheses, and misleading, in that the partial explanation given tended to be seductive and to close the mind to contrary evidence.[100] What was needed, then, was something that avoided the pitfalls of either approach:[101]

> We must therefore discover some method of investigation which allows the mind at every step to lay hold of a clear physical conception, without being committed to any theory founded on the physical science from which that conception is borrowed, so that it is neither drawn aside from the subject in pursuit of analytical subtleties, nor carried beyond the truth by a favourite hypothesis.

This was the method of physical analogy, or 'that partial similarity between the laws of one science and those of another which makes each of them illustrate the other.'[102] By such analogies, and only by such analogies, could physical ideas be brought to bear on the subject without the adoption of unwarranted physical theories.

In order to clarify his notion of physical analogies, Maxwell gave some examples. He began with 'the most universal of all analogies', by which exact physical science was itself made possible, the analogy between physical laws and the laws of numbers. Epistemologically this might be an analogy, or rather an identity, between nature and the mind, but methodologically it provided an extreme case of a complete physical analogy through which all branches of exact science were related.[103] Of more practical significance was Maxwell's second example, of the 'very partial'

[100] Maxwell (1890 and 1965), volume 1, pp. 155–6.
[101] Maxwell (1890 and 1965), volume 1, p. 156.
[102] Maxwell (1890 and 1965), volume 1, p. 156.
[103] Maxwell (1890 and 1965), volume 1, p. 156. According to Maxwell the 'aim of exact science is to reduce the problems of nature to the determination of quantities by operations with numbers.' Obvious as this seems, its clear perception and application, as for example by Dirac in his development of quantum mechanics, is remarkably rare.

analogies between the behaviour of light on one hand and those of waves or corpuscles on the other. Both analogies were valid physical analogies, and both were useful as such, but both were misleading if taken as physical hypotheses. At the time Maxwell wrote the wave analogy between light and the vibrations of an elastic medium appeared to be a far reaching one and many held that light was a wave motion in the ether. But Maxwell explained that the analogy was only a partial one and that it could be applied strictly only if stripped of its physical content and reduced to a mathematical expression, which reduction would be self-defeating:[104]

> [The analogy] is founded only on a resemblance *in form* between the laws of light and those of vibrations. By stripping it of its physical dress and reducing it to a theory of "transverse alternations", we might obtain a system of truth strictly founded on observation, but probably deficient both in the vividness of its conceptions and the fertility of its method.

As illustrative of the limitations of mathematical expression, Maxwell took yet another example of an analogy, that of the analogy between the laws of gravitational attraction at a distance and those of heat flow in a uniform medium. Each set of laws had a distinct mathematical significance that was well understood and established in the minds of men. Each was in accordance with the natural phenomena it described. Yet mathematically they were identical, and if only the mathematics were known there would be nothing to distinguish between two very different types of physical phenomenon. Hence the need for physical analogies, and for concern as to the limitations as well as the extent of those analogies.

Maxwell's description of what he meant by physical analogies was clear enough, but what was their overall place in his image of science? To what extent was the method he advocated a general one, and to what extent was it specific to the particular circumstances of electromagnetic science at the time? There are two points to be discussed here, one concerning the previous development of the science and the other its anticipated development. As regards the previous development, Maxwell was quite explicit that the method of physical analogy was the method that had been pursued by Faraday. He stated repeatedly that his method and process of reasoning were taken from Faraday and that his own role was merely to outline Faraday's theories 'as they appear from a mathematical point of view', presenting the resulting mathematical ideas to the mind in the embodied forms of the mathematically precise physical analogies, and at the same time placing the analogies Faraday himself had explored before the mathematical mind.[105]

[104] Maxwell (1890 and 1965), volume 1, p. 156.
[105] Maxwell (1890 and 1965), volume 1, pp. 157–8, 187–8.

The relevance of the method of physical analogy for the future development of the science is a slightly more difficult issue, for it has been argued that the method was a temporary one, to be replaced by the deduction of true physical theories.[106] It is, however, difficult to maintain this view. Admittedly the analogies offered by Maxwell were offered as a 'temporary theory' or 'speculation', the merit of which was that it did 'not *account* for anything'.[107] And in several places he compared this temporary theory with what he called a 'true physical theory',[108] or a 'mature theory, in which physical facts will be physically explained'.[109] By a 'physical explanation', however, Maxwell did not mean a theory based on physical hypotheses, but rather one based on a necessary connection between empirical phenomena. As in his Aberdeen lecture he insisted that physics was an 'experimental science', in which the interrogation of nature led to the establishment of physical connections.[110] The process of interrogation depended on the application of appropriate physical ideas guiding the experimenter as to what questions to ask. In this process the mathematician could also help, not by contributing anything directly to physical knowledge, but by helping the physicist arrange his own ideas.

Maxwell did not give here an example of a mature theory. But he made it quite clear that the wave theory of light, for example, was not such a theory. A better candidate, which he did use in later life as an example of what he sought,[111] would probably be Newton's theory of gravitation, in which the true physical connection was established between the falling of terrestrial bodies and the orbital motion of heavenly ones. The establishment of this connection had required physical ideas and not a little mathematics, but once established it could rest upon empirical foundations, independent of hypothesis, and could even appear as a necessary truth.

Given that a true physical theory was one of physical connections, and not one of physical hypotheses, there was nothing in Maxwell's discussion to suggest that the method of physical analogy was not intended to be quite a general one, equally appropriate to all stages in the development of physics. Given the philosophical background and underpinning of the method, there is every reason to suppose that it was so. Overall, Maxwell's method seems to come very close indeed to that advocated by Whewell, with speculative methods leading to empirically founded laws which could then be perceived as necessarily true. The fundamental incomprehensibility and unknowability of nature combined with the image of science as a search for unity, for connections, supported a methodology based on analogy as being

[106] See for example Siegel (1975 and 1981).

[107] Maxwell (1890 and 1965), volume 1, p. 207.

[108] Maxwell (1890 and 1965), volume 1, pp. 207–8, 156–9 and 189.

[109] Maxwell (1890 and 1965), volume 1, p. 159.

[110] Maxwell (1890 and 1965), volume 1, pp. 159 and 189.

[111] Maxwell (1890 and 1965), volume 2, pp. 315–16.

at once the only way forward and a precarious one. In this context Maxwell's insistence that it was important to recognise that there *were* two ways of looking at something was no mere excuse for justifying an approach differing from Weber's, but a principle based on the limitations of analogy and the need to establish divers connections, to at least see all round a phenomenon whose interior remained inscrutable. To restrict oneself to one view would be to risk mistaken identity and to limit one's knowledge unnecessarily. At the same time, however, some views were more revealing than others, and by selecting an appropriate vantage point one might hope eventually to increase one's real knowledge and to perceive clearly some of the relations (though not the underlying entities) of nature.

5

From Mechanical Lines to a Dynamical Field

In his paper on 'Faraday's lines of force', Maxwell had successfully applied the physical analogy of the geometry of lines of flow in a fluid to some of the simpler electric and magnetic phenomena. He had also made some progress towards the establishment of an analogy for the more complex phenomena of electromagnetic induction through a mathematical representation of Faraday's idea of an electrotonic state. This latter representation, however, barely amounted to a physical analogy, let alone a candidate physical theory. At the end of the first part of his paper Maxwell had expressed the hope that he would be able 'to discover a method of forming a mechanical conception of this electro-tonic state adapted to general reasoning.'[1] He hoped, in other words, to discover a physical analogy with some mechanical processes through which the phenomena of electromagnetic induction might be physically illustrated. But for the time being he could do little more than provide a mathematical representation of Faraday's speculations, which he put forward as a guide towards the further development of the ideas entailed.

Maxwell's ambitions were, however, to be fulfilled, and in the most dramatic way. For between 1859 and 1864 he developed the analyses published in the two classic papers 'On physical lines of force' and 'A dynamical theory of the electromagnetic field', to be treated in this chapter. With these two masterpieces, strongly contrasting yet intimately connected, he established the classical theory of the electromagnetic field and with it the electromagnetic theory of light. Between his completion of 'Faraday's lines of force' in the winter of 1855–6 and his commencement of its sequel, 'On physical lines of force', in the latter part of 1859, however, other interests and concerns intervened, some of which were to have a strong bearing on his electromagnetic work. First came his father's death and his

[1] Maxwell (1890 and 1965), volume 1, p. 188.

own appointment to the Aberdeen professorship, which naturally called for the preparation of teaching material, and then, competing for his time with these concerns, came his work for the Adams Prize essay on Saturn's rings.

The Adams Prize had been established in Cambridge in 1848 in honour of John Adams's prediction a few years earlier of the existence of the planet Neptune. It was awarded in alternate years for an essay in some branch of mathematics or mathematical physics, typically in astronomy, and was the nearest British equivalent to the prizes that had long been offered by the French Académie des Sciences or the Italian Società delle Scienze. As James Challis, Plumian Professor of Astronomy at Cambridge and senior examiner for the 1855 prize, explained to William Thomson, who was also an examiner in that year, the prize was not exactly hotly contested:[2]

> We have not hitherto been successful in inducing competitors to come forward. On the first occasion there was but one, who gained the prize; on the next, there was also but one, & his Essay was too imperfect for a decision. On the last occasion there were no competitors.

Despite Challis's wish to reverse this trend and to find 'some subject that will be more likely to attract candidates',[3] Maxwell too was to be a sole entrant to the competition. But he did at least get the prize, and despite the lack of interest it was sufficiently prestigious to be worth having. The subject chosen for 1855 as being that of Challis's suggestions that was most acceptable to Thomson was an investigation of the stability of Saturn's rings. This subject was announced in March 1855, the essays to be completed in 1856 for judgment in 1857. What induced Maxwell to enter is not altogether clear. He had shown no special interest in mathematical astronomy and in the summer and autumn of 1856 when the work had to be done his other commitments were considerable. Perhaps, as the editors of a recent edition of his essay have suggested, he hoped to establish his reputation and career with a piece of orthodox non-speculative mathematical physics, and perhaps he was encouraged in this by Thomson.[4] Or perhaps he just could not resist the challenge: the solution of difficult mathematical 'props' (propositions) as an exercise had long been a favourite hobby and this was a prop *par excellence*. At any rate he entered into the subject and was promptly hooked. His prize essay was submitted by December 1856, but he continued to spend a substantial part of the next two years extending and elaborating on his analysis, completing the essay as finally published only in the late summer of 1858.[5]

[2] Challis to Thomson, 28 February 1855, in Brush *et al* (1983), p. 6.
[3] Challis to Thomson, 28 February 1855, in Brush *et al* (1983), p. 6.
[4] Brush *et al* (1983).
[5] Maxwell (1859), reprinted in Brush *et al* (1983), pp. 68–158, and see Maxwell to Stokes, 7 September 1858, in Brush *et al* (1983), p. 67.

The composition of Saturn's rings had long been a subject of interest. The standard theory of the early nineteenth century was due to Laplace, who had argued for a system of irregular solid rings, but in the late 1840s and early 1850s Laplace's theory had been questioned and the whole subject opened up to debate. Maxwell responded to the problem by analysing the stability of irregular solid rings, fluid rings and rings composed of independent satellites, covering both stationary and rotating rings and including in his calculations the mutual perturbations of two rings of independent satellites. He eventually concluded that:[6]

> the rings must consist of disconnected particles; these may be either solid or liquid but they must be independent. The entire system of rings must therefore consist either of a series of many concentric rings, each moving with its own velocity, and having its own system of waves, or else of a confused multitude of revolving particles, not arranged in rings, and continually coming into collision with each other,

Throughout the period of his work on Saturn's rings Maxwell continued his research into colour vision and other subjects, including electromagnetism, but without making any distinct strides in the latter context. Further diversions, coming in the spring and summer of 1858, were his engagement and marriage to Katherine Mary Dewar.[7] Then, following swiftly on the publication of his essay on Saturn's rings, came a new and important scientific involvement with the dynamical theory of gases.

The immediate stimulus for this involvement was Maxwell's reading in early 1859 of a paper by Rudolf Clausius.[8] The orthodox theory of gases in the 1850s was still that based on the hypothesis of action at a distance between static molecules. In the 1840s, however, James Prescott Joule had argued forcibly for the convertibility of mechanical work into heat and vice versa, and had put forward the corresponding proposition that the heat of a body was due to some mechanical motion within it.[9] Following Joule's work a number of scientists, including Clausius, had advocated a dynamical as opposed to statical theory of heat, and Clausius in particular had reconciled the interconvertibility of heat and mechanical work with Sadi Carnot's analysis of the processes occurring in heat engines to provide the foundations of modern thermodynamics.[10] In his early work on the subject, published in 1850, Clausius had not attempted to analyse the nature of the motions constituting heat, and had indeed framed his principles of thermo-

[6] Brush *et al* (1983), p. 154.
[7] Campbell and Garnett (1884), pp. 190*ff*.
[8] See for example Heimann (1970a), Garber (1970 and 1972), Brush (1976) and Everitt (1975).
[9] Joule (1843, 1848 and 1850).
[10] Clausius (1850).

dynamics so as to be independent even of the general hypothesis that heat was some form of motion. In his later papers of 1857 and 1858 he had however pursued this hypothesis and had sought to develop a general theory of gases in terms of their supposed molecular motions. In the 1857 paper he had treated gas molecules as elastic spheres all moving with the same speed (but in different directions, of course), and had sought to justify this approximation by probabilistic arguments. It would, he claimed, provide an adequate representation of the average motion over a large number of molecules.[11] A Dutchman by the name of Christopher Hendrik Buijs Ballot had then objected to the analysis on the ground that the average molecular speed deduced by Clausius from the known relationship between the pressure and the volume of a gas, several hundred metres per second, failed to tie in with the empirical observation that gases diffused into each other very slowly. In his 1858 paper, Clausius had therefore given a more sophisticated analysis in which he had introduced the concept of the mean free path of a molecule before it became subject to an effective collision (i.e. before it entered the sphere of net repulsion of another molecule), and had shown that allowing for collisions the objection was fallacious.[12]

Clausius's second paper was published in English translation in the spring of 1859 and it quickly excited the interest of Maxwell. Maxwell had already become interested in the problem of analysing the effects of continual collisions between large numbers of independent particles in the course of his work on Saturn's rings. He had also been interested since his student days in the theory of probability and its applications, and he now saw a possibility of developing Clausius's analysis into a full statistical theory of gases. In his 'Illustrations of the dynamical theory of gases', read to the British Association for the Advancement of Science in September 1859 and published the following year, he derived a statistical formula for the distribution of molecular velocities in a gas at uniform pressure (since called the Maxwell distribution) and applied it to the calculation of coefficients of viscosity, diffusion and heat conduction, and to a range of other properties of gases.[13] Only when he had completed this work did his main research turn back to electromagnetic theory and to the postponed problem of a mechanical analogy for the phenomena of electromagnetic induction.

Magnetism as molecular vortices

The basis for Maxwell's new analysis of electromagnetic behaviour was a study of Thomson's completed soon after the publication of Maxwell's own paper on 'Faraday's lines of force'. Thomson's study itself drew on some

[11] Clausius (1857).
[12] Buijs Ballot (1858); Clausius (1858 and 1859).
[13] Maxwell (1860).

work by the scientist–engineer William Macquorn Rankine dating from the late 1840s and concerned, as Maxwell's own recent studies had been, with the theory of gases.

Rankine's theory of gases was contained in two papers submitted to the Royal Society of Edinburgh in December 1849 and published in 1851 and 1853.[14] It was in essence a dynamical theory of gases, in which the observed properties of the gases, including their heats, were attributed to molecular motions; and together with the earlier work of Joule on the equivalence of heat and mechanical energy and the almost contemporary work of Clausius it provided the launching pad for modern kinetic theory and statistical thermodynamics.[15] The motions assumed by Rankine were not however the simple translational motions postulated by Clausius. Instead of postulating molecules moving among themselves and colliding with each other, Rankine retained the traditional description in terms of static molecules acting at a distance, but treated the molecules themselves as being composed of elastic atmospheres revolving or oscillating around central massive nuclei, the heat being represented by the *vis viva* (kinetic energy) of the revolutions or oscillations. Using this hypothesis, he was able to derive a formula for the elasticity of a gas that corresponded more closely to the observed elasticity than did the traditional ideal gas laws, and to predict theoretically some recent experimental measurements of maximum vapour pressure. He also derived accurate specific heats for two gases, oxygen and hydrogen, and a range of other physical and engineering results. Most significantly, as far as he was concerned, the mechanism also provided an alternative basis to the traditional luminiferous aether for a wave theory of light. Rankine assumed that the vibrations of light consisted of transverse vibrations of the molecular nuclei, transmitted by their mutual attraction at a distance, and that the absorption of light and radiant heat consisted of the transfer of motion from the nuclei to their atmospheres.

For William Thomson, the interconvertibility of heat and mechanical energy and the associated dynamical theory of gases had proved something of a puzzle. Learning of Joule's ideas from Joule himself at a British Association meeting in 1847, he had been impressed by the general force of the argument, but troubled by the conflict with Carnot's claim that heat was conserved in the generation of mechanical work by heat engines.[16] This conflict had continued to trouble him for several years, but it had been partly resolved by Clausius's 1850 paper, in which Clausius extracted from Carnot's theory the fundamental principle that heat passes from a warmer to a cooler body when, for example, work is done in a heat engine cycle; and in which he had abandoned Carnot's additional assumption that the

[14] Rankine (1851 and 1853).

[15] Clausius (1850); Joule (1843 and 1850). See Hutchinson (1981) and Daub (1967).

[16] See Thomson (1872), p. 423, Thompson (1910), pp. 263–83, and Siegel (1981).

quantity of heat is conserved in the cycle in favour of Joule's conservation of the sum of heat and mechanical energy. Once this point had been cleared up Thomson had quickly adopted the dynamical theory of heat, and in 1851 he had put forward his own analysis of the foundations of thermodynamics.[17] At this stage he had naturally thought in terms of vortical motions akin to those advocated by Rankine and also, briefly, by Joule.[18] But as we shall see his principal and emerging concern had been with a dynamical approach to physics based on the general use of energy principles rather than on specific mechanical hypotheses, and during the next few years he not only developed this approach himself but also encouraged Rankine to do likewise.[19] The molecular vortex theory had thus drifted slightly into the background. At the same time, however, Thomson was also becoming increasingly conscious of the value of mechanical models in rendering less concrete theories more readily intelligible. Part of his struggle with the theory of heat had been to understand how, if mechanical energy were conserved and heat were a form of mechanical energy, some of that energy could be lost to use in the irreversible processes of imperfect engines. To give the laws of thermodynamics was not, in his view, sufficient. To understand these laws he also had to have some picture of how they could operate mechanically. More generally, since Thomson's view of energy was an essentially mechanical one, his use of energy as a unifying principle, though described by him as a 'dynamical' programme, carried with it the principle of unification through mechanics. And while cautious of mechanical hypotheses, and attracted towards a hypothesis-free approach on one hand, he also perceived the need for mechanical theories or illustrations on the other.

In 1856, Thomson saw the possibility of adapting the picture of molecular vortices to the magneto-optic effect demonstrated by Faraday (and often called the Faraday effect) and thus of bringing magnetism within his unifying mechanical framework.[20] In Faraday's experiments, made in 1845, the plane of polarisation of a linearly polarised light wave passing through a piece of heavy glass in a strong magnetic field and in the direction of the field lines had been shown to rotate by an amount proportional to both the strength of the field and the distance travelled through the glass.[21] This result together with others had encouraged the consideration of magnetism as some sort of rotational state, and in developing the elastic solid analogy of electric and magnetic phenomena in the 1840s Thomson

[17] Thomson (1851a).
[18] See Forrester (1975) and Steffens (1979).
[19] See Smith (1978).
[20] Thomson (1856 and 1857). See Knudsen (1976).
[21] Faraday (1855 and 1965), volume 3, paragraphs 2146–242, and see Chapter 3 above.

had already associated magnetism with a rotational strain in the solid.[22] In his 1856 paper he drew on a particular property of the magneto-optic effect to elaborate on the illustration of magnetism as related to molecular mechanical rotations and also to support the suggestion that this illustration could be taken as more than a mere analogy. The peculiar property was that the direction of rotation, right or left handedness, of the plane of polarisation depended on the direction of propagation of the light. So if the plane of polarisation of a light ray were turned through a certain angle, and the ray were then reflected back through the glass in the opposite direction, the rotation due to the return journey, being opposite in handedness and opposite in axial direction, would be the same as that in the original journey. So the total effect would be to double the rotation observed. If, in contrast, a light ray were passed through a naturally helicoidal material such as quartz, in which its plane of polarisation was rotated without any magnetic field present, the handedness was independent of direction and the effects on a reflected ray cancelled each other out. A related phenomenon, also noted by Thomson, was that if circularly polarised light were transmitted through magnetised glass it would be transmitted at different rates in different directions, whereas in an unmagnetised medium the rate of transmission was independent of direction.

The importance of these phenomena was that whereas the behaviour in unmagnetised media such as quartz could be explained by a naturally occurring heterogeneous rotational strain in the medium, this explanation was clearly inadequate for the magnetic case. Viewing the situation mechanically, and his programme allowed for no other type of viewing, Thomson argued that the magneto-optic rotation could only be interpreted as implying the existence of some rotational motions induced in the medium by the magnetic field, centring on the magnetic force lines as axes and with their direction determined by that of the field. Analysing the motion of circularly polarised waves through an elastic solid medium he concluded in particular that for the observed effects to be produced required the presence of microscopic or molecular vortices set up and aligned by the magnetic force lines.[23]

What was remarkable about Thomson's analysis, and what set it apart from all his earlier work, was the status he attributed to the mechanism. For he stated quite explicitly that in his view the magneto-optic effect could be explained 'only' on the assumption he proposed, that it was 'impossible to conceive any other than this dynamical explanation' (i.e. explanation through matter in motion) of the behaviour of circularly polarised rays, and that 'I believe it can be demonstrated that no other explanation of that fact is possible.'[24] He continued, moreover, to identify the rotatory component

[22] Thomson (1847a) and see Chapter 3 above.

[23] A review of Thomson's analysis is given in Knudsen (1976).

[24] Thomson (1904), pp. 569–71.

of the medium with that whose motion constituted heat on Rankine's theory, and to argue that all electromagnetic phenomena should be attributed to motions in this same medium:[25]

> The explanation of all phenomena of electro-magnetic attraction or repulsion, and of electro-magnetic induction, is to be looked for simply in the inertia and pressure of the matter of which the motions consitute heat. Whether this matter is or is not electricity, whether it is a continuous fluid interpermeating the spaces between molecular nuclei, or is itself molecularly grouped; or whether all matter is continuous, and molecular heterogeneousness consists in finite vortical or other relative motions of contiguous parts of a body; it is impossible to decide, and perhaps in vain to speculate, in the present state of science.

Despite leaving open the precise nature of the medium, Thomson clearly identified it with electricity or an electrical aether, and he suggested that 'Faraday's optical discovery effects a demonstration of the reality of Ampère's explanation of the ultimate nature of magnetism.'[26]

Coming from an established opponent of mechanical hypotheses and leading advocate of a hypothesis-free physics based on the energy principle, Thomson's claims and assertions seem at first remarkable. He was, however, drawing conclusions, not framing hypotheses. The underlying assumption of his programme was that through the energy principle all the phenomena of physics could be mechanically interpreted, and whereas before he had been able to fit electromagnetic phenomena into the mechanical framework only in terms of their overall energetic properties, through his concept of 'total mechanical effect' of an electromagnetic system, he now felt able to delve deeper by arguing that if the magneto-optic effect were mechanically explicable, then the molecular vortices must exist. In a talk given in 1860 he insisted that:[27]

> Whatever electricity is, it seems quite certain that electricity in motion IS *heat*; and that a certain alignment of axes of revolution in this motion IS *magnetism*. Faraday's magneto-optic experiment makes this not a hypothesis, but a demonstrated conclusion.

Whether or not Maxwell shared Thomson's general viewpoint, and that is something we shall discuss later in this chapter, his analysis must have been provocative. At the very least it pointed the way towards a possible mechanical analogy of electromagnetic behaviour such as Maxwell had already sought but had so far been unable to find. In November 1857

[25] Thomson (1904), p. 571.
[26] Thomson (1904), p. 571.
[27] Thomson (1872), p. 224. The talk was a Royal Institution Friday Evening Lecture, delivered on 18 May 1860.

Maxwell referred at the end of a letter to Faraday to 'questions relating to the connection between magneto-electricity and certain mechanical effects which seem to me to be opening up quite a new road to the establishment of principles in electricity, and a possible confirmation of the physical nature of magnetic lines of force. Professor Thomson', he added, 'seems to have some new lights on this subject.'[28] Sometime after completing his paper on the dynamical theory of gases he took up this challenge in earnest. Once again external events intervened, as Maxwell's chair of natural philosophy at Marischal College was axed in the course of a merger of the Aberdeen colleges. In 1860, having failed to get the chair at Edinburgh, which had become vacant due to Forbes's retirement for health reasons and to which his old friend and rival Tait was appointed, Maxwell was appointed to the vacant chair at King's College London. Before taking up the new post in the autumn of 1860 he also went down with smallpox.[29] By early 1861, however, he had been able to complete the first two parts of his new investigation and these were published under the title 'On physical lines of force' between March and May of that year. Later in the year he added two further parts to the paper and these were published in 1862.[30]

Just as Maxwell's earlier paper could be viewed as a development of Thomson's heat analogy, so the new investigation could also be seen as a development of Thomson's elastic solid analogy and molecular vortex theory. Maxwell did indeed describe it this way in a letter to Thomson of December 1861:[31]

> I have not heard from you for some time except through Balfour Stewart who told me he had seen you lately. ... Since I saw you I have been trying to develope the dynamical theory of magnetism as an affection of the whole magnetic field according to the views stated by you in the Royal Society's proceedings 1856 ...and elsewhere.

As before, however, it was much more than just an extension of another man's work.

Maxwell started his new paper by picking up some of the ideas of his earlier work on 'Faraday's lines of force', and by setting out his aims in much the same terms as he had before. Having outlined Faraday's notion of lines of force and their representation by iron filings he expressed himself dissatisfied with the action-at-a-distance theories of magnetism. While admitting that such theories were in fact 'in strict accordance' with the phenomena, he '[could not] help thinking that in every place where we find these lines of force, some physical state or action must exist in sufficient

[28] Maxwell to Faraday, 9 November 1857, in Campbell and Garnett (1884), p. 204.
[29] Campbell and Garnett (1884), p. 234.
[30] Maxwell (1861 and 1862).
[31] Maxwell to Thomson, 10 December 1861, in Larmor (1937), p. 34.

energy to produce the actual phenomena.'[32] As before, his stated aim was not to contribute any new scientific knowledge himself but to draw on a physical analogy and its mathematical expression so as to assist the physicist in the development of his speculations. In particular he hoped to throw light on what a theory based on the hypothesis of action through a medium would have to entail if it were to tie in with the established empirical laws:[33]

> My object in this paper is to clear the way for speculation in this direction, by investigating the mechanical results of certain states of tension and motion in a medium, and comparing these with the observed phenomena of magnetism and electricity. By pointing out the mechanical consequences of such hypotheses, I hope to be of some use to those who consider the phenomena as due to the action of a medium, but are in doubt as to the relation of this hypothesis to the experimental laws already established, which have generally been expressed in the language of other hypotheses.

Although Maxwell did not write explicitly of a 'physical analogy', the language he did use, with its emphasis on the exploration of speculative hypotheses, set his work unambiguously in the context of physical analogies as opposed to what he had previously referred to as true physical theories. In setting out his more specific aims, however, he gave the impression that the new analogy might be taken rather further than those he had previously drawn, and that it might indeed come close to providing a true theory. Whereas he had previously used 'mechanical illustrations to assist the imagination, but not to account for the phenomena',[34] he now proposed:[35]

> to examine magnetic phenomena from a mechanical point of view, and to determine what tensions in, or motions of, a medium are capable of producing the mechanical phenomena observed. If, by the same hypothesis, we can connect the phenomena of magnetic attraction with electromagnetic phenomena and with those of induced currents, we shall have found a theory which, if not true, can only be proved to be erroneous by experiments which will greatly enlarge our knowledge of this part of physics.

Since the observed electromagnetic *phenomena* were mechanical, in that they consisted of matter in motion, it was quite natural to ask how they might be mechanically produced. And if a simple mechanical hypothesis could be found by means of which all the phenomena could be connected, then this mechanical connection could provide the basis of a theory at least as good as Weber's and indeed better, since the supposed mechanical

[32] Maxwell (1890 and 1965), volume 1, p. 452.
[33] Maxwell (1890 and 1965), volume 1, p. 452.
[34] Maxwell (1890 and 1965), volume 1, p. 452.
[35] Maxwell (1890 and 1965), volume 1, p. 452.

properties of the medium would themselves be open to experimental investigation. If experiments revealed that the medium did not behave as supposed, then something could at least be learnt from the theory. If it did behave as predicted then the *connection* would be established as a true one, even though its underlying cause might well remain unknown and a matter of speculation and hypothesis.

From this perspective the immediate problem, and the one to which Maxwell proceeded to address himself, was to find a mechanical analogy for the behaviour of a medium through which the various electromagnetic phenomena could be explained and connected. Reviewing the possibilities, Maxwell noted that 'the mechanical conditions of a medium under magnetic influence have been variously conceived of, as currents, undulations, or states of displacement or strain, or of pressure or stress.'[36] Of these, the conception of undulations or waves emitted from magnetic poles was in Maxwell's view too difficult to reconcile with the established laws of attraction and repulsion. The conceptions of magnetic currents passing between the poles, and of a strained elastic solid medium in which electromagnetic forces were represented by states of displacement of particles in the medium, led to descriptions that were more closely analogous both to each other and to the laws of attraction and repulsion, and Maxwell referred here to Thomson's development of the elastic solid analogy in 1847. He had tried already to develop this analogy himself, however, and with only limited success; in the new paper he mentioned it as a possibility, noted that Thomson's analysis had been concerned with a mathematical analogy only, and passed on without further comment to the conception of a medium under stress.

In general, the stress at any point in a medium could be represented by three orthogonal components of pressure or tension. But for the representation of a magnetic force it seemed more appropriate to assume a directed stress at any point made up of just two components along and perpendicular to the line of force there. Since the lines of force were lines of attraction between the magnetic poles, they must represent axes of maximum tension or, in other words, of minimum pressure. So far the representation was straightforward, but did not really get anywhere. The next and crucial step, then, was to develop a mechanical model by which such a distribution of stress might be explained and through which it might be related to other electromagentic phenomena. For this, Maxwell had to make a further assumption of a 'fluid or mobile medium'; but once that assumption was made then the hypothesis of molecular vortices, rotating around the lines of force as axes, provided a natural explanation of the stress distribution he required:[37]

> Let us now suppose that the phenomena of magnetism depend on the

[36] Maxwell (1890 and 1965), volume 1, p. 453.
[37] Maxwell (1890 and 1965), volume 1, p. 455.

> existence of a . . . pressure greater in the equatorial than in the axial direction: the next question is, what mechanical explanation can we give of this inequality of pressures in a fluid or mobile medium? The explanation which most readily occurs to the mind is that the excess of pressure in the equatorial direction arises from the centrifugal force of vortices or eddies in the medium having their axes in directions parallel to the lines of force.

The vortices also suggested a way of representing the dipolar character of magnetic force, which was not incorporated in the strain analogy itself and was indeed, as Maxwell pointed out, not needed there, since the phenomena of magnetic attraction and repulsion were themselves isotropic. Any vortex was intrinsically dipolar, being left handed from one end and right handed from the other end of its axis. For convenience, Maxwell defined the direction of the vortex as that in which one type of electricity (vitreous) would have to flow to produce magnetic force lines running in the same direction as those to be represented.

Having introduced the hypothesis of molecular vortices, Maxwell's next step was to work out the effect of many such vortices, assumed to be parallel to each other, in terms of the resultant force on a small unit volume element of the medium. For this he derived the expressions

$$\begin{aligned} X &= \frac{1}{4\pi}\left(\frac{\mathrm{d}}{\mathrm{d}x}(\mu\alpha^2 - p_1) + \frac{\mathrm{d}}{\mathrm{d}y}(\mu\alpha\beta) + \frac{\mathrm{d}}{\mathrm{d}z}(\mu\alpha\gamma)\right) \\ Y &= \frac{1}{4\pi}\left(\frac{\mathrm{d}}{\mathrm{d}y}(\mu\beta^2 - p_1) + \frac{\mathrm{d}}{\mathrm{d}z}(\mu\beta\gamma) + \frac{\mathrm{d}}{\mathrm{d}x}(\mu\beta\alpha)\right) \\ Z &= \frac{1}{4\pi}\left(\frac{\mathrm{d}}{\mathrm{d}z}(\mu\gamma^2 - p_1) + \frac{\mathrm{d}}{\mathrm{d}x}(\mu\gamma\alpha) + \frac{\mathrm{d}}{\mathrm{d}y}(\mu\gamma\beta)\right) \end{aligned} \tag{5.1}$$

for the forces X, Y and Z acting in the x, y and z directions. μ was a measure of the density of the fluid medium and p_1 the pressure at the circumference of a vortex. α, β and γ were defined by

$$\alpha = \nu l \qquad \beta = \nu m \qquad \gamma = \nu n \tag{5.2}$$

with ν the velocity at the circumference of a vortex and l, m and n the direction cosines of the axes of the vortices with respect to x, y and z. From this, he deduced the expressions

$$\begin{aligned} X = {} & \frac{\alpha}{4\pi}\left(\frac{\mathrm{d}}{\mathrm{d}x}(\mu\alpha) + \frac{\mathrm{d}}{\mathrm{d}y}(\mu\beta) + \frac{\mathrm{d}}{\mathrm{d}z}(\mu\gamma)\right) + \frac{1}{8\pi}\mu\frac{\mathrm{d}}{\mathrm{d}x}(\alpha^2+\beta^2+\gamma^2) \\ & - \mu\beta\frac{1}{4\pi}\left(\frac{\mathrm{d}\beta}{\mathrm{d}x} - \frac{\mathrm{d}\alpha}{\mathrm{d}y}\right) + \mu\gamma\left(\frac{\mathrm{d}\alpha}{\mathrm{d}z} - \frac{\mathrm{d}\gamma}{\mathrm{d}x}\right) - \frac{\mathrm{d}p_1}{\mathrm{d}x} \end{aligned} \tag{5.3}$$

and similarly for Y and Z. In order to fulfil his objective, Maxwell next had to interpret these expressions electromagnetically, and to do this he identified μ with the magnetic inductive capacity of the medium and α, β and

γ with the components of magnetic force acting at any point. The quantity of magnetic induction was then given by ($\mu\alpha$, $\mu\beta$, $\mu\gamma$), and by consideration of the induction through a closed surface surrounding a magnetic pole it was an easy matter to deduce a relationship between the quantity of magnetic induction and the strength of the pole. In modern notation,

$$\oiint (\mu\boldsymbol{\alpha}) \cdot (\mathrm{d}\boldsymbol{\omega}_1 \times \mathrm{d}\boldsymbol{\omega}_2) = \iiint m \, \mathrm{d}\omega^3 \tag{5.4}$$

or

$$\boldsymbol{\nabla} \cdot (\mu\boldsymbol{\alpha}) = 4\pi m$$

with m representing the strength of the pole or, more generally, the quantity of magnetic matter per unit volume.

Now the first term of each expression in (5.2) could be rewritten as αm and interpreted as the force acting in the appropriate direction on a magnetic pole. The interpretation of the second term in each expression was also straightforward. Depending only on the magnetic inductive capacity and scalar intensity of magnetic force, not on the direction of that force, it represented the force acting by magnetic induction on paramagnetic or diamagnetic media, by which any body placed in a magnetic field was urged towards an area of stronger magnetic intensity in proportion to its magnetic inductive capacity. In Faraday's interpretation of his experiments, we may recall, paramagnetics responded more strongly in this sense than a surrounding medium of air, while diamagnetics, responding less strongly than the medium, appeared to go towards areas of weaker intensity.

Analysing the third and fourth terms, Maxwell noted that $(\mathrm{d}\beta/\mathrm{d}x - \mathrm{d}\alpha/\mathrm{d}y)$ and $(\mathrm{d}\alpha/\mathrm{d}z - \mathrm{d}\gamma/\mathrm{d}x)$ corresponded to the work that would be done on poles travelling in small closed curves round units of area in the xy and zx planes respectively, and therefore represented the effects of electric currents passing through the axes of such circuits. Defining (p, q, r) as the quantities of electric current per unit area flowing in the (x, y, z) directions, the third and fourth terms reduced in the first expression to $-\mu\beta r$ and $+\mu\gamma q$ respectively, and could therefore be interpreted as the total force exerted on a current element by the magnetic field. The final term, $-\mathrm{d}p_1/\mathrm{d}x$, represented the effect on an element of the medium of the variations in simple hydrostatic pressure, which were assumed to exist only at a microscopic level and not to effect the observed macroscopic behaviour. Summarising, Maxwell could write down the components of the force on a unit volume of the medium as

$$\begin{aligned} X &= \alpha m + \frac{1}{8\pi}\mu\frac{\mathrm{d}}{\mathrm{d}x}(\nu^2) - \mu\beta r + \mu\gamma q - \frac{\mathrm{d}p_1}{\mathrm{d}x} \\ Y &= \beta m + \frac{1}{8\pi}\mu\frac{\mathrm{d}}{\mathrm{d}y}(\nu^2) - \mu\gamma p + \mu\alpha r - \frac{\mathrm{d}p_1}{\mathrm{d}y} \\ Z &= \gamma m + \frac{1}{8\pi}\mu\frac{\mathrm{d}}{\mathrm{d}z}(\nu^2) - \mu\alpha q + \mu\beta p - \frac{\mathrm{d}p_1}{\mathrm{d}z} \end{aligned} \tag{5.5}$$

asserting that:[38]

> The first term of each expression refers to the force acting on magnetic poles.
> The second term to the action on bodies capable of magnetism by induction.
> The third and fourth terms to the force acting on electric currents.
> And the fifth to the effects of simple pressure.

In the absence of any electric current, the third and fourth terms would disappear with $\alpha \, dx + \beta \, dy + \gamma \, dz$ an exact differential or, in modern notation, $\boldsymbol{\alpha} = \nabla\phi$ for some ϕ. In a medium of constant capacity for magnetic induction (constant μ) and no electric currents, the force expression gave, again in modern notation,

$$\begin{aligned} \nabla^2\phi &= 4\pi m/\mu \quad &\text{at a pole of strength } m \\ \nabla^2\phi &= 0 \quad &\text{elsewhere} \end{aligned} \tag{5.6}$$

giving

$$\phi = -m/\mu r \tag{5.7}$$

at distance r from a pole, or

$$\frac{d\phi}{d\gamma} = \left(\frac{m}{\mu}\right)\frac{1}{r^2} \tag{5.8}$$

Coulomb's inverse square law for magnetic attraction and repulsion. As Maxwell noted, this form of Coulomb's law suggested that the attraction or repulsion between poles should be greater in diamagnetic media ($\mu < 1$) than in air, but since the range of μ appeared to be very small an experiment to confirm this result would require tremendous precision. Further simple calculations gave the effects of electrical currents on magnetic poles and on each other as determined by Ampère, and these calculations completed the first part of Maxwell's paper.

Idle wheels and electricity

In the introduction to the second part of 'On physical lines of force', Maxwell summarised the results of the first part taking care to distinguish between the different levels of hypothesis used. Although he had calculated the stress behaviour of the medium on the basis of molecular vortices, he wished to distinguish between the stress behaviour observed and the mechanism by which it was derived. The principal question he had asked was whether the observed electromagnetic phenomena could be accounted for by any hypothesis as to the mechanical condition of the medium. And

[38] Maxwell (1890 and 1965), volume 1, p. 463.

the conclusion drawn from his analysis was that they could be so accounted for, by a medium in which the lines of force defined lines of minimum pressure. But this conclusion was, he stressed, independent of any particular hypothesis as to the cause of the medium's condition. His statement here is worth quoting in full:[39]

> We have already shewn that all the forces acting between magnets, substances capable of magnetic induction, and electric currents, may be mechanically accounted for on the supposition that the surrounding medium is put into such a state that at every point the pressures are different in different directions, the direction of least pressure being that of the observed lines of force, and the difference of greatest and least pressures being proportional to the square of the intensity of the force at that point.
>
> Such a state of stress, if assumed to exist in the medium, and to be arranged according to the known laws regulating lines of force, will act upon the magnets, currents, &c. in the field with precisely the same resultant forces as those calculated on the ordinary hypothesis of direct action at a distance. This is true independently of any particular theory as to the *cause* of this state of stress, or the mode in which it can be sustained in the medium. We have therefore a satisfactory answer to the question, "Is there any mechanical hypothesis as to the condition of the medium indicated by lines of force, by which the observed resultant forces may be accounted for?" The answer is, the lines of force indicate the direction of *minimum pressure* at every point of the medium.

Having established this, Maxwell wrote, 'the second question must be, "What is the mechanical cause of this difference of pressure in different directions?"' But whereas the first question had received a definite answer, the second had been answered only by a supposition:[40]

> We have supposed, in the first part of this paper, that this difference of pressure is caused by molecular vortices, having their axes parallel to the lines of force.

Whereas 'mechanical deductions . . . resolved the first question, . . . the hypothesis of vortices . . . gave a probable answer to the second.'[41] The vortex model was, in Maxwell's earlier terminology, a physical analogy, and the next step required was clearly to explore the limits and possibilities of this analogy, to connect it with the phenomena of electricity (only the magnetic effects of currents had so far been covered) and to answer the

[39] Maxwell (1890 and 1965), volume 1, p. 467.
[40] Maxwell (1890 and 1965), volume 1, p. 467.

questions:[42]

> "How are these vortices set in rotation?" and "Why are they arranged according to the known laws of lines of force about magnets and currents?"

These questions, Maxwell observed, 'are certainly of a higher order of difficulty than either of the former', and he again distinguished explicitly between the 'suggestions I may offer by way of provisional answer to them' and his answers to the first two questions.[43]

The key problem was to establish the connection with electricity. As far as statical electricity was concerned, however, Maxwell seems to have been unable to make any marked progress at this stage, and he therefore restricted his attention to electric currents. For most physicists, electricity was something far better understood than magnetism, with statical electricity the best understood of all. But from Maxwell's perspective, in which the magnetic field was the primary conception, the reverse was the case. The nature of electricity was something as yet unknown, to be elucidated by the analogy, and not something established to be reconciled with it.[44]

> We have, in fact, now come to inquire into the physical connexion of these vortices with electric currents, while we are still in doubt as to the nature of electricity, whether it is one substance, two substances, or not a substance at all, or in what way it differs from matter, and how it is connected with it.
>
> We know that the lines of force are affected by electric currents, and we know the distribution of those lines about a current; so that from the force we can determine the amount of the current. Assuming that our explanation of the lines of force by molecular vortices is correct, why does a particular distribution of vortices indicate an electric current? A satisfactory answer to this question would lead us a long way towards that of a very important one, "What is an electric current?"

In order to tackle this problem, Maxwell first raised a difficulty with the vortex analogy that neither he nor Thomson had previously mentioned. The analogy was all very well as a means of describing and calculating the states of strain in a magnetic medium, but if it were to be taken seriously as a mechanical analogy in its own right it ran into one great difficulty. Since all the vortices were assumed to rotate in the same sense round the lines of force the contiguous parts of vortices round adjacent lines of force must be moving in opposite directions. This either did not occur to or did not trouble Thomson, but it did concern Maxwell. The only way he could

[41] Maxwell (1890 and 1965), volume 1, p. 468.
[42] Maxwell (1890 and 1965), volume 1, pp. 467–8.
[43] Maxwell (1890 and 1965), volume 1, p. 468.
[44] Maxwell (1890 and 1965), volume 1, p. 468.

conceive in which it might be mechanically possible to maintain such a combination of motions was through something corresponding to what in engineering were termed idle wheels, lying between the vortices.[45]

> In mechanism, the idle wheel is generally made to rotate about a *fixed* axle; but in epicyclic trains and other contrivances, as, for instance, in Siemens's governor for steam-engines, we find idle wheels whose centres are capable of motion. In all these cases the motion of the centre is the half sum of the motions of the circumferences of the wheels between which it is placed.

The arrangement was illustrated in the famous figure reprinted here in a corrected form as figure 5.1 (some of the arrows got pointed in reverse in the original print). The hexagonal parts represent vortices, also called 'cells', the circles idle wheels.

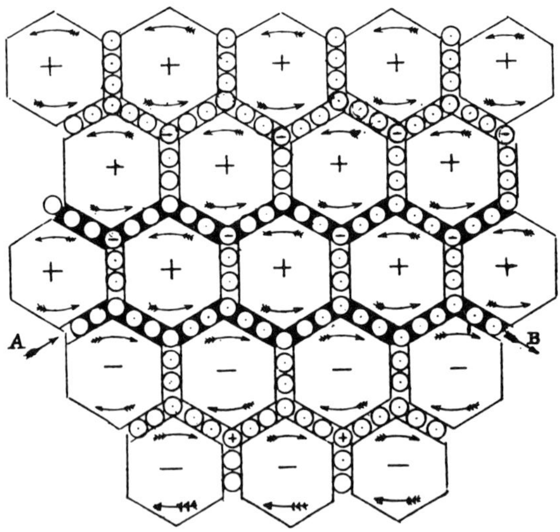

Figure 5.1 Maxwell's model of vortices and idle wheel particles, showing the vortex motions set up by an electric current (flux of particles) along AB. In the diagram as originally printed two of the vortices below AB rotated clockwise and one anticlockwise, while the fourth had its two arrows in opposite directions. The correct directions given here are deduced from the text and the + and − signs, indicating direction of magnetic field lines.

Having introduced the idle wheels so as to complete his vortex mechanism, Maxwell proceeded to calculate the effects of such a mechanism. Whereas Rankine and Thomson had talked of molecular vortices,

[45] Maxwell (1890 and 1965), volume 1, pp. 468–9.

he assumed that 'a great many vortices, with their surrounding particles, are contained in a single complete molecule of the medium.'[46] He also assumed that the particles acting as idle wheels were very small compared with the size of a vortex, with the total mass of these particles also very small compared with that of the vortices. The particles were further assumed to roll without sliding between the vortices, and not to be in contact with each other—had they been so the same problem would have arisen as with the vortices themselves. Under these assumptions the mechanical energy would be conserved so long as the particles remained within a complete molecule, but Maxwell suggested that resistance might be experienced, and mechanical energy lost to heat, in the transfer of particles from one molecule to another. Such a transfer would occur when the velocities of adjacent vortices differed, giving the particles a net rolling motion along the channel between lines of force.

Calculating the flow of particles across a unit area in unit time, Maxwell showed that this was given by the same expression as he had previously identified with the effect of a magnetic field on a current element, and he concluded that an electric current could be represented by the transfer of the particles from one vortex to another. In the absence of any externally applied force the current in a medium would disappear, and in the equilibrium state the vortical axes would be defined according to the observed lines of magnetic force. Maxwell next analysed the force exerted on the particles by a change in the motion of the vortices, deducing from this a set of equations of the form

$$\frac{\mathrm{d}Q}{\mathrm{d}z}-\frac{\mathrm{d}R}{\mathrm{d}y}=\mu\frac{\mathrm{d}\alpha}{\mathrm{d}t}\qquad\frac{\mathrm{d}P}{\mathrm{d}y}-\frac{\mathrm{d}Q}{\mathrm{d}x}=\mu\frac{\mathrm{d}\gamma}{\mathrm{d}t}\qquad\frac{\mathrm{d}R}{\mathrm{d}x}-\frac{\mathrm{d}P}{\mathrm{d}z}=\mu\frac{\mathrm{d}\beta}{\mathrm{d}t}\tag{5.9}$$

or in modern notation

$$\nabla\times\boldsymbol{P}=\mu\frac{\mathrm{d}\boldsymbol{\alpha}}{\mathrm{d}t}\tag{5.10}$$

with $\boldsymbol{P}$ or (P, Q, R) the force exerted on the layer of particles, $\boldsymbol{\alpha}$ or (α, β, γ) the circumferential velocity of a vortex and μ the density of the vortex medium. Since μ had already been identified with the quantity of magnetic induction this formula related a change in the state of the magnetic field to the electromotive force produced thereby. Defining $\boldsymbol{F}$ or (F, G, H) as the components of the electrotonic intensity, labelled $\boldsymbol{\alpha}_0$ in 'Faraday's lines of force', then from the result obtained in that paper

$$\nabla\times\boldsymbol{F}=\mu\boldsymbol{\alpha}\tag{5.11}$$

giving

$$\boldsymbol{P}=\frac{\mathrm{d}\boldsymbol{F}}{\mathrm{d}t}.\tag{5.12}$$

[46] Maxwell (1890 and 1965), volume 1, p. 471.

At last Maxwell had a mechanical conception of the electrotonic state such as he had sought in his earlier paper, with the phenomenon of induced currents appearing as part of the process by which a change in the angular velocity of the vortices was communicated from one part of the field to another, this process setting up an electromotive force or change in the electrotonic state manifest wherever the electrical resistance did not prevent the formation of a sensible current. Mechanically speaking, the induced electromotive force corresponded to the pressure on the axle of a wheel in a machine, when the velocity of the driving wheel was altered. The electrotonic state corresponded to the impulse that would act on the axle of a wheel if the velocity of the driving wheel were instantaneously changed by a finite amount.

In establishing the relationship between the vortex motion and the motion of the interspersed particles, Maxwell had so far assumed that the centres of the vortices were at rest in the medium. To continue his analysis he next generalised to a medium subject to 'all varieties of fluid motion', from which could be deduced the electromotive forces in a moving body:

$$\begin{aligned} P &= \mu\gamma\frac{\mathrm{d}y}{\mathrm{d}t} - \mu\beta\frac{\mathrm{d}z}{\mathrm{d}t} + \frac{\mathrm{d}F}{\mathrm{d}t} - \frac{\mathrm{d}\psi}{\mathrm{d}x} \\ Q &= \mu\alpha\frac{\mathrm{d}z}{\mathrm{d}t} - \mu\gamma\frac{\mathrm{d}x}{\mathrm{d}t} + \frac{\mathrm{d}G}{\mathrm{d}t} - \frac{\mathrm{d}\psi}{\mathrm{d}y} \\ R &= \mu\beta\frac{\mathrm{d}x}{\mathrm{d}t} - \mu\alpha\frac{\mathrm{d}y}{\mathrm{d}t} + \frac{\mathrm{d}H}{\mathrm{d}t} - \frac{\mathrm{d}\psi}{\mathrm{d}z}\,. \end{aligned} \tag{5.13}$$

Here the first two terms were identifiable as the effect of the motion of a body on the magnetic field, and the third term as that due to any changes in the field itself. That left the term in ψ, which had emerged as an arbitrary variable in the calculation. From consideration of the special case in which the other terms were zero, this had clearly to be identified as the electric tension or potential at any point.

In terms of its mathematical laws, Maxwell's new analysis corresponded completely with that he had already given in 'Faraday's lines of force', the symbols used being identified (using modern vector notation) as follows:

Electromotive force or electric intensity	$\boldsymbol{P}$	or	$\boldsymbol{\alpha}_2$.
Electrotonic intensity	$\boldsymbol{F}$	or	$\boldsymbol{\alpha}_0$
Electric current or quantity of electricity	$\boldsymbol{p}$	or	$\boldsymbol{a}_2$
Quantity of magnetic induction	$(\mu\boldsymbol{\alpha})$	or	$\boldsymbol{a}_1$
Intensity of magnetic induction	$\boldsymbol{\alpha}$	or	$\boldsymbol{\alpha}_1$.

$\boldsymbol{P}$ or $\boldsymbol{\alpha}_2$ may be readily identified as the modern $\boldsymbol{E}$, $\mu\boldsymbol{\alpha}$ or $\boldsymbol{a}_1$ as $\boldsymbol{B}$ and $\boldsymbol{F}$ or $\boldsymbol{\alpha}_0$ as $\boldsymbol{A}$. Equations (5.10, 5.11 and 5.12) are then recognisable as equations of the modern theory. But other parallels are harder to draw.

The new representation had not led to any significant development of the theory beyond that given a few years earlier, at least so far. In summarising his assumptions and conclusions, moreover, Maxwell again stressed the provisional and artificial nature of his model, which he did not propose as a true representation of nature, or even as an 'electrical hypothesis':[47]

> The conception of a particle having its motion connected with that of a vortex by perfect rolling contact may appear somewhat awkward. I do not bring it forward as a mode of connexion existing in nature, or even as that which I would willingly assent to as an electrical hypothesis.

The model did however provide a 'mechanically conceivable and easily investigated' way of connecting the various electromagnetic phenomena, and provided that the 'provisional and temporary character of [the] hypothesis' was understood this had in Maxwell's view to help rather than hinder the development of a true theory. For those already inclined to accept a mechanical hypothesis of the type adduced, the analysis would provide 'the conditions which must be fulfilled in order to give it mathematical coherence, and a comparison, so far satisfactory, between its necessary results and known facts.'[48] Others could benefit from comparing 'this theory with that of the existence of currents flowing freely through bodies, and with that which supposes electricity to act at a distance with a force depending on its velocity and therefore', Maxwell still thought, 'not subject to the law of conservation of energy.'[49] As in 'Faraday's lines of force' he had emphasised the importance of recognising that there might be two ways of looking at something, each corresponding to a different extensive but incomplete analogy, so now Maxwell argued that:[50]

> The facts of electro-magnetism are so complicated and various, that the explanation of any number of them by several different hypotheses must be interesting, not only to physicists, but to all who desire to understand how much evidence the explanation of phenomena lends to the credibility of a theory, or how far we ought to regard a coincidence in the mathematical expression of two sets of phenomena as an indication that these phenomena are of the same kind.

In Maxwell's view, such coincidences of mathematical expression, corresponding to physical analogies, were generally only partial. But it was only by comparing different analogies and developing them to their limits so as to detect the points at which they broke down that ever closer analogies

[47] Maxwell (1890 and 1965), volume 1, p. 486.
[48] Maxwell (1890 and 1965), volume 1, p. 488.
[49] Maxwell (1890 and 1965), volume 1, p. 488.
[50] Maxwell (1890 and 1965), volume 1, p. 488.

could be developed and an understanding of the true nature of the phenomena reached:[51]

> We know that partial coincidences of this kind have been discovered; and the fact that they are only partial is proved by the divergence of the laws of the two sets of phenomena in other respects. We may chance to find, in the higher parts of physics, instances of more complete coincidence, which may require much investigation to detect their ultimate divergence.

Magneto-optics, electrostatics and the theory of light

There were two striking omissions from the first two parts of 'On physical lines of force', one being electrostatics and the other, ironically, the magneto-optic effect that had prompted the introduction of vortices in the first place. Neither was mentioned explicitly by Maxwell, and it would seem that both had caused problems that he had so far been unable to solve.[52]

In the case of the magneto-optic effect, the problem was essentially the same as that which had already plagued Faraday in his attempt to build up a theory of magnetism. Were magnetic media to be considered, as Faraday had eventually concluded, as being all essentially similar, with diamagnetic media having a smaller magnetic inductive capacity than the vacuum and the vacuum a smaller capacity than paramagnetic bodies? Or were diamagnetic and paramagnetic media to be viewed as opposites, with the vacuum essentially neutral? In developing his vortex model, Maxwell had opted unambiguously for the former alternative, identifying the magnetic inductive capacity, μ, with the density of the vortex medium, necessarily always positive. Diamagnetics were represented by vortices of density less than 1 but greater than 0, the vacuum by density 1, and paramagnetics by density greater than 1. In the same magnetic field the three types of vortices would always rotate in the same direction. From some experiments published in 1858, however, Emile Verdet had concluded that the direction of the magneto-optic rotation in some paramagnetic substances was opposite to that in diamagnetic substances, a result that was completely at odds both with Faraday's theory and with Maxwell's assumptions about vortex behaviour.[53]

[51] Maxwell (1890 and 1965), volume 1, p. 488.
[52] See for example Siegel (1975 and 1981), Knudsen (1976), Heimann (1970b), Bromberg (1967 and 1968) and Chalmers (1973). In discussing 'On physical lines of force', however, in which there are a number of arithmetic errors, most of these writers have managed to introduce some small confusion that does not exist in the original. Their accounts are all important and useful, but should all be read with care.
[53] Verdet (1854–63).

In electrostatics, the problem was the more straightforward one of extending the model. Maxwell had already identified the motion of the idle wheel particles as corresponding to that of electricity in currents, but his description was as yet limited, as he had noted explicitly in 'Faraday's lines of force', to the case of closed current circuits.[54] In particular it rested on Ampère's law for the relation between electric flux and magnetic intensity,

$$\boldsymbol{a}_2 = \frac{1}{4\pi}\,\nabla \times \boldsymbol{\alpha}_1 \qquad \text{or} \qquad \boldsymbol{p} = \frac{1}{4\pi}\,\nabla \times \boldsymbol{\alpha} \tag{5.14}$$

which implied $\nabla \cdot \boldsymbol{a}_2 = \nabla \cdot \boldsymbol{p} = 0$, so that there could be no accumulation of electric charge. The phenomena of electrostatics also raised problems concerning the mechanical details of the model and in particular the interaction between the vortex medium and ordinary matter. Since the magnetic field extended throughout the vacuum, the vortex medium would have to do likewise. But in describing the differences between conductors and insulators Maxwell seems to have treated the vortices as contained within material molecules, and the conducting power of the medium as determined in some way by the ease of transfer of idle wheel particles between molecules. There was no necessary inconsistency here, but nor was there any clear way of visualising how the mechanism might operate so as, for example, to make electrical transfer possible in a material substance but not in the vacuum.

It is not clear whether Maxwell found the electrostatic problem temporarily intractable, as most historians have assumed, or whether the commitments created by his new job at King's College London and his presence in London simply left him insufficient time to explore the problem. The fact that part II of his paper was presented as a conclusion without any mention of a sequel appears to suggest the former, but the latter may well have been a contributing factor. At any rate, once he was away from his London commitments and in Glenlair for the summer vacation, Maxwell very quickly developed an extension of the model to electrostatics, reporting on his results in a letter to Faraday in October and publishing them in part III of the paper, which appeared a few months later in the spring of 1862.[55]

In looking for an extension of the vortex mechanism to embrace the phenomena of electrostatics, Maxwell had two natural leads. He could look at the inadequacies of the mechanism as so far described and he could look at the physical ideas on statical electricity developed by Faraday. He no longer claimed explicitly to be merely mathematising Faraday's ideas, as he had in his earlier paper, but to a very large extent this was still what he was doing. His treatment was still based on Faraday's suggestions of a magnetic

[54] Maxwell (1890) and 1965), volume 1, p. 195.

[55] Maxwell to Faraday, 19 October 1861, in Campbell and Garnett (1884), pp. 243–5. See also Maxwell to Thomson, 10 December 1861, in Larmor (1937), pp. 34–6.

medium, lines of force and an electrotonic state, and the mathematical analogy between 'Faraday's lines of force' and 'On physical lines of force' was so far complete. He had also opted for Faraday's theory of diamagnetism, and in extending his representation of electromagnetic phenomena it was natural for him to look towards Faraday's concepts of electrostatics and dielectric media as a starting point.

Faraday, we may recall, had viewed the phenomena of electrostatic induction in terms of a polarisation of the particles of a dielectric.[56] He had viewed all material particles as being 'as wholes conductors', capable of being thrown instantaneously and 'more or less readily' into an 'electrically polar state by neighbouring particles.' Faraday's conception of the particles of a dielectric medium being polarised in the presence of an electric field had also been taken up by the Italian, O F Mossotti. In a series of papers written between 1846 and 1850 Mossotti had incorporated Faraday's conception in an electrical aether theory, attributing the polarisation to a displacement of the aetherial particles in the electrical atmospheres supposed to surround material molecules.[57] He had also developed this theory mathematically and had shown that the phenomenon of induced electric polarisation could be represented mathematically by a theory completely analogous to Poisson's theory of induced magnetism.

The question facing Maxwell was whether Faraday's conception could be incorporated in the vortex model, and the work of Mossotti suggested that it could be, with Maxwell's idle wheel particles taking the place of Mossotti's atmospheric particles. Maxwell had already identified the motion of the idle wheel particles with that of electricity, and he had assumed that the particles were mobile within but not between the molecules of an insulating material. The particles could not themselves represent electricity, as they were distributed throughout space; but, just as in Mossotti's theory, an excess of the particle density over that in non-electrified media could represent electricity of one type, with the opposite type characterised by a corresponding density defect. A state of electrical polarisation could thus be represented by a displacement of the particles in each molecule to one side or another, giving an excess density on one side and a corresponding density defect on the opposite side. All that was required to incorporate dielectric media in the vortex model was accordingly a mechanism for creating and maintaining a differential displacement of the particles in a molecule.

Viewing the problem from the other end, the main inadequacies in the existing mechanical model were the absence of any mechanism for the interaction between vortices in adjacent molecules and the absence of any

[56] See Chapter 3 above, references in note 85.

[57] Mossotti (1847a, 1847b and 1850), reprinted in Mossotti (1951), pp. 321–59, the mathematical analysis being on pp. 333–59.

prescription for the nature of the vortex medium. Of these, the former is the more striking. Maxwell had indicated that the difference between conductors and insulators lay in the ability of the idle wheel particles to cross from one molecule to another in conductors and not in insulators, but he had offered no picture of how this difference might be represented mechanically, and no indication of how his model was to tie in with a theory of matter and in particular of the vacuum. It was not, however, this inadequacy but the other which was to provide him with the scope for incorporating Faraday's theory of dielectrics. In the earlier parts of 'On physical lines of force' Maxwell had described the vortex medium as 'fluid or mobile', passing by without comment the alternative possibility of an elastic solid medium. Throughout his discussion he had adopted the imagery of fluid motion, and he had even written of 'vortices or eddies'.[58] As the model had been developed however, it had required the vortices to act rather as solids. In particular, the motion of a vortex having been imparted to it at a point on its circumference, it was supposed to be transmitted instantaneously throughout the vortex, the whole of which was supposed to rotate with the same angular velocity. This transmission of motion could not occur in a fluid medium.

Analysing the mechanical behaviour of the vortices required by his model, Maxwell saw that this actually corresponded to an elastic solid medium within each vortex. And this in turn pointed clearly towards a possible mechanism for electrostatic induction. Writing to Faraday in October 1861 he described 'the conception I have hit on' as follows:[59]

> My theory of electrical forces is, that they are called into play in insulating media by *slight* electric displacements, which put certain small portions of the medium into a state of distortion, which, being resisted by the *elasticity* of the medium, produces an electromotive force. A spherical cell would, by such a displacement, be distorted thus—
>
> 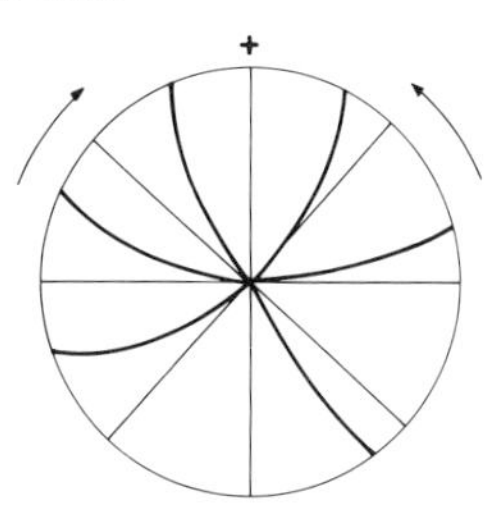
>
>
> where the curved lines represent diameters originally straight, but now curved.
>
> I suppose the elasticity of the sphere to react on the electrical matter surrounding it, and press it downwards.

[58] Maxwell (1890 and 1965), volume 1, p. 455.
[59] Maxwell to Faraday, 19 October 1861, in Campbell and Garnett (1884), p. 244.

The inclusion of the figure reminds us that the study of the distortion of elastic solids, both in theory and in practice, had been one of Maxwell's earliest scientific occupations: he was on familiar ground.

In part III of 'On physical lines of force', Maxwell spelled out his argument more clearly. He first summed up briefly the hypotheses of parts I and II, including the transmission of motion from one vortex to another by tangential action between the vortices and idle wheel particles. He noted that he had not previously attempted to explain the tangential action mechanically, but suggested that, in order to explain it,[60]

> it is necessary to suppose, in order to account for the transmission of rotation from the exterior to the interior parts of each cell, that the substance in the cells possesses elasticity of figure, similar in kind, though different in degree, to that observed in solid bodies.

Maxwell also suggested that since an elastic solid medium was also required for the luminiferous aether, to account for the transverse vibrations of the wave theory of light, 'we need not ... be surprised if the magneto-electric medium possesses the same property'.[61] But as we shall see, his reasons for making this connection may well have come later in the argument. He next summarised the ways in which electric current, electric potential or tension, and electromotive force were represented in the model, and set out the problem of incorporating electrostatic phenomena as well:[62]

> According to our theory, the particles which form the partitions between the cells consitute the matter of electricity. The motion of these particles constitutes an electric current; the tangential force with which the particles are pressed by the matter of the cells is electromotive force, and the pressure of the particles on each other corresponds to the tension or potential of the electricity.
>
> If we can now explain the condition of a body with respect to the surrounding medium when it is said to be "charged" with electricity, and account for the forces acting between electrified bodies, we shall have established a connexion between the principal phenomena of electrical science.

In order to solve this problem Maxwell first discussed the relationship between the passage of electricity in conductors and the transmission of electric action through insulators or dielectrics. On one hand, he noted the independence of the two phenomena, the capacity of a dielectric being a quite different quantity from the resistance of a conducting medium. On the other hand he also noted their connection. Electric tension or potential was the same thing, whether manifest in the potential difference between two

[60] Maxwell (1890 and 1965), volume 1, p. 489.
[61] Maxwell (1890 and 1965), volume 1, p. 489.
[62] Maxwell (1890 and 1965), volume 1, p. 490.

insulated conductors, in which case it was related to the properties of the intervening dielectric, or in that between two parts of a conductor, in which case it was related to a current flowing between these parts. A Leyden jar could be statically charged using the current generated by a dynamo. To describe the properties of a dielectric, Maxwell then noted the analogy demonstrated by Mossotti between the effect of an electrostatic force on a dielectric and that of a magnet on iron filings in its field, and deduced that the behaviour of a dielectric could be described, as it had been by Faraday and Mossotti, in terms of a state of polarisation, 'every particle [having] its poles in opposite conditions'.[63] In a dielectric medium under electrostatic induction,[64]

> We may conceive that the electricity in each molecule is so displaced that one side is rendered positively, and the other negatively electrical, but that the electricity remains entirely connected with the molecule, and does not pass from one molecule to another.

The effect of such an action on the whole mass of a dielectric would then be 'to produce a general displacement of the electricity in a certain direction.'[65]

Maxwell observed that this electric displacement did not amount to a current. Once it had reached a certain extent it would stay constant, with no passage of electricity between molecules, and with the force producing it balanced by the elastic reaction of the medium. But the displacement was, in Maxwell's words, 'the commencement of a current',[66] in the sense that any change in displacement did constitute a current, given for a displacement h in the z direction by r,

$$r = \frac{\mathrm{d}h}{\mathrm{d}t} \tag{5.15}$$

The displacement was related to the electromotive force in the z direction, R, by Hooke's law, giving

$$R = -4\pi\epsilon^2 h \tag{5.16a}$$

with ϵ a coefficient of elasticity.

The inclusion of the negative sign in equation (5.16a) has caused a lot of confusion, with some historians attributing it to a fundamental inconsistency in Maxwell's conceptions while others maintain its correctness, given his definitions. It cannot in fact be correct, for Maxwell wrote quite clearly on the previous page that the electromotive force corresponded to the

[63] Maxwell (1890 and 1965), volume 1, p. 491.
[64] Maxwell (1890 and 1965), volume 1, p. 491.
[65] Maxwell (1890 and 1965), volume 1, p. 491.
[66] Maxwell (1890 and 1965), volume 1, p. 491.

tangential force exerted by the vortex cells on the idle wheel particles, which force cannot but be in the same direction as the displacement it is supposed to produce. He was also quite consistent throughout in treating the current flow produced by the electromotive force as having the same sign as that force.[67] There is no need, however, to postulate any fundamental inconsistency in Maxwell's thought. The situation was very confusing, for whereas an electromotive force was described in terms of an effect of the vortices on the particles, it was also envisaged as the consequence of a potential difference across the medium, which is to say the consequence of pressures exerted between electric particles and by them on the vortices. Moreover, in the same paragraph as that in which he gave his equation, Maxwell wrote of 'electromotive force producing electric displacement in a dielectric' *and* of 'the dielectric recovering from its state of displacement with an equal [and of course opposite] electromotive force.'[68] The point was that the electrical energy of a dielectric was retained, whereas that of an imperfectly conducting medium was lost to heat; and as the mechanism for this retention Maxwell had in mind the analogy between the vortices and elastic bodies, yielding to the pressure from the displaced particles and recovering from it when that pressure was removed. As he explained the mechanical analogy:[69]

> According to our hypothesis, the magnetic medium is divided into cells, separated by partitions formed by a stratum of particles which will play the part of electricity. When the electric particles are urged in any direction, they will, by their tangential action on the elastic substance of the cells, distort each cell, and call into play an equal and opposite force arising from the elasticity of the cells. When the force is removed, the cells will recover their form, and the electricity will return to its former position.

Thus although Maxwell was putting forward an equation for a displacement caused by an electromotive force, he also had in mind the balancing force that was thereby induced and that acted to limit the displacement of the electric particles and return them to their original positions when the externally applied electromotive force ceased. His picture of a dielectric in equilibrium under the influence of a constant external force actually incorporated two equal and opposite electromotive forces, both exerted by the vortices on the particles, as well as the original force on the vortices. Given this confusion the inclusion of the minus sign in equation (5.16a) can be explained quite simply as a consequence of a simple arithmetic error

[67] See Bromberg (1967) and Chalmers (1973): Bromberg treated Maxwell as being fundamentally confused; Chalmers realised that this confusion was of Bromberg's own making, but gave a justification for the minus sign that is itself unsound.
[68] Maxwell (1890 and 1965), volume 1, p. 492.
[69] Maxwell (1890 and 1965), volume 1, p. 492.

elsewhere in Maxwell's analysis. Like Kepler and Newton before him, Maxwell was far from immune from such slips, and this particular one led to the requirement that R be negative; it is easy to see how Maxwell, if pressed, might have incorporated this rather than locate the original error.[70] Had that error not existed, he would have had, as he should, R positive and

$$R = +4\pi\epsilon^2 h \tag{5.16b}$$

in correspondence with the modern equivalent

$$\boldsymbol{E} = 4\pi\epsilon^2 \boldsymbol{D}. \tag{5.17}$$

Analysing the relationship between force and displacement according to this elastic vortex model, on the simplifying assumption that the vortices or cells were spherical, Maxwell derived his equation (5.16a) with the constant ϵ^2 (Maxwell used 'E^2') given by $3\pi m/(1+5m/3n)$, m being the coefficient of rigidity and n (Maxwell used 'μ') that of cubical elasticity of the vortex medium. Since he now had a mechanism for the accumulation of charge, his analysis was no longer restricted to closed currents and Ampère's equation therefore had to be modified. He had already noted that a change of displacement $\mathrm{d}h/\mathrm{d}t$ constituted a current, and given the relationship between displacement and electromotive force this could be expressed in terms of a change in electromotive force $-(4\pi/\epsilon^2)\,\mathrm{d}R/\mathrm{d}t$. Adding this as an extra term in the existing equations for the electric current gave, in Maxwell's notation,

$$\begin{aligned} p &= \frac{1}{4\pi}\left(\frac{\mathrm{d}\gamma}{\mathrm{d}y} - \frac{\mathrm{d}\beta}{\mathrm{d}z} - \frac{1}{\epsilon^2}\frac{\mathrm{d}P}{\mathrm{d}t}\right) \\ q &= \frac{1}{4\pi}\left(\frac{\mathrm{d}\alpha}{\mathrm{d}z} - \frac{\mathrm{d}\gamma}{\mathrm{d}x} - \frac{1}{\epsilon^2}\frac{\mathrm{d}Q}{\mathrm{d}t}\right) \\ r &= \frac{1}{4\pi}\left(\frac{\mathrm{d}\beta}{\mathrm{d}x} - \frac{\mathrm{d}\alpha}{\mathrm{d}y} - \frac{1}{\epsilon^2}\frac{\mathrm{d}R}{\mathrm{d}t}\right) \end{aligned} \tag{5.18}$$

or in vector notation,

$$\boldsymbol{p} = \frac{1}{4\pi}\,\nabla\times\boldsymbol{\alpha} - \frac{1}{4\pi\epsilon^2}\frac{\mathrm{d}\boldsymbol{P}}{\mathrm{d}t}. \tag{5.19}$$

Finally the equation of continuity, $\nabla\cdot\boldsymbol{P}=0$ in the absence of any accumulated charge, also had to be modified. Taking e as the 'quantity of electricity in unit of volume', or excess density of idle wheel particles, $\mathrm{d}e/\mathrm{d}t$

[70] The slip occurred in Maxwell's equation 104 which should have had a minus sign so as to read $R = -4\pi^2 m[(e+2f)/e]h$. Since $(e+2f)/e = -E^2/\pi m$, with m positive, R should have been positive but was with the error negative (ϵ^2 was of course positive). To add to the confusion there are also two other mutually cancelling mistakes of sign, one of which again relates to the tangential force: equation 88 has the wrong sign, and a similar error in equation 103 compensates for this.

gave the number of particles leaving or entering that volume per second, otherwise expressible as the divergence of the total current at that point,[71]

$$\frac{\mathrm{d}e}{\mathrm{d}t} = -\left(\frac{\mathrm{d}p}{\mathrm{d}x} + \frac{\mathrm{d}q}{\mathrm{d}y} + \frac{\mathrm{d}r}{\mathrm{d}z}\right) = -\ \nabla \cdot p. \tag{5.20}$$

Equation (5.19) then gave

$$\frac{\mathrm{d}e}{\mathrm{d}t} = \frac{1}{4\pi\epsilon^2}\frac{\mathrm{d}}{\mathrm{d}t}(\nabla \cdot P) \tag{5.21}$$

implying, since e was zero in the absence of electromotive force,

$$e = \frac{1}{4\pi\epsilon^2}\ \nabla \cdot P. \tag{5.22}$$

To complete his analysis, Maxwell derived a formula for the force between two electrified bodies in terms of the properties of the intervening dielectric medium. Expressing the energy of the medium in terms of the electric tension ψ corresponding to its displacement, and equating this tension with that due to the presence of point charged bodies of charges e_1 and e_2 at a distance r from each other he derived Coulomb's law in the form

$$\text{Force} = -\ \epsilon^2 \frac{e_1 e_2}{r^2}. \tag{5.23}$$

It is at this point of the argument that the significance of Maxwell's earlier comment on the equivalence of electric tension in the electrostatic and galvanic cases becomes apparent, for the key part of his derivation of the electrostatic force was his identification of the two definitions of electric tension, one the electrostatic tension due to the presence of a charged body and the other the galvanic tension associated with an electromotive force. Thus although the equation he had derived was the familiar one from electrostatics, the quantities in it were essentially electrodynamic and thus, in Maxwell's model, electromagnetic, with e_1 and e_2 being interpreted in terms of their magnetic effects. A unit charge e was defined as that which, passing across a unit area in unit time, would constitute a unit current, and a unit current was that which,[72]

> circulating round a ring whose area is unity, produces the same effect on a

[71] This is another area of confusion in the secondary literature. A number of writers have mistakenly treated Maxwell's displacement current as adding to the conduction current to give a closed total current, and reflecting this confusion Bromberg (1967) has contrived to see a confusion between total and conduction current in Maxwell's paper. But as Chalmers (1973) points out this confusion is Bromberg's. Maxwell's conduction current is closed, his total current not so, and in this respect he meant precisely what he wrote.

[72] Maxwell (1890 and 1965), volume 1, p. 498.

distant magnet as a magnet would produce whose strength is unity and length unity placed perpendicular to the plane of the ring.

If Coulomb's law were expressed in terms of normal electrostatic charge measures, η_1 and η_2, as

$$\text{Force} = -\frac{\eta_1\eta_2}{r^2} \tag{5.24}$$

then these would be related to the electromagnetic charges e_1 and e_2 as

$$\eta_1 = \epsilon e_1 \qquad \eta_2 = \epsilon e_2. \tag{5.25}$$

So Maxwell had, in his formula for ϵ, a theoretical measure of the ratio between electrostatic and electromagnetic charge, in terms of the properties of the vortex medium. And since this ratio had been measured by Kohlrausch and Weber he also had the means available to deduce some of the properties of the supposed medium.[73] Maxwell had already assumed the medium would behave as a perfect elastic solid, and this had allowed him to reduce his initial two variables, the coefficients of cubical elasticity and rigidity, to a single variable, the coefficient of rigidity, also called the coefficient of transverse elasticity. Denoting this by m, he had

$$\epsilon^2 = \pi m. \tag{5.26}$$

There then came the question: could the elastic solid medium be the same as that which seemed to be required for the wave theory of light? The first suggestion that it might be so was given by Maxwell in his letter of 19 October to Faraday:[74]

> From the determination by Kohlrausch and Weber of the numerical relation between the statical and magnetic effects of electricity, I have determined the *elasticity* of the medium in air, and assuming that it is the same with the luminiferous aether, I have determined the velocity of propagation of transverse vibrations.
>
> The result is 193,088 miles per second (deduced from electrical and magnetic experiments). Fizeau has determined the velocity of light = 193,118 miles per second, by direct experiment.

The result attributed to Fizeau was taken from Galbraith and Haughton's manual of astronomy, and when Maxwell checked up on Fizeau's own report he found a figure of 195 647 miles per second, giving a less perfect but still very good agreement with Weber's measurements. In his paper Maxwell assumed that the velocity of propagation of transverse vibrations in a perfect elastic solid was given by

$$v = \sqrt{m/\rho} \tag{5.27}$$

[73] Weber and Kohlrausch (1857).

[74] Maxwell to Faraday, 19 October 1861, in Campbell and Garnett (1884), p. 244.

with ρ the density of the medium. Since the density was on his model equivalent to $1/\pi$ times the coefficient of magnetic induction, which was itself unity in air or the vacuum, this gave

$$v = \sqrt{m\pi} = \epsilon. \tag{5.28}$$

Maxwell explained in his letter to Faraday and again in a letter to Thomson that he had worked out this relationship between v and ϵ at Glenlair, before seeing Weber's figure for ϵ, and 'before I had any suspicion of the nearness between the two values of the velocity of propagation of magnetic effects and that of light.'[75] He had then found, on his return to London, that Weber's figure for the ratio of the units, which had the dimension of velocity, corresponded to within $1\frac{1}{2}\%$ to Fizeau's value for the velocity of light, and more closely still to other measures of that velocity. To Faraday, Maxwell wrote that 'we have now strong reason to believe, whether my theory is a fact or not, that the luminiferous and electromagnetic medium are one.'[76] His letter to Thomson was worded almost identically,[77] and in his paper he wrote that:[78]

> We can scarcely avoid the inference that *light consists in the transverse undulations of the same medium which is the cause of electric and magnetic phenomena.*

There is one problem with Maxwell's conclusion, for, as Duhem pointed out many years ago, the correct formula for the velocity using Maxwell's definitions is in fact[79]

$$v = \sqrt{m/2\rho} \tag{5.29}$$

giving

$$v^2 = \epsilon^2/2. \tag{5.30}$$

There was also, however, some confusion in the reading of Weber's results, which used Ampèrean electrodynamic units rather than the electromagnetic ones used by Maxwell. The value measured by Weber was roughly half the speed of light, and was interpreted by Maxwell as corresponding to $\epsilon/2$.[80] In fact, though, it should have corresponded, allowing for the difference in units, to $\epsilon/2\sqrt{2}$, and once again Maxwell's two mistakes cancelled each other

[75] Maxwell to Thomson, 10 December 1861, in Larmor (1937), p. 35, and see also Maxwell to Faraday, 19 October 1861, in Campbell and Garnett (1884), p. 244.
[76] Maxwell to Faraday, 19 October 1861, in Campbell and Garnett (1884), p. 244.
[77] Maxwell to Thomson, 10 December 1861, in Larmor (1937), p. 35.
[78] Maxwell (1890 and 1965), volume 1, p. 500.
[79] Duhem (1902), pp. 211–12, and see Chalmers (1973).
[80] Maxwell to Thomson, 10 December 1861, in Larmor (1937), p. 35: 'Weber's number is really, as it appears to be, one half the velocity of light.'

out. Which error came first we cannot say, but having postulated a magnetic medium of precisely the same kind as was required for the wave theory of light, and having found the speed of propagation of transverse vibrations in this medium to correspond to that of light, even if only to within a factor of $\sqrt{2}$, Maxwell can have had few doubts that the correspondence must be a true one, with the constant factor arising from some error in the analysis. Where precisely this error lay may not have worried him unduly, and it would have been natural to attribute it to his formula for velocity, and to adapt this accordingly.

Once Maxwell had arrived at his relationship between the magnetic medium and that of light, it was only natural that he should have gone back to the other phenomenon omitted from the earlier parts of his paper, the magneto-optic effect. This was after all an interaction between magnetism and light, and was therefore an obvious testing ground for their proposed unification. The first indication that he had followed this route was again given in the letter to Faraday:[81]

> I have also examined the theory of the passage of light through a medium filled with magnetic vortices, and find that the rotation of the plane of polarisation is in the same direction with that of the vortices, that it varies inversely as the *square* of the wave length (as is shown by experiment), and that its amount is proportional to the *diameter* of the vortices.

In a fourth and final part of 'On physical lines of force', published like the third in the spring of 1862, Maxwell first reflected on some of the general arguments behind his adoption of the vortex hypothesis. The relationship between electric current and magnetic intensity,

$$\boldsymbol{a}_2 = \nabla \times \boldsymbol{\alpha}_1 \qquad \text{or} \qquad \boldsymbol{p} = \nabla \times \boldsymbol{\alpha} \tag{5.31}$$

had the same mathematical form as that generally existing between a linear and a rotatory phenomenon. Challis and Helmholtz had developed analogies in which magnetism assumed a linear and electricity a rotatory character. But Faraday, Thomson, Ampère and Weber had all treated magnetism as the rotatory phenomenon, and it was this latter view which fitted better with experiment, in which an electric current produced a linear transfer of electrolytes and a magnetic force acted to rotate the plane of polarisation of light:[82]

> The transference of electrolytes in fixed directions by the electric current, and the rotation of polarized light in fixed directions by magnetic force, are the

[81] Maxwell to Faraday, 19 October 1861, in Campbell and Garnett (1884), pp. 244–5.

[82] Maxwell (1890 and 1965), volume 1, p. 505. Maxwell's analysis is reviewed in detail by Knudsen (1976).

> facts the consideration of which has induced me to regard magnetism as a phenomenon of rotation, and electric currents as phenomena of translation, instead of following out the analogy pointed out by Helmholtz, or adopting the theory propounded by Professor Challis.
>
> The theory that electric currents are linear, and magnetic force rotatory phenomena, agrees so far with that of Ampère and Weber; and the hypothesis that the magnetic rotations exist wherever magnetic force extends, that the centrifugal force of these rotations accounts for magnetic attractions, and that the inertia of the vortices accounts for induced currents, is supported by the opinion of Professor W. Thomson. In fact the whole theory of molecular vortices developed in this paper has been suggested to me by observing the direction in which those investigators who study the action of the media are looking for the explanation of electro-magnetic phenomena.

In particular, Thomson had 'pointed out that the cause of the magnetic action on light must be a real rotation going on in the magnetic field.'[83]

The problem was, could the specific hypothesis adopted by Maxwell account for the observed characteristics of the magneto-optic effect, as established by Verdet and others? Analysing the effect of vortex rotation on the polarisation of a plane light wave propagated as a transverse vibration in the vortex medium, Maxwell was able to conclude that:[84]

> the only effect which the rotation of the vortices will have on the light will be to make the plane of polarization rotate in the *same* direction as the vortices, through an angle proportional—
>
> (A) to the thickness of the substance,
> (B) to the resolved part of the magnetic force parallel to the ray,
> (C) to the index of refraction of the ray,
> (D) inversely to the square of the wave-length in air,
> (E) to the *mean radius* of the vortices,
> (F) to the capacity for magnetic induction.

(A) and (B) agreed completely with Verdet's results. (D) also corresponded to the accepted empirical behaviour, but with enough uncertainty to allow for the possibility, in Maxwell's view the probability, that (C), which had not been properly tested yet, would also hold. (E) could not be tested, but allowed for a variation in rotating power between different but otherwise similar substances, and certainly did not threaten the accuracy of the hypothesis. The only problem was (F). On Maxwell's theory as so far developed, the capacity for magnetic induction, corresponding to the density of the vortex medium, was always positive; so the theory implied a rotating effect that was always in the same direction, diamagnetics, paramagnetics and the vacuum being distinguished only by the relative

[83] Maxwell (1890 and 1965), volume 1, p. 505.
[84] Maxwell (1890 and 1965), volume 1, p. 506.

amount of rotation. According to Verdet's experiments, however, the effect was zero in a vacuum, and acted in opposite directions in diamagnetic and paramagnetic substances. In these circumstances Maxwell had little option but to abandon Faraday's theory of diamagnetism, on which he had based his model, in favour of Weber's, in which paramagnetic and diamagnetic bodies were characterised by rotatory characteristics in opposite directions as required:[85]

> On our theory, the direction of the rotation of the plane of polarization depends on that of the mean moment of momenta, or *angular momentum*, of the molecular vortices; and since M. Verdet has discovered that magnetic substances have an effect on light opposite to that of diamagnetic substances, it follows that the molecular rotation must be opposite in the two classes of substances.
>
> We can no longer, therefore, consider diamagentic bodies as being those whose coefficient of magnetic induction is less than that of space empty of gross matter. We must admit the diamagnetic state to be the *opposite* of the paramagnetic; and that the vortices, or at least the influential majority of them, in diamagnetic substances, revolve in the direction in which positive electricity revolves in the magnetizing bobbin, while in paramagnetic substances they revolve in the opposite direction.
>
> This result agrees so far with that part of the theory of M. Weber which refers to the paramagnetic and diamagnetic conditions.

This small change, however, was sufficient to wreck Maxwell's entire model, for by implying a zero magnetic capacity and thus a zero rotation in the vacuum it removed any mechanism for the transmission of magnetic force across the vacuum, which transmission was however observed to take place. All was not entirely lost, for as Maxwell hinted in the above quotation, it would be sufficient to have the average rotation zero in the vacuum: adjacent vortices could then rotate in opposite directions at equal speeds without any requirement for idle wheels, which were in some respects a nuisance there anyway. But at the very least the changes required to adapt the model would be formidable. Not surprisingly, Maxwell did not discuss this problem.

Fortunately, given Maxwell's heuristic attitude towards the development of analogical models, problems such as these were not necessarily critical. And the inadequacies of his model were more than made up for by his success in incorporating electrostatic phenomena and light waves in a magnetically based synthesis. In place of the laws given at the end of 'Faraday's lines of force' and quoted on p. 141–2 above, he now had a new extended set of laws, which could be written mathematically, using modern notation and correcting for the error of sign in the displacement term, as follows:

[85] Maxwell (1890 and 1965), volume 1, p. 507.

Symbols as in 'Faraday's lines of force'	Symbols as in 'On physical lines of force'
$\boldsymbol{a}_1 = \nabla \times \boldsymbol{\alpha}_0$	$\mu\boldsymbol{\alpha} = \nabla \times \boldsymbol{F}$
$\boldsymbol{\alpha}_1 = k_1\boldsymbol{a}_1$	$\left[k_1 = \dfrac{1}{\mu}\right]$
$\boldsymbol{a}_2 = \dfrac{1}{4\pi}\,\nabla \times \boldsymbol{\alpha}_1 + \dfrac{1}{4\pi\epsilon^2}\,\dfrac{\mathrm{d}\boldsymbol{\alpha}_2}{\mathrm{d}t}$	$\boldsymbol{p} = \dfrac{1}{4\pi}\,\nabla \times \boldsymbol{\alpha} + \dfrac{1}{4\pi\epsilon^2}\,\dfrac{\mathrm{d}\boldsymbol{P}}{\mathrm{d}t}$
$\boldsymbol{\alpha}_2 = k_2\boldsymbol{a}_2$	$\sigma\boldsymbol{P} = \boldsymbol{p}$
$\boldsymbol{\alpha}_2 = \left(\dfrac{\mathrm{d}\boldsymbol{x}}{\mathrm{d}t} \times \boldsymbol{a}_1\right) - \dfrac{\mathrm{d}\boldsymbol{\alpha}_0}{\mathrm{d}t} - \nabla\psi$	$\boldsymbol{P} = \left(\dfrac{\mathrm{d}\boldsymbol{x}}{\mathrm{d}t} \times \mu\boldsymbol{\alpha}\right) - \dfrac{\mathrm{d}\boldsymbol{F}}{\mathrm{d}t} - \nabla\psi$
giving	giving
$\nabla \times \boldsymbol{\alpha}_2 = -\dfrac{\mathrm{d}\boldsymbol{\alpha}_1}{\mathrm{d}t}$	$\nabla \times \boldsymbol{P} = -\dfrac{\mathrm{d}(\mu\boldsymbol{\alpha})}{\mathrm{d}t}$
$\nabla \cdot \boldsymbol{a}_1 = m$ or 0	$\nabla \cdot (\mu\boldsymbol{\alpha}) = 4\pi m$ or 0
$\nabla \cdot \boldsymbol{a}_2 = 4\pi\epsilon^2 e$ or 0	$\nabla \cdot \boldsymbol{p} = 4\pi\epsilon^2 e$ or 0.

By this stage it is possible to identify all of Maxwell's principal symbols with their modern equivalents:

$\boldsymbol{F}$	or	$\boldsymbol{\alpha}_0$	corresponds to	$\boldsymbol{A}$
$\mu\boldsymbol{\alpha}$	or	$\boldsymbol{a}_1$	corresponds to	$\boldsymbol{B}$
$\boldsymbol{\alpha}$	or	$\boldsymbol{\alpha}_1$	corresponds to	$\boldsymbol{H}$
$\boldsymbol{p}$	or	$\boldsymbol{a}_2$	corresponds to	$\boldsymbol{J} + \dfrac{\partial \boldsymbol{D}}{\mathrm{d}t}$, with $\boldsymbol{J}$ closed
$\boldsymbol{P}$	or	$\boldsymbol{\alpha}_2$	corresponds to	$\boldsymbol{E}$
$\boldsymbol{f}$			corresponds to	$\boldsymbol{D}$

This gives Maxwell's equations in the form

$$\boldsymbol{B} = \nabla \times \boldsymbol{A}$$

$$\mu\boldsymbol{H} = \boldsymbol{B}$$

$$\frac{1}{4\pi}\,\nabla \times \boldsymbol{H} = \boldsymbol{J}$$

$$\sigma\boldsymbol{E} = \boldsymbol{J} \qquad \text{(for conductor, } \partial\boldsymbol{D}/\partial t = 0\text{)}$$

$$\nabla \times \boldsymbol{E} = -\frac{\mathrm{d}\boldsymbol{B}}{\mathrm{d}t}$$

$$\nabla \cdot \boldsymbol{B} = 4\pi m \quad \text{or} \quad 0$$
$$\nabla \cdot \boldsymbol{D} = 4\pi e \quad \text{or} \quad 0$$
$$\boldsymbol{E} = 4\pi\epsilon^2 \boldsymbol{D} \quad \text{(for dielectric).}$$

Energy conservation and the rise of energy physics

In 'On physical lines of force', Maxwell had drawn on a specific type of mechanism previously postulated by Rankine for the explanation of heat energy and by Thomson for that of the magneto-optic effect. As we have already intimated, however, this work of Rankine's and Thomson's was part of a much broader development, the overall effect of which was to bring about something of a revolution in physical science. And in order to understand the further evolution of Maxwell's electromagnetic theory we must first paint in a bit more of this revolutionary background picture.

We have already discussed how in the first half of the nineteenth century, when the dynamistic approach to nature was in the ascendant, the idea of the ultimate unity and interconvertibility of the forces of nature had been very much 'in the air'.[86] In the context of electromagnetic theory this was most clearly apparent in the work of Oersted and Faraday, but it also had many other manifestations, among which was the important work of Joule we have already mentioned. In the early 1840s Joule had tried to develop an electrical theory of chemistry along lines proposed by Faraday and Davy, and in so doing to demonstrate the unity between the phenomena of electricity, chemical exchange and heat.[87] In order to study the relationship between different forces, Joule first used an electric engine in which mechanical work was used to generate electricity, which in turn generated heat. Although he continued to advance an electrical theory of nature, according to which thermal and chemical effects were interpreted in terms of the behaviour of electrical atmospheres supposed to surround the atoms of matter, his work soon led him, however, to focus on the direct production of heat from mechanical work through the friction of a paddle wheel rotating in water. From measurements of the mechanical work expended and of the temperature change of the water he was able to show that the quantity of heat generated was directly proportional to the mechanical work expended, and thus to establish a mechanical equivalent for heat and to demonstrate, to his own satisfaction at least, the interconvertibility of heat and mechanical energy.[88] After an objection by Faraday, who refereed

[86] For a fuller discussion of the background to energy conservation see the classic paper by Kuhn (1959 and 1972) and the important works by Hiebert (1962), Cardwell (1967) and Elkana (1974).

[87] See Forrester (1975) and Steffens (1979).

[88] See for example Joule (1850) and Smith (1976b).

Joule's important 1850 paper, to the effect that he had demonstrated only a mechanical equivalence for heat and not an interconvertibility between heat and mechanical work, Joule's claim to the latter conclusion was dropped from the paper as published.[89] But the inference was easily drawn, and Joule's work was soon taken with that of Clausius as the basis for a dynamical theory of heat which then provided the immediate context for the molecular vortex proposals of Rankine and Thomson.

Despite his success in relating heat to mechanical work, Joule was not able to extend his unification to cover any measurable equivalence of electrical or chemical forces. But in 1847 Hermann von Helmholtz published a remarkable paper 'On the conservation of force' in which a general law of energy conservation was established.[90] The background to Helmholtz's work was not the unification of physics itself so much as that of physiology with physics and chemistry, and partly as a result of this his paper is not easy to understand. He seems to have used the word 'force' or '*Kraft*' in at least two distinct ways, and he combined a mechanistic form of reductionism, in which the forces of life were supposed reducible to physical laws of central attraction and repulsion, with a justification for this in terms of necessary modes of thought that seems to have found its origins in the dynamism of Kant.[91] The results, however, were striking. He started from the postulate, derived from his reductionist view of physiology, that it was impossible to obtain an unlimited amount of 'work force' or '*Arbeitskraft*', and he attempted to show that this was equivalent to the postulate that all actions in nature were reducible to attractive or repulsive central forces dependent only on the distance between the points between which they acted. (Here was the origin of Maxwell's claim against Weber that velocity-dependent forces were inconsistent with the conservation of energy.) From these postulates he deduced the law of the 'conservation of force', expressed as the conservation of the sum of 'living force' or *vis viva* (corresponding to kinetic energy) and 'tensional force' (corresponding to potential energy). In the context of mechanics this could be seen as a generalisation of the traditional law of the conservation of *vis viva* to apply to phenomena such as inelastic collisions in which, Helmholtz argued, the lost *vis viva* was taken up by the colliding objects in the form of a tensional force. But familiar with the writings of Joule and others, and concerned himself with a reductionist unification of the forces of nature, Helmholtz also indicated how his new result could be applied across the range of physical phenomena. Thus part of the *vis viva* of inelastically colliding

[89] Smith (1976b).

[90] Helmholtz (1847).

[91] Heimann (1974) has made a valiant attempt to come to grips with the paper, but the problem of Helmholtz's attitude to nature and science remains a very difficult one and we shall not treat it here.

bodies would be transformed into heat, and the concepts of living and tensional energies could also be invoked in other thermal phenomena as well as in the phenomena of electricity.

The word 'energy' was introduced to this context of conservation and convertibility by Thomson in a footnote to a paper on Carnot's theory of heat engines in 1849,[92] and it was Thomson who converted the insights of Joule and Helmholtz into the basis of a new physics.[93] At the time of writing his 1849 paper Thomson was still grappling with the reconciliation of Joule's work on the equivalence of heat and mechanical energy with Carnot's work on irreversible processes, and with the problem of how something could be lost and conserved at the same time. But although he had not fully solved this problem he had accepted Joule's conclusion, which he expressed in terms of a conservation of energy:[94]

> Nothing can be lost in the operations of nature—no energy can be destroyed. What effect then is produced in place of the mechanical effect which is lost [in the conduction of heat through a solid]? A perfect theory of heat imperatively demands an answer to this question.

The lost mechanical effect was the work which would have been produced by a temperature differential in a perfect heat engine, but was not so produced in the irreversible process of an imperfect one, and Thomson was still some way from visualising the dissipation of heat energy as part of an energy conserving process. But he had clearly accepted the principle of energy conservation, and at about the same time he had also given an indication of how this could be used in electromagnetic theory, introducing as we have seen the 'equivalent mechanical effect' of an electrical or magnetic system.[95]

From Thomson's point of view, Joule's work seems to have provided the fundamental insight into the possibility of treating phenomena such as heat in terms of their equivalent mechanical effects and so bringing them into the framework of general dynamical theory. Helmholtz's work then provided a formalisation of the mechanical effect (or total energy) of a mechanical system in terms of which this possibility could be developed. Thomson's original justification for developing purely mathematical analogies to electromagnetic phenomena had been concerned largely with the reconciliation of rival theoretical viewpoints. But with the introduction of the conceptions of mechanical effect and the conservation of energy the analogies took on a new significance, as representations of the energetic properties of a

[92] Thomson (1849).
[93] For my discussion of the rise of energy physics I have drawn heavily on Smith (1978). See also Moyer (1977).
[94] Thomson (1882–1911), volume 1, p. 118.
[95] See page 105 above.

system. Moreover, if all physical phenomena could be represented, through application of the principle of energy conservation, by equivalent mechanical effects, then the whole of physics could be united under a generalised dynamics such as that of Lagrange, which was based solely on the analysis of energy variations.

By the time he wrote his paper on 'The dynamical theory of heat' (1851) and a follow-up paper on the dissipation of heat (1852),[96] Thomson was clearly committed to a dynamical and even dynamistic programme of Lagrangian energy physics based on the conservation principle. But, despite the elucidation of Carnot's work provided by Clausius, he was still concerned with the problem of visualising the conversion and dissipation processes. His work in this period was therefore focused on the provision of 'dynamical illustrations' or hypothetical models rather than on the development of a general dynamical theory, and it was in fact Rankine who first set forward the latter programme explicitly. The precise relationship between the papers of Rankine and Thomson in this period is not altogether clear, but the two men do seem to have been in close communication and pursuing closely related themes, with Rankine's work apparently infuenced quite strongly by Thomson.[97] Both published on the kinetic theory of heat in 1851 (Rankine putting forward his molecular vortex hypothesis); and in response to Thomson's 1852 paper on heat dissipation, in which he had stressed the conservation of energy in dissipation processes and introduced the terms 'statical energy' and 'dynamical energy' for Helmholtz's tensional and living forces, Rankine wrote a short speculative paper 'On the reconcentration of the mechanical energy of the universe' in which he set out the principle of energy conservation with unprecedented clarity:[98]

> ...all the different kinds of physical energy in the universe are mutually convertible; ... the total amount of physical energy, whether in the form of visible motion and mechanical power, or of heat, light, magnetism, electricity or chemical agency, or in other forms not yet understood, is unchangeable, the transformations of its different portions from one of those forms of power into another, constituting the phenomena which are the objects of experimental physics.

The following year Rankine made the energy principle the explicit subject of a paper, introducing the terms 'potential energy' and 'actual energy'.[99] Then in 1855 he published his 'Outlines of the science of energetics', in which he proposed a methodological programme for the physical sciences based on the laws of energy.[100] Rankine himself had already sought a

[96] Thomson (1851a and 1852).
[97] See Smith (1976a and 1978).
[98] Rankine (1852). Quotation from reprint in Rankine (1881), p. 200.
[99] Rankine (1853).
[100] Rankine (1855), reprinted in Rankine (1881), pp. 209–28.

unification of physics in terms of the mechanical hypothesis of molecular vortices, and he noted that:[101]

> The fact that the theory of motions and motive forces is the only complete physical theory, has naturally led to the adoption of *mechanical hypotheses* in the theories of other branches of physics.

But he now joined those such as Reid and Whewell who had earlier drawn attention to the dangers of hypotheses, which were widely misused and which tended to take on 'in the minds of the public generally, as well as in those of many scientists even, that authority which belongs to facts alone.'[102] He therefore suggested an alternative method, based on empirical observations and free from the uncertainty of hypotheses:[103]

> Instead of supposing the various classes of physical phenomena to be constituted, in an occult way, of modifications of motion and force, let us distinguish the properties which those classes possess in common with each other, and so define more extensive classes denoted by suitable terms. For axioms, to express the laws of those more extensive classes of phenomena, let us frame propositions comprehending as particular cases the laws of the particular classes of phenomena comprehended under the more extensive classes. So shall we arrive at a body of principles, applicable to physical phenomena in general, and which, being framed by induction from facts alone, will be free from the uncertainty which must always attach, even to those mechanical hypotheses whose consequences are most fully confirmed by experiment.

The general thrust of Rankine's argument was a commonplace within the dynamistic tradition we have outlined in earlier chapters, but in the generalised energy concept there now existed a property that was at once empirically defined and applicable over the whole range of physical phenomena:[104]

> Energy, or the capacity to effect change, is the common characteristic of the various states of matter to which the several branches of physics relate; if then, there be general laws respecting energy, such laws must be applicable *mutatis mutandis* to every branch of physics, and must express a body of principles as to physical phenomena in general.

This was precisely what was needed to transform the traditional dynamist ideal into a realistically feasible approach, and in the bulk of his paper

[101] Rankine (1881), p. 211.
[102] Rankine (1881), p. 212.
[103] Rankine (1881), p. 213.
[104] Rankine (1881), p. 213.

Rankine accordingly built up a body of general definitions and laws relating to energy, from which, he hoped, the laws of particular phenomena could be deduced without recourse to hypothesis.

The new approach to physics did not receive its definitive expression until the completion of Thomson and Tait's *Treatise of Natural Philosophy* in 1867, and in the meantime it was far from universally accepted. In the late 1850s both Rankine (in public) and Maxwell (in private) had cause to chide Faraday for continuing to speak loosely and ambiguously of the 'conservation of force'.[105] Others of the older generation, whether mechanists such as Brewster or dynamists such as Whewell, also remained largely uninterested in the energy conceptions,[106] while John Herschel attacked the concept of energy conservation as being essentially a useless truism. On his view *vis viva* was sometimes conserved and sometimes not, and to introduce a potential energy defined, in effect, as that which had to be added to the *vis viva* for the total to be conserved seemed to get one nowhere. It was the concept of force, grounded in the metaphysics of volition, that had in his opinion to be taken as primary.[107] On the other hand, however, Maxwell could write of the conservation of energy in 1857 as something which 'every student of dynamics learns';[108] and as early as 1855, in 'Faraday's lines of force', he could cite Helmholtz on the conservation of energy in a way that assumed some acquaintance with the principle on the part of his readers. In 1857 Lagrangian dynamics, which had never previously received much attention in Britain (William Rowan Hamilton apart), but which was perfectly adapted to the formulation of energy physics, was brought to the general attention of British mathematicians by a report of Arthur Cayley to the British Association.[109] And throughout the 1860s the approach of energy physics also featured strongly in the writings of P G Tait.[110] In 1864 the first productive application of the new approach outside thermodynamics was given by Maxwell in a paper to the Royal Society on 'A dynamical theory of the electromagnetic field'.[111]

A dynamical theory of the field

In both 'Faraday's lines of force' and 'On physical lines of force' Maxwell had explained the phenomena of electromagnetism by means of physical

[105] Maxwell to Faraday, 9 November 1857, in Campbell and Garnett (1884), p. 202. Rankine (1859a and 1859b).
[106] Smith (1976a).
[107] Herschel (1865) and see Smith (1978).
[108] Maxwell to Faraday, 9 November 1857, in Campbell and Garnett (1884), p. 204.
[109] Cayley (1857).
[110] Tait (1860 and 1864b); Tait and Steele (1865).
[111] Maxwell (1865 and 1982).

analogies. But in both cases he had emphasised the limitations of such analogies, and although he seems to have embarked on the exploration of the molecular vortex hypothesis with fairly high expectations his failure to reconcile it with the magneto-optic effect must have quickly shattered any excessive optimism he may have had. Yet the results of his analysis, including the unification of electrodynamics and electrostatics and the beginnings of an electromagnetic theory of light, were far too impressive for the subject to be abandoned. Through the pursuit of a mechanical analogy Maxwell had succeeded in glimpsing the framework of a true physical theory, or true physical connection between a range of diverse phenomena. According to the philosophy of science he had already expounded the next step must be to seek to establish that theory independent of the heuristic hypotheses by which he had arrived at it, and the energy physics approach of Rankine and Thomson provided him with the perfect tool with which to do this. In a letter to Thomson of 17 December 1861 he announced that 'I have more time now to work', and set out an experimental programme aimed at confirming some of the basic results of his analysis in 'On physical lines of force' and at establishing the empirical foundations of the theory he sought.[112] In the same letter he also began to explore some of the properties of his model in terms of the transfer between potential and kinetic energy,[113] and in a letter of 28 December to his friend H R Droop he reported that[114]

> I am trying to form an exact mathematical expression for all that is known about electromagnetism without the aid of hypothesis.

Over the next few years divers interests and commitments vied for Maxwell's attention.[115] His teaching load at King's College was apparently a relatively heavy one, and his extramural lecturing commitments were also greater in London than they had been in Aberdeen. With his wife as both subject and assistant he continued his experiments on colour vision and he also continued his struggle with the problems of gas theory. Developing the work of Clausius he had deduced that the statistical distribution of energy between the rotational and translational motions of roughly spherical particles was one of equality (an example of what became known as the law of equipartition of energy). This, however, had led to the conclusion that the specific heat of a gas made up of spherical molecules should be 1.333 compared with an experimental value of 1.408, and the discrepancy, which seemed to him important enough to threaten the whole dynamical theory of gases, was a recurring subject of concern throughout the 1860s.[116] It was

[112] Maxwell to Thomson, 17 December 1861, in Larmor (1937), pp. 37–9
[113] Maxwell to Thomson, 17 December 1861, in Larmor (1937), p. 38.
[114] Maxwell to Droop, 28 December 1861, in Campbell and Garnett (1884), p. 246.
[115] Campbell and Garnett (1884), chapter 10.
[116] See for example Everitt (1974), pp. 219–20; Maxwell to Droop, 28 January 1862 , in Campbell and Garnett (1884), p. 248.

however electromagnetic theory that dominated his research throughout the first half of the decade. By the summer of 1864 he could write to a friend that he had 'cleared the electromagnetic theory of light from all unwarrantable assumption',[117] and by the beginning of December he had written up his paper on a dynamical theory of the electromagnetic field.

In order to progress from the analogy of 'On physical lines of force' to something approaching a true physical theory, Maxwell had to do two things. He had to express the specific dynamical relationships previously deduced from his vortex model in the form of general energetic relationships, independent of any particular dynamical hypothesis or illustration; and he also had to restructure the theory so as to make it rest firmly on empirical phenomena. In 'On physical lines of force' he had argued from the details of the model and from the laws established in 'Faraday's lines of force' to a revised and refined set of laws, the consequences of which were empirically testable. The laws adopted from 'Faraday's lines of force' had themselves rested partly on observation and partly on the analogies used. He now had to test the empirical consequences of the model, and reverse the line of argument so as to go as far as possible from the empirical observations to the laws through which these were connected.

In his letter of 17 December 1861 to Thomson, Maxwell was already beginning to attack this problem from both ends. Having used Thomson's method of electric images to analyse the behaviour of magnetic poles and electric currents in diamagnetic and paramagnetic media, and having reverted in the process to Faraday's theory of magnetism with the coefficient of induction having the same sign for diamagnetics and paramagnetics, he concluded that[118]

> It is remarkable that the spontaneous movements of magnets tend to diminish their potentials, but the spontaneous movements of currents tend to increase their potentials and the whole energetic value of the field they move in.

He then asked whether this result could be expressed as a general dynamical one, independent of the particular mechanism being considered, by which the behaviour of something that was being driven by a motive power (as was electric current) could be distinguished from that of something that (like a magnet) was not. He next turned to experiment and set out a list of electrostatic experiments he wished to perform, concerned mainly with the establishment of the behaviour and effects of dielectrics. Finally he wanted 'to put Verdet's results into absolute measure', separating out the effects of the earth's magnetic field from those of the laboratory field, as a means of establishing empirically the values of some of the variables in the vortex model.

[117] Maxwell to Hockin, 7 September 1864, in Campbell and Garnett (1884), p. 255. See also Maxwell to Stokes, October 1864, in Larmor (1907), p. 26.
[118] Maxwell to Thomson, 17 December 1861, in Larmor (1937), p. 38.

Ten days later, having moved up to Glenlair for the Christmas vacation, Maxwell wrote to Droop, 'to arrange my own thoughts by imagining myself speaking to you',[119] that he was trying to establish a hypothesis-free generalisation of Ampère's formula for the force between current elements:[120]

> I am trying to form an exact mathematical expression for all that is known about electro-magnetism without the aid of hypothesis, and also what variations of Ampère's formula are possible without contradicting his expressions. All that we know is about the action of *closed* currents—that is, currents through closed curves. Now, if you make a hypothesis (1) about the mutual action of the elements of two currents, and find it agrees with experiments on closed circuits, it is not proved for—
>
> If you make another hypothesis (2) which would give *no action* between an element and a *closed* circuit, you may make a combination of (1) and (2) which will give the same result as (1). So I am investigating the most general hypothesis about the mutual action of elements, which fulfils the condition that the action between an element and a closed circuit is null. This is the case if the action between two elements can be reduced to forces between the extremities of those elements depending only on the distance and + or − according as they act between similar or opposite ends of the elements. If the force is an attraction
>
> $$= \phi(r)ss'\,(\cos\omega + 2\cos\theta\cos\theta')$$
>
> where ω is the angle between s and s', r the distance of s and s' and θ and θ' the angles s and s', the elements, make with r, then the condition of no action will be fulfilled.

By the time of his next letter to Droop, on 24 January 1862, he had concluded that Ampère's own formula was in fact the most general one consistent with experiment, and had begun to study the relationship between Ampère's hypothesis of direct action at a distance between elements and his own formulation in terms of an intervening magnetic field:[121]

> I want to see if there is any evidence from the mathematical expressions as to whether element acts on element, or whether a current first produces a certain effect in the surrounding field, which afterwards acts on any other current.
>
> Perhaps there may be no mathematical reasons in favour of one hypothesis rather than the other.
>
> As a fact, the effect on a current at a given place depends solely on the direction and magnitude of the magnetic force at that point, whether the magnetic force arises from currents or from magnets. So that the theory of the effect taking place through the intervention of a medium is consistent with fact, and

[119] Maxwell to Droop, 24 January 1862, in Campbell and Garnett (1884), p. 247.
[120] Maxwell to Droop, 28 December 1861, in Campbell and Garnett (1884), p. 246.
[121] Maxwell to Droop, 24 January 1862, in Campbell and Garnett (1884), p. 247.

(to me) appears the simplest in expression; but I must prove either that the direct action theory is completely identical in its results, or that in some conceivable case they may be different.

We unfortunately have little evidence concerning the development of Maxwell's private research between January 1862 and the completion of his paper in the summer or autumn of 1864, but we may assume that the process of generalising, questioning and refining his analysis continued. Meanwhile a call to public duty provided the context for a clarification of his overall aims. Whatever reservations Maxwell, Thomson and others might have had about Weber's electrodynamic theory, there could be no denying the value of the German physicist's work in establishing an absolute system of electrodynamically defined electromagnetic units. His theory had indeed been put forward in the course of a series of papers on 'Electrodynamic measurements',[122] and it was for his precise measurements and his establishment of a consistent system of units that he was chiefly famed. With such a system of units the accurate comparison of electromagnetic measurements by different researchers became a realistic possibility for the first time, and in 1861 the British Association for the Advancement of Science set up a committee under Thomson to determine a set of internationally acceptable electrical standards. The following year Maxwell was appointed to the committee and set to work with Fleeming Jenkin to determine a standard of electrical resistance.[123]

This project inevitably took up much of Maxwell's time, but it tied in remarkably well with the development of his own interests. With Thomson chairing the committee it was agreed to adopt a system of units similar to Weber's but based on the application of general energy principles rather than on Weber's electrodynamic theory, so Maxwell's target of an energy-based electromagnetic theory was in a sense incorporated in the aims of the committee. And since a fundamental feature of any system of electromagnetically defined units would have to be its relationship to the established system of electrostatic units, the establishment of a set of units was inextricably linked to the testing of Maxwell's electromagnetic theory of light. In their 1863 report to the British Association, Maxwell and Jenkin put forward two parallel sets of definitions of electromagnetic quantities, one based on electrostatically determined and the other on electromagnetically determined units, and this led to five different ways in which the ratio between the two types of unit, associated by Maxwell with the velocity of light, could be experimentally measured.[124]

In the introduction to 'A dynamical theory of the electromagnetic field', Maxwell sketched out the overall structure of the argument he was now

[122] Weber (1846 and 1852a,b,c).
[123] See for example Everitt (1974), p. 209.
[124] Maxwell and Jenkin (1863).

going to employ. The fundamental postulate of his theory was the same as in both of his earlier papers: that electromagnetic action was propagated through a medium and not, as Weber's theory assumed, by direct action at a distance between electric and magnetic bodies. He conceded as he had before that Weber's theory, recently developed by Carl Neumann, was 'exceedingly ingenious, and wonderfully comprehensive in its application to the phenomena of statical electricity, electromagnetic attractions, induction of currents and diamagnetic phenomena.'[125] It also carried the authority of a master experimentalist. As before, however, Maxwell noted his unease with 'the assumption of particles acting at a distance with forces which depend on their velocities,'[126] and expressed his own preference for action through a medium, for 'a theory of the *Electromagnetic Field,* ... to do with the space in the neighbourhood of the electric or magnetic bodies.'[127] Only whereas before he had talked of the mathematisation of Faraday's ideas, and of the importance of having a second way of looking at things, he now seemed a little more confident of his ground. In effect, the identification of magnetic and luminiferous media that had followed as an apparently unexpected *consequence* from his vortex model analysis, now provided a *foundation* for the new theory. For the phenomena of light and, especially, radiant heat, provided clear evidence, independent of the subject being treated, of the existence of a pervasive aetherial medium of just the kind his theory assumed:[128]

> We have therefore some reason to believe, from the phenomena of light and heat, that there is an etherial medium filling space and permeating bodies, capable of being set in motion and of transmitting that motion from one part to another, and of communicating that motion to gross matter so as to heat it and affect it in various ways.
>
> ... Now the energy communicated to the body in heating it must have formerly existed in some moving medium, for the undulations had left the source of heat some time before they reached the body, and during that time the energy must have been half in the form of motion of the medium and half in the form of elastic resilience.

Of course, the electromagnetic theory of light itself was still a consequence of the theory, to be derived at a later stage. But the fact that it could be derived meant that instead of hypothesising the existence of a magnetic medium Maxwell could take as his starting point the luminiferous medium, the existence and properties of which were, though essentially hypothetical, empirically well supported. The supposed medium was pervasive, of small but finite density, and capable of transmitting motion at large but finite

[125] Maxwell (1982), p. 34.
[126] Maxwell (1982), p. 34.
[127] Maxwell (1982), p. 34.
[128] Maxwell (1982), pp. 34–5.

velocity. And having some elastic resilience it could receive and store potential as well as kinetic energy.

With the existence of the luminiferous medium established as an empirically well supported hypothesis, Maxwell's next step was to propose that this medium was also the seat of electromagnetic phenomena. Again the proposition was hypothetical, but it was an hypothesis that there were 'warrantable grounds' for exploring.[129] It was basically reasonable to suppose that if the luminiferous medium existed, it[130]

> may be capable of other kinds of motion and displacement than those which produce the phenomena of light and heat, and some of these may be of such a kind that they may be evidenced to our senses by the phenomena they produce.

The phenomenon of magneto-optic rotation provided empirical evidence 'that the luminiferous medium is in certain cases acted on by magnetism.'[131] Thomson's analysis of the effect had shown, moreover, that it could not be deduced without assuming 'the existence of a motion in the medium depending on the magnetization, in addition to the vibratory motion which constitutes light.'[132] As Maxwell concluded,[133]

> We have therefore warrantable grounds for inquiring whether there may not be a motion of the ethereal medium going on wherever magnetic effects are observed, and we have some reason to suppose that this motion is one of rotation, having the direction of the magnetic force as its axis.

The evidence from electrical phenomena was also encouraging. Maxwell observed that 'when a body is moved across the [empirically defined] lines of magnetic force it experiences what is called an electromotive force.'[134] Depending on the nature of the body and the power of this force, its effect was either to produce a current and heat the body, or to decompose the body electrolytically, or if it could do neither of these to put the body in a state of electric polarisation—'a state of constraint in which opposite extremities are oppositely electrified, and from which the body tends to relieve itself as soon as the disturbing force is removed.'[135] From an empirical viewpoint what was called an electromotive force was simply something invoked to link the initial motion of a body across the field with the resulting motions of current, chemical decomposition or electric

[129] Maxwell (1982), pp. 36 and 82.
[130] Maxwell (1982), p. 35.
[131] Maxwell (1982), p. 35.
[132] Maxwell (1982), p. 36.
[133] Maxwell (1982), p. 36.
[134] Maxwell (1982), p. 36.
[135] Maxwell (1982), p. 37.

displacement, and according to Maxwell's theory it had therefore to be a manifestation of the communication of motion from one part of the medium to another, or the means by which motion in one part caused that in the other.

Maxwell next considered more carefully the effect of an electromotive force on a dielectric. This effect was manifest only as a macroscopic polarisation or displacement of electric charge; but it could be imagined and described, as by Faraday and Mossotti, as a state of microscopic polarisation or displacement, existing throughout the dielectric but with the effects on adjacent molecules cancelling out so that there was no indication of any electrification inside the medium. The effect was that of a 'kind of elastic yielding' of the medium. Dielectrics also exhibited two other phenomena: a small degree of conductivity and the phenomenon known as electric absorption. When a dielectric was exposed to an electromotive force the resulting displacement was set up only gradually, and when the force was removed the medium also retained a temporary residual polarisation. Both of these phenomena seemed to suggest the notion of an electromagnetic medium, subject to complex forms of elastic yielding and in which potential energy could be stored.

Altogether, both magnetic and electrical phenomena seemed to tie in well with the assumption of an electromagnetic medium of the same type as that required for the theory of light, but subject to 'a vast variety of motion' besides that corresponding to the simple transmission of light waves. How the behaviour of this medium might be mechanically represented was unknown, but from Maxwell's current perspective it did not matter. It was not even necessary, indeed, that a consistent mechanical representation should be possible. All he wished to assume for the construction of his dynamical theory of the electromagnetic field was that there was a medium through which electromagnetic effects were transmitted and the observed phenomena connected, and that this medium, being composed of matter in motion, was subject to the general laws of dynamics. From these very general and very reasonable hypotheses, and from the observed relationships between electromagnetic motions, he proposed to derive the general dynamical behaviour of the medium, and with it the dynamical connections between the different electromagnetic quantities observed.

Maxwell began his analysis by considering the phenomena of electromagnetic induction. It was known experimentally that magnetic effects were excited in the field of an electric current and that these effects were proportional to the strength of the current. It was also known that the effect due to two currents in the field was the sum of the effects of the individual currents. Assuming that the effects were dependent on some unspecified motion of the medium, the combination of currents and medium could be considered as a connected dynamical system. Any change in the force represented by one current would lead to a change in the motion of the medium and this in turn would exert a force on the other current. To explain this linkage, Maxwell used a dynamical illustration. The medium could be seen as a body of mass C, and the currents as independent driving points, A and B, connected to the body. If u, v, w, represented the velocities of A, B, C, with the linkage defined by

$$w = pu + qv \qquad \frac{\mathrm{d}w}{\mathrm{d}t} = p\frac{\mathrm{d}u}{\mathrm{d}t} + q\frac{\mathrm{d}v}{\mathrm{d}t} \tag{5.32}$$

and if X and Y represented the forces applied at A and B respectively, then the elementary laws of dynamics gave, in the absence of any friction,

$$X = C\frac{\mathrm{d}}{\mathrm{d}t}(p^2a + pqv) \qquad Y = C\frac{\mathrm{d}}{\mathrm{d}t}(pqu + q^2v) \tag{5.33}$$

where $(Cp^2u + Cpqv)$ and $(Cpqu + Cq^2v)$ were termed the momenta of C referred to A and B respectively. Generalising to the case of a number of bodies or media, each characterised by different values of C, p, q, and writing

$$L = \sum(Cp^2) \qquad M = \sum(Cpq) \qquad N = \sum(Cq^2)$$

gave

$$X = \frac{\mathrm{d}}{\mathrm{d}t}(Lu + Mv) \qquad Y = \frac{\mathrm{d}}{\mathrm{d}t}(Mu + Nv). \tag{5.34}$$

If in addition the motions of A and B were resisted by forces proportional to their velocities, Ru and Sv, then the total applied forces ζ and η were given by

$$\begin{aligned} \zeta &= X + Ru = Ru + \frac{\mathrm{d}}{\mathrm{d}t}(Lu + Mv) \\ \eta &= Y + Sv = Sv + \frac{\mathrm{d}}{\mathrm{d}t}(Mu + Nv). \end{aligned} \tag{5.35}$$

Returning to the language of electromagnetic phenomena, u and v represented the currents at A and B, which Maxwell now wrote confusingly as x and y, R and S the electrical resistances there, and ζ and η the electromotive forces. With steady currents the electromotive forces would just balance the resisting forces,

$$\zeta = Rx \qquad \eta = Sy$$

but with a variable current there would be resultant forces, corresponding to the change in what could be called the electromagnetic momentum of the system,

$$\zeta - Rx = \frac{\mathrm{d}}{\mathrm{d}t}(Lx + My) \qquad \eta - Sy = \frac{\mathrm{d}}{\mathrm{d}t}(Mx + Ny).$$

Stressing the generality of his argument, Maxwell noted that the term 'electromotive force' did not correspond to any ordinary mechanical force moving any supposed body of electricity in a conductor. In full accordance with his limited assumptions the analogy was rather with an unknown complex connected system in which the current elements acted merely as driving points.

Using his dynamical equations, Maxwell could easily derive the effects of the simple induction of one current by another and of a current by the relative motion of two conductors. Thus if the current at A increased over a period from 0 to x, the total current induced in B was given by[136]

$$y_1 = -\frac{Mx}{S}. \tag{5.36}$$

If the current at A remained constant at x but the conductors moved so as to alter their mutual linkage from M to M', the induced current was given by

$$y_1 = \frac{-(M' - M)x}{S}. \tag{5.37}$$

Maxwell next turned to the consideration of the energy of the system under the action of the electromotive forces ζ and η, given by the rate of work done:

$$\zeta x + \eta y = Rx^2 + Sy^2 + x\frac{\mathrm{d}}{\mathrm{d}t}(Lx + My) + y\frac{\mathrm{d}}{\mathrm{d}t}(Mx + Ny). \tag{5.38}$$

Here $Rx^2 + Sy^2$ represented the rate of work done against resistance, or energy converted into heat, while the remainder of the right-hand side of equation (5.36) could be rewritten as two terms

$$x\frac{\mathrm{d}}{\mathrm{d}t}(Lx + My) + y\frac{\mathrm{d}}{\mathrm{d}t}(Mx + Ny) = \frac{1}{2}\frac{\mathrm{d}}{\mathrm{d}t}(Lx^2 + 2Mxy + Ny^2) + \left(\frac{1}{2}\frac{\mathrm{d}L}{\mathrm{d}t}x^2 + \frac{\mathrm{d}M}{\mathrm{d}t}xy + \frac{1}{2}\frac{\mathrm{d}N}{\mathrm{d}t}y^2\right).$$

If the relative position of the currents in the medium remained constant, so that L, M, N were constants, then the whole energy must be contained in

[136] Maxwell himself used Y for my y_1, but this leads to possible confusion with his use of Y for electromotive force just two pages earlier. His use of x and y rather than u and v for currents just two pages after using them for displacements is also potentially confusing, but since x and y as displacements were used only fleetingly while he persisted with the notation of x and y for currents (at least until changing again in part III of the paper to p and q!) I have chosen to retain the latter.

the currents, so that

$$E = \tfrac{1}{2}Lx^2 + Mxy + \tfrac{1}{2}Ny^2$$

represented the intrinsic energy of the currents.

The remaining terms represented energy due to variations in the forms or positions of the conducting circuits, or to the effects of ordinary mechanical forces (since they produced mechanical motions) on the conducting bodies. If, in particular, the two conductors were allowed to move along the line joining them, so as to increase M to M', the work done would be $(M - M')xy$, representing an attraction if the currents were in the same direction (i.e. x and y having the same sign) and a repulsion if they were in opposite directions. So the attraction and repulsion of current elements followed from the general formulae for electromagnetic induction. In order to complete the first part of his analysis, Maxwell proceeded to show how the variables L, M and N could be determined explicitly, L and N representing the self-inductions of the circuits, given by the formulae

$$\xi - Rx = \frac{\mathrm{d}}{\mathrm{d}t}(Lx) \qquad \eta - Sy = \frac{\mathrm{d}}{\mathrm{d}t}(Ny) \tag{5.39}$$

and manifest as counter currents delaying the increase of current in response to the application of an electromotive force, or the decrease of current in response to the breaking of a circuit.

So far, Maxwell's theory had entailed no more than the simplest of applications of general dynamical principles. But this was, amazingly, all that was needed, for he had already established the rest of his electromagnetic theory on the basis of the phenomena of electromagnetic induction in 'On physical lines of force'. All he had to do now was, essentially, to rehearse the process of deduction in what he termed an 'exploration of the electromagnetic field.'[137] By considering the relationship between a fixed primary circuit and a movable secondary circuit he could use the inductive effect on the secondary circuit to determine the direction of the lines of magnetic force, and the coefficient of mutual induction M to quantify these lines. Thereafter the laws of the electromagnetic field followed as before. On this occasion they were expressed by Maxwell in the form of nine sets of equations labelled A to I, the first eight of which, comprising twenty equations in all, connected twenty electromagnetic quantities, while the ninth gave an expression for the total energy of the field. Maxwell was still using cartesian components, but if we translate his symbols into vector form he had $\boldsymbol{F}$ or (F, G, H) for the electromagnetic momentum, $\boldsymbol{\alpha}$ or (α, β, γ) for the magnetic intensity, $\boldsymbol{P}$ or (P, Q, R) for electromotive force, $\boldsymbol{f}$ or (f, g, h) for electric displacement, $\boldsymbol{p}$ or (p, q, r) for conduction current, $\boldsymbol{p}'$ or (p', q', r') for total current, e for 'quantity of electricity' and ψ for the electric potential. Using modern vector notation his equations were:

[137] Maxwell (1982), p. 57.

(A)	$\boldsymbol{p}' = \boldsymbol{p} + \dfrac{\mathrm{d}\boldsymbol{f}}{\mathrm{d}t}$	equations of total currents
(B)	$\mu\boldsymbol{\alpha} = -\nabla \times \boldsymbol{F}$	equations of magnetic force
(C)	$-\nabla \times \boldsymbol{\alpha} = 4\pi\boldsymbol{p}'$	equations of electric currents
(D)	$\boldsymbol{P} = -\mu\left(\boldsymbol{\alpha} \times \dfrac{\mathrm{d}\boldsymbol{x}}{\mathrm{d}t}\right) - \dfrac{\mathrm{d}\boldsymbol{F}}{\mathrm{d}t} - \nabla\psi$	equations of electromotive force
(E)	$\boldsymbol{P} = k\boldsymbol{f}$	equations of electric elasticity
(F)	$\boldsymbol{P} = -\rho\boldsymbol{p}$	equations of electric resistance
(G)	$e = -\nabla \cdot \boldsymbol{f}$	equations of free electricity
(H)	$\dfrac{\mathrm{d}e}{\mathrm{d}t} = -\nabla \cdot \boldsymbol{p}$	equations of continuity
(I)	$\text{Energy} = \dfrac{1}{8\pi}\iiint\left(\boldsymbol{\alpha} \cdot \mu\boldsymbol{\alpha} + \dfrac{1}{2}\boldsymbol{P} \cdot \boldsymbol{f}\right)\mathrm{d}w^2$	total energy of field.

Translating as before into modern symbols Maxwell now had (using $\boldsymbol{I}$ for total current)

$$\text{(A)}\quad \boldsymbol{I} = \boldsymbol{J} + \frac{\mathrm{d}\boldsymbol{D}}{\mathrm{d}t}$$

$$\text{(B)}\quad \boldsymbol{B} = -\nabla \times \boldsymbol{A}$$

$$\text{(C)}\quad \nabla \times \boldsymbol{H} = 4\pi\boldsymbol{I}$$

$$\text{(D)}\quad \boldsymbol{E} = -\left(\boldsymbol{B} \times \frac{\mathrm{d}\boldsymbol{x}}{\mathrm{d}t}\right) - \frac{\partial \boldsymbol{A}}{\partial t} - \nabla\psi$$

$$\text{(E)}\quad \epsilon_0\boldsymbol{E} = \boldsymbol{D}$$

$$\text{(F)}\quad \boldsymbol{E} = -\rho\boldsymbol{J}$$

$$\text{(G)}\quad e = -\nabla \cdot \boldsymbol{D}$$

$$\text{(H)}\quad \frac{\mathrm{d}e}{\mathrm{d}t} = -\nabla \cdot \boldsymbol{J}.$$

Implicit in Maxwell's notation was also

$$\boxed{\boldsymbol{B} = \mu \boldsymbol{H}.}$$

Having set out his equations of the field, to the analysis of which we shall return shortly, Maxwell next considered the mechanical actions in the field, namely the motions of current-carrying conductors and the motions due to magnetostatic and electrostatic attractions and repulsions. The force exerted by the field on a movable conducting element carrying a current $\boldsymbol{p}'$ was easily derivable as

$$\text{(J)} \qquad \boldsymbol{X} = -(\mu \boldsymbol{\alpha} \times \boldsymbol{p}').$$

The force of a field characterised by a magnetic intensity $\boldsymbol{\alpha}_1$ on a magnetic pole m_2 came out as

$$\text{(K)} \qquad \boldsymbol{X} = m_2 \boldsymbol{\alpha}_1$$

giving a force between two magnetic poles m_1 and m_2 at distance r of

$$\text{Force} = m_1 m_2 / \mu r^2. \tag{5.40}$$

Similarly the force between two electric conductors of charges e_1 and e_2 in a dielectric medium characterised by k (as in equations (E)) was

$$\text{Force} = \left(\frac{k}{4\pi}\right) e_1 e_2 / r^2. \tag{5.41}$$

According to Maxwell's theory both electrostatic and magnetostatic effects were derived from the dynamical properties of the intervening medium, and he next inquired whether gravitational attraction might not also be traced to the action of a medium. He deduced, however, that gravitational attraction would have to be represented by a diminishment of the intrinsic energy of the medium, which, to be always positive, would have to be effectively infinite. 'As I am unable to understand in what way a medium can possess such properties', he concluded, 'I cannot go any further in this direction in searching for the cause of gravitation.'[138]

Maxwell finished his paper with two short sections, one on the theory of condensers, in which he derived the phenomena of electric absorption and secondary discharge discussed in the introduction to the paper, and the other on the electromagnetic theory of light. In 'On physical lines of force' Maxwell had derived the speed of a light wave as that of the propagation of transverse vibrations through his hypothetical vortex medium. In 'A dynamical theory of the electromagnetic field' the mechanical properties of the electromagnetic medium were no longer specified, and he could not

[138] Maxwell (1982), p. 77.

therefore repeat his previous calculations. But otherwise the situation was the same. Although he had drawn on the evidence of optical phenomena to justify his hypothesis of a pervading medium, the field equations at which he had arrived were deduced from electromagnetic phenomena alone. The question was thus, as before, whether the properties of the electromagnetic medium were 'sufficient to explain the propagation of light through the same substance.'[139]

To answer this question, Maxwell considered the propagation of a plane wave, defined by direction cosines (l, m, n) and velocity V, through the medium. He argued that in these circumstances all the electromagnetic functions of the field would become functions of the displacement

$$w = lx + my + nz - Vt.$$

Expressions such as $\mathrm{d}F/\mathrm{d}y$ could then be rewritten as $(\mathrm{d}w/\mathrm{d}y)\,(\mathrm{d}F/\mathrm{d}w)$ or $m\,\mathrm{d}F/\mathrm{d}w$ and equations (B) gave

$$l\mu\alpha + m\mu\beta + n\mu\gamma = \boldsymbol{l} \cdot \mu\boldsymbol{\alpha} = 0$$

so that the direction of magnetisation must be in the plane of the wave. The next step was to combine the equations of the electromagnetic field so as to produce a wave equation. Introducing the symbol J for $\boldsymbol{\nabla} \cdot \boldsymbol{F}$, and William Rowan Hamilton's operator ∇^2 for $\mathrm{d}^2/\mathrm{d}x^2 + \mathrm{d}^2/\mathrm{d}y^2 + \mathrm{d}^2/\mathrm{d}z^2$, equations (B) and (C) gave, in modern vector form

$$4\pi\mu\boldsymbol{p}' = \boldsymbol{\nabla} J - \nabla^2\boldsymbol{F}. \tag{5.42}$$

Assuming there was no conduction in the medium, equations (A) gave $\boldsymbol{p}' = \mathrm{d}\boldsymbol{f}/\mathrm{d}t$, while $\boldsymbol{P} = k\boldsymbol{f}$, as in equations (E). With no motion of the conductors through space, equations (D) simplified to

$$\boldsymbol{P} = -\frac{\mathrm{d}\boldsymbol{F}}{\mathrm{d}t} - \boldsymbol{\nabla}\psi. \tag{5.43}$$

Substituting in equation (5.40) then gave

$$-4\pi\mu\frac{\mathrm{d}}{\mathrm{d}t}\left(\frac{\mathrm{d}\boldsymbol{F}}{\mathrm{d}t} + \boldsymbol{\nabla}\psi\right) = k\boldsymbol{\nabla}\,J - k\,\nabla^2\boldsymbol{F}. \tag{5.44}$$

Eliminating J and ψ by taking the curl of both sides, and substituting for $\boldsymbol{F}$ from equations (B),

$$\frac{k}{4\pi\mu}\,\nabla^2(\mu\boldsymbol{\alpha}) = \frac{\mathrm{d}^2}{\mathrm{d}t^2}(\mu\boldsymbol{\alpha}) \tag{5.45}$$

gave a wave equation for the propagation of magnetic disturbances $(\mu\boldsymbol{\alpha})$.

Combining this conclusion with his earlier analysis of a plane wave, Maxwell deduced that if magnetic disturbances were to be propagated

[139] Maxwell (1982), p. 83.

through the medium as plane waves characterised by $w = lx + my + nz - Vt$, they would have to be propagated as transverse vibrations (direction of magnetism in the plane of the wave) and with velocity V given by the velocity term in the wave equation (5.45) as

$$V = \sqrt{\frac{k}{4\pi\mu}} \tag{5.46}$$

with $V = \sqrt{k/4\pi}$ in air, for which $\mu = 1$. Magnetic disturbances propagated as plane waves in the electromagnetic medium were thus of the same kind as light waves and had a velocity given by $\sqrt{k/4\pi}$, which was from equation (5.39) given by the ratio between electrostatic and electromagnetic units, which was of course within a few per cent of the velocity of light. Moreover, as Maxwell showed next, no disturbances other than transverse vibrations could be propagated through a perfectly insulating electromagnetic medium. The experiments by which the velocity of light was measured made no use of electricity or magnetism, and those by which the ratio of units was determined made no essential use of light. Maxwell concluded that:[140]

> The agreement of the results seems to show that light and magnetism are affections of the same substance, and that light is an electromagnetic disturbance propagated through the field according to electromagnetic laws.

To conclude his paper Maxwell looked briefly, and inconclusively, at the relationships between the optical and electromagnetic properties of bodies, and gave a further account of the calculation of the coefficients of electromagnetic induction, L, M and N, based on the work he had done with Fleeming Jenkin on the determination of a standard for electrical resistance. He did not analyse the magneto-optic effect.

'A dynamical theory of the electromagnetic field' is probably the most difficult of Maxwell's three long papers on electromagnetism, but the achievement it represents is remarkable. Maxwell himself, in a short passage following his derivation of the field equations, compared the structure of the argument with that in 'On physical lines of force'. In the earlier paper he had had to assume a hierarchy of hypotheses as to the nature of the motions and strains existing in the medium. In the new paper, in contrast, he 'avoided any hypothesis of this kind'.[141] Some of his expressions, such as 'electromagnetic momentum' and 'electric elasticity', were suggestive of underlying mechanical properties. But they were not defined by such prop-

[140] Maxwell (1982), p. 86.
[141] Maxwell (1982), p. 70.

erties and Maxwell stressed that their retention in the new treatment was [142]

> merely to direct the mind of the reader to mechanical phenomena which will assist him in understanding the electrical ones. All such phrases in the present paper are to be considered as illustrative, not as explanatory.

Only 'speaking of the energy of the field' did he 'wish to be understood literally', [143] and this corresponded to his fundamental assumption that an electromagnetic medium existed and that its behaviour was conformable to the general laws of dynamics including the conservation of energy. The theory required that the energy of the field reside in states of what he called magnetic and electric polarisation, but it did not specify any mechanical representations of these states.

On the basis of his broad and 'warrantable' hypothesis of a dynamical medium, and on the basis of experimental data relating to electromagnetic and electrostatic induction and the distribution of magnetic force, Maxwell had been able to establish a complete set of connections between electromagnetic quantities and so demonstrate the physical connection of the divers phenomena covered. Although his theory of light still lacked experimental confirmation, he had provided the strongest possible theoretical grounds for assuming the identity of light waves and the propagation of magnetic disturbances. In terms of his own earlier discussions he had progressed from analogy to theory, from a complex hypothesis by which the phenomena could be represented as being related to each other to an empirically based demonstration that, granted a simple and reasonable assumption, the phenomena really were physically connected.

Having said this, however, it must also be said that the analysis was not flawless and that the assumptions were not quite so minimal as Maxwell was tempted to maintain. The first and most striking weakness of the new theory was that it was still, like its predecessor, incompatible with Verdet's observations of the magneto-optic effect. Maxwell still cited this effect as evidence of a connection between magnetic and luminiferous phenomena, but throughout his analysis he continued to adopt Faraday's theory of magnetism according to which the coefficient of magnetic induction was always of the same sign, with that for the vacuum being $+1$. As we noted above, it is difficult if not impossible to reconcile this with Verdet's observation of rotation in paramagnetics being in the opposite direction to that in diamagnetics and Maxwell did not try. Nor did he even mention, in this paper, that there was a problem.

The second weakness of the new theory concerned the theory of electric charge and of dielectric polarisation. Maxwell's treatment has often been criticised on the grounds that his assumption of molecular polarisation in

[142] Maxwell (1982), p. 70.
[143] Maxwell (1982), p. 70.

the dielectric, with the consequent introduction of electric displacement and displacement current to the field description, was not in fact sanctioned by experiment.[144] The situation is not as straightforward as it might at first appear, for there were in fact two steps in the argument. The first was to claim that the dielectric medium was subject to macroscopic electric polarisation and the second to deduce that, given the assumption that action was transmitted through a medium rather than at a distance, the macroscopic polarisation must be a manifestation of a state of microscopic polarisation existing throughout the medium: this latter step corresponded to that taken by Fourier in his heat theory. Given the existence of an electric polarisation or displacement in the medium, any change in this displacement could then not but be reflected in a contribution to the total current. The basic criticism seems, however, to be valid, and the problem it concerns is intimately connected to that of electric charge itself.

There can be little doubt that in dealing with electric charge Maxwell was both confused and inconsistent. The clearest manifestation of this lies in the fact that his four equations (A), (C), (G) and (H) are blatantly self-contradictory. (A) and (G) give

$$\frac{\mathrm{d}e}{\mathrm{d}t} = -\frac{\mathrm{d}}{\mathrm{d}t}(\boldsymbol{\nabla}\cdot f) = -\boldsymbol{\nabla}\cdot\frac{\mathrm{d}f}{\mathrm{d}t} = -\boldsymbol{\nabla}\cdot(\boldsymbol{p}'-\boldsymbol{p})$$

while (C) gives

$$\boldsymbol{\nabla}\cdot\boldsymbol{p}' = 0$$

so that

$$\frac{\mathrm{d}e}{\mathrm{d}t} = \boldsymbol{\nabla}\cdot\boldsymbol{p}$$

while from (H)

$$\frac{\mathrm{d}e}{\mathrm{d}t} = -\boldsymbol{\nabla}\cdot\boldsymbol{p}$$

with $\boldsymbol{\nabla}\cdot\boldsymbol{p}$ generally not equal to zero. Moreover, unlike the inconsistencies in 'On physical lines of force', this cannot be attributed to a simple mistake of sign or other mathematical error. The quantity e represents 'free' or accumulated electric charge, with f the displacement of electric charge and $\boldsymbol{p}$ the conduction current of electric charge. On any self-consistent definition of signs for e, f and $\boldsymbol{p}$ (for example, in the one-dimensional case, a positive charge with displacement and current positive in the direction of x increasing) it is easy to show that all the signs of the equations concerned are correct.

To see where Maxwell's confusion lay, we need only compare his

[144] See for example Chalmers (1973), p. 143.

formulae in 'A dynamical theory of the electromagnetic field' with those in 'On physical lines of force'. Apart from corrections to his earlier mistakes in sign, there is one striking difference. In the earlier paper the conduction current was assumed closed, with the total current open, while in the new treatment the reverse was the case. In the notation of 'A dynamical theory of the electromagnetic field', his earlier analysis had had

$$\nabla \times \boldsymbol{\alpha} = 4\pi \boldsymbol{p} \tag{5.47}$$

in place of equations (C). If we now reinstate this form, and if we also make the corresponding change to the equations of continuity (H), which must now apply to the open current $\boldsymbol{p}'$ rather than to the closed current $\boldsymbol{p}$, for which $(\mathrm{d}e/\mathrm{d}t)$ is zero, so that

$$\frac{\mathrm{d}e}{\mathrm{d}t} = -\nabla \cdot \boldsymbol{p}' \tag{5.48}$$

the inconsistency is removed.

The question now arises, why did Maxwell change his analysis so as to make the total current closed, and why, in physical terms, should this have led to a contradiction? Any answer to the first part of this question must be somewhat speculative, but there are various clues. In particular, it appears that the change may have been needed in order to derive the electromagnetic theory of light. This theory rested on the derivation of a wave equation for a dielectric medium characterised by the presence of displacement currents only, and by the absence of any moving conductors. These conditions could only obtain together if the displacement currents were themselves assumed to be closed in this case, leading to the general requirement of a closed total current. Perhaps more significantly, in terms of the historical sequence of events, the assumption of a closed total current also followed from Maxwell's more careful consideration of electrostatic phenomena, and especially the charging and discharging of a condenser, following his completion of 'On physical lines of force'. Considering, as he did in 'A dynamical theory of the electromagnetic field', a closed electric circuit containing a condenser, it must have been clear that the closed current in this case included the displacement current in the dielectric region between the plates of the condenser. The total closed system in this case included three possible elements, one being a current in the circuit, another the accumulation of charge on the plates, and the third the corresponding displacement in the electric. The conduction current alone was patently not closed, but the total current was.

Once Maxwell had decided to treat the total current as closed, there was no fundamental reason why this decision, firmly based as it was on empirical observation, should have led to contradictions in his analysis. The fact that it did so can only reflect, it would seem, some confusion on his part, and the location of this confusion is not hard to find. For although the assumption of a closed total current entailed the consideration of a complete system, including both static conductors and the dielectric medium between them, Maxwell was also inclined to treat the system under analysis as comprising the medium *only,* with the conductors merely defining the boundaries of this medium. In his discussion of electrostatics he wrote that:[145]

> The energy, by the expenditure of which electrical attractions and repulsions are produced, we suppose to be stored up in the dielectric medium which surrounds the electrified bodies, and not on the surfaces of those bodies themselves, which on our theory are merely the bounding surfaces of the air or other dielectric in which the true springs of action are to be sought.

This viewpoint was consistent with the analysis of 'On physical lines of force', for in that case all charge accumulation had been attributed to displacement currents and the conductors themselves really had been treated as outside the system. It was not however consistent with the new assumption of a closed total current and open conduction currents, for this assumption could only be made if the conductors were included in the system. If we now go back to the inconsistencies in Maxwell's equations we can see that his equations of free electricity (G) apply only to the accumulation of charge due to displacement in a dielectric medium and not to the accumulation due to an open conduction current. In contrast the equations of continuity (H) apply only to an open conduction current and not to an open displacement current in the medium. The two equations are therefore inconsistent both with each other, the charge e being interpreted differently in the two cases, and with the other equations, in which a closed total current is assumed.

In more general terms, Maxwell would seem to have been confused about the nature of electric charge and, above all, about the relationship between a charged conductor and the surrounding medium. Did the electric displacement of the medium alongside a charged conductor balance the opposite charge on the conductor? Or was the displacement of the medium the property which, on the field theory, *replaced* the charge on the conductor? Did the energy of a current-carrying circuit lie within the body of that circuit, with a compensating reaction in the adjacent field? Or did it lie solely in the field, the disturbance of which was merely observed as a current in the body? Did electric charge exist as an independent entity, or was all charge a manifestation of polarisation? If we focus on the case of a 'charged' conductor and the surrounding dielectric medium, most writers before Maxwell had no hesitation in attributing the phenomenon entirely to the presence of electric charge on the conductor. Faraday, pioneering what became known as a field theory, had in contrast attributed it entirely to the

[145] Maxwell (1982), p. 76.

polarisation of the medium. Thomson and Mossotti, however, had assumed the existence *both* of electric charge on the conductor *and* of a polarisation of the medium. Maxwell's explicit statements in both 'On physical lines of force' and 'A dynamical theory of the electromagnetic field' make it quite clear that he intended to follow Faraday and attribute electric phenomena entirely to properties of the medium. But he was never as happy with the phenomena of electricity as he was with those of magnetism, and in 'A dynamical theory of the electromagnetic field' this showed. He clearly upheld the viewpoint of Faraday, but he also strayed repeatedly into the adoption of that of Thomson and Mossotti, and it was this fundamental confusion that underlay the inconsistencies of his equations.

Energy physics and the role of mechanics

In this chapter we have described 'A dynamical theory of the electromagnetic field', in accordance with Maxwell's own early statements of his methodology and epistemology, as being a development of his earlier, more hypothetical, more temporary representations. He himself wrote of the new theory to a cousin that:[146]

> I have also a paper afloat, with an electromagnetic theory of light, which, till I am convinced to the contrary, I hold to be great guns.

The editor of his scientific papers, a former student, described it as giving his 'mature thoughts' on the subject.[147] In contrast his biographers, one of whom was a former student and the other a close friend, described 'On physical lines of force' as presenting a 'semi-popular' form of the theory. It is only fair to note, however, that not all commentators have taken this view, and that Maxwell's successors were divided as to which of the two papers, both of which were undoubtedly brilliant, was the more significant. We shall postpone a proper discussion of this point until after we have considered Maxwell's later writings on electromagnetism and other subjects, but a few comments may appropriately be made here.

We have interpreted Maxwell's paper 'On physical lines of force' in accordance with his methodological statements of five years earlier and with the qualifications he included in the paper itself, as an attempt to explore the nature and above all the connections of electromagnetic phenomena through their purely heuristic representation by a partial physical analogy. But despite what we know of Maxwell's youthful philosophy of science, and despite his own explicit qualifications, a great many people reading 'On physical lines of force' have concluded that Maxwell took his hypothesis

[146] Maxwell to Cay, 5 January 1865, in Campbell and Garnett (1884), p. 257.
[147] Maxwell (1890 and 1965), p. xxi.

much more seriously than that. In particular his confident claim to be putting forward 'a theory, which, if not true, can only be proved to be erroneous by experiments which will greatly enlarge our knowledge of this part of physics'[148] has suggested to people that he really believed in the vortex medium as something that existed in nature and not as a merely heuristic analogy. And although all the evidence we have found so far as to Maxwell's philosophy of science places him quite firmly in what we have here called the dynamistic tradition, the common impression of him, based largely on 'On physical lines of force' and especially on his introduction of the idle wheel mechanism, is of someone with a thoroughly mechanistic approach.

There is, unfortunately, no explicitly methodological study of Maxwell's contemporary with 'On physical lines of force'. But there is ample evidence both in the paper and elsewhere that his philosophy and methodology were unchanged from the earlier period, that the model he put forward was not intended as a description of the real world, and that he was no more a mechanist than he had ever been. We have already noted the evidence from the paper itself. The existence of a medium, of a strain distribution within that medium, of a vortex motion underlying that strain and of idle wheels facilitating the vortex motion, were all put forward explicitly as hypotheses, each one less certain than the one before. The quotation concerning 'a theory, which, if not true . . .' is slightly ambiguous, but it is certainly not contrary to Maxwell's earlier dynamistic proclamations. His concept of a 'true theory', we may remember, was one of established 'connections', such as the connection of earthly and planetary gravitation, and not one of the causes supposed to underlie these connections. And if we read the quotation carefully we see that the same concept is again present. Maxwell does not in fact equate the hypotheses with the theory, but states simply that if the hypotheses should lead to a *connection* of the phenomena ('If . . . we can connect the phenomena . . .'), then a theory will have been found.

Turning to other sources, we also know that in later years Maxwell himself took the same view of 'On physical lines of force' as we have, noting in a review of Thomson's 1872 *Reprint of Papers on Electrostatics and Magnetism* that:[149]

> In 1861 and 1862 appeared Maxwell's "theory of molecular vortices applied to magnetism, electricity &c." which may be considered as a development of Thomson's idea in a form which, though rough and clumsy compared with the realities of nature, may have served its turn as a provisional hypothesis.

We also know, finally, that Maxwell's overall approach to science at the time he was writing 'On physical lines of force' was still very much that

148 Maxwell (1890 and 1965), volume 1, p. 452.
149 Maxwell (1890 and 1965), volume 2, p. 306.

of his earlier years. In his inaugural lecture at King's College London, delivered in the autumn of 1860, he returned to some of his favourite themes. Much of the address, appropriately enough, was a call for careful and painstaking experiments and calculations. But dominating it in terms of force of expression was a rather less orthodox sermon on Maxwell's pet theme, physical science as an aid to mental development. 'I know', he wrote, 'the tendency of the human mind to do anything rather than think.'[150] But thinking, which he distinguished clearly from mere 'mental labour', was what he called for from his students, and thinking about physics not as an end in itself but as an exercise and training for higher problems:[151]

> I shall not now enter upon the question whether the fundamental truths of Physics are to be regarded as mere facts discovered by experiment, or as necessary truths, which the mind must acknowledge as true as soon as its attention has been directed to them. Questions of this kind belong to Metaphysics. In this class we do not pretend to study Metaphysics in a formal and direct manner, but if by the careful study of the laws of nature and their dependence on each other we have been trained into watchfulness over the processes of our own minds, and clear habits of thought, we shall come all the better prepared for the study of higher problems, whether they are presented to us in a metaphysical shape, or as they occur sooner or later to every thinking man. ...
>
> Physical Science affords the exercise which has developed the powers of the greatest and most original thinkers.

And again,[152]

> We shall find that it is the peculiar function of physical science to lead us, by the steps of rigid demonstration, to the confines of the incomprehensible, and to encourage us to apply our minds to that which we do not yet understand, since it is only to those who labour patiently and think steadily, that such mysteries are ever opened. The higher laws of nature are hid from us at present, but we, and those who come after us, will find in the search for them that which will prepare our minds for the next stage of human knowledge; and the discovery of each new law will not only open up new regions of science, but will alter men's expectations of what the laws of nature ought to be.

Throughout his lecture, Maxwell strayed into the topic of particular interest to us now only twice, but both times his comments served to play down rather than exalt the significance of hypotheses such as those of 'On physical lines of force'. At one point he called for humility in the contemplation of scientific laws through which men deemed to judge the laws

[150] Maxwell (1979), p. 931.
[151] Maxwell (1979), p. 930.
[152] Maxwell (1979), p. 931.

of creation by the principles of reason, and he noted there that 'Man has indeed a very partial knowledge of the simplest real thing'.[153] Then, immediately following the second of the long quotations above, he turned to the danger, inherent in any form of progressive learning, of assuming that the unknown conformed to the laws of the known:[154]

> New discoveries must be consistent with the old, for all *facts* are consistent with each other, but there is a rest mass of opinion about scientific facts, which I am certain is susceptible of modification, when the light of new truths is brought to bear upon it. We must beware of "anticipating nature" and reasoning from the supposed existence in a particular form of laws of which we have no distinct idea, and assuming that the higher laws which we do not yet know are capable of being stated under the same forms as the lower ones which we do know.

We may reasonably ask whether it is remotely conceivable that the man who wrote this could also have believed that in using a contrived mechanical model to probe the unknown nature of electromagnetism he was describing what was really happening.

We may safely conclude that Maxwell's ideas had not changed, and that his progress from the specific mechanical analogy of the vortex medium to the connections of the dynamical theory was indeed in his own view a progression, and not a temporary retreat. But what stimulated this progress, and how, in particular, did the dynamical theory of the field relate to the developing energy physics of Thomson and Rankine? Unfortunately we have no way of knowing whether Maxwell would have reached the approach of 'A dynamical theory of the electromagnetic field' without the stimulus of energy physics. He could well have done so, though. The combination of the outstanding achievement of 'On physical lines of force' with the blatant failings of the vortex model hypothesis provided very strong grounds indeed for trying to reformulate the argument in more general terms, independent of the hypothesis. And the new energy physics was not essential to this process. Maxwell could have turned directly to the existing generalised dynamics of Lagrange and Hamilton, or, perhaps more likely, to the generalised potential theory of Green. As it was, however, the approach of Thomson and Rankine fitted his needs perfectly. The possibilities of unification inherent in the generalisation of the energy concept and the associated principle of energy conservation matched perfectly his own desire to establish unifying connections. The complete freedom of the approach from specific mechanical hypotheses and its emphasis upon general properties common to all physical phenomena provided a perfect response to his concern as to the dangers and limitations of partial

[153] Maxwell (1979), p. 931.
[154] Maxwell (1979), p. 931.

analogies. The roots of the approach in Lagrangian dynamics also placed it in sympathy with his own emphasis of the importance of analogies between nature and the mind. And although Thomson's philosophy and methodology do not seem to have corresponded to his own, some of the arguments in Rankine's paper on energetics, such as those quoted earlier in this chapter, could almost have been written by Maxwell. In the circumstances in which he found himself after completing 'On physical lines of force' it would have been remarkable indeed if Maxwell had not adopted the energy physics approach.

6

Maxwell's Maturity: *A Treatise on Electricity and Magnetism* and Other Writings

A simplified formulation of the theory of light

With the dynamical theory of the electromagnetic field, Maxwell's electromagnetic theory was more or less completed in its mature form. But within Maxwell's epistemological and methodological framework completeness was relative. All analogies broke down at some point and progress was achieved by finding and exploring that point. To rest content with any theory would have been unthinkable, a sign either of defeatism or of arrogance. Maxwell's investigations into electromagnetism consequently continued, and although he achieved nothing further to compare with the unification of electromagnetic and electrostatic phenomena or the electromagnetic theory of light his work was none the less important, both for the development of his own understanding and for the communication of this understanding to a wider audience.

Following the completion of 'A dynamical theory of the electromagnetic field', Maxwell turned back to gas theory and, with the help of his wife, to an experimental study of the relationship between viscosity, temperature and pressure.[1] In his earlier theory he had assumed that the gas particles behaved as elastic spheres, but he already had reason to doubt this from comparison of the experimental specific heats with those predicted by the equipartition theorem, and he now demonstrated that it was in fact inconsistent with viscosity measurements. Whereas the theory required the viscosity to vary as the square root of temperature, the measurements showed an almost linear dependence on the temperature.

[1] See Everitt (1974), p. 220 and Campbell and Garnett (1884), p. 233. Mrs Maxwell appears to have stoked the furnace.

Soon after completing these experiments, which were conducted in London in the summer of 1865, Maxwell suffered an attack of erysipelas (St Anthony's fire) following a scratch on his head in a minor riding accident. Also in the summer of 1865 he resigned his post at King's College and, after honouring his obligations to lecture to working men the following winter, he retired to Glenlair. By May 1866, however, he had completed a new paper 'On the dynamical theory of gases', which was read to the Royal Society the same month.[2] In this he replaced the assumption of elastic sphere molecules by that of molecules as 'small bodies or groups of smaller molecules repelling one another with a force whose direction always passes very nearly through the centres of gravity of the molecules, and whose magnitude is represented very nearly by some function of the distance of the centres of gravity.'[3] Here then was Maxwell's version of action at a distance—as an explicitly approximate description only. With straight trajectories replaced by orbits the concept of mean free path was replaced by one of relaxation time, defining the relationship between elasticity and viscosity in the gas. The resulting revised theory of gases need not concern us here, but it was to be of the utmost importance for the development of kinetic theory.

Maxwell never stated explicitly his reasons for retirement from King's, but it is not difficult to infer what they might have been. Financially speaking he had no need of his professorship, and with the maintenance of his home in Kensington's Palace Gardens Terrace and the social and professional obligations of London life it may even have been an encumbrance. It certainly detracted from the time available for research and writing, and he does not seem to have found London generally conducive to serious thought. From another angle, the estate at Glenlair needed attention, and there is no doubt that both he and Mrs Maxwell were always at their happiest and most content there. Besides, he had a project.

That project was, of course, *A Treatise on Electricity and Magnetism*, to the preparation of which, and to that of the lighter *Theory of Heat* as a counterpoint and relaxation, he largely devoted the five years he was to spend at Glenlair. We shall be largely concerned in this chapter with the *Treatise*, but while working towards it Maxwell also published one other significant work on electromagnetic theory, a short 'Note on the electromagnetic theory of light' that he submitted to the Royal Society in June 1868.[4]

Maxwell's 'Note' was appended to an account of a direct experimental comparison of electrostatic and electromagnetic units, and its inclusion appears to have been prompted by the appearance of two articles relating

[2] Maxwell (1867).
[3] Maxwell (1890 and 1965), volume 2, p. 29.
[4] Maxwell (1868).

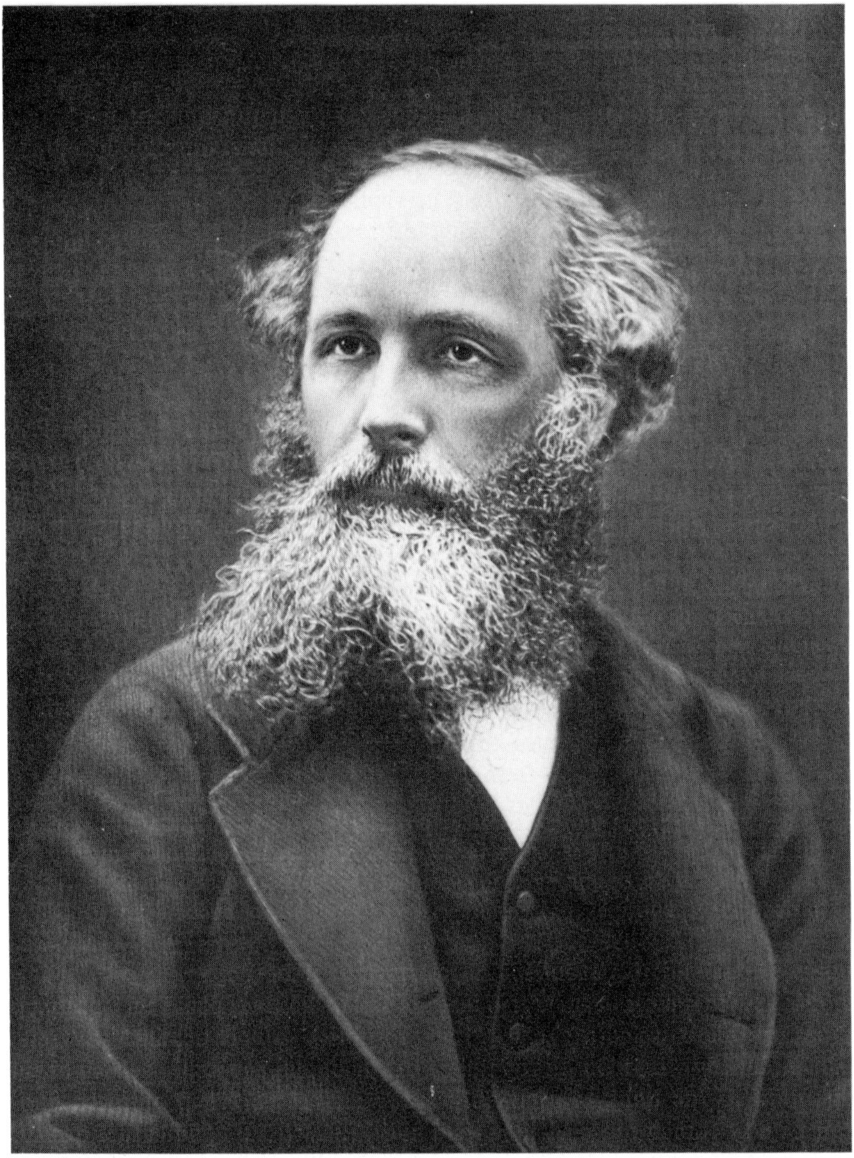

James Clerk Maxwell 1870-9. Courtesy the Cavendish Laboratory, University of Cambridge.

to the electromagnetic theory of light. Both articles had appeared in the German *Annalen der Physik* in 1867. One had originally been written in 1858 by Bernhard Riemann but was now published for the first time the year after his death.[5] The other was by Ludwig Lorenz.[6] Riemann put forward a modification of Laplace's equation to describe the transmission of electric potential at a finite velocity, which he showed must approximate to the velocity of light. Lorenz showed that according to Weber's theory electric disturbances could be propagated with the velocity of light. Neither author explicitly admitted the existence of a medium through which the propagation might take place, however, and both treatments rested on the assumption of a time-dependent force law. In Maxwell's view this made them inconsistent not only with the conservation of energy but also with the Newtonian law of action and reaction.[7] Far from adding to the force of Weber's theory, the new contributions seemed to him to point through their weaknesses to the need to assume the action of a medium if electrical phenomena were to be satisfactorily explained, and thus to support his own theory. But Maxwell was also aware that this theory was not itself easily understood, the identification of light with electromagnetic disturbances having been tied up in 'A dynamical theory of the electromagnetic field' with many other aspects of electromagnetism. He therefore proposed:[8]

> to state [the theory] in what I think the simplest form, deducing it from admitted facts and shewing the connexion between the experiments already described and those which determined the velocity of light.

Basically, Maxwell restricted himself to the consideration of a medium in which there was displacement current only (no conduction currents), and in which there were no electrical or magnetic sources. In a discussion that is in some ways reminiscent of his earliest paper on 'Faraday's lines of force' he then described the properties of such a medium in terms of simple observations and the physical ideas introduced by Faraday. The first of his four laws or 'theorems' followed from the experiments of Oersted and corresponded to his earlier 'Law III':[9]

> THEOREM A,— If a closed curve be drawn embracing an electric current, then the integral of the magnetic intensity taken round the closed curve is equal to the current multiplied by 4π.

The difference from the earlier paper was that he now had the concept of displacement and so the current, being in this case a displacement current,

[5] Riemann (1867).
[6] Lorenz (1867).
[7] Maxwell (1890 and 1965), volume 2, p. 137.
[8] Maxwell (1890 and 1965), volume 2, p. 138.
[9] Maxwell (1890 and 1965), volume 2, p. 138.

could be expressed as the time derivative of an electrical quantity (displacement) rather than just as a quantity itself (current), giving in modern notation and in the modern symbols

$$\boxed{\nabla \times H = 4\pi \frac{\mathrm{d}D}{\mathrm{d}t}.}$$

The second theorem, the discovery of which he attributed to Faraday, corresponded to the earlier 'Law VI':[10]

> THEOREM B.— If a conducting circuit embraces a number of lines of magnetic force, and if, from any cause whatever, the number of these lines is diminished, an electromotive force will act round the circuit, the total amount of which will be equal to the decrement of the number of lines of magnetic force in unit of time.
>
> The number of lines of magnetic force may be otherwise defined as the integral of the magnetic intensity resolved perpendicular to a surface, multiplied by the element of surface, and by the coefficient of magnetic induction, the integration being extended over any surface bounded by the conducting circuit.

In modern notation and symbols,

$$\boxed{\nabla \times \boldsymbol{E} = -\frac{\mathrm{d}\boldsymbol{B}}{\mathrm{d}t}.}$$

The third theorem concerned static electricity, and was again drawn from Faraday, but this time from his ideas on dielectric polarisation rather than from strictly demonstrated facts. It gave the energy of a dielectric medium, as determined in 'A dynamical theory of the electromagnetic field':[11]

> THEOREM C.— When a dielectric is acted on by electromotive force it experiences what we may call electric polarisation. If the direction of the electromotive force is called positive, and if we suppose the dielectric bounded by two conductors, A on the negative, and B on the positive side, then the surface of the conductor A is positively electrified, and that of B negatively.
>
> If we admit that the energy of the system so electrified resides in the polarised dielectric, we must also admit that within the dielectric there is a displacement of electricity in the direction of the electromotive force, the amount of this displacement being proportional to the electromotive force at each point, and depending also on the nature of the dielectric.

[10] Maxwell (1890 and 1965), volume 2, p. 138.
[11] Maxwell (1890 and 1965), volume 2, p. 139.

> The energy stored up in any portion of the dielectric is half the product of the electromotive force and electric displacement, multiplied by the volume of that portion.
>
> It may also be shewn that at every point of the dielectric there is a mechanical tension along the lines of electric force, combined with an equal pressure in all directions at right angles to these lines, the amount of this tension on unit area being equal to the amount of energy in unit of volume.

Finally, theorem D stated simply that the effect of an increase or decrease in the electric displacement was equivalent to that of an electric current in the positive or negative direction.

From these theorems, the electromagnetic theory of light followed much as in 'A dynamical theory of the electromagnetic field'. The demonstration was not quite, perhaps, as Maxwell claimed, 'deduc[ed] from admitted facts',[12] but it was deduced, as before, from a minimum of hypothesis, and the paper also served to show the theory in a relatively straightforward and easily assimilable way. Maxwell's discussion also sheds a little more light on the confusion noted in the last chapter in respect of electric charge and open and closed currents, on which his position seems to have remained unchanged from 'A dynamical theory of the electromagnetic field'. For his derivation of the theory of light, Maxwell defined a system consisting of a dielectric medium only, in which all currents were closed displacement currents. But in his discussion of the electrostatic postulates he reintroduced the dual perspective of his earlier work. When he talked of electric charge or current it was in the context of a system made up of two conductors, the medium between them and, when appropriate, the wire joining them. The conductors were unambiguously described as 'electrified', and the total current during discharge, composed of a conduction current through the wire and a displacement current in the medium, was taken as closed. On the other hand, though, he attributed the electrical energy of a system of two charged conductors, equally unambiguously, to the medium between them, which could in that respect be treated as a system in itself, with the conductors merely defining its boundaries. He had talked in 'A dynamical theory of the electromagnetic field' of the energy of a conduction current not being spatially coincident with the current-carrying wire, but his discussion there had been somewhat obscure. In the new paper it became quite clear that he was distinguishing localised charge and current on one hand from their electrical energy on the other, in a way that is strongly reminiscent of Faraday's distinction between matter as a localised entity and matter as a gravitational field.

This aspect of a field theory is now relatively familiar, if still a cause of great difficulty, but in Maxwell's time it was not so. Thus Faraday, moving towards a force field theory, had tended to *replace* particle matter by field

[12] Maxwell (1890 and 1965), volume 2, p. 139.

matter and, in his work on electrostatics, to *replace* the charge on a conductor by a polarisation in the medium. Thomson and Mossotti, on the other hand, developing Faraday's ideas but in the very different context of an aetherial or fluid concept of electricity, had simply kept *both* the charge on the conductor *and* the polarisation in the field. In Maxwell's theory, the overall thrust was in sympathy with Faraday, and the theory was essentially an energetic theory of the field. But seeking a total and exact unified theory of electromagnetic phenomena he had not been able to draw out from each situation the field-theoretic perspective as Faraday had, His field theory had to account, in detail, for observations of localised conductors and current-carrying wires, and it was in mixing the two types of description, in terms of field concepts and local observations, that he repeatedly got into confusion. This situation also shows up again an important distinction between Maxwell and Thomson. Despite being a founder of field theory and of energy physics, Thomson's physical conception was essentially a mechanical one in which the presence, for example, of electricity, produced a disturbance in the medium. Maxwell himself accepted and used such a description as a physical analogy, but his theory was a field theory in which, in line with Faraday's ideas, the presence of electricity was described as a disturbance of the medium: the electricity *was* the disturbance. This was a very different view from Thomson's and, in any complex situation, as evidenced by Maxwell's confusion, a very difficult one to maintain. For Thomson this difficulty was reason enought to militate against it in favour of a more easily visualised model. For Maxwell it was reason only to supplement it by illustrations that *could* be visualised.

A Treatise on Electricity and Magnetism

Maxwell's 1868 paper was of considerable historical importance, for it set forward his theory in the simple form in which it was taken up and developed by others. In the context of his own research, however, it was only incidental, and the great achievement of his period of retirement at Glenlair was of course *A Treatise on Electricity and Magnetism.*[13] This was finally finished in 1872, after Maxwell had come out of retirement to set up the new Cavendish Laboratory in Cambridge. But the bulk of the work was put in during the Glenlair years,[14] and bulky it certainly was, running to about a thousand pages in two volumes. Soon after publication of the *Treatise* Maxwell also began to write a short and relatively popular account of electricity, apparently intended for publication but used only, in his lifetime, as the basis of some of his Cambridge lectures. After his death this

[13] Maxwell (1873 and 1954).
[14] Campbell and Garnett (1884), p. 285.

was prepared for publication by William Garnett, his student and biographer, and it eventually appeared in 1881 as the *Elementary Treatise on Electricity*.

Surprisingly, perhaps, for such a major historical text, there was little new in Maxwell's *Treatise on Electricity and Magnetism*. It was in effect a definitive and comprehensive survey of the state of electromagnetic theory rather than a pioneering work on that subject. But it was nevertheless pioneering in certain methodological aspects, and because of its definitive and comprehensive character it also offers a very clear portrayal of Maxwell's mature views both on the electromagnetic theory itself and on a range of related physical and methodological questions. Taken in conjunction with the *Elementary Treatise on Electricity* and other semi-popular writings of the period, it also allows us to form a clear impression of Maxwell's views on a still broader range of topics, including for example the communication of scientific understanding and the status of the popular physical concepts of his day. In this section we shall outline very briefly some of the content of the *Treatise*, relating both its aims and its results to those of Maxwell's earlier papers. In the following sections we shall then close the main narrative of our account of Maxwell's work by looking more specifically at a number of points of particular interest.

Maxwell's aims in writing the *Treatise on Electricity and Magnetism* were set out in a preface, the main themes of which were already familiar from his earlier writings. The specific aim of the *Treatise* was however rather different from those of his major papers in that he was concerned with a comprehensive presentation of the theory as developed rather than with any particular development. The study of electromagnetism had, he observed, made tremendous strides in recent years. And as a result of the relations that had been developed between electromagnetism and, on the one hand, dynamics, and on the other, heat, light, chemical action etc, it had assumed a position 'of the first importance as a means of promoting the progress of science.'[15] But despite all this, the effect had been only to open up the field, and not to exhaust it:[16]

> What has been hitherto done, however, has by no means exhausted the field of electrical research. It has rather opened up that field, by pointing out subjects of enquiry, and furnishing us with means of investigation.

Given this situation, Maxwell suggested that there was a serious problem in that what had been written on the subject so far did not provide a suitable starting point for those wishing to develop it. The introductory works did not go far enough, and the higher mathematical works remained disjointed,

[15] Maxwell (1954), p. vi.
[16] Maxwell (1954), p. vii.

of uneven quality and beyond the reach of many would-be physicists:[17]

> There are several treatises in which electrical and magnetic phenomena are described in a popular way. These, however, are not what is wanted by those who have been brought face to face with quantities to be measured, and whose minds do not rest satisfied with lecture-room experiments.
>
> There is also a considerable mass of mathematical memoirs which are of great importance in electrical science, but they lie concealed in the bulky Transactions of learned societies; they do not form a connected system; they are of very unequal merit, and they are for the most part beyond the comprehension of any but professed mathematicians.

The *Treatise* was intended to fill this gap and to provide a comprehensive and mathematical treatment of the subject that would start from first principles but would do full justice both to its theoretical subtlety and to its experimental details:[18]

> I have therefore thought that a treatise would be useful which should have for its principal object to take up the whole subject in a methodical manner, and which should also indicate how each part of the subject is brought within the reach of methods of verification by actual measurement.

With this aim established, Maxwell turned next to consider the nature of his exposition, and it was here that the familiar themes re-emerged. Though comprehensive in scope, the *Treatise* was not comprehensive in the sense of giving equal coverage to the different theoretical viewpoints, and in describing the theoretical stance preferred Maxwell returned to his original justification of a field-theoretic approach. This approach was, he asserted, that of Faraday, and not just in its empirical dependence or physical ideas. Even the mathematical theory of potentials was described as 'belonging essentially to the method which I have called that of Faraday'.[19] Later, in a preface written for his *Elementary Treatise on Electricity*, Maxwell adopted an approach still closer to Faraday's and suggested that since writing the *Treatise* his conviction in this approach had increased:[20]

> In this smaller book I have endeavoured to present, in as compact a form as I can, those phenomena which appear to throw light on the theory of electricity, and to use them, each in its place, for the development of electrical ideas in the mind of the reader.
>
> In the larger treatise I sometimes made use of methods which I do not think the best in themselves, but without which the student cannot follow the

[17] Maxwell (1954), p. viii.
[18] Maxwell (1954), p. viii.
[19] Maxwell (1954), p. ix.
[20] Maxwell (1881), p. viii.

investigations of the founders of the Mathematical Theory of Electricity. I have since become more convinced of the superiority of methods akin to those of Faraday, and have therefore adopted them from the first.

But the difference lay only in the way he presented the work of Ampère and other key figures in the history of the subject, the *Elementary Treatise* making no attempt to retrace the historical evolution of the mathematical theory. In this historical sense the *Treatise* was a comprehensive work, and methods other than Faraday's accordingly played a significant part. But the exploration of the mature theory was nevertheless presented very much in tune with Maxwell's own developments, which here as before he described repeatedly as developments of Faraday's ideas and methods. Later in the *Treatise* he wrote indeed that:[21]

It is only with the hope of making [Faraday's] ideas the basis of a mathematical method that I have undertaken this treatise.

Also as before, he justified sticking to this approach in the face of the admitted success of the German action-at-a-distance school of Weber in terms of the importance of a 'second view':[22]

These physical hypotheses [of Weber], however, are entirely alien from the way of looking at things which I adopt, and one object that I have in view is that some of those who wish to study electricity may, by reading this treatise, come to see that there is another way of treating the subject, which is no less fitted to explain the phenomena, and which, though in some parts it may appear less definite, corresponds, as I think, more faithfully with our actual knowledge, both in what it affirms and in what it leaves undecided.

In a philosophical point of view, moreover, it is exceedingly important that two methods should be compared, both of which have succeeded in explaining the principal electromagnetic phenomena, and both of which have attempted to explain the propagation of light as an electromagnetic phenomenon and have actually calculated its velocity, while at the same time the fundamental conceptions of what actually takes place, as well as most of the secondary conceptions of the quantities concerned, are radically different.

Towards the very end of the *Treatise*, Maxwell gave a brief description of Weber's theory, and mentioned some new objections that Helmholtz had brought to bear on it,[23] but he did not introduce these criticisms into his discussion in the preface. The value of having two different theories for comparison appears to have outweighed in this context the value of an argument against his opponents' theory.

[21] Maxwell (1954), volume, 2, p. 176.
[22] Maxwell (1954), p. x.
[23] Maxwell (1954), volume 2, pp. 484–5.

The main bulk of the *Treatise*, following a preliminary discourse on the measurement of quantities, was divided into four parts, each dealing with a separate subject, and each following a similar self-contained pattern of a set of elementary chapters describing the phenomena and simple theory followed by a more advanced theoretical and mathematical development of the subject. The first part dealt with electrostatics, Maxwell's treatment of which was based explicitly on Faraday's theory of dielectric polarisation. From our present context the main interest of this part lies in the discussion of charge and its relation to the properties of the medium, and we shall return to this later in the chapter. The second part dealt with electrokinematics, or the theory of electrical conductivity and of entire circuits, and was relatively straightforward. The third part dealt with magnetism and the fourth, which is of most interest to us, with electromagnetism.

Maxwell's treatment of electromagnetism essentially followed that in 'A dynamical theory of the electromagnetic field'. Once again the basis was a dynamical theory of the medium, the ideas of which Maxwell introduced through the consideration of electromagnetic self-induction. The effects of self-induction indicated that an electric current 'has something very like momentum, that it resists being suddenly stopped, and that it can exert, for a short time, a great electromotive force.' But 'the momentum is certainly not that of the electricity in the wire, because the same wire, carrying the same current, exhibits effects which differ according to its form; and even when its form remains the same, the presence of other bodies, such as a piece of iron or a closed metallic circuit, affects the result.'[24] Besides something like momentum, moreover, a conducting circuit in which a current flowed also had the power of doing work in virtue of the current, 'and this power cannot be said to be something very like energy, for it is really and truly energy.'[25] It could be transformed into mechanical work, in the moving of magnets, or into heat, when decreased by the resistance of the circuit. In view of these observations Maxwell felt able to conclude that:[26]

> a system containing an electric current is a seat of energy of some kind; and since we can form no conception of an electric current except as a kinetic phenomenon, its energy must be kinetic energy, that is to say, the energy which a moving body has in virtue of its motion.

But since the electricity could not be considered as the moving body in which such kinetic energy was located, it was natural to look for the energy in the field of the wire, in which the electromagnetic effects of the current were manifest. This was the basis of the dynamical approach:[27]

[24] Maxwell (1954), volume 2, p. 197.
[25] Maxwell (1954), volume 2, p. 197.
[26] Maxwell (1954), volume 2, p. 197.
[27] Maxwell (1954), volume 2, p. 198.

> What I propose now to do is to examine the consequences of the assumption that the phenomena of the electric current are those of a moving system, the motion being communicated from one part of the system to another by forces, the nature and laws of which we do not yet even attempt to define, because we can eliminate these forces from the equations of motion by the method given by Lagrange for any connected system.

Maxwell admitted frankly that the dynamical assumption, general as it was, was an hypothesis. But it was, he claimed, more satisfactory, and more consistent with the general approach of Faraday that he had adopted, than the rival hypotheses based on action at a distance.

To build up his dynamical theory Maxwell began by establishing the generalised equations of motion of a system in the Lagrangian and Hamiltonian forms, taking as his basic assumption the conservation of energy. He then followed the general pattern established in 'A dynamical theory of the electromagnetic field', coming out as before with a set of general equations connecting the various electromagnetic variables. For his derivation of these equations he used cartesian notation and more or less the same symbols he had in his earlier papers. But he also introduced vector symbols, from which have derived those we now use. If we make some changes to the vector symbols he used, writing them in bold type rather than gothic script and replacing those of his letters which are no longer used by their more common equivalents already introduced in the last chapter, we may write Maxwell's new set of equations in two forms as follows:

(A) Equations of magnetic induction $\boldsymbol{a} = -\,\boldsymbol{\nabla}\times\boldsymbol{F}$	$\boldsymbol{B} = -\,\boldsymbol{\nabla}\times\boldsymbol{A}$
(B) Equations of electromotive force $\boldsymbol{P} = \left(\frac{\mathrm{d}\boldsymbol{x}}{\mathrm{d}t}\times\boldsymbol{a}\right) - \frac{\mathrm{d}\boldsymbol{F}}{\mathrm{d}t} - \boldsymbol{\nabla}\psi$	$\boldsymbol{E} = -\left(\boldsymbol{B}\times\frac{\mathrm{d}\boldsymbol{x}}{\mathrm{d}t}\right) - \frac{\mathrm{d}\boldsymbol{A}}{\mathrm{d}t} - \boldsymbol{\nabla}\psi$
(C) Equations of electromagnetic force $\boldsymbol{X} = \boldsymbol{u}\times\boldsymbol{a} + e\boldsymbol{P} - m\boldsymbol{\nabla}\Omega$	$\boldsymbol{F} = \boldsymbol{I}\times\boldsymbol{B} + eE - m\boldsymbol{\nabla}\Omega$
(D) Equations of magnetisation $\boldsymbol{a} = \boldsymbol{\alpha} + 4\pi\boldsymbol{A}$	$\boldsymbol{B} = \boldsymbol{H} + 4\pi\boldsymbol{M}$
(E) Equations of electric currents $4\pi\boldsymbol{u} = -\,\boldsymbol{\nabla}\times\boldsymbol{\alpha}$	$4\pi\boldsymbol{I} = -\,\boldsymbol{\nabla}\times\boldsymbol{H}$

(F) Equations of electric displacement

$$\boldsymbol{f} = \left(\frac{K}{4\pi}\right)\boldsymbol{P} \qquad\qquad \boldsymbol{D} = \epsilon \boldsymbol{E}$$

(G) Equations of conductivity

$$\boldsymbol{p} = C\boldsymbol{P} \qquad\qquad \boldsymbol{J} = \sigma \boldsymbol{E}$$

(H) Equations of true currents

$$\boldsymbol{u} = \boldsymbol{p} + \frac{\mathrm{d}\boldsymbol{f}}{\mathrm{d}t} \qquad\qquad \boldsymbol{I} = \boldsymbol{J} + \frac{\mathrm{d}\boldsymbol{D}}{\mathrm{d}t}$$

(J) Electric volume density

$$\rho = \nabla \cdot \boldsymbol{f} \qquad\qquad \rho = \nabla \cdot \boldsymbol{D}$$

(L) Equations of induced magnetisation

$$\boldsymbol{a} = \mu \boldsymbol{\alpha} \qquad\qquad \boldsymbol{B} = \mu \boldsymbol{H}.$$

There were also equations for magnetic volume density and for the expression of $\boldsymbol{H}$ in terms of the magnetic potential Ω.

Here ρ has been introduced by Maxwell for his previous e, $\boldsymbol{a}$ for $\mu\boldsymbol{\alpha}$, and $\boldsymbol{u}$ for $\boldsymbol{p}'$. The constants have also changed, with C for the old $(-\rho)$ and $(K/4\pi)$ for the old $(1/k)$. Maxwell chose his vector symbols by listing the variables concerned and labelling the first one $\boldsymbol{A}$, the second $\boldsymbol{B}$, and so on (only in gothic script of course). Thus were the modern $\boldsymbol{A}$, $\boldsymbol{B}$, $\boldsymbol{D}$, $\boldsymbol{E}$, $\boldsymbol{F}$ and $\boldsymbol{H}$ born. He used $\boldsymbol{C}$ for total current (we have used $\boldsymbol{I}$) and $\boldsymbol{K}$ for conduction current (our $\boldsymbol{J}$).

Comparing Maxwell's new equations with those in 'A dynamical theory of the electromagnetic field', we may see that although set out, confusingly, in a different order, they were fundamentally the same. The new mechanical force equation (C) contained electrostatic and magnetostatic terms, equation (D) with its 'intensity of magnetisation' $\boldsymbol{A}$ or $\boldsymbol{M}$ was new, and the continuity equation was dropped, but otherwise the two sets of equations are identical apart from a change of sign in the equation (J) relating charge and displacement. This and the continuity equation were of course two of those that had led to contradictions in the earlier set, and the changes, for which there is no other apparent explanation, may well have been related to an attempt to remove that contradiction. But the resulting situation is still unsatisfactory, for the new sign in equation (J), in which positive charge is related to an increasing displacement along the x axis, is in contradiction with the conventions of charge and displacement adopted elsewhere.

Also unresolved was the problem of the magneto-optic effect. This had continued to puzzle Maxwell and in 1867, while he was working on the *Treatise*, he had mentioned the subject in a letter to Tait, noting that while Faraday's theory of diamagnetism was 'a pretty doctrine', he did not think that Faraday himself had thought it certain, and Verdet's observations seemed to go strongly against it. But he also admitted that 'I am myself sorry to part with Faraday's theory', and in none of his writings did he in fact depart from it.[28]

In the *Treatise*, however, Maxwell did re-analyse the magneto-optic effect in terms of the angular momentum of the medium, through which he was led back to the molecular vortex representation. He noted as before that Verdet's results showed 'that the difference between ferromagnetic and diamagnetic substances does not arise merely from the "magnetic permeability" being in the first case greater, and in the second less, than that of air, but that the properties of the two classes of bodies are really opposite.'[29] But he no longer suggested that Faraday's theory must be wrong—only that it was not sufficient, that the effect could not be derived 'merely' from it. He was, moreover, careful to stress the hypothetical and provisional nature of the theory of the magneto-optic effect as compared with that of light itself, though in a long note he also made it clear that the molecular vortex hypothesis on which it depended, though quite unproven, still held a considerable attraction for him.[30]

The problem of the magneto-optic effect and the confusion over open and closed currents, charge and displacement, were obviously important flaws in Maxwell's theory. But this theory, as presented in the *Treatise*, was nevertheless impressive. To the opposing theory of action at a distance he devoted only a few pages at the very end of the book, but this was sufficient for him to make the point that all the recent variants of the theory, in which the electromagnetic theory of light was derived, seemed to demand, though not to admit, some kind of medium for the propagation of the energy:[31]

> Hence all these theories lead to the conception of a medium in which the propagation takes place, and if we admit this medium as an hypothesis, I think it ought to occupy a prominent place in our investigations, and that we ought to endeavour to construct a mental representation of all the details of its action, and this has been my constant aim in this treatise.

With that he finished.

[28] Maxwell to Tait, 23 December 1867, quoted by Heimann (1970b), p. 195. Heimann interprets Maxwell as having gone over from Faraday's theory to Weber's between parts I and III of 'On physical lines of force', but this simply does not fit with his later writings.

[29] Maxwell (1954), volume 2, p. 453.

[30] Maxwell (1954), volume 2, pp. 468–70.

[31] Maxwell (1954), volume 2, p. 493.

Energy physics and vector analysis

Maxwell's *Treatise* is an immense and immensely rich work, to which a brief and partial summary such as that given above cannot begin to do justice. The development of the general equations of the field, for example, comprised just thirty pages out of the thousand that made up the work, and the development of the formulae for the mechanical forces due to the field and of the electromagnetic theory of light just thirty pages more. But Maxwell's basic theory had been developed in his earlier papers, and to go into further details of the analysis of the *Treatise* would only take us out of our core concern with this theory into a multitude of relatively minor issues. There are, however, a number of fairly specific aspects of the *Treatise*, and of other writings by Maxwell contemporary with it, which do impinge on our general concern with Maxwell's method and approach to science and with the general historical significance of his work. Prominent among these aspects is Maxwell's use of mathematical methods, and in particular of the methods of energy physics and vector analysis.

We have already noted the importance of the emerging concept of energy physics for Maxwell's paper on 'A dynamical theory of the electromagnetic field', which he wrote up in 1864; and the close linkage between Thomson's work on the methods of mathematical physics and Maxwell's work on their application was maintained in the *Treatise*. Following the pioneering papers by Rankine and Thomson, the new energy physics received its definitive exposition in Thomson and Tait's *Treatise on Natural Philosophy*.[32] This was published in 1867, but had been conceived many years earlier, when Tait had been appointed (in preference to Maxwell) to what had been Forbes's chair of natural philosophy at Edinburgh. He had then become acquainted with Thomson, who was professor at Glasgow, and together they had conceived the plan, in Thomson's words, of 'writing a book on Natural Philosophy, beginning with a purely geometrical preliminary chapter on kinematics, and going on thence instantly to Dynamics, and the science of force, as foundation of all that was to follow.'[33] In contrast with the existing textbooks, statics was to come only after dynamics. The initial, uniquely ambitious, plan was to cover the whole of natural philosophy, including heat, light, electricity and magnetism, within a series of highly advanced textbook treatises based on the energetic viewpoint. In fact only the first volume, dealing with dynamics itself, ever appeared. But this was still sufficient to revolutionise the practice of mathematical physics and to establish the procedures based on general dynamics and the conservation of energy with which we are familiar today. Starting with a definition of a 'conservative' system (one, effectively, in which all processes were reversible, with no dissipation of energy as through friction), Thomson and Tait developed the established results of dynamics from the principle of energy

[32] Thomson and Tait (1867 and 1879–83). See also Smith (1978) and Moyer (1977).
[33] Thomson (1899–1911), 499–500.

conservation. Consideration of energy conservation in the perturbations of a system from equilibrium gave them Lagrange's principle of virtual velocities. They then deduced the general equations of motion of a system in both Lagrangian and Hamiltonian forms. In 1872 the same authors also published a short version of their treatise, without any higher mathematics, as the *Elements of Natural Philosophy. Part 1.*[34]

Maxwell himself does not seem to have been a party to the overall conception of Thomson and Tait's works. But he was in regular correspondence with both men throughout their enterprise, and indeed the familiar nickname for their book, TT′, derives from the shorthand signatures used in this correspondence, much of it conducted in miniscule hands on postcards: Maxwell signed himself $\mathrm{d}p/\mathrm{d}t$ (from an equation in one of Tait's books, $JCM = \mathrm{d}p/\mathrm{d}t$), Thomson was T and Tait T′. Maxwell was also highly sympathetic to the enterprise, to the extent that when Thomson was asked why the project had never got beyond the first book he could quite reasonably reply that others had done it for him, citing as the first of these continuations Maxwell's *Treatise.*[35] A few years later Rayleigh and Lamb, both of whom were also working within the general framework of Thomson and Tait's approach, supplied further extensions to sound and hydrodynamics respectively.[36] In 1877 Maxwell himself also gave a much simplified exposition of the new dynamics in his popular book *Matter and Motion.*[37]

We have already seen that Maxwell's attraction to the energy dynamics of Thomson and Tait was quite natural, in that they were progressing in very general terms in the same direction that he wished to. But from Maxwell's *Treatise* and his other writings of the 1870s we can also see some of the more specific aspects of this attraction. In particular we can see that the new approach had at least four characteristics to which Maxwell was drawn. The first, to which we have already referred, was the unifying power of the energy principle. Maxwell stated in the *Treatise* that:[38]

> Capacity for performing work is nothing else than energy, in whatever way it arises, and all energy is the same kind, however it may differ in form.

But his clearest discussions of this point were in his more popular works. Thus in *Matter and Motion* he emphasised the importance of the principle of energy conservation as being the one physical statement that was applicable across the whole range of physical phenomena.[39]

[34] Thomson and Tait (1872).
[35] Thompson (1910), volume 1, p. 476–7.
[36] Lord Rayleigh (1877); Lamb (1879).
[37] Maxwell (1877 and 1920).
[38] Maxwell (1954), volume 2, p. 211.
[39] Maxwell (1920), pp. 54–5.

> The progress of physical science has led to the discovery and investigation of different forms of energy, and to the establishment of the doctrine that all material systems may be regarded as conservative systems, *provided* that all the different forms of energy which exist in these systems are taken into account.
>
> This doctrine, considered as a deduction from observation and experiment, can, of course, assert no more than that no instance of a non-conservative system has hitherto been discovered.
>
> As a scientific or science-producing doctrine, however, it is always acquiring additional credibility from the constantly increasing number of deductions which have been drawn from it, and which are found in all cases to be verified by experiment.
>
> In fact the doctrine of the Conservation of Energy is the one generalised statement which is found to be consistent with fact, not in one physical science only, but in all.
>
> When once apprehended it furnishes to the physical inquirer a principle on which he may hang every known law relating to physical actions, and by which he may be put in the way to discover the relations of such actions in new branches of science.
>
> For such reasons the doctrine is commonly called the Principle of the Conservation of Energy.

The same passage also appears, with very slight alterations, in his *Elementary Treatise on Electricity.*[40]

Associated with the power to connect and unify was, as we have mentioned before, the property of being fundamental, and the fundamental nature of the energy concept and of dynamical explanation in general also appealed to Maxwell. Thomson and Tait both seem to have been confident that all physical phenomena would ultimately prove reducible to microscopic motions in which all processes were reversible and conservative.[41] Maxwell was less sanguine on the mechanistic aspect of this hope, but he does seem to have shared his colleagues' belief in the fundamental nature of the energy principle it implied. He also argued that while not everything might prove reducible to an explanation in terms of specific matter in specific motions, such an explanation was nevertheless a reasonable goal and one, in particular, that was well matched to the powers of the human mind. Thus, for example, in a lecture to the Chemical Society, 'On the dynamical evidence of the molecular constitution of bodies', he declared that,[42]

> when a physical phenomenon can be completely described as a change in the configuration and motion of a material system, the dynamical explanation of

[40] Maxwell (1881), p. 22.
[41] See for example Smith (1978).
[42] Maxwell (1880 and 1965), volume 2, p. 418.

> that phenomenon is said to be complete. We cannot conceive any further explanation to be either necessary, desirable or possible, for as soon as we know what is meant by the words configuration, motion, mass, and force, we see that the ideas which they present are so elementary that they cannot be explained by means of anything else.

This time, however, it is the *Treatise* that gives the thrust of the argument most clearly. In the course of introducing the idea of an energy-based description through the discussion of the self-induction phenomenon Maxwell wrote that:[43]

> It is difficult . . . for the mind which has once recognised the analogy between the phenomena of self-induction and those of the motion of material bodies, to abandon altogether the help of this analogy, or to admit that it is entirely superficial and misleading. The fundamental dynamical idea of matter, as capable by its motion of becoming the recipient of momentum and of energy, is so interwoven with our forms of thought that whenever we catch a glimpse of it in any part of nature, we feel that a path is before us leading, sooner or later, to the complete understanding of the subject.

We shall return to the role of understanding in Maxwell's philosophy of science in the context of his continued discussion and use of physical analogies. But it seems clear from the above quotation that whatever his views on the ultimate constitution of nature, the intimate connection between dynamical explanation and the forms of thought gave dynamics in his view a fundamental role closely related to that postulated by Thomson and Tait.

Maxwell's view of the relation between dynamics and the mind also carries echoes of the traditional relationship, discussed in the early chapters of this book, between analytic dynamics and the dynamistic attitude to science that we have associated with Maxwell. In Maxwell's earlier writings there was little to associate him explicitly with this mathematical dynamical tradition, but by the time he wrote the *Treatise* he was prepared to set himself firmly in the tradition of Lagrange and William Rowan Hamilton,[44] a tradition he recognised as being concerned with *a priori* abstract dynamics or 'the necessary laws of dynamical systems', quite independent of 'real bodies or portions of matter.'[45] Apart from the necessary or mental aspect of Lagrangian dynamics, Maxwell was also strongly drawn to its power to treat a system parts of which were unknown, a power that had two related facets. On one hand it provided a way of circumventing temporary ignorance without resorting to arbitrary hypotheses. In the context of his own

[43] Maxwell (1954), volume 2, p. 196.
[44] Maxwell (1954), volume 2, pp. 199–200.
[45] Maxwell (1890 and 1965), volume 2, p. 781.

work on electromagnetic theory the Lagrangian approach of describing a system by its overall energetic properties and its overall response to external forces allowed him to leave the inner workings of the electromagnetic medium unspecified and, in particular, to proceed in complete ignorance of the nature of electric charge and current. On the other hand it also provided a check on unwarranted and unnecessary hypotheses concerning those elements of a system beyond observation, through the application of what Thomson and Tait called, in the second edition of their *Treatise on Natural Philosophy*, the 'Ignoration of Coordinates'. As Maxwell wrote in his review of this edition,[46]

> We may regard this investigation as a mathematical illustration of the scientific principle that in the study of any complex object, we must fix our attention on those elements of it which we are able to observe and to cause to vary, and ignore those which we can neither observe nor cause to vary.
>
> In an ordinary belfry, each bell has one rope which comes down through a hole in the floor to the bellringers' room. But suppose that each rope, instead of acting on one bell, contributes to the motion of many pieces of machinery, and that the motion of each piece is determined not by the motion of one rope alone, but by that of several, and suppose, further, that all this machinery is silent and utterly unknown to the men at the ropes, who can only see as far as the holes in the floor above them.
>
> Supposing all this, what is the scientific duty of the men below? They have full command of the ropes, but of nothing else. They can give each rope any position and any velocity, and they can estimate its momentum by stopping all the ropes at once, and feeling what sort of tug each rope gives. If they take the trouble to ascertain how much work they have to do in order to drag the ropes down to a given set of positions, and to express this in terms of these positions, they have found the potential energy of the system in terms of the known co-ordinates. If they then find the tug on any rope arising from a velocity equal to unity communicated to itself or to any other rope, they can express the kinetic energy in terms of the co-ordinates and velocities.
>
> These data are sufficient to determine the motion of every one of the ropes when it and all the others are acted on by any given forces. This is all that the men at the ropes can ever know. If the machinery above has more degrees of freedom than there are ropes, the co-ordinates which express these degrees of freedom must be ignored. There is no help for it.

It was not until the advent of quantum mechanics in the 1920s that the observability criterion came to be recognised as necessary if contradictions were to be avoided, but it would be hard to find a clearer expression of this criterion as a general scientific principle than that given by Maxwell here.

Finally, while Maxwell traced the basic method of the new dynamics to Lagrange and Hamilton, he also considered the way in which Thomson and Tait had reformulated it through the energy principle to be of the utmost

[46] Maxwell (1890 and 1965), volume 2, pp. 783–4.

importance for the development of physical understanding. In the review just cited he wrote that it was 'remarkable how slow natural philosophers at large have been to make use' of the methods of Lagrange, Hamilton and Jacobi; that despite having been well known to mathematicians for nearly a century Lagrange's methods had only recently been widely used in physics and that the credit for the recent change in this respect 'belongs in great measure to Thomson and Tait.'[47] The point was that the techniques concerned had been lost in the obscure and technical language of higher mathematics, and had been brought to fruition only through their clear expression in terms of dynamical concepts, and in particular the energy concept:[48]

> The two northern wizards [Thomson and Tait] were the first who, without compunction or dread, uttered in their mother tongue the true and proper names of those dynamical concepts which the magicians of old were wont to invoke only by the aid of muttered symbols and inarticulate equations. And now the feeblest among us can repeat the words of power and take part in dynamical discussions which but a few years ago we should have left for our betters.

He also made this point forcibly in the *Treatise*, where he observed that while in the execution of Lagrangian analysis *qua* mathematics 'the mind is exercised in calculation, and should therefore be kept free from the intrusion of dynamical ideas', the aim of physicists, and of the work in hand, was precisely 'to cultivate our dynamical ideas.'[49] This required the 're-translation' of the mathematical results into the language of physical dynamics, the clarification of which language, with energy as its central concept, was largely due to Thomson and Tait.[50]

If Maxwell's *Treatise* was important for providing the first application of the new dynamics (and, incidentally, the first important application of Hamilton's dynamics, which was to become central to the physics of the twentieth century), it was no less so for another methodological innovation, also linked with the achievements of William Rowan Hamilton and with the advocacy of Tait. This was Maxwell's use of quaternion or vector analysis. Like the concept of energy, that of a vector seems so fundamental to our view of physics today that it is hard to imagine working without it. Yet vector analysis as used today dates only from the work of Heaviside and

[47] Maxwell (1890 and 1965), volume 2, p. 782.
[48] Maxwell (1890 and 1965), volume 2, p. 782.
[49] Maxwell (1954), volume 2, pp. 199–200.
[50] Maxwell (1954), volume 2, p. 200.

Gibbs at the very end of the nineteenth century, and both men took up the subject as a result of reading Maxwell's *Treatise*.[51]

The origins of vector analysis lie firmly in the dynamistic tradition, in the quaternion calculus developed by William Rowan Hamilton in the 1840s. In 1835 Hamilton had written a remarkable two-part paper on the 'Theory of conjugate functions, or algebraic couples; with a preliminary and elementary essay on algebra as the science of pure time'.[52] The relationship between the two parts of this paper is not altogether clear, and its details need not concern us here, but crudely speaking the preliminary essay was a thoroughly metaphysical attempt to derive number from the pure intuition (in the Kantian sense) of time. In this derivation pairs of moments in time were used to define steps, and pairs of steps or step couples were then related to give the integers as multipliers of, and real numbers as ratios between, step couples. Complex couples were then derived as pairs of real numbers acting as operators, and the theory of couples itself was a theory of complex number operators, the number $a + ib$ being represented (following its traditional geometrical representation by cartesian coordinates in two dimensions) as an ordered couple (a, b).

Part of Hamilton's concern with complex numbers had been with their 'imaginary' or unintuitable nature, and by combining the development of algebra from time with the formulation of complex numbers as operators he had succeeded in achieving his aim of rendering the imaginaries intuitable. But he had also been concerned with the geometric aspects of the problem, and having established an algebra of couples he sought for several years to extend this to triplets, and so to provide a connection between algebra and the geometry of space. The triplet problem proved intractable, but in 1843, while pursuing the possibility of triplets based on two distinct square roots of -1 (since imaginary numbers were defined as operators there was nothing to rule out such a possibility), he realised that to get a workable algebra he actually needed three such roots, and that the triplets should really be quaternions, (a, b, c, d) corresponding to $a + b\mathrm{i} + c\mathrm{j} + d\mathrm{k}$, with i, j, k, three distinct roots of -1 such that $\mathrm{ij} = \mathrm{k}$, $\mathrm{jk} = \mathrm{i}$, $\mathrm{ki} = \mathrm{j}$ and $\mathrm{ji} = -\mathrm{k}$, $\mathrm{kj} = -\mathrm{i}$, $\mathrm{ik} = -\mathrm{j}$. If the quaternions were portrayed geometrically, any unit vector in the i, j, k space was also a square root of -1, so that this space had the homogeneity required for a representation of ordinary three-dimensional space. Hamilton then distinguished between this directed spatial or vector part of the quaternion, and its 'real' one-dimensional non-spatial part, for which he introduced the word 'scalar'. In his 1853 *Lectures on Quaternions* he developed an analysis of quaternions treated as operators upon vectors.[53]

[51] Gibbs (1881–4) and Heaviside (1892 and 1893). See also Crowe (1967).

[52] Hamilton (1837). For the origins of this paper see Hankins (1976) and Hendry (1984a). For Hamilton's work in general see Hankins (1980) and Graves (1882–9).

[53] Hamilton (1853). See Graves (1882–9), volume 2, pp. 432*ff.*

Besides his *Lectures on Quaternions*, Hamilton also wrote an *Elements of Quaternions*, published shortly after his death in 1865.[54] Both works were extremely difficult and went largely unread, but the *Lectures* did excite the interest of the young Tait, then professor of mathematics at Belfast. Tait was intrigued by the quaternion methods and he prepared his own *Elementary Treatise on Quaternions*, which was eventually published in 1867.[55] He also prepared a longer *Introduction to Quaternions* with Kelland, and this was published in 1873.[56] All of these works followed the same basic format, with the vectors being introduced first and the quaternions then introduced as their operators or quotients, and all contained the elements of vector analysis, including definitions of vector and scalar products ($V.\alpha\beta$ for our modern $\boldsymbol{\alpha} \times \boldsymbol{\beta}$ and $S.\alpha\beta$ for our $\boldsymbol{\alpha} \cdot \boldsymbol{\beta}$) and of the three types of vector differentials, using the operator symbol $\boldsymbol{\nabla}$ for

$$\left(\mathbf{i}\frac{\mathrm{d}}{\mathrm{d}x} + \mathbf{j}\frac{\mathrm{d}}{\mathrm{d}y} + \mathbf{k}\frac{\mathrm{d}}{\mathrm{d}z}\right).$$

In retrospect it is clear that Hamilton's quaternion calculus and the vector analysis it incorporated constituted an enormous step forward in the mathematical methods of physics. The concept of a vector was not new, but vectors had only previously been expressed in terms of their cartesian (or other linear) coordinates and the concept of a vector analysis was quite new. To an audience accustomed only to cartesian analysis, however, and quite unused to working with vectors, let alone with quaternions, it was forbiddingly difficult. Even Tait had come unstuck with the more advanced parts of the *Lectures*, and it is easy to see why.[57] The work began with a 60 page metaphysical preface (Tait, who was no friend of metaphysics and became renowned, indeed, for his opposition to it, seems simply to have passed this over) and ended with a single 'lecture' of over 300 pages in which the differential quaternion calculus was developed—without recourse to infinitesimals. A further difficulty was that in developing and applying the elements of vector analysis, Hamilton insisted on working throughout with the entire quaternion, even when it was only the vector or scalar part that was relevant. This meant, for example, that the scalar product of two vectors, being a product of imaginaries, was always negative, and that the familiar Laplacian operator

$$\left[\left(\frac{\mathrm{d}}{\mathrm{d}x}\right)^2 + \left(\frac{\mathrm{d}}{\mathrm{d}y}\right)^2 + \left(\frac{\mathrm{d}}{\mathrm{d}z}\right)^2\right]$$

was expressed in quaternion notation by the operator $-\nabla^2$. Both seemed counter to common sense, and so indeed they were. For it was not common

[54] Hamilton (1865).
[55] Tait (1867).
[56] Kelland and Tait (1873).
[57] Tait to Hamilton, 19 August 1858, in Knott (1911), pp. 119–20.

sense with which Hamilton, seeking to penetrate beyond the restricted mechanistic understanding of everything in terms of quantities and to develop an exact metaphysic of quality, was concerned.

Hamilton realised that his *Lectures* were not easy reading, and his *Elements* were designed to remedy this. Tait's *Treatise* was intended to simplify the treatment of the *Elements*, and that of Kelland and Tait was intended to simplify that of Tait. But even the last named work, intended specifically for students, was prodigiously difficult. Moreover, since Tait, who was philosophically quite out of sympathy with Hamilton's aims, concentrated on using the new calculus for the routine rederivation of existing results rather than on developing the quaternions as the creative tool that Hamilton had intended, there was little reason for anyone to brave their complexity. Maxwell, however, when introduced to quaternions by Tait, took a different view. He did not himself try to master all the details of quaternion analysis, and he did not expect others to, but he was enormously inspired by the basic physical concepts of vector analysis as he saw it in Hamilton's work. And in 1870 he determined, as he wrote to Tait, to bring something of these concepts into his *Treatise*:[58]

> With regard to my dabbling in Hamilton I want to leaven my book with Hamiltonian ideas without casting the operations into Hamiltonian form for which neither I nor I think the public are ripe. Now the value of Hamilton's idea of a vector is unspeakable, and so are those of the addition and multiplication of vectors. I consider the form into which he put these ideas, such as the names Tensor, Versor, Quaternion, etc., important and useful, but subject to the approval of the mathematical world.

In another letter of the same period Maxwell noted that he looked forward with enthusiasm to the possibility (not in fact to be) that Tait would be able to 'cause the Quaternion ideas to overflow all their mathematical symbols and to become embodied in ordinary language so as to give their form to the thoughts of all mankind.'[59] As his work on the *Treatise* progressed he wrote of the quaternion as 'a flaming sword', the virtue of which lay 'in enabling us to see the meaning of the question and its solution' when struggling with physical problems. He even defended its apparent quirks, such as the negative sign of the Laplacian, against Thomson's tendency to adopt Hamilton's symbol with the more natural positive sign interpretation.[60]

What, then, did Maxwell see in the quaternions? The answer lies partly in his *Treatise* and partly in a contemporary paper on the mathematical classification of physical quantities, inspired by his study of the quaternions.[61] In this paper he drew attention to Hamilton's distinction between

[58] Maxwell to Tait, 14 November 1870, in Knott (1911), p. 144.
[59] Maxwell to Balfour, 28 November 1870, in Knott (1911), pp. 149–50.
[60] Maxwell to Tait, 2 November and 21 December 1871, in Knott (1911), p. 150.
[61] Maxwell (1890 and 1965), volume 2, pp. 257–66.

vectors and scalars and proclaimed the quaternion calculus as the most important step since Descartes's introduction of coordinate systems towards our understanding of spatial quantities:[62]

> A most important distinction was drawn by Hamilton when he divided the quantities with which he had to do into Scalar quantities, which are completely represented by one numerical quantity, and Vectors, which require three numerical quantities to define them.
>
> The invention of the calculus of Quaternions is a step towards the knowledge of quantities related to space which can only be compared for its importance, with the invention of triple co-ordinates by Descartes. The ideas of this calculus, as distinguished from its operations and symbols, are fitted to be of the greatest use in all parts of science.

More significantly, though, he also connected Hamilton's achievements with his own efforts in the development of electromagnetic theory. He began by noting the importance in the development of physics of analogies such as those used by Thomson (between action-at-a-distance theories and theories of heat conduction) and Mossotti (between the quantities in electrostatics and those in magnetostatics), both of which had of course played a part in his own work. He next observed that since these were mathematical analogies between divers physical phenomena there must be some mathematical classification of physical quantities underlying them. If there existed a true mathematical classification of quantities then it would be possible to detect at once 'the analogy between any system of quantities presented to us and other systems of quantities in known sciences, so that we should lose no time in availing ourselves of the mathematical labours of those who had already solved problems essentially the same.'[63]

Maxwell did not think that Hamilton's distinction solved this problem, for he saw the quaternions as being mainly associated with spatial or geometric quantities and not with those of dynamics, and he felt that 'in the higher sciences the ideas might receive a still higher development if they could be expressed in language as appropriate to dynamics as Hamilton's is to geometry.'[64] But Hamilton's work nevertheless went a long way towards achieving clarification in a direction in which Maxwell had himself long sought it. Thus, for example, Rankine had observed that the quantity energy could be represented as the product of two factors in many different ways, but some of these such as [half of] 'mass × square of velocity' had made no physical sense to Maxwell. What was 'square of velocity'? If, however, one contemplated energy as the scalar product (or scalar part of the quaternion product) of two vectors rather than as the product of two scalars, this always gave 'results capable of a satisfactory interpretation'.

[62] Maxwell (1890 and 1965), volume 2, p. 259.
[63] Maxwell (1890 and 1965), volume 2, p. 258.
[64] Maxwell (1890 and 1965), volume 2, p. 259.

Of the two factors in such a product, for example momentum and velocity, one could always be 'conceived as a tendency towards a certain change, and the other as that change itself.'[65] If, moreover, one made the additional distinction that Maxwell himself had introduced in 'Faraday's lines of force', between 'forces', or vector quantities related to a unit of length and corresponding to intensities, and 'fluxes', or those related to a unit of area and corresponding to simple quantities, then the vector constituents of energy were always one force and one flux.

Despite Maxwell's earlier work, the distinction between forces and fluxes had still not been widely recognised, and he accordingly devoted a part of his paper to stressing its importance, both generally and in electromagnetic theory. But he then turned to another important physical distinction, between vectors defined with reference to translation and those defined with reference to rotation. This distinction was fundamental to electromagnetic theory, in which Maxwell, following Ampère and Thomson, had treated the electric force as linear and the magnetic as rotational, while Helmholtz had adopted the opposite identification. And once again the quaternion analysis contributed something to its understanding. For the vector part of the quaternion differential operator on a vector, which Maxwell christened the 'curl' ($\nabla \times \boldsymbol{\alpha}$) always converted a vector of translation into one of rotation and vice versa. The operation of vector differentiation thus had a physically meaningful interpretation, and so did its scalar counterpart, christened by Maxwell the 'convergence' (the term divergence followed the later abandonment of the imaginary nature of the components with its resulting negative sign), and the Laplacian operator or 'concentration'.

The association of physical meaning with mathematical operations that the quaternion calculus afforded must have appealed to Maxwell in much the same way as did Thomson and Tait's rederivation of abstract dynamics from the energy principle. In both cases the task of selecting the appropriate mathematical formulation for the physical phenomena and ideas to be treated was much simplified, and the use of mathematical forms and analogies to extend the physical theory also become much more straightforward and feasible. Vectors also provided, as he observed in the *Treatise*, a 'mode of contemplating geometrical and physical quantities that is more primitive and more natural than' that of cartesian coordinate representations.[66]

For the main analysis of the *Treatise*, Maxwell retained the methods of Descartes as being both 'the most familiar to students of science' and 'really the most useful for purposes of calculation'.[67] But he also observed that:[68]

> I am convinced, however, that the introduction of the ideas, as distinguished

[65] Maxwell (1890 and 1965), volume 2, p. 260.
[66] Maxwell (1954), volume 1, p. 9.
[67] Maxwell (1954), volume 1, p. 9.
[68] Maxwell (1954), volume 1, p. 9.

> from the operations and methods of Quaternions, will be of great use to us in the study of all parts of our subject, and especially in electrodynamics, where we have to deal with a number of physical quantities, the relations of which to each other can be expressed far more simply by a few expressions of Hamilton's, than by the ordinary equations.

He accordingly introduced the concepts of vectors, of the quaternion relations between them, and of the quaternion differential operators on them, much as in his paper on the mathematical classification of quantities. Using gothic script to denote vectors he also expressed the main results of the work in the differential vector form with which we are familiar today.

How far Maxwell understood the quaternions as Hamilton had intended them is not clear. He seems to have taken up the important idea of the quaternion as an operator as well as the more straightforward ideas of vectors and scalars, and he insisted on retaining the peculiarities arising from the origins of the quaternion in the analysis of the square roots of -1. But he never referred to, and may never have read, Hamilton's metaphysical preface. He always framed his discussion in terms of quantities and his emphasis in the *Treatise* was very much on the vector concept rather than on the far more complex concept of the quaternion.

Matter, charge and aether

A second subject of particular interest in the context of Maxwell's mature writings is his attitude towards the principal physical concepts of the physics of his time, and especially towards the concepts of matter, charge and aether. We have argued in general that Maxwell's attitude towards such ontological elements was strongly conditioned by his philosophy of analogy, and that his frequent references to them must not be taken as implying the view that they necessarily existed in any of the forms in which they were commonly represented. We shall return in the next section to Maxwell's general views on the use of analogy and the nature of scientific explanation and understanding, but it is also worth addressing more specifically his use of the individual concepts mentioned.

Given Maxwell's emphasis upon dynamical explanation the concept of matter in particular would seem to have been fundamental to his physics. And so in a very important sense it was. As we noted in the last section, the fundamental idea of matter was in his view so interwoven with the laws of thought as to be in some sense irreducible and fully understood.[69] But as he stressed in his review of the second edition of Thomson and Tait's *Treatise on Natural Philosophy*, to assert this was very different indeed from asserting anything about the nature of matter itself. Thomson and

[69] Maxwell (1890 and (1965), volume 2, p. 418, and (1954), volume 2, pp. 196–7.

Tait, he observed, took what seemed to him a rather strange view of matter:[70]

> Our authors, one of whom [Tait] never misses an opportunity of denouncing metaphysical reasoning, except when he has occasion to expound the peculiarities of the Unconditioned, make the following somewhat pusillanimous statement:—
>
> "We cannot, of course, give a definition of *Matter* which will satisfy the metaphysician, but the naturalist may be content to know matter as *that which can be perceived by the senses, or as that which can be acted upon by, or can exert, force.*" ...
>
> Again, ..., the capacity of the student is called upon to accept the following statement:—
>
> "Matter has an innate power of resisting external influences, so that every body, as far as it can, remains at rest or moves uniformly in a straight line."

All of this struck Maxwell as being 'very much out of place' in a treatise on abstract dynamics, in which mass was in his view merely something with which bodies were supposed endowed. In this abstract context it was no less absurd to say that matter had the power, innate or otherwise, of resisting external influences than it would have been to say that tea had the power of resisting the sweetening influence of sugar, by virtue of which it refused to turn sweet unless sugar was actually put into it. Nor was mass in the abstract sense dependent on sense perception, any more than were abstract space and time. Physical matter, on the other hand, was in Maxwell's view something the properties of which were entirely unknown—and largely irrelevant in the context of dynamical explanation:[71]

> The phenomena of real bodies are found to correspond so exactly with the necessary laws of dynamical systems, that we cannot help applying the language of dynamics to real bodies, and speaking of the masses in dynamics as if they were real bodies or portions of matter.
>
> We must be careful, however, to remember that what we sometimes, even in abstract dynamics, call matter, is not that unknown substratum of real bodies, against which Berkeley directed his arguments, but something as perfectly intelligible as a straight line or a sphere.
>
> Real bodies may or may not have such a substratum, just as they may or may not have sensations, or be capable of happiness or misery, knowledge or ignorance, and the dynamical transactions between them may or may not be accompanied with the conscious effort which the word force suggests to us when we imagine one of the bodies to be our own, but so long as their motions are related to each other according to the conditions laid down in dynamics, we call them, in a perfectly intelligible sense, dynamical or material systems.

[70] Maxwell (1890 and 1965), volume 2, pp. 778–9.
[71] Maxwell (1890 and 1965), volume 2, p. 781.

Here the dynamistic elements of Maxwell's philosophy are clearly apparent. The laws of dynamics were discovered from observation, and their elements, space, time, matter and cause, were all recognised empirically. But once discovered the laws were recognised as necessary, *a priori*, laws independent of their observation. And just as the ideas of space, time and cause were all located in the mind, so was that of matter. In *Matter and Motion*, Maxwell asserted repeatedly that 'we are acquainted with matter only as that which may have energy communicated to it from other matter, and which may in its turn communicate energy to other matter'.[72] Matter was merely the undefined recipient of energy, or that which conformed to the laws of dynamics. Of course there were questions one could ask about matter, in the sense of gross observed matter rather than ultimate matter, and on such questions Maxwell had his views. He subscribed, in particular, to the view that matter was atomic, that there would be some smallest parts beyond which it could not be divided.[73] But whenever he talked of particulate matter in a scientific context it was either in the abstract sense of mathematical point-centres, or in the physical sense of bodies that could be approximated by point-particles in the context of the problem to be solved, or in the sense of chemical molecules. And even in the latter context he was careful to designate what were generally called the hydrogen and oxygen atoms (and what we still call atoms, despite having split them) as hydrogen and oxygen molecules, leaving open the question as to whether they were or were not ultimate atoms.[74]

Maxwell's view of matter has led to considerable difficulties on the part of his commentators, many of whom have treated him as more or less a traditional mechanist. His view of charge has caused even more problems. We have already discussed the confusion introduced by his advocacy of a field interpretation in which static or current charge was replaced by its effect on the energetic properties of the medium, alongside his continued use of the more familiar language of charged conductors and current-carrying wires. As a result of this confusion in 'A dynamical theory of the electromagnetic field' he himself got into a tangle from which he was unable, even in the *Treatise*, to extricate himself, and it is no wonder that many of his readers were baffled. Heinrich Hertz, for example, claimed that the *Treatise* incorporated several quite different concepts of electricity.[75] We have already seen, however, that Maxwell had at least a clear view of what he intended, and that this was to describe charge, in the context of a field theory, by the dynamical properties of the field. Whether and in what form electricity existed on a conductor or in a conducting wire he did not claim

[72] Maxwell (1920), p. 89.
[73] See for example Maxwell (1890 and 1965), volume 2, p. 362.
[74] See for example Maxwell (1890 and 1965), volume 2, p. 363.
[75] Hertz (1914), volume 2, pp. 28–9. See Knudsen (1976), p. 254.

to know, and the field theory did not require him to know it. In his *Elementary Treatise* he was more explicit on this latter point, stressing that people were still ignorant of the ultimate nature of charge and should take care to remember this. In particular, they should not be led astray by the popular but misleading language of electric fluids:[76]

> And here we may introduce once for all the common phrase The Electric Fluid for the purpose of warning our readers against it. It is one of those phrases, which, having been at one time used to denote an observed fact, was immediately taken up by the public to connote a whole system of imaginary knowledge. As long as we do not know whether positive electricity, or negative, or both, should be called a substance or the absence of a substance, and as long as we do not know whether the velocity of an electric current is to be measured by hundreds of thousands of miles a second or by an hundredth of an inch in an hour, or even whether the current flows from positive to negative or in the reverse directions, we must avoid speaking of the electric fluid.

From the very beginning Maxwell's own work had been based on the phenomena of magnetism and this had helped him to avoid the problem posed by the nature of electricity. Once he had the dynamical theory, however, this evasion, dictated by ignorance, also became justified by the dynamical approach. His work, as we have seen, still contained serious inconsistencies; but his concepts did not.

Finally in this section, a third issue that has engaged and confused Maxwell's commentators is that of his attitude to the aether. Here again we find a situation similar to those for matter and charge. In offering a dynamical theory of the field, Maxwell inevitably hypothesised the existence of a material aether, and it is tempting therefore to set him in the same tradition as Thomson and other aether-theorists of the period. But once again Maxwell's attitude was much more cautious than that of his principal contemporaries, and when he discussed the aether at length, in a Royal Institution lecture on action at a distance, he was careful to dissociate himself from anything other than the minimal hypothesis that there was 'something there'.[77] He drew a parallel, as had others before him, with Newton:[78]

> When Newton demonstrated that the force which acts on each of the heavenly bodies depends on its relative position with respect to other bodies, the new theory met with violent opposition from the advanced philosophers of the day, who described the doctrine of gravitation as a return to the exploded method of explaining everything by occult causes, attractive virtues, and the like.

[76] Maxwell (1881), p. 8.
[77] Maxwell (1890 and 1965), volume 2, pp. 311–23.
[78] Maxwell (1890 and 1965), volume 2, pp. 315–16.

> Newton himself, with that wise moderation which is characteristic of all his speculations, answered that he made no pretence of explaining the mechanism by which the heavenly bodies act on each other. To determine the mode in which their mutual action depends on their relative position was a great step in science, and this step Newton asserted that he had made. To explain the process by which this action is effected was a quite distinct step, and this step Newton, in his *Principia*, does not attempt to make.

Just as Newton refrained from making any claim as to *how* gravitational effects were propagated, but yet admitted, as in a letter to Bentley, that he could not conceive of action at a distance through a vacuum, without some sort of mediation, so Maxwell also required a medium while at the same time remaining strictly agnostic as to its nature. His electromagnetic investigations had led him to the conclusion that 'there are several different kinds of work to be done by the electro-magnetic medium if it exists', and that the properties that would be required of such a medium also corresponded to those that would be required of a medium for the transmission of light waves.[79] The hypothesis of a medium thus made it possible 'to reduce several kinds of action at a distance into actions between contiguous parts of a continuous substance', and this represented, in his view, a distinct gain in scientific understanding. But he recognised that his hypothesis was nevertheless just that, and that it was ultimately a metaphysical question 'whether the resolution is of the nature of explication or complication'.[80] And he had nothing but blunt condemnation for those who took the hypotheses of aetherial media too lightly:[81]

> And as for those who introduce aetherial, or other media, to account for these actions, without any direct evidence of the existence of such media, or any clear understanding of how the media do their work, and who fill all space three or four times over with aethers of different sorts, why the less these men talk about their philosophical scruples about admitting action at a distance the better.

The aims and methods of physical science

Everything we have encountered so far tends to support the view that the main features of Maxwell's methodology and epistemology remained essentially the same as those to which he had been committed in his youth. It would nevertheless be reassuring if, in closing our account of his work, we could demonstrate that this was in fact the case, and that the traditional

[79] Maxwell (1890 and 1965), volume 2, p. 321.
[80] Maxwell (1890 and 1965), volume 2, p. 323.
[81] Maxwell (1890 and 1965), volume 2, p. 315.

picture of a simple-minded mechanist was as incorrect for the mature scientist as it was for the youthful metaphysician. Fortunately, there is ample evidence that this is so, with many of the motifs of Maxwell's youthful writings reappearing prominently in those of his maturity. His notion of the aim of science, for example, as being concerned with self-development through the communication between mind and nature as well as with the training of the mind for more important things is reflected in a discussion of the history of science in his 'Introductory lecture on experimental physics' at Cambridge, and again in his review of Thomson and Tait's *Elements of Natural Philosophy.*[82] In the former context his aim was to emphasise the close connection that should exist between the study of nature and the study of man. He admitted, following Socrates and others, that 'the proper study of mankind is man', but put forward science and the history of science as part of that study, arguing that the actions and thoughts of great men of science, 'being more free from the influence of passion, and recorded more accurately than those of other men, are all the better materials for the study of the calmer parts of human nature.'[83] In the review he compared the 'great work of subduing the earth to our use', the utilitarian motive for science, with 'the still greater work of strengthening [our] reason and developing new powers of thought',[84] and wrote of science as providing 'the opportunity of awakening the powers of thought which each fresh revelation of nature is fitted to call forth.'[85] The same review also provided the occasion for a brief resumé of the nature of fundamental ideas as the media through which the phenomena of nature were ordered in accordance with the laws of mind:[86]

> Every science must have its fundamental ideas—modes of thought by which the process of our minds is brought into the most complete harmony with the process of nature—and these ideas have not attained their most perfect form as long as they are clothed with the imagery, not of the phenomena of the science itself, but of the machinery with which mathematicians have been accustomed to work problems about pure quantities.

And in his *Elementary Treatise on Electricity* Maxwell's old concept of physical analogies reappeared in a section entitled, explicitly 'On the use of physical analogies'.[87] Here he rehearsed his arguments both on the need for physical analogies and illustrations to develop and convey physical ideas and on the limitations of these analogies, which referred only to partial

[82] Maxwell (1890 and 1965), volume 2, pp. 241–55 and 324–8.
[83] Maxwell (1890 and 1965), volume 2, p. 251.
[84] Maxwell (1890 and 1965), volume 2, p. 324.
[85] Maxwell (1890 and 1965), volume 2, p. 325.
[86] Maxwell (1890 and 1965), volume 2, p. 325.
[87] Maxwell (1881), pp. 51*ff.*

similarities, and only to similarities between relations, and which must not be taken to imply any real physical similarity between the phenomena related.

Maxwell's main methodological work of this period was an address to the mathematical and physical section of the British Association for the Advancement of Science in 1870, and this is of interest on two counts. On one hand it again reflects his earlier concerns, with discussions of the relationship between physics and metaphysics and of the use of physical analogies. On the other hand it also goes beyond his earlier writings in considering explicitly what was apparently becoming an increasingly important problem for him, that of the communication of scientific understanding. Maxwell had always viewed physical science itself as being concerned with the development of the mind through its communication with nature, and he had always been aware of the value of illustrations and analogies for the communication of physical ideas. In his later work he also stressed the importance of the communication of mathematical ideas, and of physical ideas mathematically expressed. Against this, however, he had always tended to resist the mechanistic claim that nature of itself must be visualisable and its properties thus easily communicable, and to view this as an unwarrantable assumption. Unfortunately he never gave a full and explicit account of his views on visualisation, but he did begin in his address to treat the general problem of communication.

Maxwell took as the theme for his address the relationship between mathematics and physics. He deliberately refrained from plunging into the deeper realms of metaphysics, 'where Thought weds Fact, where the mental operation of the mathematician and the physical action of the molecules are seen in their true relation.' But when he referred to the 'very den of the metaphysician, strewed with the remains of former explorers, and abhorred by every man of science', it was with obvious humour.[88] For mathematics was concerned with mental operations and physics with natural phenomena, and even in their 'daily work' both mathematicians and physicists were 'led up to questions the same in kind with those of metaphysics.'[89] According to Maxwell the aim of the man of science, whether mathematician or physicist, was 'to acquire and develope clear ideas of the things he deals with', and in practice this was most fruitfully done through 'trying to understand the subject by means of well-chosen illustrations derived from subjects with which he is more familiar.'[90] Such illustrations could be of different kinds, but if an illustration was both 'truly scientific' and mathematically 'correct' then the form of mathematical and physical ideas it embodied could lead, in Maxwell's view, to a knowledge

[88] Maxwell (1890 and 1965), volume 2, p. 216.
[89] Maxwell (1890 and 1965), volume 2, p. 216.
[90] Maxwell (1890 and 1965), volume 2, p. 219.

of both the related subjects that was more perfect than any that could be obtained by their separate study:[91]

> Now a truly scientific illustration is a method to enable the mind to grasp some conception or law in one branch of science, by placing before it a conception or law in a different branch of science, and directing the mind to lay hold of that mathematical form which is common to the corresponding ideas in the two sciences, leaving out of account for the present the difference between the physical nature of the real phenomena.
>
> The correctness of such an illustration depends on whether the two systems of ideas which are compared together are really analogous in form, or whether, in other words, the corresponding physical quantities really belong to the same mathematical class. When this condition is fulfilled, the illustration is not only convenient for teaching science in a pleasant and easy manner, but the recognition of the formal analogy between the two systems of ideas leads to a knowledge of both, more profound than could be obtained by studying each system separately.

Maxwell reached this conclusion by analysing the connection between mathematics and physics made possible by the mathematical classification of physical quantities, or, in effect, by the mental classification of natural phenomena. But he quickly applied it to the problem of the communication of scientific understanding. For whereas some minds might be able to 'go on contemplating with satisfaction pure quantities presented to the eye by symbols, and to the mind in a form which none but mathematicians can conceive',[92] others might gain more from geometrical forms and yet others from dynamical or mechanical illustrations. In the light of this psychological fact, and of the possibility of developing alternative illustrations all conformable to the requirements imposed by the mathematical classification of quantities, Maxwell was led to a significant extension of his old idea that it was important to have more than one way of looking at things. 'For the sake of persons of these different types', he argued, 'scientific truth should be presented in different forms, and should be regarded as equally scientific, whether it appears in the robust form and vivid colouring of a physical illustration, or in the tenuity and paleness of a symbolic expression.'[93] In essence this assertion was no different from what he had always maintained concerning the use of physical analogies, but it does seem to provide a strengthening of the argument. Physical analogies or illustrations were still viewed as partial analogies only, the limitations of which must be accepted. But as well as being heuristically valuable in the development of science they were now presented as essential for its communication. Maxwell was still no more a mechanist than he had ever been,

[91] Maxwell (1890 and 1965), volume 2, p. 219.
[92] Maxwell (1890 and 1965), volume 2, p. 220.
[93] Maxwell (1890 and 1965), volume 2, p. 220.

but if other people viewed the world in a mechanical way, he now implied that it was up to him to communicate the truths of science through their way of looking at things, and not just up to them to view things his way. Communication, and communication as the means of development, was thus given the same primary place in his methodology of science that it had always had in his philosophy of personal development. And of course the analogies retained their function as a means of developing physics as well. Physical research was constantly revealing new features of natural processes, and men were 'thus compelled to search for new forms of thought appropriate to these features.'[94] And it was through the development of analogies, constrained again by the principles of the mathematical classification of quantities, that ideas would be extended from familiar contexts and developed to meet this challenge.

Finally, having stressed also the importance of comparing rival theories such as those of particles and waves in optics, or of fields and action at a distance in electromagnetic theory, and of asking the question how such different theories could lead to the same results, Maxwell turned explicitly to the relationship between mind and matter and to the very question of disturbing causes that had provided the foundation, in his talk to the Apostles, for his youthful philosophy of analogy. Physical theories were formed from partial data and it was customary to treat any deviations from the theory as due to disturbing causes. But such disturbances were, Maxwell noted, features of our minds, of our neglect or ignorance of certain circumstances relevant to the phenomena. They were not facts of nature:[95]

> I shall only make one more remark on the relation between Mathematics and Physics. In themselves, one is an operation of the mind, the other is a dance of molecules. The molecules have laws of their own, some of which we select as most intelligible to us and most amenable to our calculation. We form a theory from these partial data, and we ascribe any deviation of the actual phenomena from this theory to disturbing causes. At the same time we confess that what we call disturbing causes are simply those parts of the true circumstances which we do not know or have neglected, and we endeavour in future to take account of them. We thus acknowledge that the so-called disturbance is a mere figment of the mind, not a fact of nature, and that in natural action there is no disturbance.

Similarly the mind of the mathematician was subject to disturbing causes which were in fact due to physical or physiological factors and which led to thought processes we recognised as wrong. On one hand, therefore, there were laws of thought that we could recognise as absolute. But on the other hand the same laws were constantly violated and observed as being so. So wherein lay their absoluteness? It originated, for Maxwell, in precisely the

[94] Maxwell (1890 and 1965), volume 2, p. 227.
[95] Maxwell (1890 and 1965), volume 2, pp. 228–9.

same source as did the absoluteness of the laws of nature, an absoluteness that our own limitations of mind never allowed us to see but that we were nevertheless convinced was there. And that source, though fundamental to science, lay beyond its realm:[96]

> One of the most profound mathematicians and thinkers of our time, the late George Boole, when reflecting on the precise and almost mathematical character of the laws of right thinking as compared with the exceedingly perplexing though perhaps equally determinate laws of actual and fallible thinking, was led to another of those points of view from which Science seems to look out in a region beyond her own domain.
>
> "We must admit," he says, "that there exist laws" (of thought) "which even the rigour of their mathematical forms does not preserve from violation. We must ascribe to them an authority, the essence of which does not consist in power, a supremacy which the analogy of the inviolable order of the natural world in no way assists us to comprehend.

How many of Maxwell's audience were able to make sense of this concluding passage to his address we do not know, but we can at least be sure that its inclusion was due to conviction, and not to convention. One does not write as Maxwell did without meaning it.

[96] Maxwell (1890 and 1965), volume 2, p. 229.

7

After Maxwell

Late in 1870 the Duke of Devonshire, Chancellor of the University of Cambridge, had offered to build and furnish a physics laboratory for the university. A chair of experimental physics was promptly founded in connection with this offer. Maxwell was invited to stand for it (Thomson declined) and was elected unopposed in March 1871. The next few years were largely spent supervising the construction and equipment of the new laboratory, which was named the Cavendish Laboratory after Henry Cavendish, an eighteenth-century pioneer of electrical science and great uncle to the Duke of Devonshire. Thereafter, Maxwell continued to work at electricity and other subjects but devoted most of his energies to teaching, running the laboratory and editing a volume of previously unpublished electrical researches by Henry Cavendish. This volume was published in October 1879,[1] and Maxwell died on 5 November the same year, after a long illness. He was only 48. His childhood education had been leisurely and he had been doing relatively little in the way of original research since his middle or late thirties, but his achievement, crammed as it was into such a short space of time, was immense. There was scarcely a branch of the physical sciences in which he had not made his mark, and he had completely transformed no fewer than four such branches, those of colour vision, the kinetic theory of gases, and electricity and magnetism, now united with optics.

In electromagnetic theory, as in other areas, Maxwell rested heavily on the work of his predecessors, and especially in this case on the work of Faraday. There is a sense, indeed, in which his entire work on the subject may be seen as a commentary on Faraday's *Experimental Researches in Electricity*. But though the concepts on which he built his theory were not original, the way in which he used them, and the way in which he combined them with higher mathematics, were. Similarly with the methods of mathematical physics. Maxwell did not himself invent vector analysis or energy physics, but he did show how to use them.

[1] Cavendish (1879).

In this concluding chapter we shall look at how Maxwell's theory and the approach to physics on which it was based fared in the hands of his successors. We shall review briefly the relationship between his approach and that dominant in present day physics. And we shall review also the historical framework we introduced at the beginning of the book, to see how far the perspective we have adopted has proved its value in terms of the events recounted.

Electromagnetic theory after Maxwell

Maxwell's electromagnetic theory was not immediately well received. The ideas it embodied, though fairly simple in themselves, were difficult to grasp, and the unifying power of the theory was marred by the inconsistencies surrounding the nature of electric charge and current. In England, the mechanical analogy of 'On physical lines of force' held greater appeal than did the dynamical theory of the electromagnetic field. On the Continent, the inadequate representation of charge and the apparently gratuitous hypothesis of an electromagnetic medium were both seen as arguments for rejecting the theory, which did nothing that the action-at-a-distance theories could not be made to do, by appropriate manipulation of their hypothetical force laws.

The action-at-a-distance theories had their own flaws, however, and in 1870 Hermann von Helmholtz renewed his earlier attack on Weber's theory from the standpoint of energy conservation and energetic behaviour. This time he claimed that according to Weber's theory it was possible under certain conditions for a system of two charged points, one negative and the other positive, to accelerate spontaneously and acquire an ever increasing kinetic energy. Weber's pupils responded vigorously to this charge, and the debate continued throughout the decade without reaching a definite conclusion. But the overall effect was to undermine confidence in Weber's theory. Meanwhile, Helmholtz also put forward a theory of his own, based on a generalisation of Neumann's potential theory, and showed that for the treatment of all closed currents his own theory embraced all the earlier rival theories. In particular he was able, by introducing a polarisation term in the potential, to derive an equation for the transmission of light waves as electromagnetic disturbances, and he showed that mathematically speaking Maxwell's theory could be seen as a special case of his own. During the mid 1870s Helmholtz sought to distinguish experimentally between the different theories, carrying out research into the properties of open currents. By the end of 1876, though he had failed to find any conclusive argument to support his case, he was confident that a dielectric medium such as Maxwell supposed was in fact essential for a satisfactory theory. Conceptually he was still a long way from accepting Maxwell's viewpoint. His own theory, though it incorporated a medium, was still based on action at a distance between discrete electric charges, and Maxwell's theory was in his view no more than a special mathematical case of this, with additional physical hypotheses. But his conclusion in favour of a dielectric medium nevertheless did much to bolster Maxwell's theory as compared with the older action-at-a-distance theory of Weber, which had generally been viewed as its main rival.[2]

After 1876 Helmholtz ceased to devote much of his time to electromagnetic theory, but he continued to encourage others, and particularly his pupil Heinrich Hertz, to pursue the topic. In 1878 he set as the subject for the Berlin Philosophical Society prize an experimental investigation of Weber's theory. Hertz, at whom the subject was specifically aimed, duly won, and in so doing demonstrated further the implausibility of Weber's theory. When Helmholtz continued by setting as the subject for the 1879 Berlin Academy prize an experimental investigation of the critical assumptions of Maxwell's theory, however, Hertz declined to enter, and it was not until the mid 1880s that he picked up the subject again.[3] Meanwhile, however, Maxwell's theory was gaining ground in another context.

The real strength of Maxwell's theory lay not so much in his derivation of electromagnetic properties as in the new foundation he provided for the theory of light, and it was on this foundation that the success of his theory ultimately rested. Fresnel's wave theory of light had of course been enormously successful, but all attempts to found this upon a model of the luminiferous aether had run into severe difficulties. In particular, whereas experiment revealed only transverse vibrations and not longitudinal ones, most aetherial models allowed for the possibility of both types. And the models also failed to reproduce Fresnel's results for the double refraction and reflection of polarised light at the interface of two optical media.[4] In contrast Maxwell's theory, as presented in 'A dynamical theory of the electromagnetic field', predicted that only transverse vibrations could be propagated through the electromagnetic medium and led to a simple derivation of Fresnel's results. Maxwell did not himself publish this derivation, but he pointed the way towards it. Then in 1875, in his doctoral thesis, Hendrik Antoon Lorentz derived Fresnel's results from the Maxwell–Helmholtz theory, and showed explicitly how this theory accounted for the absence of longitudinal light waves.[5] Later in the decade he extended his analysis into dispersion theory, where once again the aether models failed but the Maxwell–Helmholtz electromagnetic theory succeeded.[6] In the

[2] See Turner (1972) and Helmholtz (1897–1907), volume 5.
[3] McCormmach (1972).
[4] See Everitt (1974), p. 213, and McCormmach (1973).
[5] Lorentz (1875) and see McCormmach (1973).
[6] Lorentz (1878).

1880s Lord Rayleigh and Josiah Willard Gibbs showed that Maxwell's system of optical equations was the only one to give a self-consistent set of formulae for reflection, refraction and dispersion in agreement with experiment.[7] Meanwhile, back in the early 1870s, Ludwig Boltzmann had shown that the relationship between the refractive index and specific inductive capacity of a gas predicted by Maxwell's theory was experimentally confirmed.

The optical researches of Lorentz and others provided an increasing weight of evidence in support of Maxwell's electromagnetic theory of light. But it was not conclusive and the theory of electricity and magnetism *per se* had still to overcome the opposition of the continental action-at-a-distance theories. In a very real sense, as we shall see, it never did so. But to the extent that it did, a critical factor was the research of Heinrich Hertz in the 1880s, as a result of which the electromagnetic theory of light was finally established.

Although Hertz had not taken up Helmholtz's challenge of an empirical investigation of the critical assumptions of Maxwell's theory in 1879, he did not forget this problem entirely and in the middle of the 1880s he moved gradually towards it. In 1884 he conducted a theoretical study of the rival electromagnetic theories and concluded that Maxwell's equations were compatible with the physical assumptions of all the action-at-a-distance theories, which, strange as it may seem, was more than could be said for the equations of these theories themselves.[8] Hertz still viewed Maxwell's theory in a physical sense as resting on an unproven and unwarrantable hypothesis in the form of the assumed medium, and he also took as Maxwell's equations a simplified set corresponding to those given in the 1868 'Note' rather than the full set of the dynamical theory or the *Treatise*. But his conclusion did encourage him to take up the problem of analysing the assumption of the medium experimentally. In 1886 he tried unsuccessfully to determine the influence of dielectrics on the induction of sparks between a primary circuit and a secondary detection circuit. The following year he turned his attention to the induction of sparks through air but across a relatively large distance, and to the measurement of the velocity of propagation of the electric waves concerned. If this velocity were found to be finite, he reasoned, it would provide strong evidence for the existence of a medium such as Maxwell hypothesised.

Helmholtz had already tried to measure the velocity of a transient electric wave in air, and had been unsuccessful. Once he had hit on the project, however, Hertz was very soon successful. His transmission apparatus

[7] Lord Rayleigh (1881) and Gibbs (1888).

[8] Hertz (1884). My account of Hertz draws heavily on McCormmach (1972). See also Heimann (1971b).

consisted of an induction coil connected to a pair of copper plates, and his receiving apparatus of a simple open circuit. The electric waves were produced in the spark gap between the copper plates and detected in the form of sparks across the gap in the receiving circuit. The apparatus allowed Hertz to measure the wavelength of the waves, and thus, knowing the frequency of the primary oscillator, to calculate their velocity. This he found to be equal to the velocity of light. He then followed up the initial experiment with a series in which he demonstrated the reflection, refraction and interference of electric waves, as well as their polarisation effects, and as a result of these further experiments he was able to conclude that the electric waves behaved in every way as light waves. The two types of waves were, he deduced, the same.[9]

Hertz's experiments could not strictly be said to distinguish between the rival electromagnetic theories, since these had mostly been adapted, in the wake of Maxwell's work, to provide for the transmission of electrical disturbances at the finite speed of light. Moreover, if arguments in support of Maxwell's postulate of an electromagnetic medium were required then those deriving from optics and based on the identification of the proposed electromagnetic medium with the accepted luminiferous one were already strong. The psychological force of Hertz's demonstration was however immense. An electric spark in one part of a room could be seen to induce another spark, a finite time later, in another part of the room, with the transmission taking place at the speed of light. There must be a medium. Maxwell must have been right.

Hertz himself was quickly converted to Maxwell's theory, but not to all of it. Whereas before he had tended towards accepting Maxwell's equations but had rejected his hypothesis of a medium, he now accepted the medium, but not the equations. For analysing the physical content of these equations, confused as it was by Maxwell's ambivalent treatment of electric charge, he simply could not understand it. Moreover, while he now accepted the medium as an empirical fact he was still unhappy with it as a fundamental hypothesis. Over the next few years, Hertz completed a reformulation of Maxwell's theory in simplified, axiomatic form.[10] He eliminated Maxwell's vector potential A, which struck him as a carry over from the action-at-a-distance theories, and he eliminated the distinction between electric displacement and electric force in the free aether, which again seemed intelligible only on the basis of action at a distance. He then reduced Maxwell's full system of equations as presented in 'A dynamical theory of the electromagnetic field' and the *Treatise* to a symmetric system of equations for the electromagnetic aether similar to those presented by

[9] Hertz (1887, 1888a and 1888b).
[10] Hertz (1890a, 1890b, 1892, 1893 and 1962).

Maxwell himself in his 1868 'Note'. In modern notation and symbols Hertz had, for velocity of light c,

$$\frac{1}{c}\frac{\partial \boldsymbol{H}}{\partial t} = -\nabla \times \boldsymbol{E} \tag{7.1}$$

$$\frac{1}{c}\frac{\partial \boldsymbol{E}}{\partial t} = \nabla \times \boldsymbol{H} \tag{7.2}$$

$$\nabla \cdot \boldsymbol{H} = 0 \tag{7.3}$$

$$\nabla \cdot \boldsymbol{E} = 0. \tag{7.4}$$

He also developed a theory of moving bodies in the aether, assuming for simplicity that the aether was dragged along by the bodies.

In the introduction to a collection of his papers on electricity, published in 1892, Hertz wrote that 'Maxwell's theory is Maxwell's system of equations'.[11] By Maxwell's system of equations he actually meant his own simplified version of that system, but his general point was an important one. For whereas Maxwell had based his theory upon physical assumptions and principles, Hertz took the equations as axiomatic and left their physical significance to be worked out thereafter. This was partly a consequence of Hertz's own attitude to physics, which was uncompromisingly mechanistic. In his *Principles of Mechanics*, published posthumously in 1894, he set out a programme for the deduction of the whole of physics from the motions of rigid masses, bound to one another by rigid constraints, without either force or energy as fundamental concepts.[12] Since this was completely opposed to Maxwell's own dynamistic approach, the success of Maxwell's theory left him little option but to adopt an axiomatic stance. But this stance was also justified by the inconsistencies in Maxwell's theory. The full theory was of course far richer than Hertz's simplistic formulation, but it was clearly flawed in its treatment of charge, and the obvious way to remove the flaw was to start from the equations and attempt to find a self-consistent physical interpretation of them.

Quite independently of Hertz, the simplified symmetric form of Maxwell's equations was also developed in the mid 1880s by the English electrical engineer Oliver Heaviside.[13] But the next significant development of Maxwell's theory, which phrase now covered (the ultimate accolade) a variety of sins, came in the 1890s. Then Emil Wiechert, Joseph Larmor and Hendrik Antoon Lorentz all put forward what were to become known as

[11] Hertz (1893), p. 21.
[12] Hertz (1894, 1899 and 1956).
[13] Heaviside (1892).

electron theories. The most significant of these theories historically was the one due to Lorentz, and like Lorentz's earlier work on Maxwell's theory this was founded on the analysis of its optical consequences.[14]

The central problem was that of aether drag.[15] The question as to whether there was any relative motion between matter, such as a planet, and the aether adjacent to it had arisen in the context of the explanation of stellar aberration according to the wave theory of light. Fresnel had assumed that the earth and other bodies passed unhindered through the stationary luminiferous aether, but that moving transparent bodies dragged a part of the aether along with them, giving an absolute velocity of light in such bodies of $c + w(1 - 1/\mu^2)$, where c was the velocity of light through the aether, w that of the body with respect to the aether, and μ the refractive index of the body. This latter result had been confirmed experimentally by Hippolyte Fizeau.[16] Fresnel's theory had provided a satisfactory account of aberration, but it had clashed with the generally accepted view that in order to convey transverse rather than longitudinal waves the aether would have to be a certain kind of elastic solid. On the basis of this assumption George Stokes had argued that there must be friction between the aether and the earth, and that the aether must therefore be dragged along by the moving earth, at least close to its surface. Stokes was also able to provide a satisfactory theory of aberration, which required total aether drag within a body, giving a velocity of light in moving bodies of $c + w$, and so clashed with the empirically confirmed Fresnel drag term.[17]

In the early 1860s, Maxwell had read of Fizeau's experiments in confirmation of the Fresnel drag term and had himself considered the problem of detecting the motion of the aether relative to the earth that Fresnel's theory required.[18] He did not succeed in carrying out a suitable experiment himself, but his electromagnetic theory brought the problem of the relationship between aether and matter to the fore. In an article written in the last year of his life, and in a letter published after his death, he discussed in detail the experimental problem of detecting relative motion.[19]

Prompted by Maxwell's comments, an American, Albert Michelson, attempted to detect the relative motion of earth and aether using an optical

[14] My discussion of Lorentz draws heavily on McCormmach (1970a, 1970b and 1973) and Hirosige (1966 and 1969). See also Rosenfeld (1957), Goldberg (1969) and Swenson (1972).

[15] Summaries of this problem are to be found in Hirosige (1976) and Swenson (1972).

[16] Fresnel (1818); Fizeau (1851).

[17] Stokes (1849).

[18] See Everitt (1974), p. 214.

[19] Everitt (1974), pp. 214–15. See also *Philosophical Transactions of the Royal Society* **158** (1868), 532, *Nature* **21** (1880), pp. 314,315, and Maxwell (1890 and 1965), volume 2, p. 763.

interferometer.[20] To his surprise he could detect no motion, and Stokes's theory seemed to be vindicated. But in 1885 Lorentz, who had already been convinced of the superiority of the electromagnetic over the elastic solid theory of light, picked out a flaw in Stokes's theory. He also pointed out a flaw in Michelson's analysis of his experiment, which had the effect of halving the observed magnitude of the effect to be expected if Fresnel's theory were right, thus making the null result appear less conclusive than it had.[21] Michelson then repeated his experiment in collaboration with Edward Morley, and also repeated Fizeau's experimental test of Fresnel's theory.[22] The outcome was that he confirmed Fizeau's result, but again failed to detect any motion of the earth through the aether.

In his analysis of the electromagnetism of moving bodies in 1890, Hertz assumed that the aether was dragged along according to Stokes's theory. But he acknowledged the inadequacy of his assumption. Then, in 1892, Lorentz turned his attention to the subject, and to electromagnetic theory in general. In his earlier analyses, Lorentz had adopted the Maxwell–Helmholtz theory of electromagnetism, using Helmholtz's rather than Maxwell's derivation of the theory. Following Hertz's demonstration of the propagation of electromagnetic waves he was won over to Maxwell's aetherial assumption, but remained unhappy with both Maxwell's and Hertz's versions of the theory. He disliked Hertz's axiomatic formulation, preferring like Maxwell to derive the theory from physical principles. And drawing on his own earlier work in optics he also rejected Hertz's assumption of a dragged aether. But he was also unhappy, as Hertz had been, with Maxwell's treatment of the relationship between aether and matter, and especially with the place of electric charge and current in this.[23]

Whereas Maxwell had sought a pure field theory, Lorentz set about the construction of a dual theory, in which the free aether was treated as in Maxwell's theory, through a dynamical theory of the field, but in which matter, in the form of positively and negatively charged particles (later called electrons) was present as a separate entity. Assuming that the aether was stationary everywhere he identified the potential energy of the aether as its electrical energy and the kinetic energy as its magnetic energy, and derived Maxwell's equations of the free aether from Lagrangian dynamics in the form

$$\nabla \cdot \boldsymbol{D} = 0 \quad \text{or} \quad \rho \tag{7.5}$$

$$\nabla \cdot \boldsymbol{H} = 0 \tag{7.6}$$

[20] Michelson (1881).

[21] Lorentz (1886). For analysis of this paper see Hirosige (1976).

[22] Michelson and Morley (1886 and 1887).

[23] Lorentz (1892a and 1892b)

$$\nabla \times \boldsymbol{H} = -4\pi\left(\rho \boldsymbol{v} + \frac{\partial \boldsymbol{D}}{\partial t}\right) \tag{7.7}$$

$$4\pi c^2 \nabla \times \boldsymbol{D} = \frac{\partial \boldsymbol{H}}{\partial t}. \tag{7.8}$$

$\boldsymbol{D}$ was the electric displacement, $\boldsymbol{H}$ the magnetic force, ρ the charge density and $\boldsymbol{v}$ the charge velocity. He then postulated for the force of the aether on matter containing unit charge:

$$\textbf{Force} = 4\pi^2 c^2 \boldsymbol{D} + \boldsymbol{v} \times \boldsymbol{H}. \tag{7.9}$$

In conformity with his basic assumptions, Lorentz derived the Fresnel drag coefficient as an interference effect between the incident light and that produced by the consequent vibrations of electrons in the optical body, rather than as a mechanical dragging effect. And in a second paper of 1892 he interpreted the null result of the Michelson–Morley experiment as being due to a contraction effect. If the molecular forces in a body behaved in the same way with respect to the aether as did the electrical forces, a fairly reasonable hypothesis, then a body moving through the aether must contract, and this contraction would be such as to compensate for the optical Fresnel drag effect due to the same motion through the aether, giving the observed null result. The Irish mathematician George Fitzgerald had already come up with the same hypothesis, though Lorentz did not know it, a few years earlier.[24]

In his major treatise on the electron theory, published in 1895, Lorentz finally followed Hertz in putting forward an axiomatic formulation of electromagnetic theory.[25] But whereas Hertz had placed this in the context of a mechanistic ideal Lorentz sought to build physics upon purely electromagnetic concepts. With the particulate electron playing a central part in his theory, however, he moved right away as Hertz had done from Maxwell's field theoretic approach. Joseph Larmor, who developed a theory similar to Lorentz's but with the electrons identified as centres of rotational strain in the medium (a notion derived from Thomson's vortex atom concept), kept much closer to Maxwell's ideal of a field theory.[26] Emil Wiechert, author of yet another electron theory in this period, also avoided Lorentz's blatant dualism.[27] But it was Lorentz's electron theory that gained the widest acceptance, especially after the experimental identification of the negative electron by J J Thomson in the late 1890s. As Hertz had said, however, Maxwell's theory was Maxwell's system of equations—

[24] Fitzgerald (1889).
[25] Lorentz (1895).
[26] Larmor (1894, 1895, 1897 and 1900).
[27] Wiechert (1896 and 1898).

or at least a system related to it—and the equations of Lorentz's theory corresponded closely to those of Maxwell's *Treatise*, with the vector potential $\boldsymbol{A}$ eliminated and the pairs of electric and magnetic variables, $\boldsymbol{B}$ and $\boldsymbol{H}$, and $\boldsymbol{D}$ and $\boldsymbol{E}$, conflated. The so-called Lorentz force for the action of the field on an electron was Maxwell's equation (C). Moreover, though Lorentz's theory differed critically from Maxwell's in its treatment of charge, it was, like Maxwell's, a theory of an electromagnetic medium. The assumption of such a medium had been what most obviously characterised Maxwell's theory as compared with its rivals, and that assumption was also characteristic of its successors. However far they differed from Maxwell's field theoretical approach, they could still claim to be versions of 'Maxwell's theory'.

Quantum and relativity theories

Even if Maxwell's work in electromagnetism had done no more than provide the foundations for the modern classical theories of electromagnetism and optics it would have been a remarkable achievement. In fact, however, the consequences of his work reached far deeper into physics than that, and it was beyond the classical theories, in the formation of the modern theories of relativity and quanta, that some of the more fundamental aspects of his approach to the electromagnetic theory bore fruit.

The story of special relativity theory is quite well known. By introducing the contraction hypothesis, Lorentz was able to account reasonably well for the Michelson–Morley results. His theory was also able to explain a wide range of optical phenomena, and even provided the basis for a consistent explanation of the magneto-optic effect that had caused Maxwell such problems. Paramagnetic substances could be interpreted as possessing permanent electron dipole moments responding to a magnetic field in one sense, with diamagnetism being characterised by an induced dipole moment in the opposite sense. The reconciliation with the rest of the electromagnetic theory then came about through the recognition of paramagnetism and diamagnetism as distinct effects, so that all substances responded diamagnetically, in the same sense, with the coefficient of diamagnetic induction always possessing the same sign just as Maxwell had assumed. However, in the case of paramagnets this diamagnetic response was swamped by the stronger paramagnetic effect. The problems with the electron theory arose when Lorentz, seeking a consistent theory that could act as an electromagnetic basis for the whole of physics, reformulated his theory axiomatically. Between 1899 and 1904 he rewrote the theory on a completely axiomatic basis, attributing the behaviour he had formerly postulated for matter subject to intermolecular forces to all matter, in all its interactions. The Fitzgerald–Lorentz contraction became a coordinate transformation applicable within as well as between the molecules of matter. The mass of any particle became a function of its motion through the aether, and the mass of an electron was attributed entirely to the electromagnetic self-reaction of the electron with the field. A moving electron became subject to deformation, and all forces, of whatever kind, became motion-dependent. The velocity of light became an upper limit to the velocity of any material particles.[28]

This new formulation allowed Lorentz to derive the laws of classical mechanics from those of the electron theory, and so to provide an electromagnetic unification of physics akin to the mechanical unification sought by Hertz. But it quickly ran into serious difficulties. The aim of the theory was to explain all phenomena in terms of electromagnetic properties, for the description of which the electron was a primitive entity. But the energy of deformation of an electron could not, by definition, be so explained. Nor could the structure of an electron of finite dimensions, which was needed if the problem of an infinite self-energy of the field, which arose if the electron were treated as a point charge, were to be avoided. These difficulties had far more to do with Lorentz's goal of an electromagnetic world view than with his theory of electromagnetism *per se*, but they were sufficiently acute to play a major part in leading Albert Einstein to his reformulation of physics in terms of the special theory of relativity and the hypothesis of quanta of light.[29]

Einstein's starting point was in fact the kinetic theory of gases. He was strongly attracted to this theory, but was also concerned that it rested on an unproven molecular hypothesis, and he set about testing this hypothesis by analysing the thermal energy fluctuations (Brownian motion) whose existence it implied. In the course of this analysis he realised that nothing in the theory of fluctuations depended on the material nature of the body possessing the thermal energy, and this prompted him to consider the fluctuations of pure radiant energy, or black-body radiation. But when he applied the kinetic theory to black-body radiation, drawing on the equipartition theorem, he reached a law for the black-body radiation energy distribution which was patently incorrect. He was not the first to realise this, for the law had already been derived by Rayleigh from the wave theory of light and the equipartition principle, and its failings had been recognised not only by Rayleigh but by others, including Planck. Indeed it was through a comparison of Rayleigh's law with a rival one due to Wien, and based on the assumption of particulate radiation, that Planck had derived his own law in which the quantum constant was first introduced.[30] But Einstein's

[28] Lorentz (1904 and 1909).

[29] For Einstein's early work I draw mainly on McCormmach (1970a). See also Pais (1982).

[30] See for example Kuhn (1978), Klein (1977).

interest in the subject was tied up with an interest in Drude's work on the kinetic theory of electrons, which was in turn tied up with Lorentz's electron theory. Einstein saw that while the kinetic theory was based on particulate assumptions, and radiation theory on wave assumptions, Lorentz's theory combined both. And looking at Lorentz's theory in this way he saw rather more clearly than did his contemporaries just what its problems were. Convinced of the need for consistency and simplicity in physical theory he saw two choices: to go for a self-consistent continuous field theory, or to go for a self-consistent particle theory; and, influenced by his work on fluctuations and the confidence this inspired in the particulate theory, he went for the latter. In 1905 he published four classic papers. One introduced the concept of particulate light quanta, which he supported as an heuristic hypothesis by empirical evidence from the photoelectric and optical absorption effects. Another developed the theory of Brownian motion. A third explored the relationship between mass and energy implied by the hypothesis of light quanta. And a fourth introduced the special theory of relativity, according to which Lorentz's coordinate transformations were interpreted as observational consequences of the relative motion of the observer and the object being observed, rather than as physical changes due to motion through a stationary luminiferous aether.[31]

The relationship between Maxwell's theory and the special theory of relativity is a strange one. In one sense special relativity followed on as a consequence of Maxwell's theory. Maxwell's equations were actually inconsistent with the classical, Galilean, principle of relativity, and if taken as applicable at a submolecular level they required that coordinate transformations take place according to the Lorentz–Einstein transformation laws and not the Galilean ones. Viewed another way, however, it could also be said that by abandoning any reference to an aetherial medium Einstein actually rejected the hypothesis on which Maxwell based his theory. But then, in a deeper sense that Einstein himself recognised, this was itself a development of Maxwell's own field-theoretic approach. After 1905 Einstein continued to champion the light-quantum hypothesis as absolutely necessary for the explanation of experimental results concerning the absorption of light. But he also became quickly convinced that this hypothesis would itself have to be derived, ultimately, from a pure field theory. The wave theory of light remained as necessary for the explanation of interference effects as the quantum theory was for that of absorption effects. Moreover the special theory of relativity incorporated Lorentz's requirement of a maximum speed c for all actions and so did not allow for the instantaneous action at a distance that seemed to be required for a particulate theory of matter and light. From as early as 1907 Einstein therefore sought to derive the light

[31] Einstein (1905a,b,c and d).

quanta as singularities from a pure field theory, and also to bring gravitational theory, which had so far been based on instantaneous action at a distance, within the scope of field theory—a possibility that Maxwell had considered but quickly abandoned.[32] Einstein never succeeded in the first of these endeavours, but he did in the second, and what we generally refer to as the general theory of relativity was more strictly speaking a relativistic field theory of gravitation—a realisation, in effect, of the field theory of matter that both Faraday and Maxwell had advocated.

Given Maxwell's talk of a 'medium', and his use of mechanical analogies, it may fairly be questioned to what extent his theory really was the forerunner of modern field theory, as encapsulated in particular by Einstein's general relativity theory. When it came down to it, though, Maxwell was quite clear that his medium was nothing more than the recipient of energetic properties. It could be interpreted as a mechanical aether, but such an interpretation was not strictly part of Maxwell's theory, and even though he talked of a medium the concept entailed was essentially that of the modern field. At the centenary of Maxwell's birth Einstein wrote that:[33]

> Before Maxwell people thought of physical reality—in so far as it represented events in nature—as material points, whose changes consist only in motions which are subject to total differential equations. After Maxwell they thought of physical reality as represented by continuous fields, not mechanically explicable, which are subject to partial differential equations. This change in the conception of reality is the most profound and the most fruitful that physics has experienced since Newton.

For 'after Maxwell' one should read 'quite a long time after Maxwell', and one should also stress, as Einstein indeed did, the important part played before Maxwell by Faraday. The statement as it stands is simplistic, but the basic historical insight is sound.

Maxwell's theory itself led on to the special theory of relativity, and his field-theoretic approach led on to general relativity. If, finally, we look at the history of the greatest of the revolutions in twentieth-century physics, that of quantum mechanics, we find a tenuous but still deeper connection with his thought. The key problem in this context is that of visualisation. We noted in the early chapters of this book a contrast between the mechanistic assumption that nature is visualisable and the dynamistic rejection of that assumption as arrogant and unfounded. In reviewing Maxwell's mature writings we also noted how he followed in the dynamistic tradition, but yet remained acutely aware of the value of mechanism. There was in his view no reasons why nature should conform to our visualisation and every reason to assume that our visual analogies of nature were limited and

[32] For the history of the duality problem see Hendry (1980).
[33] J C Maxwell (1982), p. 31.

partial. But such visualisations were nevertheless necessary, both for understanding and for the communication of that understanding. In the decades after Maxwell's death physics seems to have been dominated by the mechanistic attitude, and by the early 1920s there were few physicists not committed to the ideal of visualisation, even though the wave–particle duality of light presented them with an immensely strong *prima facie* case against that view.[34] The creation of quantum mechanics came about, however, through the work of two physicist–philosophers who rejected the ideal of visualisation, and it came about because they rejected it. Wolfgang Pauli argued that our visual conceptions were patently inadequate to cope with the wave–particle and field–particle dualities, and that physics must be based upon a replacement set of concepts, themselves founded upon what was in principle observable. Niels Bohr argued, much like Maxwell, that our visual concepts were inadequate, but that we were nevertheless restricted to them. And the quantum mechanics that resulted from the dialogue between Bohr and Pauli, and also from the genius of men like Heisenberg, prepared to follow Bohr and Pauli's lead and able to do so far better than they were themselves, was characterised by a final rejection of the visualisation criterion for nature.[35] Of course, visualisations have continued to play an important and indeed crucial part in the development of physics. We have only to think, for example, of Feynman's visualisation of elementary particle interactions. But the picture can no longer be confused with the reality in the way that it was before the acceptance of quantum mechanics.

Maxwell's legacy: the aims and methods of modern physics

It hardly needs stressing that Maxwell's electromagnetic field theory and the ideas on which it was based have continued to play an important part in physics since the advent of quantum mechanics. The favoured approach of theoretical physicists has varied substantially during the intervening half century, but at the time of writing a field-theoretic approach, in the form of gauge theory, is once again ascendent.[36] The methodological tools of energy conservation, Hamiltonian dynamics and vector analysis, all pioneered by Maxwell in his electromagnetic theory, remain central. Following the quantum-mechanical rejection of space–time visualisations, indeed, energy has become the basic building block of physics.

It would also be fair to say that Maxwell's method of analogy, though not known by that name, is the practical methodology characteristic of modern physics. The contrasting notion of a single 'true' description of the

[34] Hendry (1980).
[35] For support of this interpretation of the creation of quantum mechanics see Hendry (1984b) and see also MacKinnon (1983).
[36] See Pickering (1984).

physical world now seems quite outdated, and the relativity and incompleteness of physical theory appear to be widely accepted. Amongst philosophers of science, the social relativity of scientific knowledge as proclaimed by Whewell has also become conventional wisdom, though Whewell's own advocacy of this has long been forgotten. It is still a matter for historical investigation, however, to what extent this situation has developed as a result of problems encountered within physics itself raising the sensitivity or eroding the self-confidence or arrogance of the physicists; to what extent it reflects the practice of modern research schools and laboratories, largely developed in the late nineteenth century, among others by Maxwell at the Cavendish Laboratory; and to what extent its roots lie in societal changes essentially extrinsic to physical practice, in particular those which transformed the world and the place of science in that world during and between the two world wars.

What is striking about the aims and methods of modern physics when compared with those characteristic of Maxwell is that while the 'cautious' side of Maxwell's dynamism has been widely adopted (albeit, perhaps from other sources), and physicists' claims for the objective content of their theories modified accordingly, the more positive side of the dynamical philosophy underlying Maxwell's approach seems to have been almost completely rejected. Its place has been taken, moreover, by what was to Maxwell as to Whewell the most objectionable of all philosophies, that of positivism. This may not be the strict positivism of Comte: it does not stifle the development of hypotheses or analogies. But it does deprive that development of any metaphysical underpinning or direction. To quote an eminent modern scientist, Emilio Segré, 'Most modern physicists are satisfied that their art, as practiced [*sic*], gives answers that can be validated by experiment and are of great predictive power, technically prolific, and aesthetically satisfying. They leave the deeper roots to philosophers.'[37] The role of society or convention in determining what is or is not accepted as scientific knowledge is becoming increasingly recognised, but that of the human mind in shaping observation of the phenomena rationally into intelligible form has, at the very least, been put to one side.

Maxwell's insistence on science as a training for more important things, as a means of communication through which the individual can grow and develop, also seems quite alien to present day scientific culture. The intimate connection between science, morality and religion on which his philosophy of science was built almost invites contempt from the viewpoint of modern positivism, and was indeed greeted with contempt, and not a little anger, when expressed in the interwar period by Eddington, who was in this respect one of Maxwell's closest followers.[38] Again, though, this

[37] Segré (1984), p. ix.

[38] See for example Eddington (1928, 1939 and 1958), especially the penultimate paragraph of the 1958 work, p. 222.

whole subject is one that requires considerable historical study if the roots of the phenomenon and its connection with the wider realms of social and intellectual life are to be historically comprehended.

8

Conclusions

In his classic work of 1926 on *Science and the Modern World* the mathematician and philosopher A N Whitehead characterised and criticised classical physics as being uncompromisingly mechanistic and as having developed in complete isolation from the development of philosophy.[1] And to a very large extent that characterisation has stuck. It has not gone unchallenged. In 1965 L P Williams, in his monumental biography of Faraday, drew attention to the links between Faraday's scientific ideas and aspects of German dynamical philosophy.[2] In 1975 R G Olson, following an earlier work by G E Davie, related the approaches of a number of nineteenth-century British physicists, most notably Maxwell, to the dynamical elements of Scottish common-sense philosophy.[3] But following the discovery of one or two errors in Williams's analysis his claims were first disputed and then quite widely rejected. And since Olson did not carry his analysis into the heart of the physics, his work too could be easily dismissed. It was not in fact totally dismissed, and it is now customary, indeed, to allude to the influence of Scottish philosophy, and especially of William Hamilton, on Maxwell and his contemporaries. This has done little to affect the general perception of nineteenth-century physics, however, or even that of Maxwell himself.

Nineteenth-century physics is still treated as being largely contained within a thoroughly mechanistic tradition and Maxwell himself is still treated, despite all the evidence to the contrary, as a mechanist. If Hamilton is mentioned it is in order to explain away Maxwell's philosophical writings as being due to his 'influence', rather than to any thoughts of Maxwell's own, and so as irrelevant to Maxwell's physics. Where the dynamical elements of Maxwell's thought intrude too obviously into his physics to be

[1] Whitehead (1926).

[2] Williams (1965). The errors referred to below were unfortunate, for even with them this book remains a classic study, and model scientific biography.

[3] Olson (1975) and Davie (1964).

dismissed in this way they are typically accounted for, not by any questioning of the presumption that he was a mechanist, but by the assumption that he must have been a vacillating or inconsistent mechanist. Thus, to take just one example:[4]

> If Maxwell, in his work on the theory of molecular vortices in 1861–2, had been a leader in the movement towards a definite, concrete, and realistically intended mechanical account of the universal ether, he also very soon, beginning in 1864, played a central role in the subsequent retreat from that kind of ether theory. As we shall see, it was a tactical retreat that Maxwell undertook in 1864, but this soon developed into a long-term strategy, a strategy of concentration on *dynamical theories* of ether, which involved much less commitment to specific mechanical pictures.

It is a bit unfair to quote this particular author, for he is in fact one of the more sober Maxwell scholars, and has contributed substantially to our understanding of a number of aspects of Maxwell's work. His crime lies in his quotability rather than in the relative severity of his error. But the point must be made. We have seen in the course of this book that Maxwell was remarkably consistent in his philosophical and methodological approach to physics, and that his development of electromagnetic theory was a progressive, quite unidirectional process. We have seen too that he was a thoughtful and very careful writer. He was a competent poet, a skilled essayist, and acutely aware of the problem of communicating his own understanding, depending as this did upon his own mental reference frame of attitudes, concepts and experiences, to someone with a completely different frame of reference. But ignoring or failing to realise all this the author of the passage quoted has contrived to conflate the message and the medium in such a way as to make Maxwell appear confused, inconsistent and, so far as can be made out, a mechanist. He has taken the analogy of 'On physical lines of force' for a realistically intended mechanical representation, which Maxwell was quite clear it was not. And he has mistaken Maxwell's use of analogy itself, as a medium of communication of a partial understanding, for a true reflection of the whole of Maxwell's own understanding.

Throughout what has been a fairly detailed analysis of Maxwell's writings we have found no evidence whatsoever of any change in his philosophical or methodological stance, and ample evidence of his consistency in this respect. This consistency would indeed appear astonishing, were it not for the fact that we know him to have worked out his position with great thoroughness and at a very early age. And whatever name or characterisation we may choose to give it, this position was certainly not a mechanistic one. In the terminology I have adopted in this book, it was quite clearly and

[4] Siegel (1981), p. 259.

uncompromisingly dynamistic. To summarise very briefly some of what it entailed, Maxwell based his science, as he did his whole life, upon a concept of growth through communication and understanding through analogy. Physical science was for him a means of communication with nature through which one could learn not only about nature, but also about oneself. One's knowledge, be it scientific, moral or religious, could never be complete; but through the method of analogy it could be progressively developed. In Maxwell's view this method of analogy was based ultimately on the identity of mind and matter. He drew evidence for this view from the realm of moral science, but recognised that it rested essentially upon religious faith. In practice the method rested upon the existence of analogies between the processes of mind and those of matter, through which one could recognise analogies between material relations themselves. All analogies open to human comprehension were partial analogies, and there was always more than one possible way of looking at things, each way capturing a different analogy, or different part of the unknowable whole. Science, or any other form of understanding, proceeded by extending and comparing analogies, and by exploring the points at which they differed or broke down. Generally this might lead to further analogies of a similar kind, but one could also hope to attain a more certain type of knowledge, in the form of true physical connections, subsuming different phenomena under some single set of laws. Such, for example, was the law of gravitation, connecting terrestrial fall and planetary orbits. And such would be the laws of the electromagnetic field, connecting the phenomena of electricity, magnetism and light. Although they possessed a greater degree of certainty than ordinary analogies, of course, such laws were still fundamentally analogical. Moreover the law itself was to be distinguished carefully from any physical embodiment of it, mechanical or otherwise. In the case of the electromagnetic theory, for example, an explanation in terms of a medium of a particular kind might be used as an aid to one's own understanding, to the further development of science, or to the communication of understanding to others, but it must never be taken *too* seriously.

A proper understanding of Maxwell's philosophical framework, and in particular of his concept of partial analogies, enables us to understand the development of his electromagnetic theory for what it was: not, as has sometimes been assumed, a series of disjunct theories, but a representation of the continuous and progressive development through succesive analogies of his own thought. And although Maxwell's methodological control and self-awareness are not perhaps typical of physicists as a whole, these characteristics of his scientific programme are probably typical of a great deal of scientific activity. To most people today, the dominant image of scientific development is still that of discovery: at three o'clock on such and such a date a scientist discovered something and scientific knowledge advanced. T S Kuhn, in his famous work on *The Structure of Scientific*

Revolutions,[5] has observed that discovery is rarely a simple event, and has suggested that it be treated more as a process. But even with this improvement the image of discovery still fails to capture some of the most significant aspects of scientific activity. There is a sense in which Maxwell discovered the electromagnetic theory of light, and we might even time this discovery to the moment he calculated that the speeds of electrical and luminiferous propagation were the same. But as a description of what he was doing, and of what he achieved, that seems to miss the whole point. For it was not the discovery itself that mattered so much as the understanding through which it was reached and that to which it led. It is quite artificial to extract just one point of Maxwell's research from the whole endeavour, extending over many years, of which it was a part. And so too with much else in the history of science. It is the process of understanding that is characteristic, not the event of discovery.[6]

In concentrating on the development of Maxwell's electromagnetic theory and setting it in the biographical context of his other scientific and philosophical writings, I have sought in this book to improve our understanding both of Maxwell himself and of the process of scientific understanding he exemplifies. But I have also sought at the same time to address the wider historical question of the development of classical electromagnetic theory and, through this, the development of nineteenth-century physics in general. Here too the analysis seems to lead to some important conclusions, for it was not only in Maxwell's work that physics and philosophy were brought together and a dynamistic approach to physics pursued.

Of course the categories of mechanism and dynamism themselves remain somewhat artificial. The human mind is far too complex and subject to far too many influences and variations to be classified so crudely, and we have met examples in the course of this book—Thomson, and perhaps Helmholtz—who seem to defy even a tentative description in these terms. The categories must also be taken relative to each other to an extent that makes their consistent use over a long period of time or across a wide range of intellectual activities difficult. The writings of Whewell, Ampère and

[5] Kuhn (1970).

[6] I have explored this point further in Hendry (1983a). Strangely enough, though the dynamism of people like Maxwell and Whewell is completely out of fashion today, many of their leading ideas are incorporated in precisely what is most fashionable. Kuhn writes of the conventionality of scientific knowledge and many sociologists have followed his lead, little realising that their relativism on this point would have been wholly acceptable to Whewell, who made the very same point himself, to Maxwell, or to anyone else in the same tradition. The difference between the two viewpoints, relating to the existence or otherwise of an absolute, is profound, but its profundity places it well beyond what is virtually a shared analysis of scientific activity.

Maxwell have all been described here as falling within a predominantly dynamistic tradition, and this description seems appropriate in respect of their attitudes relative to those of some of their predecessors and older contemporaries. But it would be folly to assert that ideas drawn from a more mechanistic tradition were absent from their works, and one could indeed make out a very strong case for affording them the middle ground in which the tendencies we have described as mechanistic and dynamistic were relatively balanced. Since the terms are relative anyway it does not really matter where we attempt to draw the line. But the fact that it could be redrawn, and indeed reoriented to take account of different combinations of ideas from those considered here, is important. Human beings simply do not sit comfortably in boxes.

It must also be recognised that because of their relative nature the categories have a status somewhere between objective historical categories and subjective actors' categories. One definition of the dynamistic tradition, as that phrase has been used here, might be that tradition of thought with which Maxwell found himself in sympathy (actor's category), as understood and interpreted by the author (attempted historical category). But the mix is necessarily a fuzzy one, and the categories are ultimately heuristic. Finally, it should perhaps be stressed that, used in this way, the categories neither need nor are intended to carry any implications for the origins of the tendencies described. Some will view them as innately psychological, others as socially determined. My own view is that it would be foolish to dismiss either source and that any attempted analysis should take account of both, at least as possibilities. But that is not something that is at issue here.

These qualifications are awesome, but for the historian, who must necessarily be something of a pragmatist, they are necessary. They do not seem to me to be sufficient or severe enough to undermine the whole enterprise. There is, I believe, a cohesion within the tendencies as described, and they do seem to reflect well Maxwell's own impressions and those of his teachers, most especially Whewell. There is moreover a sufficient conformity between the perceptions of the different actors (not just Maxwell and those close to him) to give the categories some kind of objective validity. Given all this, their heuristic value for anyone seeking to comprehend the development of Maxwell's work and of nineteenth-century physics in general seems to be immense.

What were the relationships between the school of Laplacian physics in the early nineteenth century, the pioneering works of Fourier and Ampère and the British energy physics of mid century? What was the relationship, at the practical level of hard physics, between common-sense philosophy and Maxwell's electromagnetic theory? On what was Maxwell's immense sympathy with Faraday's physics based? What role did Whewell play in the development of nineteenth-century physics? What was the significance of

William Rowan Hamilton's dynamics in this period? Or of German Kantian philosophy? How did Maxwell's pioneering of vector analysis tie in with the rest of his programme in the *Treatise?* The history of physical thought in the nineteenth century as it stands has too many disjunctions to be convincing. People, even physicists, are not isolated islands. The degree of interaction between physicists themselves and between physicists, philosophers and other intellectuals, both directly through their writings and indirectly through the media of shared cultures and societies, cannot but have been enormous. And while it is historically rather dangerous to adduce too much direct influence from one individual to another, especially when we are dealing with highly original thinkers, we should nevertheless expect some common threads, some conceptual commensurability. This is what the framework used here provides.

In Maxwell's *Treatise,* three aspects of the recent development of physics were brought together. First there was the use of a dynamical theory in the Lagrangian sense, a mathematical dynamics of a system that was independent of the detailed mechanical structure of that system. After Lagrange this approach had been developed by William Rowan Hamilton and introduced to the mainstream of physics by Thomson and Tait: Maxwell's was its first sustained application to a problem in physics rather than in applied mathematics. Secondly, there was the use of energy conservation as a fundamental postulate. Introduced by Joule and Helmholtz and developed by Rankine this had also been fundamental to the method of Thomson and Tait. Thirdly there was the limited use of vector analysis, extracted by Maxwell himself from the quaternion analysis of William Rowan Hamilton.

That these three developments were in some ways related is apparent. It was indeed the principle of energy conservation that made the dynamics of Lagrange, formulated in terms of a system's energy, the powerful tool for physics that it was, and that induced Thomson, Tait and Maxwell to base their methods upon that dynamics. The presence of Hamilton as a prime author of both the dynamics and the quaternion analysis is itself evidence of some link there. But it is when we think in terms of the dynamistic tradition in physics that the force of the links really becomes apparent. For energy conservation, Lagrangian dynamics and quaternion analysis were all conceived and developed within this one tradition. So too, at the hands of Oersted, Ampère, Faraday, Thomson and Maxwell, was the theory of electromagnetism. This in turn drew on the works of Fourier and Fresnel, through which the impact of the tradition was first felt in theoretical physics.

Finally, if we take all these developments together, and if we consider the development of physics as a whole from the pioneering works of Fourier, Fresnel, Faraday, Oersted and Ampère in the 1820s through to the masterly synthesis of Maxwell in the 1860s, it might not be going too far to talk of a dynamical revolution. Of course, some aspects of this revolution stand out more than others. The introduction of the principle of energy conservation was in itself sufficient to delineate two periods in physics, the fundamental physical conceptions of which were barely commensurate. But the developments are so intimatey related in their origins, and so intricately connected in the physics in which they resulted, that to talk of a single revolution seems to me to be wholly justifiable. And if that is accepted there seems little doubt that its principle unifying characteristic, apart from that of unification itself, is the approach that I have described as dynamism.

Appendix

Alternative interpretations of Maxwell's methodology: a review of further reading

By using selective quotations it is possible to make out a case for Maxwell's advocacy of almost any methodology, and it is no surprise that quite diverse philosophers have claimed him for their camps. In this book I have taken an essentially biographical view. Rather than deriving my interpretation from a study of disjoint and disembodied texts, I have tried to establish what Maxwell himself believed he was doing, and in this way I have, I hope, been able, if nothing else, to lay to rest once and for all the image of Maxwell as a traditional mechanist. Whether or not one agrees with Maxwell's dynamical philosophy of life, personal development and scientific enquiry, one must I think admit its presence, and admit too that it was well thought out and held with both consistency and conviction.

It is less easily established, however, that Maxwell's philosophy of science was really followed closely in his practice of science, or even indeed that it was of particular relevance in the practical context. It is my view that it was, and so far as seemed possible within the limits of the book I have tried to demonstrate this. But I have painted the picture of Maxwell's scientific work only with a relatively broad brush, and cannot claim that my demonstration is complete. I should therefore like to draw attention here to a selection of the more important studies of Maxwell's physics which either differ from the interpretation I have offered or go deeper than I have into the detailed analysis of his scientific work.

Of the purely historical studies of Maxwell's methodology in electromagnetic theory, two are of particular importance. In a substantial paper on 'Maxwell and the modes of consistent representation' Peter Heimann has looked at Maxwell's choice of models or analogies in the successive formulations of his theory, and has identified what he sees as a 'fundamental conceptual dichotomy in Maxwell's thought'.[1] Some of Maxwell's presen-

[1] Heimann (1970b).

tations were, he notes, based on Faraday's concept of lines of force ('Faraday's lines of force', the 'Note' of 1868 and the *Elementary Treatise*), while others were based on the concept of polarisation as in Faraday's electrotonic state ('On physical lines of force', 'A dynamical theory of the electromagnetic field' and the *Treatise*). Heimann's argument is, in my view, put much too strongly. It is quite misleading to talk as he does of Maxwell 'believing in' his physical models, and oscillating between one belief and another, when his choice of model was always made, as we have seen, for a reason, in the context of the particular work being written, its aims and its intended audience. As noted in Chapter 3, Heimann has also argued, again it seems quite erroneously, that Faraday himself abandoned one of the viewpoints concerned for the other, and he seems in general far too ready to interpret a conscious 'way of looking at things' as a belief that that was what they objectively looked like. Despite these qualifications, however, the paper is certainly essential reading for anyone wishing to probe deeper than I have done here into the details of Maxwell's physics and, in particular, his choice of models.

The second purely historical paper worth noting here is Dan Siegel's 'Thomson, Maxwell and the universal ether'.[2] As noted in Chapter 8, Siegel is, like Heimann, inclined to read far too much into Maxwell's use of models and to mistake the medium for the message. He interprets Maxwell's hopes or expectations as to what forms future theories might take as 'convictions' as to what form they must take. He does however give a fairly full discussion of a very important side to Maxwell's scientific hopes that I have not discussed in this book. The line of reasoning represented by the hypothesis of molecular vortices led, in the 1860s, to the advocacy by Thomson of a theory of vortical molecules in which the molecules were supposed to exist as stable vortical motions in an aetherial fluid. In his mature period, by when the rise of spectroscopy was beginning to have an impact on molecular theory, Maxwell was strongly attracted to Thomson's theory. It afforded to molecules the complexity of internal motions that seemed necessary if spectral phenomena were to be explained, combined with the stability and uniformity of the chemical molecules. Had it proved successful it would also have established a true connection (the essence of a successful theory in Maxwell's terms) between the phenomena of matter and of light, and this was in Maxwell's view a possibility well worth exploring. Unfortunately Siegel does not get involved with the implications of the theory for a connection between matter and light, and he does therefore tend to misread, in my view, Maxwell's interest in it. But he does open up the question of the relationship between Maxwell's work and that of contemporary aether-theorists, and in so doing he treats an important dimension to Maxwell's thought beyond those treated here.

[2] Siegel (1981).

Besides these two purely historical papers, there is one other very important work lying somewhere between the history and the philosophy of science, and that is A F Chalmers's paper on 'Maxwell's methodology and his application of it to electromagentism'.[3] The overall argument of Chalmers's paper is fairly crude. He treats Maxwell's methodology as consisting simply of an opposition to hypotheses and an aim of reducing everything to mechanics, and he argues that this methodology hindered rather than helped Maxwell's science. In particular he claims that the displacement current, which he sees as Maxwell's principal contribution to electromagnetic theory, was hypothetical and so contrary to his philosophy, while the field theory that emerged after Maxwell and for the creation of which he is often given credit, was actually contrary to his own aims. Historically speaking this argument deserves little attention, for Maxwell's methodology was patently not what Chalmers assumes, the displacement current was not an independent hypothesis in the way he describes it, and while Maxwell's desire for a more complete theory than his own field theory is obviously of relevance for the history of field theories it certainly does not place him against the field-theoretic approach. In presenting this argument, however, Chalmers does give a fairly full account of Maxwell's work on electromagnetism, and one that goes in some ways beyond that given here.

Besides these three papers there is of course an immense further literature on Maxwell, both historical and philosphical, though much of this serves more to confuse than to enlighten. Among the historical works Norton Wise's analysis of Maxwell's use of the visual image of interlocking lines of electric and magnetic force is worth reading.[4] He also has forthcoming a work on Maxwell's use of the flow analogy, following on from his important discussion of Thomson's use of this analogy on which I drew heavily in Chapter 3. I have not however seen this. The work of Joan Bromberg should also be mentioned, as should works by Siegel, Knudsen, Kargon, Everitt and Olson.[5] For a modern philosopher's reinterpretation of Maxwell's method the work of Mary Hesse is also of considerable interest.[6]

[3] Chalmers (1973).

[4] Wise (1979).

[5] Bromberg (1967 and 1968), Siegel (1975), Knudsen (1976), Kargon (1969), Everitt (1975) and Olson (1975).

[6] Hesse (1973).

Recollections of Dreamland

Cambridge, June 1856

ROUSE ye! torpid daylight-dreamers, cast your carking cares away!
As calm air to troubled water, so my night is to your day;
All the dreary day you labour, groping after common sense,
And your eyes ye will not open on the night's magnificence.
Ye would scoff were I to tell you how a guiding radiance gleams
On the outer world of action from my inner world of dreams.

When, with mind released from study, late I lay me down to sleep,
From the midst of facts and figures, into boundless space I leap;
For the inner world grows wider as the outer disappears,
And the soul, retiring inward, finds itself beyond the spheres.
Then, to this unbroken sameness, some fantastic dream succeeds,
Vague emotions rise and ripen into thoughts and words and deeds.
Old impressions, long forgotten, range themselves in Time and Space,
Till I recollect the features of some once familiar place.
Then from valley into valley in my dreaming course I roam,
Till the wanderings of my fancy end, where they began, at home.

Calm it lies in morning twilight, while each streamlet far and wide
Still retains its hazy mantle, borrowed from the mountain's side;
Every knoll is now an island, every wooded bank a shore,
To the lake of quiet vapour that has spread the valley o'er.
Sheep are couched on every hillock, waiting till the morning dawns,
Hares are on their early rambles, limping o'er the dewy lawns.
All within the house is silent, darkened all the chambers seem,
As with noiseless step I enter, gliding onwards in my dream.

What! has Time run out his cycle, do the years return again?
Are there treasure-caves in Dreamland where departed days remain?
I have leapt the bars of distance—left the life that late I led—
I remember years and labours as a tale that I have read;

Yet my heart is hot within me, for I feel the gentle power
Of the spirits that still love me, waiting for this sacred hour.
Yes,—I know the forms that meet me are but phantoms of the brain,
For they walk in mortal bodies, and they have not ceased from pain.
Oh! those signs of human weakness, left behind for ever now,
Dearer far to me than glories round a fancied seraph's brow.
Oh! the old familiar voices! Oh! the patient waiting eyes!
Let me live with them in dreamland, while the world in slumber lies!
For by bonds of sacred honour will they guard my soul in sleep
From the spells of aimless fancies, that around my senses creep.
They will link the past and present into one continuous life,
While I feel their hope, their patience, nerve me for the daily strife.

For it is not all a fancy that our lives and theirs are one,
And we know that all we see is but an endless work begun.
Part is left in Nature's keeping, part is entered into rest,
Part remains to grow and ripen, hidden in some living breast.
What is ours we know not, either when we wake or when we sleep,
But we know that Love and Honour, day and night, are ours to keep.

What though Dreams be wandering fancies, by some lawless force entwined,
Empty bubbles, floating upwards through the current of the mind?
There are powers and thoughts within us, that we know not, till they rise
Through the stream of conscious action from where Self in secret lies.
But when Will and Sense are silent, by the thoughts that come and go,
We may trace the rocks and eddies in the hidden depths below.

Let me dream my dream till morning; let my mind run slow and clear,
Free from all the world's distraction, feeling that the Dead are near,
Let me wake, and see my duty lie before me straight and plain.
Let me rise refreshed, and ready to begin my work again.

James Clerk Maxwell

Bibliography

d'Alembert J 1921 *Traité de Dynamique* (Paris: Gauthiers-Villars) reprint of 1758 edition

—— 1929 *Discours Préliminaire de l'Encyclopédie* (Paris: Colin)

Ampère A M 1822 *Recueil d'Observations Électro-dynamiques* (Paris)

—— 1826 *Théorie des Phénomènes Électrodynamiques* (Paris)

—— 1885–7 *Collection de Mémoires Relatifs à la Physique, Tômes II et III: Mémoires sur l'Électrodynamique, par A M Ampère* 2 volumes (Paris: Société Française de Physique)

Appleton E V *et al* 1963 *Clerk Maxwell and Modern Science: Six Commemorative Lectures* (London: Athlone Press)

Arago F 1826 Note concernant les phénomènes magnétiques auxquels le mouvement dont naissance *Ann. Chim. Phys* **32** 213–23

Arnold D H 1983 The Mécanique Physique of Siméon Denis Poisson *Arch. Hist. Exact Sci.* **28** 243–368 and **29** 27–94

Babbage C and Herschel J F W 1825 Account of the repetition of M Arago's experiments on the magnetism manifested by various substances during the act of rotation *Phil. Trans. R. Soc.* **115** 467–96

Becher H W 1980 William Whewell and Cambridge mathematics *Hist. Stud. Phys. Sci.* **11** 1–48

Bechler Z (ed) 1982 *Contemporary Newtonian Research* (Dordrecht: Reidel)

Benton E 1974 Vitalism in nineteenth-century scientific thought: a typology and reassessment *Stud. Hist. Phil. Sci.* **5** 17–48

Berzelius J J 1821 Letter from Berzelius to Berthollet *Ann. Chim. Phys.* **16** 116–19

Biot J B 1804 Mémoire sur la propagation de la chaleur *Bibliothèque Britannique* **37** 310–29

—— 1809 Review article in *Mercure de France* **38** 327–8

—— 1816 *Traité de Physique Expérimentale et Mathématique* (Paris)

—— 1819 Article on magnetism in *Edinburgh Encyclopedia* **13**

—— 1820 Sur le magnétisme de la pile de Volta *Ann. Chim. Phys.* **15** 222–3

—— 1821a in *Journal de Savants* (April) 221

—— 1821b *Précis Elementaire de Physique* 2nd edn (Paris)

—— 1824 *Précis Elementaire de Physique* 3rd edn (Paris)

Blondel C 1982 *Ampère et la Création de l'Électrodynamique* (Paris: Bibliotheque Nationale)

Boas M 1952 The establishment of the mechanical philosophy *Osiris* **10** 412–541

Boole G 1847 *The Mathematical Analysis of Logic* (Cambridge). Reprinted 1948 (Oxford: Basil Blackwell)

—— 1851 On the theory of probability and in particular on Mitchell's problem of the distribution of the fixed stars *Phil. Mag.* **1** 521–30

—— 1854 *An Investigation into the Laws of Thought* (London). Reprinted 1958 (New York: Dover)

Bork A M 1967 Maxwell and the vector potential *Isis* **58** 201–22

Boscovich R J 1922 *A Theory of Natural Philosophy* transl. J M Child (Chicago: Open Court)

Bromberg J 1967 Maxwell's displacement current and his theory of light *Arch. Hist Exact Sci.* **4** 218–34

—— 1968 Maxwell's electrostatics *Am. J. Phys.* **36** 142–51

Brown T 1969 The electric current in early nineteenth-century French physics *Hist. Stud. Phys. Sci.* **1** 61–103

Brown T M 1974 From mechanism to vitalism in eighteenth century England *J. Hist. Biol.* **7** 179–216

Brush S G 1976 *The Kind of Motion we call Heat: a History of the Kinetic Theory of Gases in the Nineteenth Century* 2 volumes (Amsterdam: Elsevier)

Brush S G, Everitt C W F and Garber E (eds) 1983 *Maxwell on Saturn's Rings* (Cambridge, MA: MIT Press)

Buchwald J Z 1976 William Thomson, Baron Kelvin of Largs *Dict. Sci. Biog.* **13** 374–88

—— 1977 William Thomson and the mathematization of Faraday's electrostatics *Hist. Stud. Phys. Sci.* **8** 101–36

Buijs Ballot C H D 1858 Über die Art von Bewegung, welche wir Wärme und Elektricität nennen *Ann. Phys., Lpz.* **103** 240–59

Burckhardt J J *et al* 1983 *Leonhardi Euler. Beiträge zur Leben und Werke* (Basel: Birkhäuser)

Campbell L and Garnett W 1882 *The Life of James Clerk Maxwell* (London: Macmillan). Reprinted 1969 (New York: Johnson Reprint)

—— 1884 *The Life of James Clerk Maxwell* 2nd edn (London: Macmillan)

Caneva K L 1978 From Galvanism to electrodynamics: the transformation of German physics and its social context *Hist. Stud. Phys. Sci.* **9** 63–159

—— 1980 Ampère, the etherians, and the Oersted connexion *Br. J. Hist. Sci.* **13** 121–38

Cantor G N 1983 *Optics after Newton. Theories of Light in Britain and Ireland, 1704–1840* (Manchester: Manchester University Press)

Cantor G N and Hodge M J S (eds) 1981 *Conceptions of Ether: Studies in the History of Ether Theories, 1740–1900* (Cambridge: Cambridge University Press)

Cardwell D S L 1967 Some factors in the early development of the concepts of power, work and energy *Br. J. Hist. Sci.* **3** 209–24

—— 1971 *From Watt to Clausius: the Rise of Thermodynamics in the Early Industrial Age* (London: Heinemann)

—— 1983 The origins and consequences of certain of J P Joule's scientific ideas. In *Springs of Scientific Creativity. Essays on the Founders of Modern Science* ed R Aris *et al* (Minneapolis: University of Minnesota Press) 44–70

Cauchy A L 1830 Mémoire sur la théorie de la lumière *Mémoires de l'Académie* **10** 293–316

Cavendish H 1879 *The Scientific Papers of the Honourable Henry Cavendish. Volume 1. The Electrical Researches* ed J C Maxwell (Cambridge: Cambridge University Press). Reprinted 1979 (London: Cass)

Cayley A 1857 Report on the recent progress of theoretical dynamics *Rep. Br. Assoc. Adv. Sci.* **27** 1–42

Chalmers A F 1973 Maxwell's methodology and his application of it to electromagnetism *Stud. Hist. Phil. Sci.* **4** 107–64

Charleton W 1966 *Physiologia Epicuro–Gassendo–Charletoniana* (New York: Johnson Reprint) reprint of 1655 edition

Clarke D M 1982 *Descartes' Philosophy of Science* (Manchester: Manchester University Press)

Clausius R 1850 Über die bewegende Kraft der Wärme und die Gesetze welche sich daraus für die Wärmelehre selbst ableiten lassen *Ann. Phys., Lpz.* **79** 368–97 and 500–24

—— 1857 Über die Art der Bewegung, welche wir Wärme nennen *Ann. Phys., Lpz.* **100** 353–80

—— 1858 Über die mittlere Länge der Wege, welche bei der Molecularbewegung gasförmigen Körper von den einzelnen Molecülen zurückgelegt werden; nebst einigen anderen Bemerkungen über die mechanische Wärmetheorie *Ann. Phys., Lpz.* **105** 239–58

—— 1859 On the mean length of the paths described by the separate molecules of gaseous bodies on the occurrence of molecular motion; with some other remarks upon the mechanical theory of heat *Phil. Mag.* **17** 81–91

Clavelin M 1974 *The Natural Philosophy of Galileo* (Cambridge, MA: MIT Press)

Cohen I B 1956 *Franklin and Newton* (Philadelphia: American Philosophical Society)

—— 1980 *The Newtonian Revolution: with Illustrations of the Transformations of Scientific Ideas* (Cambridge: Cambridge University Press)

Coleman W 1977 *Biology in the Nineteenth Century. Problems of Form, Function and Transformation* (Cambridge: Cambridge University Press)

Coleridge S T 1818 *The Friend* 3 volumes (London)

—— 1848 *Hints Towards the Formation of a More Comprehensive Theory of Life* (London)

—— 1949 *Philosophical Lectures* ed K Coburn (London: Pilot Press)

—— 1956 *Biographia Literaria* (London: J M Dent) reprint of the 1817 edition

—— 1972 *The Statesman's Manual* volume VI of *Collected Works of Samuel Taylor Coleridge* ed R J White (London: Routledge and Kegan Paul)

Collingwood R G 1945 *The Idea of Nature* (Oxford: Oxford University Press)

Comte A 1830–42 *Cours de Philosophie Positive* 6 volumes (Paris)

Coulomb C A 1884 *Mémoires de Coulomb. Collection de Mémoires Relatif à la Physique, Tôme I* (Paris)

Cranefield P F 1954 Clerk Maxwell's corrections to page proofs of 'A dynamical theory of the electromagnetic field' *Ann. Sci.* **10** 359–62

Crombie A C 1959 *Augustine to Galileo* (London: Heinemann)

Crosland M P 1967 *The Society of Arcueil: A View of French Science at the Time of Napoleon I* (London: Heinemann)

Crowe M J 1967 *A History of Vector Analysis: the Evolution of the Idea of a Vectorial System* (Notre Dame: University of Notre Dame Press)
Culotta E 1973 German biophysics, objective knowledge, and romanticism *Hist. Stud. Phys. Sci.* **4** 3–38
Dalton J 1808–10 *A New System of Chemical Philosophy* (London)
Daub E E 1967 Atomism and thermodynamics *Isis* **58** 293–303
Davie G E 1964 *The Democratic Intellect: Scotland and her Universities in the Nineteenth Century* (Edinburgh: Edinburgh University Press)
Davy H 1821 On the magnetic phenomena produced by electricity *Phil. Trans. R. Soc.* **111** 7–19
Debus A G 1978 *Man and Nature in the Renaissance* (Cambridge: Cambridge University Press)
Descartes R 1664 *Le Monde* (Paris)
—— 1897–1910 *Oevres de Descartes* ed C A and P Tannery (Paris)
—— 1983 *Principles of Philosophy* ed and transl. V R and R P Miller (Dordrecht: Reidel)
Dibner B 1961 *Oersted and the Discovery of Electromagnetism* (New York: Blaisdell)
Dijksterhuis E J 1961 *The Mechanisation of the World Picture* transl. C Dikshoorn (Oxford: Oxford University Press)
Doran B G 1974 Origins and consolidation of the field theory in nineteenth-century Britain: from the mechancial to the electromagnetic view of nature *Hist. Stud. Phys. Sci.* **6** 132–260
Drake S 1978 *Galileo at Work. His Scientific Biography* (Chicago: Chicago University Press)
Duhem P 1902 *Les Théories Électriques de J. Clerk Maxwell: Étude Historique et Critique* (Paris: Hermann)
Eddington A S 1928 *The Nature of the Physical World* (Cambridge: Cambridge University Press)
—— 1938 *The Philosophy of Physical Science* (Cambridge: Cambridge University Press). Reprinted in 1958 (Michigan: Michigan University Press)
Einstein A 1905a Über einen die Erzeugung and Verwandlung des Lichtes betreffenden heuristischen Gesichtspunkt *Ann. Phys., Lpz.* **17** 132–48
—— 1905b Über die von der molekular-kinetischen Theorie der Wärme gefordete Bewegung von in ruhenden Flüssigkeiten suspendierten Teilchen *Ann. Phys., Lpz.* **17** 549–60
—— 1905c Zur Elektrodynamik bewegter Körper *Ann. Phys., Lpz.* **17** 891–921
—— 1905d Ist die Trägheit eines Körpers von seinem Energieinhalt abhängig? *Ann. Phys., Lpz.* **18** 639–41
Elkana Y 1974 *The Discovery of the Conservation of Energy* (London: Hutchinson)
Everitt C W F 1974 James Clerk Maxwell *Dict. Sci. Biog.* **9** 198–230
—— 1975 *James Clerk Maxwell: Physicist and Natural Philosopher* (New York: Scribner)
Faraday M 1821–57 *Experimental Researches in Chemistry and Physics* (London: Taylor and Francis). Collected edition in 1859
—— 1821 New electromagnetic apparatus *Q. J. Sci.* **12** 186–7
—— 1846a On the magnetization of light and the illumination of magnetic lines of force *Phil. Trans. R. Soc.* **136** 1–20

—— 1846b Thoughts on ray vibrations *Phil. Mag.* **28** 345–50

—— 1851 On the magnetic and diamagnetic conditions of bodies *Phil. Trans. R. Soc.* **141** 7–28

—— 1932–6 *Faraday's Diary, being the Various Philosophical Notes of Experimental Investigations Made by Michael Faraday* ed T Martin, 8 volumes (London: G Bell)

—— 1965 *Experimental Researches in Electricity* 2 volumes (New York: Dover). Reprint of 3-volume edition of 1839–55

—— 1971 *Selected Correspondence* ed L P Williams, 2 volumes (Cambridge: Cambridge University Press)

Fitzgerald G F 1889 The ether and the earth's atmosphere *Science* **13** 390

Fizeau H 1851 Sur les hypothèses relatives à l'éther lumineux, et sur une expérience qui paraît démontrer que les mouvements des corps change la vitesse avec laquelle la lumière so propage dans leur intérieur *Comptes Rendus* **33** 349–55

Forbes J D 1835 On the refraction and polarization of heat *Phil. Mag.* **6** 134–42, 205–14, 284–91 and 366–71

Forrester J 1975 Chemistry and the conservation of energy: the work of James Prescott Joule *Stud. Hist. Phil. Sci.* **6** 273–313

Fourier J 1955 *The Analytical Theory of Heat* transl. A Freeman (New York Dover). Reprint of the 1878 edition

Fox R 1974 The rise and fall of Laplacian physics *Hist. Stud. Phys. Sci.* **4** 89–136

Frankel E 1977 J. B. Biot and the mathematization of experimental physics in Napoleonic France *Hist. Stud. Phys. Sci.* **8** 33–72

Fraser C G 1983 J.L. Lagrange's early contributions to the principles and methods of mechanics *Arch. Hist. Exact Sci.* **28** 197–242

Fresnel A 1818 Letter to Arago *Ann. Chim. Phys.* **9** 57*ff*. Reprinted in A Fresnel (1866–70) vol 2 627–36

—— 1819 Mémoire sur la diffraction de la lumière *Ann. Chim. Phys.* **11** 246–96 and 337–78

—— 1866–70 *Oevres Complètes d'Augustin Fresnel* 3 volumes (Paris)

Galileo Galilei 1974 *Two New Sciences* transl. S Drake (Madison: University of Wisconsin Press)

Galvani L 1791 *De Viribus Electricitatis in Motu Musculari Commentaris* (Bologna)

Garber E 1970 Clausius and Maxwell's kinetic theory of gases *Hist. Stud. Phys. Sci.* **2** 299–319

—— 1972 Aspects of the introduction of probability into physics *Centaurus* **17** 11–39

Gassendi P 1972 *The Selected Writings of Pierre Gassendi* ed and transl. C B Brush (New York: Johnson Reprint)

Gaukroger S (ed) 1980 *Descartes: Philosophy, Mathematics and Physics* (Brighton: Harvester)

Gauss C F 1843 General theorems relating to attractive and repulsive forces *Scientific Memoirs* **3** 153–96. Translation of German article of 1839

Gibbs J W 1881–4 *Elements of Vector Analysis* 2 volumes (New Haven). Reprinted in J W Gibbs (1906) **2** 17–117

—— 1888 A comparison of the elastic and the electrical theories of light with respect to the law of double refraction and the disperson of colors *Am. J. Sci.* **35** 467–75. Reprinted in J W Gibbs (1906) **2** 223–31

—— 1889 A comparison of the electric theory of light and Sir William Thomson's theory of a quasi-labile ether *Am. J. Sci.* **37** 129–44. Reprinted in J W Gibbs (1906) **2** 232–45

—— 1906 *The Scientific Papers of J. Willard Gibbs* ed H A Bumstead and R G Van Name, 2 volumes (New Haven: Yale University Press). Reprinted in 1961 (New York: Dover)

Gillispie C G *et al* (eds) 1970–80 *Dictionary of Scientific Biography* 16 volumes (New York: Scribner)

Gillmor C S 1971 *Coulomb and the Evolution of Physics and Engineering in Eighteenth Century France* (Princeton: Princeton University Press)

Goldberg S 1969 The Lorentz theory of electrons and Einstein's theory of relativity *Am. J. Phys.* **37** 982–94

Goldman M 1983 *The Demon in the Aether. The Story of James Clerk Maxwell* (Edinburgh: Paul Harris)

Gooding D 1978 Conceptual and experimental bases of Faraday's denial of electrostatic action at a distance *Stud. Hist. Phil. Sci.* **9** 117–49

—— 1980a Metaphysics versus measurement: the conversion and conservation of force in Faraday's physics *Ann. Sci.* **37** 1–29

—— 1980b Faraday, Thomson and the concept of the magnetic field *Br. J. Hist. Sci.* **13** 91–120

—— 1981 Final steps to the field theory: Faraday's study of magnetic phenomena, 1845–1850 *Hist. Stud. Phys. Sci.* **11** 231–75

—— 1982 Empiricism in practice: teleology, economy and observation in Faraday's physics *Isis* **73** 46–67

Graves R P 1882–9 *Life of Sir William Rowan Hamilton* 3 volumes (London: Longman)

Grattan-Guinness I with Ravetz J R 1972 *Joseph Fourier 1768–1830: a Survey of his Life and Work, based on a Critical Edition of his Monograph on the Propagation of Heat, Presented to the Institut de France in 1807* (Cambridge, MA: MIT Press)

Green G 1828 *Essay on the Application of Mathematical Analysis to the Theories of Electricity and Magnetism* (Nottingham). Reprinted in G Green (1871) 1–115

—— 1839 Memoir on ordinary refraction *Trans. Camb. Phil. Soc.* **7** 1–25 and 113–20

—— 1871 *Mathematical Papers* (London: Macmillan). Reprinted in 1970 (New York: Chelsea Publishing)

Guerlac H 1975 *Antoine-Laurent Lavoisier: Chemist and Revolutionary* (New York: Scribner)

Hall A R 1962 *The Scientific Revolution, 1500–1800* (London: Longman)

—— 1983 *The Revolution in Science, 1500–1750* (London: Longman)

Hamilton W 1865 *Lectures on Metaphysics and Logic* ed H C Mansel and J Veitch (Edinburgh)

Hamilton W R 1834 On a general method in dynamics *Phil. Trans. R. Soc.* **124** 247–308

—— 1835 Second essay on a general method in dynamics *Phil. Trans. R. Soc.* **125** 95–144

—— 1837 Theory of conjugate functions or algebraic couples, with a preliminary and elementary essay on algebra as the science of pure time *Trans. R. Irish Acad.* **17** 293–422

—— 1853 *Lectures on Quaternions* (Dublin: Hodges and Smith)
—— 1865 *Elements of Quaternions* (London: Longman, Green)
Hankins T 1970 *Jean d'Alembert: Science and the Enlightenment* (Oxford: Clarendon Press)
—— 1976 Algebra as pure time: William Rowan Hamilton and the foundations of algebra. In *Motion and Time, Space and Matter* ed P J Machamer and R G Turnbull (Columbus: Ohio State University Press) 327–59
—— 1980 *Sir William Rowan Hamilton* (Baltimore: Johns Hopkins University Press)
Harman P M 1982 *Energy, Force and Matter. The Conceptual Development of Nineteenth-Century Physics* (Cambridge: Cambridge University Press)
Harré R 1964 *Matter and Method* (London: Macmillan)
Heaviside O 1892 *Electrical Papers* (London: Macmillan)
—— 1893–1912 *Electromagnetic Theory* 3 volumes (London: 'The Electrician')
Heilbron J L 1979 *Electricity in the 17th and 18th Centuries: a Study of Early Modern Physics* (Berkeley: University of California Press)
Heimann P M 1970a Molecular forces, statistical representation, and Maxwell's demon *Stud. Hist. Phil. Sci.* **1** 189–211
—— 1970b Maxwell and the modes of consistent representation *Arch. Hist. Exact Sci.* **6** 171–213
—— 1971a Faraday's theories of matter and electricity *Br. J. Hist. Sci.* **5** 235–57
—— 1971b Maxwell, Hertz and the nature of electricity *Isis* **62** 149–57
—— 1974 Helmholtz and Kant: the metaphysical foundations of 'Über die Erhaltung der Kraft' *Stud. Hist. Phil. Sci.* **5** 205–38
Heimann P M and McGuire J E 1971 Newtonian forces and Lockean powers: concepts of matter in eighteenth-century thought *Hist. Stud. Phys. Sci.* **3** 233–306
von Helmholtz H 1847 *Über die Erhaltung der Kraft* (Berlin: Reimer)
—— 1853 On the conservation of force *Scientific Memoirs in Natural Philosophy* **1** 114–62. A revised version of this translation of H von Helmholtz (1847) is in *Scientific Writings of Herman von Helmholtz* ed R Kahl (Middleton, CT: Weslyan University Press, 1971) 3–55
—— 1897–1907 *Vorlesungen über Theoretische Physik* 6 volumes (Leipzig: Barth)
Hendry J 1980 The development of attitudes to the wave–particle duality of light and quantum theory, 1900–1920 *Ann. Sci.* **37** 59–79
—— 1983a Understanding science *Hist. Sci.* **21** 415–24
—— 1983b Monopoles before Dirac *Stud. Hist. Phil. Sci.* **14** 81–7
—— 1984a The evolution of William Rowan Hamilton's view of algebra as the science of pure time *Stud. Hist. Phil. Sci.* **15** 63–81
—— 1984b *The Creation of Quantum Mechanics and the Bohr–Pauli Dialogue* (Dordrecht: Reidel)
Herivel J W 1966 Aspects of French theoretical physics in the nineteenth century *Br. J. Hist. Sci.* **3** 121–4
—— 1975 *Joseph Fourier. The Man and the Physicist* (Oxford: Clarendon)
Herschel J F W 1830 *A Preliminary Discourse on the Study of Natural Philosophy* volume 1 of the *Cabinet Cyclopedia* (London)
—— 1865 On the origin of force *Fortnightly Review* **1** 435–42
Hertz H 1880 Versuche zur Feststellung einer oberen Grenze für die kinetische Energie der elektrischen Strömung *Ann. Phys., Lpz.* **10** 414–48
—— 1884 Über die Beziehungen zwischen den Maxwell'schen elektrodynamischen

Grundgleichungen und den Grundgleichungen der gegnerischen Elektrodynamik *Ann. Phys., Lpz.* **23** 84–103

—— 1887 Über sehr schnelle elektrische Schwingungen *Ann. Phys., Lpz.* **31** 421*ff.* Reprinted in H Hertz (1892) 32–58

—— 1888a Über die Ausbreitungsgeschwindigkeit der elektromagnetischen Wirkungen *Sitz. ber. Preuss. Akad. Wiss. Berlin* 197–210

—— 1888b Die Kräfte elektrischer Schwingungen behandelt nach der Maxwell'schen Theorie *Ann. Phys., Lpz.* **36** 1–22

—— 1890a Über die Grundgleichungen der Elektrodynamik für ruhende Körper *Ann. Phys., Lpz.* **40** 577–624

—— 1890b Über die Grundgleichungen der Elektrodynamik für bewegte Körper *Ann. Phys., Lpz.* **41** 369–99

—— 1892 *Untersuchung über die Ausbreitung der Elektrischen Kraft* (Leipzig: Barth). Translated as H Hertz (1893)

—— 1893 *Electric Waves* transl. D E Jones (London: Macmillan). Reprinted in 1962 (New York: Dover)

—— 1894 *Die Principien der Mechanik, in Neuem Zusammenhange* (Leipzig: Barth). Translated as H Hertz (1899)

—— 1899 *The Principles of Mechanics* (London: Macmillan). Reprinted in 1956 (New York: Dover)

—— 1914 *Gesammelte Werke* 3 volumes (Leipzig: Barth)

Hesse M 1961 *Forces and Fields: the Concept of Action at a Distance in the History of Physics* (London: Nelson)

—— 1973 Logic of discovery in Maxwell's electromagnetic theory. In *Foundations of Scientific Method: the Nineteenth Century* ed R N Giere and R S Westfall (Bloomington: Indiana University Press)

Hiebert E 1962 *Historical Roots of the Principle of Conservation of Energy* (Madison: University of Wisconsin Press)

Hirosige T 1966 Electrodynamics before the theory of relativity, 1890–1905 *Jpn. Stud. Hist. Sci.* **5** 1–49

—— 1969 Origins of Lorentz's theory of electrons and the concept of the electromagnetic field *Hist. Stud. Phys. Sci.* **1** 151–209

—— 1976 The ether problem, the mechanistic world view, and the origins of the theory of relativity *Hist. Stud. Phys. Sci.* **7** 3–82

Holton G J 1973 *Thematic Origins of Scientific Thought: Kepler to Einstein* (Cambridge, MA: Harvard University Press)

Home R W 1983 Poisson's memoirs on electricity: academic politics and a new style in physics *Br. J. Hist. Sci.* **16** 239–60

Hume D 1975 *Enquiries Concerning Human Understanding and Concerning the Principles of Morals* (Oxford: Oxford University Press)

—— 1978 *A Treatise of Human Nature* (Oxford: Oxford University Press)

Hutchinson K 1981 W J M Rankine and the rise of thermodynamics *Br. J. Hist. Sci.* **14** 1–26

Hutton J 1794 *An Investigation of the Principles of Knowledge, and of the Progress of Reason from Sense to Science and Philosophy* (Edinburgh)

James W 1907 *Pragmatism: a New Name for Some Old Ways of Thinking* (London: Longman)

Jones H B 1870 *Life and Letters of Faraday* 2 volumes (London)

Jones R V 1973 James Clerk Maxwell at Aberdeen, 1856–1860 *Notes Rec. R. Soc.* **28** 57–81

Joule J P 1843 On the calorific effects of magneto-electricity and the mechanical value of heat *Phil. Mag.* **23** 263–76, 347–55 and 435–43. Reprinted in J P Joule (1884–7) **1** 123–59

—— 1848 On the mechanical equivalent of heat and on the constitution of electric fluids *Rep. Br. Assoc. Adv. Sci.* **21**. Printed in full in J P Joule (1884–7) **1** 288–97

—— 1850 On the mechanical equivalent of heat *Phil. Trans. R. Soc.* **140** 61–82. Reprinted in J P Joule (1884–7) **1** 298–328

—— 1884–7 *The Scientific Papers of James Prescott Joule* 2 volumes (London: Physical Society). Reprinted in 1963 (London: Physical Society)

Jung C G 1923 *Psychological Types* transl. H G Baynes (London: Routledge and Kegan Paul)

Kant I 1770 *De Mundi Sensibilis* (Königsberg)

—— 1883 *Prolegomena and Metaphysical Foundations of Natural Science* transl. E B Bax (London: George Bell)

—— 1902 Metaphysicae cum geometria iunctae usus in philosophia naturali, cuius specimen I continet monadologiam physicam in *Gesammelte Schrifften, Band I* (Berlin) 473–88

—— 1933 *Critique of Pure Reason* transl. N K Smith (London: Macmillan)

Kargon R H 1965 William Rowan Hamilton and Boscovichean atomism *J. Hist. Ideas* **26** 137–40

—— 1969 Model and analogy in Victorian science: Maxwell's critique of the French physicists *J. Hist. Ideas* **30** 423–36

Kelland P and Tait P G 1873 *Introduction to Quaternions* (London)

Klein M J 1977 The beginnings of quantum theory. In *History of Twentieth Century Physics* ed C Weiner (New York: Academic)

Knott C G 1911 *Life and Scientific Work of Peter Guthrie Tait* (Cambridge: Cambridge University Press)

Knudsen O 1972 From Lord Kelvin's notebook: ether speculations *Centaurus* **16** 41–53

—— 1976 The Faraday effect and physical theory *Arch. Hist Exact Sci.* **15** 235–81

Koyré A 1973 *The Astronomical Revolution* transl. R E W Maddison (London: Methuen)

—— 1978 *Galilean Studies* transl. J Mepham (Brighton: Harvester)

Koyré A and Cohen I B 1962 Newton and the Leibniz–Clarke correspondence *Arch. Int. Hist. Sci.* **15** 63–126

Kuhn T S 1959 Energy conservation as an example of simultaneous discovery. In *Critical Problems in the History of Science* ed M Clagett (Madison: University of Wisconsin Press). Reprinted in T S Kuhn (1972) 66–104

—— 1970 *The Structure of Scientific Revolutions* 2nd edn (Chicago: University of Chicago Press)

—— 1972 *The Essential Tension. Selected Studies in Scientific Tradition and Change* (Chicago: University of Chicago Press)

—— 1978 *Black-Body Theory and the Quantum Discontinuity 1894–1912* (Oxford: Oxford University Press)

Lagrange J L 1788 *Mécanique Analytique* (Paris)

Laita L M 1979 Influences on Boole's logic: the controversy between William Hamilton and Augustus de Morgan *Ann. Sci.* **36** 45–65

Lamb H 1879 *A Treatise on the Mathematical Theory of the Motion of Fluids* (Cambridge: Cambridge University Press)

de Laplace P S 1799 *Traité de Mécanique Celeste* (Paris)

—— 1809 *The System of the World* (London)

—— 1878–1912 *Oevres Complètes* 14 volumes (Paris: Gauthier-Villars)

Larmor J 1894, 1895 and 1897 A dynamical theory of the electric and luminiferous medium *Phil. Trans. R. Soc.* **185** 719–822, **186** 695–743 and **190** 205–300

—— 1900 *Aether and Matter* (Cambridge: Cambridge University Press)

—— (ed) 1907 *Memoir and Scientific Correspondence of the late Sir George Gabriel Stokes* 2 volumes (Cambridge: Cambridge University Press). Reprinted in 1971 (New York: Johnson Reprint)

—— (ed) 1937 *Origins of Clerk Maxwell's Electric Ideas, as Described in Familiar Letters to William Thomson* (Cambridge: Cambridge University Press)

Lavoisier A L 1802 *Elements of Chemistry* (Edinburgh)

Leibniz G W 1898 *The Monadology* (Oxford: Oxford University Press)

Lenoir T 1980 The Göttingen school and the development of transcendental Naturphilosophie in the Romantic era *Stud. Hist. Biol.* **5** 111–205

—— 1981 Kant, Blumenbach, and vital materialism in German biology *Isis* **71** 77–108

—— 1982 *The Strategy of Life: Teleology and Mechanics in Nineteenth-Century German Biology* (Dordrecht: Reidel)

Levere T H 1968 Faraday, matter and natural theology—reflections on an unpublished manuscript *Br. J. Hist. Sci.* **4** 95–107

—— 1971 *Affinity and Matter. Elements of Chemical Philosophy, 1800–1865* (Oxford: Oxford University Press)

—— 1981 *Poetry Realised in Nature: Samuel Taylor Coleridge and Early Nineteenth-Century Science* (Cambridge: Cambridge University Press)

Locke J 1979 *An Essay Concerning Human Understanding* ed P H Nidditch (Oxford: Oxford University Press)

Lorentz H A 1875 Sur la théorie de la reflection et de la refraction de la lumière. In H A Lorentz (1934–9) **1** 193–383

—— 1878 Concerning the relationship between the velocity of propagation of light and the density and composition of media *Verhandl. Kon. Akad. Wetensch. Amsterdam* **18** 1*ff* (in Dutch). English version in H A Lorentz (1934–9) **2** 1–119

—— 1886 De l'influence du mouvement de la terre sur les phénomènes lumineux *Verslagen Kon. Akad. Wetensch. Amsterdam* **2** 297–372 (in Dutch). French version in H A Lorentz (1934–9) **4** 153–214

—— 1892a La théorie électromagnétique de Maxwell et son application aux corps mouvants *Archives Néerlandaises des Sciences* **25** 363–551

—— 1892b The relative motion of the earth in the aether *Verslagen Kon. Akad. Wetensch. Amsterdam* **1** 74–9 (in Dutch). English version in H A Lorentz (1934–9) **4** 219–23

—— 1895 *Versuch einer Theorie der Electrischen und Optischen Erscheinungen in Bewegten Körpern* (Leyden: E J Brill)

—— 1904 Electromagnetic phenomena in a system moving with any velocity smaller than that of light *Proc. Kon. Akad. Wetensch. Amsterdam* **6** 809–31

—— 1909 *The Theory of Electrons and its Application to the Phenomena of Light and Radiant Heat* (Leipzig: Teubner)
—— 1934–9 *Collected Papers* 9 volumes (The Hague: Martinus Nijhoff)
Lorenz L 1867 On the identity of the vibration of light with electric currents *Phil. Mag.* **34** 287–304. German original in *Ann. Phys., Lpz.* **131** 243–63
McCormmach R 1970a H A Lorentz and the electromagnetic view of nature *Isis* **61** 458–97
—— 1970b Einstein, Lorentz and the electron theory *Hist. Stud. Phys. Sci.* **2** 41–87
—— 1972 Heinrich Hertz *Dict. Sci. Biog.* **6** 340–50
—— 1973 Hendrik Antoon Lorentz *Dict. Sci. Biog.* **8** 487–500
MacCullagh J 1840 An essay towards a dynamical theory of reflection and refraction *Trans. R. Irish Acad.* **21** 17–50
McGuire J E 1968 Force, active principles and Newton's invisible realm *Ambix* **15** 154–208
—— 1978 Forces, powers, aethers and fields. In *Methodological and Historical Essays in the Natural and Social Sciences* ed R S Cohen and M W Wartofsky *Boston Studies in the Philosophy of Science* **14** (Dordrecht: Reidel) 119–59
McGuire J E and Tamny M (eds) 1983 *Certain Philosophical Questions. Newton's Trinity Notebook* (Cambridge: Cambridge University Press)
MacKinnon E M 1983 *Scientific Explanation and Atomic Physics* (Chicago: Chicago University Press)
Maxwell J C 1846 On the description of oval curves, and those having a plurality of foci *Proc. R. Soc. Edinburgh* **2** 89–93. Reprinted in J C Maxwell (1890) **1** 1–3
—— 1850 On the equilibrium of elastic solids *Trans. R. Soc. Edinburgh* **20** 87–120. Reprinted in J C Maxwell (1890) **1** 30–71
—— 1856 On Faraday's lines of force *Trans. Camb. Phil. Soc.* **10** part I 27–83. Reprinted in J C Maxwell (1890) **1** 155–229
—— 1859 *On the Stability of the Motion of Saturn's Rings* (Cambridge: Macmillan). Reprinted in J C Maxwell (1890) **1** 289–374 and S G Brush *et al* (1983) 68–158
—— 1860 Illustrations of the dynamical theory of gases *Phil. Mag.* **19** 19–32 and **20** 21–37. Reprinted in J C Maxwell (1890) **1** 377–409
—— 1861 and 1862 On physical lines of force *Phil. Mag.* **21** 161–75, 281–91 and 338–48, and **22** 12–24 and 85–95. Reprinted in J C Maxwell (1890) **1** 451–513
—— 1865 A dynamical theory of the electromagnetic field *Phil. Trans. R. Soc.* **155** 459–512. Reprinted in J C Maxwell (1890) **1** 526–97 and J C Maxwell (1982)
—— 1867 On the dynamical theory of gases *Phil. Trans. R. Soc.* **157** 49–88. Reprinted in J C Maxwell (1890) **2** 26–78
—— 1868 On a method of making a direct comparison of electrostatic and electromagnetic force; with a note on the electromagnetic theory of light *Phil. Trans. R. Soc.* **158** 643–57. Reprinted in J C Maxwell (1890) **2** 125–43
—— 1873 *A Treatise on Electricity and Magnetism* 2 volumes (Oxford: Clarendon Press)
—— 1877 *Matter and Motion* (London). Reprinted in 1920 (London: Sheldon Press) and 1951 (New York: Dover)
—— 1881 *Elementary Treatise on Electricity* ed W Garnett (Oxford: Clarendon Press)
—— 1890 *The Scientific Papers of James Clerk Maxwell* ed W D Niven, 2 volumes

(Cambridge: Cambridge University Press). Reprinted in one volume in 1965 (New York: Dover)

—— 1954 *A Treatise on Electricity and Magnetism* 2 volumes (New York: Dover). Reprint of the 3rd edition of 1891 (Oxford: Clarendon Press)

—— 1979 James Clerk Maxwell's inaugural lecture at King's College London *Am. J. Phys.* **47** 928–33

—— 1982 *A Dynamical Theory of the Electromagnetic Field* ed T F Torrance (Edinburgh: Scottish Academic Press)

Maxwell J C and Jenkin F 1863 On the elementary relations of electrical quantities *Rep. Br. Assoc. Adv. Sci.* **32** 130–63

Mendelsohn E 1965 Physical models and physiological concepts: explanation in nineteenth-century biology *Br. J. Hist. Sci.* **2** 201–19

Merchant C 1980 *The Death of Nature* (San Francisco: Harper and Row)

Merz J T 1904–12 *A History of European Thought in the Nineteenth Century* (London: Blackwood)

Michelson A A 1881 The relative motion of the earth and the luminferous ether *Am. J. Sci.* **22** 120–9

Michelson A A and Morley E W 1887 On the relative motion of the earth and the luminiferous aether *Am. J. Sci.* **34** 333–45 and *Phil Mag.* **24** 449–63

Miller A I 1978 Visualisation lost and regained. In *On Aesthetics in Science* ed J Wechsler (Cambridge, MA: MIT Press)

—— 1985 *Imagery in Scientific thought. Creating 20th-Century Physics* (Boston: Birkhäuser)

Mossotti O F 1847a Recherches théoriques sur l'induction électrostatique envisagée d'après les idées de Faraday *Suppl. Bibliothèque Universelle de Genève, Arch. Sci. Phys. et Nat.* **6** 193*ff*. Reprinted in O F Mossotti (1951) 321–8

—— 1847b Sull' induzione elettrostatica *Il Cimento* **5**. Reprinted in O F Mossotti (1951) 329–32

—— 1850 Discussione analitica sull'influenza de l'azione di un mezzo dielettrico ha sulla distribuzione dell'elettricità all superfice di più corpi elettrici diseminati in esso *Mem. Società Italiana delle Science* **24** part II 49–74. Reprinted in O F Mossotti (1951) 333–59

—— 1951 *Scritti* ed L Gabba and G Polvani, 2 volumes (Pisa: Domus Galileana)

Moyer D F 1977 Energy, dynamics, hidden machinery: Rankine, Thomson and Tait, Maxwell *Stud. Hist. Phil. Sci.* **8** 251–68

—— 1978 Continuum mechanics and field theory: Thomson and Maxwell *Stud. Hist. Phil. Sci.* **9** 35–50

Murphy R 1832 *Elementary Principles of the Theories of Electricity, Heat and Molecular Atomism. Part I. On Electricity* (Cambridge)

Newton I 1730 *Opticks* 4th edn (London). Reprinted in 1952 (New York: Dover)

Oersted H C 1806 Des forces électriques considérées comme des forces chimiques *J. Physique* **62** 369–75

—— 1812 *Ansichten der Chemischen Naturgesetze* (Berlin)

—— 1813 *Recherches sur l'identité des forces chimiques et électriques* (Paris)

—— 1821a Letter to Schweigger *J. für Chemie u. Physik* **33** 123–31

—— 1821b Consideration au l'électromagnétism *Bibliothèque Universelle* **18** 11*ff*

—— 1823 Expèrience électromagnétique *Ann. Chim. Phys.* **22** 201–3

—— 1830 Thermoelectricity *Edinburgh Encyclopedia* **18** 573–89

—— 1920 *Scientific Papers* ed K Meyer (Copenhagen: A F Høst)

—— 1928 Experimenta circa effectum conflictus electrica in acum magneticum *Isis* **10** 435–44

Ohm G S 1826 *Die Galvanische Kette Mathematisch Bearbeitet* (Berlin)

Olson R G 1975 *Scottish Philosophy and British Physics 1750–1880: a Study in the Foundations of the Victorian Scientific Style* (Princeton: Princeton University Press)

Pais A 1982 *'Subtle is the Lord . . .' The Science and the Life of Albert Einstein* (Oxford: Oxford University Press)

Peierls R 1963 Field theory since Maxwell. In E V Appleton (1963)

Pickering A 1984 *Constructing Quarks. A Sociological History of Particle Physics* (Edinburgh: Edinburgh University Press)

Playfair J 1814 *Outlines of Natural Philosophy* (Edinburgh)

—— 1822 *The Works of John Playfair* (Edinburgh)

Plücker J 1852 On the relationship of magnetism to diamagnetism *Scientific Memoirs* **5** 553–78

Poisson S D 1812 Mémoire sur la distribution de l'électricité à la surface des corps conducteurs *Mém. Classe Sci. Math. de l'Institut de France, 1811* 1–92 and 163–274

—— 1815 Extrait d'un mémoire sur la distribution de la chaleur *J. Physique* **80** 434–41

—— 1826 Mémoire sur la théorie de magnétisme *Mém. Acad. Roy. des Sciences, 1821 et 1822* 247–338 and 488–533

—— 1835 *Théorie Mathématique de la Chaleur* (Paris)

Prechtl J 1822 On the fundamental magnetic phenomena of electrical conducting wire, or on the transverse electrical charge *Ann. Phil.* **4** 1–6

Priestley J 1782 *Disquisitions Relating to Matter and Spirit* 2nd edn (London)

—— 1817–31 *Theological and Miscellaneous Works* ed J T Rutt, 25 volumes (London)

Randall J 1963 Aspects of the life and work of James Clerk Maxwell. In E V Appleton (1963)

Rankine W J M 1851 On the centrifugal theory of elasticity as applied to gases and vapours *Phil. Mag.* **2** 509–42

—— 1852 On the reconcentration of the mechanical energy of the universe. Paper to the British Association for the Advancement of Science in W J M Rankine (1881) 200–2

—— 1853 On the general law of the transformation of energy *Phil. Mag.* **5** 106–17

—— 1855 Outlines of the science of energetics *Proc. Phil. Soc. Glasgow* **3**. Printed in W J M Rankine (1881) 209–28

—— 1859a On the conservation of energy *Phil. Mag.* **17** 250–3

—— 1859b Note to a letter 'On the conservation of energy' *Phil. Mag.* **17** 347–8

—— 1881 *Miscellaneous Scientific Papers* ed W J Miller (London: C Griffin)

Rayleigh Lord 1877 *Sound* 2 volumes (London: Macmillan)

—— 1881 On the electromagnetic theory of light *Phil. Mag.* **12** 81–101

Rees G 1980 Atomism and subtlety in Francis Bacon's Philosophy *Ann. Sci.* **37** 549–72

—— 1984 *Francis Bacon's Natural Philosophy: A New Source* assisted by C Upton (Chalfont St Giles: British Society for the History of Science)

Reid T 1858 *The Works* ed W Hamilton 5th edn (Edinburgh)
Riemann B 1867 A contribution to electrodynamics *Phil. Mag.* **34** 368–72. German original in *Ann. Phys., Lpz.* **131** 237–43
Rogers G A J 1983 The system of Locke and Newton. In Z Bechler (1983) 215–38
Roll-Hansen N 1976 Critical teleology: Immanuel Kant and Claude Bernard on the limitations of experimental biology *J. Hist. Biol.* **9** 59–86
Rosenfeld L 1957 The velocity of light and the evolution of electrodynamics *Supp. Nuovo Cim.* **4** 1630–69
Rossi P 1968 *Francis Bacon: From Magic to Science* (London: Routledge and Kegan Paul)
Schaffner K F (ed) 1972 *Nineteenth-Century Aether Theories* (Oxford: Pergamon)
Schelling F W 1956 *Werke. Band I. Zur Naturphilosophie* (Munich: Beck)
Schofield R E 1970 *Mechanism and Materialism: British Natural Philosophy in an age of Reason* (Princeton: Princeton University Press)
Segré E 1984 *From Falling Bodies to Radio Waves. Classical Physicists and their Discoveries* (New York: Freeman)
Shankland R S 1964 The Michelson–Morley experiment *Am. J. Phys.* **32** 16–35
Shea W R 1972 *Galileo's Intellectual Revolution* (London: Macmillan)
Sherman P D 1981 *Colour Vision in the Nineteenth Century: the Young–Helmholtz–Maxwell Theory* (Bristol: Adam Hilger)
Siegel D 1975 Completeness as a goal in Maxwell's electromagnetic theory *Isis* **66** 361–8
—— 1981 Thomson, Maxwell, and the universal ether in Victorian physics. In G N Cantor and M J S Hodge (1981) 239–68
Silliman R H 1974 Fresnel and the emergence of physics as a discipline *Hist. Stud. Phys. Sci.* **4** 137–62
Simpson T K 1966 Maxwell and the direct experimental test of his electromagnetic theory *Isis* **57** 411–32
Smith C W 1976a 'Mechanical Philosophy' and the emergence of physics in Britain, 1800–1850 *Ann. Sci.* **33** 3–29
—— 1976b Faraday as a referee of Joule's Royal Society paper 'On the mechanical equivalent of heat' *Isis* **67** 444–9
—— 1976c William Thomson and the creation of thermodynamics, 1840–1855 *Arch. Hist. Exact Sci.* **16** 231–8
—— 1978 A new chart for British natural philosophy: the development of energy physics in the nineteenth century *Hist. Sci.* **16** 231–79
—— 1980 Engineering the universe: William Thomson and Fleeming Jenkin on the nature of matter *Ann. Sci.* **37** 387–412
—— 1982 'Positivism' and 'reductionism' in early modern physics *Revista di Filosofia* nos 22–23 1–35
Snelders H A M 1975 The reception in the Netherlands of the discoveries of electromagnetism and electrodynamics *Ann. Sci.* **32** 39–54
Stauffer R C 1957 Speculation and experiment in the background of Oersted's discovery of electromagnetism *Isis* **48** 33–50
Steffens H J 1979 *James Prescott Joule and the Concept of Energy* (New York: Science History Publications)
Stewart D 1858 *Elements of the Philosophy of the Human Mind* ed W Hamilton (Edinburgh)

Stokes G G 1849 On the theories of the internal friction of fluids in motion, and of the equilibrium and motion of elastic solids *Trans. Camb. Phil. Soc.* **8** 287*ff*. Reprinted in G G Stokes (1880–1905) **1** 75–129

—— 1880–1905 *Mathematical and Physical Papers* 5 volumes (Cambridge: Cambrige University Press). Reprinted in 1966 (New York: Johnson Reprint)

Swenson L S 1972 *The Etherial Aether: A History of the Michelson–Morley–Miller Aether-Drift Experiments, 1880–1930* (Austin: University of Texas Press)

Tait P G 1860 *The Position and Prospects of Physical Science. A public Inaugural Lecture Delivered on November 7 1860* (Edinburgh: Edinburgh University)

—— 1864a The dynamical theory of heat *North British Review* **40** 40–69

—— 1864b Energy *North British Review* **40** 337–68

—— 1867 *An Elementary Treatise on Quaternions* (Oxford: Clarendon Press)

Tait P G and Steele W J 1865 *Dynamics of a Particle* 2nd edn (London: Macmillan)

Thackray A W 1970 *Atoms and Powers: An Essay in Newtonian Matter-Theory and the Development of Chemistry* (Cambridge, MA: Harvard University Press)

—— 1972 *John Dalton. Critical Assessments of his Life and Science* (Cambridge, MA: Harvard University Press)

Thompson S P 1910 *The Life of William Thomson, Baron Kelvin of Largs* 2 volumes (London: Macmillan)

Thomson W 1841a On Fourier's expansions of functions in trigonometrical series *Camb. Math. J.* **2** 258–62. Reprinted in W Thomson (1882–1911) **1** 1–6

—— 1841b Note on a passage in Fourier's Heat *Camb. Math. J.* **3** 25–7. Reprinted in W Thomson (1882–1911) **1** 7–10

—— 1842 On the uniform motion of heat in homogeneous solid bodies, and its connexion with the mathematical theory of electricity *Camb. Math. J.* **3** 71–84. Reprinted in W Thomson (1872) 1–14

—— 1842–3 Propositions in the theory of attraction *Camb. Math. J.* **3** 189–96 and 201–6. Reprinted in W Thomson (1872) 126–38

—— 1843 On the attractions of conducting and non-conducting electrified bodies *Camb. Math. J.* **3**. Reprinted in W Thomson (1872) 98–9

—— 1845a Demonstration of a fundamental proposition in the mechanical theory of electricity *Camb. Math. J.* **4** 223–6. Reprinted in W Thomson (1972) 100–3

—— 1845b On the elementary laws of statical electricity *Camb. and Dublin Math. J.* **1** 75*ff*. Reprinted in W Thomson (1872) 15–37

—— 1847a On a mechanical representation of electric, magnetic, and Galvanic forces *Camb. and Dublin Math. J.* **2**. Reprinted in W Thomson (1882–1911) **1** 76–80

—— 1847b On the forces experienced by small spheres under magnetic influence *Camb. and Dublin Math. J.* **2** 230*ff*. Reprinted in W. Thomson (1872) 493–9

—— 1848a Theorems with reference to the solution of certain partial differential equations *Camb. and Dublin Math. J.* **3**. Reprinted in W Thomson (1872) 139–41

—— 1848b On the theory of electromagnetic induction. Paper to the British Association for the Advancement of Science, printed in W Thomson (1882–1911) **1** 88–92

—— 1849 An account of Carnot's theory of the motive power of heat, with numerical results deduced from Regnault's experiments on steam *Trans. R. Soc. Edinburgh* **16** 541–74. Reprinted in W Thomson (1882–1911) **1** 113*ff*

—— 1851a On the dynamical theory of heat, with numerical results deduced from Mr Joule's equivalent of a thermal unit, and M Regnault's observations on steam *Trans. R. Soc. Edinburgh* **20** 261–88. Reprinted in W Thomson (1882–1911) **1** 174–232

—— 1851b A mathematical theory of magnetism *Phil. Trans. R. Soc.* **141** 243–85

—— 1852 On a universal tendency in nature to the dissipation of mechanical energy *Phil. Mag.* **6** 304–6

—— 1856 and 1857 Dynamical illustration of the magnetic and helicoidal rotatory effects of transparent bodies on polarized light *Proc. R. Soc.* **8** 150–8 and *Phil. Mag.* **13** 198–204

—— 1872 *Reprint of Papers on Electrostatics and Magnetism* (London: Macmillan)

—— 1882–1911 *Mathematical and Physical Papers* 6 volumes (Cambridge: Cambridge University Press)

—— 1899–1911 Professor Tait *Proc. R. Soc. Edinbugh* **23** 499–500

—— 1904 *Baltimore Lectures on Molecular Dynamics and the Wave Theory of Light* (London: C J Clay)

Thomson W and Tait P G 1867 *Treatise on Natural Philosophy* (Oxford: Clarendon Press)

—— 1872 *Elements of Natural Philosophy. Part I* (Cambridge: Cambridge University Press)

—— 1879–83 *Treatise on Natural Philosophy* 2nd edn, 2 volumes (Oxford: Clarendon Press). Reprinted in 1962 (New York: Dover)

Tricker R A R 1965 *Early Electrodynamics: The first Law of Circulation* (Oxford: Pergamon)

Turner R S 1972 Hermann von Helmholtz *Dict. Sci. Biog.* **6** 241–53

Verdet E 1854–63 Recherches sur les propriétés optiques développées dans les corps transparent par l'action du magnétisme *Ann. Chim. Phys.* **41** 370–412, **43** 37–44, **52** 129–63 and **69** 415–91

Volta A G A A 1800 On the electricity excited by the mere contact of conducting substances of different kinds *Phil. Trans. R. Soc.* **90** 403–43 and *Phil. Mag.* **7** 288–311

Weber W E 1846 Elektrodynamische Massbestimmungen. Über ein allgemeines Grundgesetz der elektrisch Wirkung *Abh. Begr. Kgl. Sächs. Ges. der Wiss. Leipzig* 211–378. Reprinted in W E Weber (1892–4) **3** 25–214

—— 1852a Elektrodynamische Massbestimmungen, insbesondere Widerstandsmessungen *Abh. Begr. Kgl. Sächs. Ges. der Wiss. Leipzig* 199–381. Reprinted in W E Weber (1892–4) **3** 301–471

—— 1852b On the measurement of electrodynamic forces *Scientific Memoirs* **5** 489–529

—— 1852c On the excitation of diamagnets according to the laws of individual currents *Scientific Memoirs* **5** 477–88

—— 1853 On the connexion of diamagnetism with magnetism and electricity *Scientific Memoirs on Natural Philosophy* **1** 114–62

—— 1892–4 *Werke* 6 volumes (Berlin: Springer)

Weber W E and Kohlrausch F W G 1857 Elektrodynamische Massbestimmungen, insbesondere Zurückführung der Stromintensitäts-Messungen auf mechanisches Mass *Abh. Begr. Kgl. Sächs. Ges. der Wiss. Leipzig* **3** 221–90. Reprinted in W E Weber (1892–4) **3** 609–76

Webster C 1983 *From Paracelsus to Newton. Magic and the Making of Modern Science* (Cambridge: Cambridge University Press)

Westfall R S 1971 *Forces in Newton's Physics* (New York: Elsevier)

—— 1977 *The Construction of Modern Science: Mechanisms and Mechanics* (Cambridge: Cambridge University Press)

—— 1980 *Never at Rest. A Biography of Isaac Newton* (Cambridge: Cambridge University Press)

Whewell W 1835 Report on the recent progress and present condition of the mathematical theories of electricity, magnetism, and heat *Rep. Br. Assoc. Adv. Sci.* **5** 1–35

—— 1837 *History of the Inductive Sciences* (London)

—— 1840 *Philosophy of the Inductive Sciences* 2 volumes (London) 2nd edn 1847

—— 1845 *The Elements of Morality* 2 volumes (London)

—— 1967 *Philosophy of the Inductive Science* 2 volumes (London: Frank Cass). Reprint of 2nd edition of 1847 (London)

Whitehead A N 1926 *Science and the Modern World* (Cambridge: Cambridge University Press)

Whittaker E T 1951 *A History of the Theories of Aether and Electricity. Volume 1. The Classical Theories* (London: Nelson)

Wiechert E 1896 Über die Grundlagen der Elektrodynamik *Ann. Phys., Lpz.* **59** 283–323

—— 1898 Hypothesen für eine Theorie der elektrischen und magnetischen Erscheinungen *Nachr. Kgl. Ges. der Wiss. Göttingen* 87–106

Wiederkehr K H 1967 *Wilhelm Eduard Weber* (Stuttgart: Wissenshaftliche Verlagsgesellschaft)

Williams L P 1965 *Michael Faraday: A Biography* (London: Chapman and Hall)

—— 1970 André Marie Ampère *Dict. Sci. Biog.* **1** 139–47

—— 1983 What were Ampère's earliest discoveries in electrodynamics? *Isis* **74** 492–508

Wise N 1979 The mutual embrace of electricity and magnetism *Science* **203** 1310–18

—— 1981 The flow analogy to electricity and magnetism: Part 1: William Thomson's reformulation of action at a distance *Arch. Hist. Exact Sci.* **25** 19–70

Wright J P 1983 *The Sceptical Realism of David Hume* (Manchester: Manchester University Press)

Young T 1807 *Course of Lectures on Natural Philosophy and the Mechanical Arts* 2 volumes (London)

Index